# THE WALLS MANUAL OF EMERGENCY AIRWAY MANAGEMENT

EDITOR-IN-CHIEF

**Calvin A. Brown III, MD**

Assistant Professor of Emergency Medicine
Director of Faculty Affairs
Department of Emergency Medicine
Brigham and Women's Hospital
Harvard Medical School
Boston, Massachusetts

ASSOCIATE EDITORS

**John C. Sakles, MD**

Professor
Department of Emergency Medicine
University of Arizona College of Medicine
Tucson, Arizona

**Nathan W. Mick, MD, FACEP**

Associate Professor
Department of Emergency Medicine
Tufts University School of Medicine
Associate Chief
Department of Emergency Medicine
Maine Medical Center
Portland, Maine



Wolters Kluwer

Philadelphia • Baltimore • New York • London
Buenos Aires • Hong Kong • Sydney • Tokyo

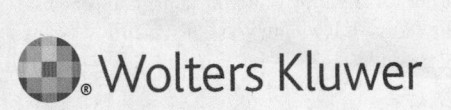

*Acquisitions Editor:* Sharon Zinner
*Developmental Editor:* Ashley Fischer
*Editorial Coordinator:* Maria M. McAvey, Annette Ferran
*Production Project Manager:* Kim Cox
*Design Coordinator:* Stephen Druding
*Manufacturing Coordinator:* Beth Welsh
*Marketing Manager:* Rachel Mante Leung
*Prepress Vendor:* S4Carlisle Publishing Services

Fifth edition



9 8 7 6 5 4 3 2 1

Printed in China

**Library of Congress Cataloging-in-Publication Data**

ISBN-13: 978-1-4963-5196-8
ISBN-10: 1-4963-5196-7

Cataloging-in-Publication data available on request from the Publisher.



LWW.com

RRS1704

# Dedication

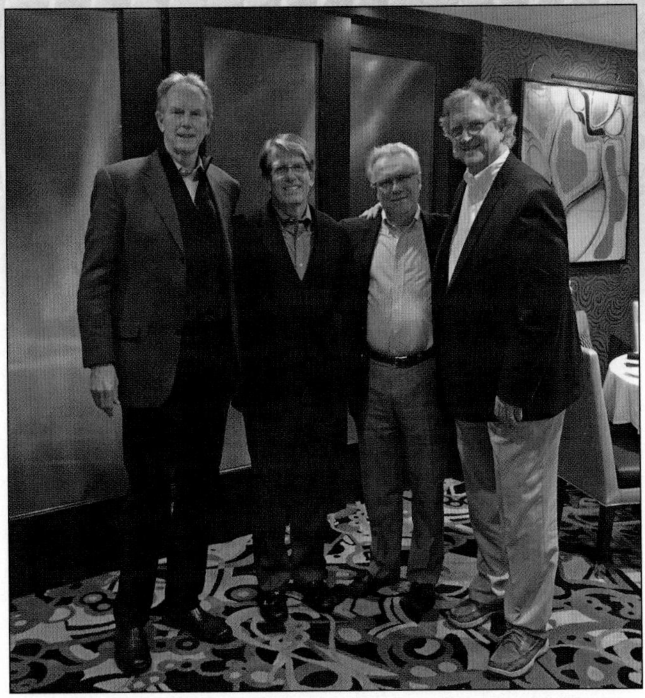

*This book is dedicated to four pioneers in emergency medicine (left to right): Drs. Robert Schneider, Ron Walls, Mike Murphy and Robert Luten. Their vision and tireless devotion to education led to the creation of The Difficult Airway Course and this comprehensive text of emergency airway management. They have defined and refined safe, evidence-based airway management practices for generations of emergency providers and, in the process, have saved countless lives."*

# Preface

It is with pride and immense joy that we present this fifth edition of *The Walls Manual of Emergency Airway Management*, from here on known simply as "*The Walls Manual*." This book has been extensively updated from cover to cover and expanded with exciting new chapters. It contains the latest in evidence-based approaches to airway management presented in a practical, yet creative style by our highly talented authors, who teach with us in The Difficult Airway Course: Emergency and The Difficult Airway Course: Anesthesia, The Difficult Airway Course: Critical Care and The Difficult Airway Course: EMS. As with previous editions, each topic has undergone a critical appraisal of the available literature to ensure the content is on the vanguard of clinical medicine.

New information sparks vigorous debate and oftentimes a departure from previous thinking. To this end, the fifth edition contains several fundamental changes. The seven Ps of rapid sequence intubation (RSI), unadulterated fixtures in previous editions, have undergone a transformative change with the elimination of *Pretreatment* as a discrete pharmacologic action, now replaced by *Preintubation Optimization*. With new information surfacing about the hemodynamic consequences of RSI in critically ill emergency department patients, this new step emphasizes the importance of maximizing cardiopulmonary physiology prior to induction and positive pressure ventilation in order to prevent hypoxic insult and circulatory collapse. A new chapter on intubating the unstable patient dovetails nicely with this approach and provides a solid framework that addresses the metabolic, physiologic, and hemodynamic factors that make emergency airway management complex and challenging. Cutting-edge information on flush flow rate oxygen for emergency preoxygenation provides us with new insight and options for maximizing the safety of RSI. Lidocaine, previously advocated as a pretreatment agent for patients with elevated intracranial pressure and reactive airways disease, no longer plays a role and has been removed from our lexicon; however, fentanyl remains as a sympatholytic option in patients with hypertensive crises, although is now considered part of a holistic approach to cardiovascular optimization and is no longer thought of as an independent pharmacologic maneuver. We present updated mnemonics for difficult airway detection with the "MOANS" mnemonic for difficult bag and mask ventilation refreshed to create "ROMAN," which better highlights our newly understood association between radiation changes (the "R" in ROMAN) and difficult bagging. In addition, we cover the latest in airway tools as old standbys like the GlideScope and C-MAC videolaryngoscopes continue to transform into more streamlined and affordable devices with improved image quality and overall performance.

This compendium embodies what we believe to be the knowledge and skill set required for emergency airway management in both the emergency department and the prehospital environment. The principles, however, are applicable to a wide array of clinical settings. As inpatient care continues to evolve and roles become redefined, we are witnessing the emergence of hospitalists and critical care physicians as primary airway managers being called upon frequently to intubate on hospital floors and in intensive care units. The concepts we present in the fifth edition can be extrapolated to any arena where urgent airway management might take place and is as relevant to inpatient clinicians as it is to emergency medicine specialists. Tapping yet again into Terry Steele's vision and creativity, we drew upon the combined knowledge base from both the anesthesia and emergency medicine courses to develop The Difficult Airway Course: Critical Care in 2016, a comprehensive and robust new curriculum to meet the educational needs of this unique group of airway managers. New chapters on intubating the unstable patient and safe extubation techniques augments this new curriculum and helps to make this latest edition the most versatile manual ever.

We are fortunate for the opportunity to provide this resource and are hopeful that the material in this book will play an important role when, late at night, faced with little information, less help, and virtually no time for debate we are called to act, make extraordinary decisions, and save lives.

**Calvin A. Brown III, MD**
Boston, Massachusetts

**John C. Sakles, MD**
Tucson, Arizona

**Nathan W. Mick, MD, FACEP**
Portland, Maine

# Acknowledgments

One of the most precious gifts in medicine is that of mentorship and I have been fortunate beyond measure. My development as an academic emergency physician would not have been possible without the frequent advice, incredible opportunities, and genuine friendship from Dr. Ron Walls. While professional aspirations are important, family is paramount. I must thank my wife Katherine and our two wonderful boys, Calvin and Caleb. Their steadfast love and support despite years of travel and long office hours has provided me with the privilege to pursue my professional goals. Finally, I would like to acknowledge the national teaching faculty of our airway courses as well as the faculty, residents, and medical students at Brigham and Women's Hospital and Harvard Medical School who help keep me energized, challenged, and intellectually honest on a daily basis.

Calvin A. Brown III, MD
**Boston, Massachusetts**

There are many people in my life, including my family, professional colleagues, and patients, who have greatly enriched my career and have made my participation in the airway course and manual possible. I thank them all for their understanding, continued support, and faith in me. I would like to dedicate this manual to all the frontline providers, of every specialty and discipline, who manage the airways of critically ill and injured patients. It is through their tireless efforts, working in uncontrolled environments and under difficult circumstances, that the lives of our loved ones are saved.

John C. Sakles, MD
**Tucson, Arizona**

Ten years ago, I was contacted by Dr. Ron Walls asking if I would be available to help teach at the Difficult Airway Course and it was with great honor and pleasure that I accepted his offer. Today, I remain immensely grateful to him for his teaching and mentorship during residency and in the early portion of my academic career. A decade has passed, and I feel blessed to have interacted with such an amazing group of airway educators and often feel as if I have received as much as I have given during those long weekends. A special thanks to Dr. Bob Luten, who has a special place in my heart as one of the founding fathers of Pediatric Emergency Medicine and a true pioneer in pediatric airway management. Thank you as well to my family, wife Kellie, daughters Gracyn and Afton, for putting up with the frequent travel, with only the occasional "snow globe" present on my return. Know that time away from the family is never easy, but we feel we are truly making a difference.

Nathan W. Mick, MD, FACEP
**Portland, Maine**

# Contributors

Jennifer L. Avegno, MD
Clinical Assistant Professor of Medicine
Section of Emergency Medicine
Louisiana State University Health Sciences Center
New Orleans, Louisiana

Aaron E. Bair, MD
Professor
Department of Emergency Medicine
University of California Davis School of Medicine
Sacramento, California

Jeff Birrer, EMT-P
Paramedic
American Medical Response
Portland, Oregon

Darren A. Braude, MD
Paramedic Chief
Division of Prehospital, Austere, and Disaster Medicine
Professor of Emergency Medicine and Anesthesiology
University of New Mexico Health Sciences Center
Medical Director, The Difficult Airway Course: EMS
Albuquerque, New Mexico

Calvin A. Brown III, MD
Assistant Professor of Emergency Medicine
Director of Faculty Affairs
Department of Emergency Medicine
Brigham and Women's Hospital
Harvard Medical School
Boston, Massachusetts

Stephen Bush, MA (Oxon), FRCS, FRCEM
Consultant in Emergency Medicine
Emergency Department
Leeds Teaching Hospitals Trust
United Kingdom

Steven C. Carleton, MD, PhD
Professor
W. Brian Gibler Chair of Emergency Medicine Education
Department of Emergency Medicine
University of Cincinnati College of Medicine
Cincinnati, Ohio

David A. Caro, MD
Associate Professor
Department of Emergency Medicine
University of Florida College of Medicine
Jacksonville, Florida

Ken Davis EMT-P, FP-C, BA
EMSRx LLC
Waxahachie, Texas

Peter M.C. DeBlieux, MD
Professor of Clinical Medicine
Section of Emergency Medicine
Louisiana State University Health Sciences Center
University Medical Center New Orleans
New Orleans, Louisiana

Brian E. Driver, MD
Assistant Professor
Department of Emergency Medicine
University of Minnesota Medical School
Faculty Physician
Department of Emergency Medicine
Hennepin County Medical Center
Minneapolis, Minnesota

Laura V. Duggan, MD
Clinical Associate Professor
Department of Anesthesiology, Pharmacology, and Therapeutics
University of British Columbia
Vancouver, British Columbia, Canada

Jan L. Eichel, RN, CFRN, BA, EMT-P
Director of Clinical Operations
West Michigan Air Care
Kalamazoo, Michigan

Frederick H. Ellinger, Jr., NRP
Flight Paramedic
MidAtlantic MedEvac
AtlantiCare Regional Medical Center
Atlantic City, New Jersey

Megan L. Fix, MD
Assistant Professor
Division of Emergency Medicine
University of Utah Hospital
Salt Lake City, Utah

Kevin Franklin, RN, EMT-P, CFRN
Flight Nurse
West Michigan Air Care
Kalamazoo, Michigan

Michael A. Gibbs, MD
Professor and Chairman
Department of Emergency Medicine
Carolinas Medical Center
Levine Children's Hospital
Charlotte, North Carolina

Steven A. Godwin, MD, FACEP
Professor and Chair
Department of Emergency Medicine
University of Florida College of Medicine
Jacksonville, Florida

Michael G. Gonzalez, MD, FACEP, FAAEM
Assistant Professor
Emergency Medicine
Baylor College of Medicine
Associate Medical Director
Houston Fire Department
Houston, Texas

Alan C. Heffner, MD
Director of Critical Care
Director of ECMO Services
Professor
Department of Internal Medicine
Department of Emergency Medicine
Carolinas Medical Center
University of North Carolina
Charlotte, North Carolina

Cheryl Lynn Horton, MD
Associate Physician
Department of Emergency Medicine
Kaiser Permanente East Bay
Oakland, California

Andy S. Jagoda, MD
Professor and System Chair
Department of Emergency Medicine
Icahn School of Medicine at Mount Sinai
New York, New York

Michael Keller, BS, NRP
Curriculum Faculty
Department for EMS Education
Gaston College
Dallas, North Carolina

Erik G. Laurin MD
Professor
Department of Emergency Medicine
Vice Chair for Education
University of California, Davis, School of Medicine
Sacramento, California

Robert C. Luten, MD
Professor
Department of Emergency Medicine
Division of Pediatric Emergency Medicine
University of Florida College of Medicine
Jacksonville, Florida

Nathan W. Mick, MD, FACEP
Associate Professor
Tufts University School of Medicine
Associate Chief
Department of Emergency Medicine
Maine Medical Center
Portland, Maine

Jarrod M. Mosier, MD
Associate Professor
Department of Emergency Medicine
Department of Medicine
Division of Pulmonary, Allergy, Critical Care, and Sleep
University of Arizona College of Medicine
Tucson, Arizona

Michael F. Murphy MD, FRCPC
Professor Emeritus
University of Alberta
Edmonton, Alberta, Canada

Joshua Nagler, MD, MHPEd
Assistant Professor
Harvard Medical School
Division of Emergency Medicine
Boston Children's Hospital
Boston, Massachusetts

Justen Naidu, MD
Anesthesiology Resident
Department of Anesthesiology, Pharmacology and Therapeutics, University of British Columbia
Vancouver, British Columbia, Canada

Bret P. Nelson, MD
Associate Professor
Department of Emergency Medicine
Icahn School of Medicine at Mount Sinai
New York, New York

Ali S. Raja, MD, MBA, MPH
Vice Chairman and Associate Professor
Department of Emergency Medicine
Massachusetts General Hospital
Harvard Medical School
Boston, Massachusetts

Robert F. Reardon, MD
Professor of Emergency Medicine
University of Minnesota Medical School
Department of Emergency Medicine
Hennepin County Medical Center
Minneapolis, Minnesota

John C. Sakles, MD
Professor
Department of Emergency Medicine
University of Arizona College of Medicine
Tucson, Arizona

Leslie V. Simon, DO
Assistant Professor
Department of Emergency Medicine
Mayo Clinic Florida
Jacksonville, Florida

Mary Beth Skarote, EMT-P, LPN
All Hazards Planner
Veteran Corps of America
Jacksonville, North Carolina

Julie A. Slick, MD
Assistant Professor
Louisiana State University Health Sciences Center
Chief, Emergency Medicine
Southeast Louisiana Veterans Health Care System
New Orleans, Louisiana

Michael T. Steuerwald, MD
Assistant Professor
Department of Emergency Medicine
University of Wisconsin School of Medicine and Public Health
Madison, Wisconsin

Eli Torgeson, MD
Assistant Professor
Department of Anesthesiology and Critical Care Medicine
University of New Mexico School of Medicine
Albuquerque, New Mexico

Katren R. Tyler, MD
Associate Professor
Associate Residency Director
Geriatric Emergency Medicine Fellowship Director
Vice Chair for Faculty Development, Wellbeing, and Outreach
Department of Emergency Medicine
University of California Davis School of Medicine
Sacramento, California

Ron M. Walls, MD
Executive Vice President and Chief Operating Officer
Brigham and Women's Health Care
Neskey Family Professor of Emergency Medicine
Harvard Medical School
Boston, Massachusetts

Richard D. Zane, MD
Professor and Chair
Department of Emergency Medicine
University of Colorado School of Medicine
University of Colorado Hospital
Denver, Colorado

# Contents

# Section I

# Principles of Airway Management

Chapter 1

# The Decision to Intubate

Calvin A. Brown III and Ron M. Walls

## INTRODUCTION

Airway management is constantly evolving. The emergence of new technology, principally the various methods of video laryngoscopy, our understanding of contributors to intubation difficulty, and a renewed focus on oxygenation and cardiovascular stability during airway management are changing our fundamental decision-making in an effort to maximize patient safety and outcome. What has not changed, however, is the critical importance of the determination of whether a patient requires intubation and, if so, how urgently. The decision to intubate is the first step in emergency airway management, and sets in motion a complex series of actions required of the clinician, before performing the actual intubation:

- Rapidly assess the patient's need for intubation and the urgency of the situation.
- Determine the best method of airway management based on assessment of the patient's predicted difficulty and pathophysiology.
- Decide which pharmacologic agents are indicated, in what order, and in what doses.
- Prepare a plan in the event that the primary method is unsuccessful, know in advance how to recognize when the planned airway intervention has failed or will inevitably fail, and clearly lay out the alternative (rescue) technique(s).

Clinicians responsible for emergency airway management must be proficient with the techniques and medications used for rapid sequence intubation (RSI), the preferred method for most emergency intubations, as well as alternative intubation strategies when neuromuscular blockade is contraindicated. The entire repertoire of airway skills must be mastered, including bag-mask ventilation, video laryngoscopy, conventional laryngoscopy, flexible endoscopy, the use of extraglottic airway devices, adjunctive techniques such as use of an endotracheal tube introducer (also known as the gum elastic bougie), and surgical airway techniques (e.g., open or Seldinger-based cricothyrotomy).

This chapter focuses on the decision to intubate. Subsequent chapters describe airway management decision-making, methods of ensuring oxygenation, techniques and devices for airway management, the pharmacology of RSI, and considerations for special clinical circumstances, including the prehospital environment and care of pediatric patients.

## INDICATIONS FOR INTUBATION

The decision to intubate is based on three fundamental clinical assessments:

1. Is there a failure of airway maintenance or protection?
2. Is there a failure of ventilation or oxygenation?
3. What is the anticipated clinical course?

The results of these three evaluations will lead to a correct decision to intubate or not to intubate in virtually all conceivable cases.

**A.** *Is there a failure of airway maintenance or protection?*

Without a patent airway and intact protective reflexes, adequate oxygenation and ventilation may be difficult or impossible and aspiration of gastric contents can occur. Both expose the patient to significant morbidity and mortality. The conscious, alert patient uses the musculature of the upper airway and various protective reflexes to maintain patency and to protect against the aspiration of foreign substances, gastric contents, or secretions. The ability of the patient to phonate with a clear, unobstructed voice is strong evidence of airway patency, protection, and cerebral perfusion. In the severely ill or injured patient, such airway maintenance and protection mechanisms are often attenuated or lost. If the spontaneously breathing patient is not able to maintain a patent airway, an artificial airway may be established by the insertion of an oropharyngeal or nasopharyngeal airway. Although such devices may restore patency, they do not provide any protection against aspiration. Patients who are unable to maintain their own airway are also unable to protect it. Therefore, as a general rule, any patient who requires the establishment of a patent airway also requires protection of that airway. The exception is when a patient has an immediately reversible cause of airway compromise (e.g., opioid overdose) and reversal of the insult promptly restores the patient's ability to maintain an open, functioning airway. The need to protect the airway requires placement of a definitive airway (i.e., a cuffed endotracheal tube), and devices that simply maintain, but do not protect, the airway, such as oropharyngeal or nasopharyngeal airways, are temporizing measures only. It has been widely taught that the gag reflex is a reliable method of evaluating airway protective reflexes. In fact, this concept has never been subjected to adequate scientific scrutiny, and the absence of a gag reflex is neither sensitive nor specific as an indicator of loss of airway protective reflexes. The presence of a gag reflex has similarly not been demonstrated to ensure the presence of airway protection. In addition, testing the gag reflex in a supine, obtunded patient may result in vomiting and aspiration. Therefore, the gag reflex is of no clinical value, and in fact may be dangerous to assess when determining the need for intubation and should not be used for this purpose.

Spontaneous or volitional swallowing is a better assessment of the patient's ability to protect the airway than is the presence or absence of a gag reflex. Swallowing is a complex reflex that requires the patient to sense the presence of material in the posterior oropharynx and then execute a series of intricate and coordinated muscular actions to direct the secretions down past a covered airway into the esophagus. The finding of pooled secretions in the patient's posterior oropharynx indicates a potential failure of these protective mechanisms, and hence a failure of airway protection. A common clinical error is to assume that spontaneous breathing is proof that protective airway mechanisms are preserved. Although spontaneous ventilation may be adequate, the patient may be sufficiently obtunded to be at serious risk of aspiration.

**B.** *Is there a failure of ventilation or oxygenation?*

Stated simply, "gas exchange" is required for vital organ function. Even brief periods of hypoxia should be avoided, if possible. If the patient is unable to ventilate sufficiently, or if adequate oxygenation cannot be achieved despite the use of supplemental oxygen, then intubation is indicated. In such cases, intubation is performed to facilitate ventilation and oxygenation rather than to establish or protect the airway. An example is the patient with status asthmaticus, for whom bronchospasm and fatigue lead to ventilatory failure and hypoxemia, heralding respiratory arrest and death. Airway intervention is indicated when it is determined that the patient will not respond sufficiently to treatment to reverse these cascading events. Similarly, although the patient with severe acute respiratory distress syndrome may be maintaining and protecting the airway, he or she may have progressive oxygenation failure and supervening fatigue that can be managed only with tracheal intubation and positive-pressure ventilation. Unless ventilatory or oxygenation failure is resulting from a rapidly reversible cause, such as opioid overdose, or a condition known to be successfully managed with noninvasive ventilation (e.g., bi-level positive airway pressure [Bi-PAP] for acute pulmonary edema), intubation is required. Even then, the clinician must be vigilant and constantly reassess the patient's condition, and if there is not an early and clear trajectory of improvement, he or she should be intubated.

C. *What is the anticipated clinical course?*

Most patients who require emergency intubation have one or more of the previously discussed indications: failure of airway maintenance, airway protection, oxygenation, or ventilation. However, there is a large and important group for whom intubation is indicated, even if none of these fundamental failures are present at the time of evaluation. These are the patients for whom intubation is likely or inevitable because their conditions, and airways, are predicted to deteriorate from dynamic and progressive changes related to the presenting pathophysiology or because the work of breathing will become overwhelming in the face of catastrophic illness or injury. For example, consider the patient who presents with a stab wound to the midzone of the anterior neck and a visible hematoma. At presentation, the patient may have perfectly adequate airway maintenance and protection and be ventilating and oxygenating well. The hematoma, however, provides clear evidence of significant vascular injury. Ongoing bleeding may be clinically occult because the blood often tracks down the tissue planes of the neck (e.g., prevertebral space) rather than demonstrating visible expansion of the hematoma. Furthermore, the anatomical distortion caused by the enlarging internal hematoma may well thwart a variety of airway management techniques that would have been successful if undertaken earlier. The patient inexorably progresses from awake and alert with a patent airway to a state in which the airway becomes obstructed, often quite suddenly, and the anatomy is so distorted that airway management is difficult or impossible.

Analogous considerations apply to the polytrauma patient who presents with hypotension and multiple severe injuries, including chest trauma. Although this patient initially maintains and protects his airway, and ventilation and oxygenation are adequate, intubation is indicated as part of the management of the constellation of injuries (i.e., as part of the overall management of the patient). The reason for intubation becomes clear when one examines the anticipated clinical course of this patient. The hypotension mandates fluid resuscitation and evaluation for the source of the blood loss, including abdominal computed tomography (CT) scan. Pelvic fractures, if unstable, require immobilization and likely embolization of bleeding vessels. Long bone fractures often require operative intervention. Chest tubes may be required to treat hemopneumothorax or in preparation for positive-pressure ventilation during surgery. Combative behavior confounds efforts to maintain spine precautions and requires pharmacologic restraint and evaluation by head CT scan. Throughout all of this, the patient's shock state causes inadequate tissue perfusion and increasing metabolic debt. This debt significantly affects the muscles of respiration, and progressive respiratory fatigue and failure often supervene. With the patient's ultimate destination certain to be the operating room or the ICU, and the need for complex and potentially painful procedures and diagnostic evaluations, which may require extended periods of time outside the resuscitation suite, this patient is best served by early intubation. In addition, intubation improves tissue oxygenation during shock and helps reduce the increasing metabolic debt burden.

Sometimes, the anticipated clinical course may necessitate intubation because the patient will be exposed to a period of increased risk on account of patient transport, a medical procedure, or diagnostic imaging. For example, the patient with multiple injuries who appears relatively stable might be appropriately managed without intubation while geographically located in the emergency department (ED). However, if that same patient requires CT scans, angiography, or any other prolonged diagnostic procedure, it may be more appropriate to intubate the patient before allowing him or her to leave the ED so that an airway crisis will not ensue in the radiology suite, where recognition may be delayed and response may not be optimal. Similarly, if such a patient is to be transferred from one hospital to another, airway management may be indicated on the basis of the increased risk to the patient during that transfer.

Not every trauma patient or every patient with a serious medical disorder requires intubation. However, in general, it is better to err on the side of performing an intubation that might not, in retrospect, have been required, than to delay intubation, thus exposing the patient to the risk of serious deterioration.

## APPROACH TO THE PATIENT

When evaluating a patient for emergency airway management, the first assessment should be of the patency and adequacy of the airway. In many cases, the adequacy of the airway is confirmed by having the patient speak. Ask questions such as "What is your name?" or "Do you know where you are?" The responses provide information about both the airway and the patient's neurologic status. A normal voice (as opposed to a muffled or distorted voice), the ability to inhale and exhale in the modulated manner required for speech, and the ability to comprehend the question and follow instructions are strong evidence of adequate upper airway function. Although such an evaluation should not be taken as proof that the upper airway is definitively secure, it is strongly suggestive that the airway is adequate *at that moment*. More important, the inability of the patient to phonate properly; inability to sense and swallow secretions; or the presence of stridor, dyspnea, or altered mental status precluding responses to questioning should prompt a detailed assessment of the adequacy of the airway and ventilation (see **Box 1-1**). After assessing verbal response to questions, conduct a more detailed examination of the mouth and oropharynx. Examine the mouth for bleeding, swelling of the tongue or uvula, abnormalities of the oropharynx (e.g., peritonsillar abscess), or any other abnormalities that might interfere with the unimpeded passage of air through the mouth and oropharynx. Examine the mandible and central face for integrity. Examination of the anterior neck requires both visual inspection for deformity, asymmetry, or abnormality and palpation of the anterior neck, including the larynx and trachea. During palpation, assess carefully for the presence of subcutaneous air. This is identified by a crackling feeling on compression of the cutaneous tissues of the neck, much as if a sheet of wrinkled tissue paper were lying immediately beneath the skin. The presence of subcutaneous air indicates disruption of an air-filled passage, often the airway

BOX 1-1

**Four key signs of upper airway obstruction.**

- Muffled or "hot potato" voice (as though the patient is speaking with a mouthful of hot food)
- Inability to swallow secretions, because of either pain or obstruction
- Stridor
- Dyspnea

The first two signs do not necessarily herald imminent total upper airway obstruction; stridor, if new or progressive, usually does, and dyspnea also is a compelling symptom.

itself, especially in the setting of blunt or penetrating chest or neck trauma. Subcutaneous air in the neck also can be caused by pulmonary injury, esophageal rupture, or, rarely, gas-forming infection. Although these latter two conditions are not immediately threatening to the airway, patients may nevertheless rapidly deteriorate, requiring subsequent airway management. In the setting of blunt anterior neck trauma, assess the larynx for pain on motion. Move the larynx from side to side, assessing for "laryngeal crepitus", indicating normal contact of the airway with the air-filled upper esophagus. Absence of crepitus may be caused by edema between the larynx and the upper esophagus.

After inspecting and palpating the upper airway, note the patient's respiratory pattern. The presence of inspiratory stridor, however slight, indicates some degree of upper airway obstruction. Lower airway obstruction, occurring beyond the level of the glottis, more often produces expiratory stridor. The volume and pitch of stridor are related to the velocity and turbulence of ventilatory airflow. Most often, stridor is audible without a stethoscope. Auscultation of the neck with a stethoscope can reveal subauditory stridor that may also indicate potential airway compromise. Stridor is a late sign, especially in adult patients, who have large-diameter airways, and significant airway compromise may develop before any sign of stridor is evident. When evaluating the respiratory pattern, observe the chest through several respiratory cycles, looking for normal symmetrical, concordant chest movement. In cases where there is significant injury, paradoxical movement of a flail segment of the chest may be observed. If spinal cord injury has impaired intercostal muscle functioning, diaphragmatic breathing may be present. In this form of breathing, there is little movement of the chest wall, and inspiration is evidenced by an increase in abdominal volume caused by descent of the diaphragm. Auscultate the chest to assess the adequacy of air exchange. Decreased breath sounds indicate pneumothorax, hemothorax, pleural effusion, emphysema, or other pulmonary pathology.

The assessment of ventilation and oxygenation is a clinical one. Arterial blood gas determination provides little additional information as to whether intubation is necessary, and may be misleading. The patient's mentation, degree of fatigue, and severity of concomitant injuries or comorbid medical conditions is more important than isolated or even serial determinations of arterial oxygen or carbon dioxide ($CO_2$) tension. Oxygen saturation is monitored continuously by pulse oximetry, so arterial blood gases rarely are indicated for the purpose of determining arterial oxygen tension. In certain circumstances, oxygen saturation monitoring is unreliable because of poor peripheral perfusion, and arterial blood gases may then be required to assess oxygenation or to provide a correlation with pulse oximetry measurements. Continuous capnography (see Chapter 8) may be used to assess changes in the patient's ability to ventilate adequately, and the measurement of arterial $CO_2$ tension contributes little additional useful information, although often a single arterial blood gas measurement is used to provide a correlation baseline with end-tidal $CO_2$ readings. A venous or arterial blood gas can provide a good general snapshot of the patient's acid–base status and baseline ventilation, but assessment of overall ventilation remains a clinical task, requiring evaluation of the patient's overall status and perceived trajectory. In patients with obstructive lung disease, such as asthma or chronic obstructive pulmonary disease (COPD), intubation may be required in the face of relatively low $CO_2$ tensions if the patient is becoming fatigued. Other times, high $CO_2$ tensions may be managed successfully with noninvasive positive-pressure ventilation instead of intubation if the patient is showing clinical signs of improvement (e.g., increased alertness, improving speech, and less fatigue).

Finally, after assessment of the upper airway and the patient's ventilatory status, including pulse oximetry, capnography (if used), and mentation, consider the patient's anticipated clinical course. If the patient's condition is such that intubation is inevitable and a series of interventions are required, early intubation is preferable. Similarly, if the patient has a condition that is at risk of worsening over time, especially if it is likely to compromise the airway itself, early airway management is indicated. The same consideration applies to patients who require interfacility transfer by air or ground or a prolonged procedure in an area with diminished resuscitation capability. Intubation before transfer is preferable to a difficult, uncontrolled intubation in an austere environment after the condition has worsened. In all circumstances, the decision to intubate should be given precedence. If doubt exists as to whether the patient requires intubation, err on the side of intubating the patient. It is preferable to intubate the patient and ensure the integrity of the airway than to leave the patient without a secure airway and have a preventable crisis occur.

## EVIDENCE

- **Are there reliable indicators of the need to intubate?** The clinician's determination regarding the need for intubation is based on the clinical scenario, pathophysiology, bedside airway assessment, and likelihood of deterioration. Some measurable data and patient characteristics can be helpful, whereas others are largely folklore. First, the gag reflex continues to be taught in some settings as a key determinant in assessing the adequacy of airway protection or the need for intubation, yet the literature does not support this claim. The patient's Glasgow Coma Scale is a better predictor of airway protection and his or her aspiration risk in overdose.[1] Inspiratory stridor, when seen in adults, is particularly ominous and typically mandates intubation. Although there is no absolute cutoff for oxygen saturation or $CO_2$ that dictates intubation, a saturation that cannot be sustained above 80%, a RR $>$ 30 or a $CO_2 >$ 100 has strong associations with intubation. Moreover, many conditions can often be managed without definitive airway management even when the patient seems, initially, to be in severe respiratory distress. COPD and acute pulmonary edema are uncommon causes of ED intubation and can typically be managed with medical therapy and noninvasive positive airway pressure.[2]

## REFERENCES

1. Elzadi-Mood N, Saghaei M, Alfred S, et al. Comparative evaluation of Glasgow Coma Score and gag reflex in predicting aspiration pneumonitis in acute poisoning. *J Crit Care*. 2009;24:470.e9–470.e15.
2. Brown CA 3rd, Bair AE, Pallin DJ, et al. Techniques, success, and adverse events of emergency department adult intubations. *Ann Emerg Med*. 2015;65(4):363–370.e1.

Chapter 2

# Identification of the Difficult and Failed Airway

Calvin A. Brown III and Ron M. Walls

## INTRODUCTION

Although both difficult and failed airways are discussed in this chapter, the two concepts are distinct. A difficult airway is one in which identifiable anatomical attributes predict technical difficulty with securing the airway. A failed airway is one for which the chosen technique has failed, and rescue must be undertaken. Obviously, there is much overlap, but it is important to keep the two notions distinct.

In addition, one can think about airway difficulty in two categories: an anatomically difficult airway and a physiologically difficult airway. The former presents anatomical or logistical barriers to successful airway management, whereas the latter requires the operator to optimize overall patient management in the context of critically low oxygen saturation, blood pressure, or metabolic derangement, such as severe metabolic acidosis. This chapter focuses on the anatomical issues related to airway management, and the term "difficult airway," throughout this manual, refers to airways with anatomical or logistical difficulties for airway management. Chapter 32 discusses the approach to the physiologically compromised patient, which some authors refer to as a physiologically difficult airway.

A difficult airway is one for which a preintubation examination identifies physical attributes that are likely to make laryngoscopy, intubation, bag-mask ventilation (BMV), the use of an extraglottic device (e.g., laryngeal mask airway [LMA]), or surgical airway management more difficult than would be the case in an ordinary patient without those attributes. Identification of a difficult airway is a key component of the approach to airway management for any patient and is a key branch point on the main airway algorithm (see Chapter 3). The key reason for this is that, depending on the degree of predicted difficulty, one should not administer a neuromuscular blocking medication to a patient unless one has a measure of confidence that gas exchange can be maintained if laryngoscopy and intubation fail. Accordingly, if an anatomically difficult airway is identified, the difficult airway algorithm is used.

A failed airway situation occurs when a provider has embarked on a certain course of airway management (e.g., rapid sequence intubation [RSI]) and has identified that intubation by that method is not going to succeed, requiring the immediate initiation of a rescue sequence (the failed airway algorithm, see Chapter 3). Certainly, in retrospect, a failed airway can be called a difficult airway because it has proven to be difficult or impossible to intubate, but the terms "failed airway" and "difficult airway" must be kept distinct because they represent different situations, require different approaches, and arise at different points in the airway management timeline. One way of thinking about this is that the difficult airway is something one anticipates and plans for; the failed airway is something one experiences (particularly if one did not assess for, and anticipate, a difficulty airway).

Airways that are difficult to manage are fairly common in emergency practice. Difficult direct laryngoscopy (DL), defined as a grade III or grade IV laryngoscopic view, occurs in approximately 10% of all adult emergency intubations. The incidence is drastically lower when a video laryngoscope is used (see Chapter 14 Video Laryngoscopy). However, the incidence of overall intubation failure is quite low, that is, less than 1%. Intubation failure can occur in a setting where the patient can be oxygenated by an alternative method, such as by BMV or using an EGD, or in a setting where the patient can be neither intubated nor oxygenated. The incidence of the "*can't* intubate, *can't* oxygenate" (CICO) situation in preselected operating room intubations is rare, estimated to occur once in 5,000 to 20,000 intubations. The true incidence is unknown in emergency intubations, but it is likely substantially more common, given patient acuity, lack of preselection, and a higher rate of difficult airway markers. Rescue cricothyrotomy most often happens in the setting of a *can't* oxygenate failed airway, but its incidence has declined with the advent of video laryngoscopy (VL) and various rescue devices. Based on large registry data of adult intubations, rescue surgical airways occur in 0.3% to 0.5% of all encounters. This chapter explores the concepts of the failed and the difficult airway in the setting of emergency intubation. Recognizing the difficult airway in advance and executing an appropriate and thoughtful plan, guided by the difficult airway algorithm (see Chapter 3), will minimize the likelihood that airway management will fail. Furthermore, recognizing the failed airway promptly allows use of the failed airway algorithm to guide selection of a rescue approach.

## THE FAILED AIRWAY

A failed airway exists when any of the following conditions is met:

1. Failure to maintain acceptable oxygen saturation during or after one or more failed laryngoscopic attempts (CICO) *or*
2. Three failed attempts at orotracheal intubation by an experienced intubator, even when oxygen saturation can be maintained *or*
3. The single "best attempt" at intubation fails in the "Forced to Act" situation (see below).

Clinically, the failed airway presents itself in two ways, dictating the urgency created by the situation:

1. ***Can't** Intubate*, ***Can't** Oxygenate:* There is not sufficient time to evaluate or attempt a series of rescue options, and the airway must be secured immediately because of an inability to maintain oxygen saturation by BMV or with an EGD.
2. ***Can't** Intubate*, ***Can** Oxygenate:* There is time to evaluate and execute various options because the patient is oxygenated.

The most important way to avoid airway management failure is to identify in advance those patients for whom difficulty can be anticipated with intubation, BMV, insertion of an EGD, or cricothyrotomy. In the "Forced to Act" scenario, airway difficulty is apparent, but the clinical conditions (e.g., combative, hypoxic, rapidly deteriorating patient) force the operator's hand, requiring administration of RSI drugs in an attempt to create the best possible circumstances for tracheal intubation, with immediate progression to failed airway management if that one best attempt is not successful (see Chapter 3).

## THE DIFFICULT AIRWAY

According to the main emergency airway management algorithm, RSI is the method of choice for any non-crash airway when airway management difficulty is not anticipated. This requires a reliable and reproducible method for identifying the difficult airway. This evaluation must be expeditious, easy to remember, and complete.

In clinical practice, the difficult airway has four dimensions:

1. Difficult laryngoscopy
2. Difficult BMV
3. Difficult EGD
4. Difficult cricothyrotomy

A distinct evaluation is required for difficult laryngoscopy, difficult BMV, difficult EGD, and difficult surgical airway management, and each evaluation must be applied to each patient before airway management is undertaken (**Fig. 2-1**).

### Difficult Laryngoscopy: LEMON

The concept of difficult laryngoscopy and intubation is inextricably linked to poor glottic view; the less adequate the glottic view, the more challenging the intubation. This concept, developed during an era when almost all intubations were done by DL, appears to hold true even in the era of VL. Nearly all research relating certain patient characteristics to difficult or impossible intubation is based on studies of DL. VL is much less affected than DL by the presence or number of difficult airway attributes. With the exception of severely reduced mouth opening such that the device is unable to be inserted or sudden unanticipated device failure, it is rare for VL to yield a Cormack and Lehane grade III (or worse) glottic view. VL accomplishes this independently of the need to align the various airway axes, as must occur during DL (see Chapters 13 and 14). Difficult laryngoscopy and intubation are uncommon, even rare, when certain video laryngoscopes are used. It follows that evidence-based guidelines for prediction of difficult VL may be challenging, or even impossible, to develop. Pending further information, however, we recommend performing a difficult laryngoscopy assessment, using the LEMON mnemonic, on all patients for whom intubation is planned, including for planned VL.

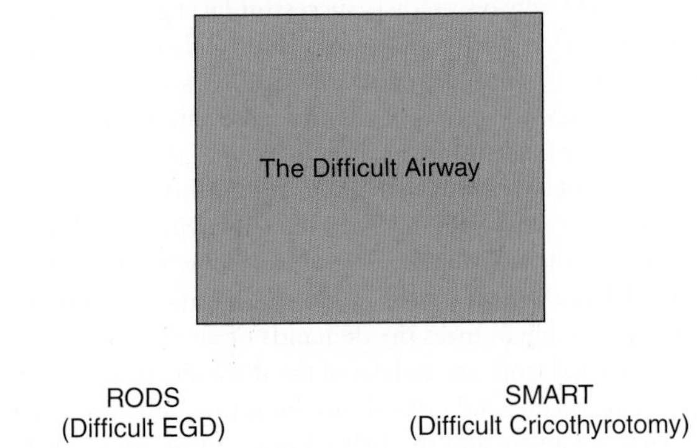


**FIGURE 2-1.** Difficult Airway Box. Note that the *four corners* represent the four dimensions of difficulty.

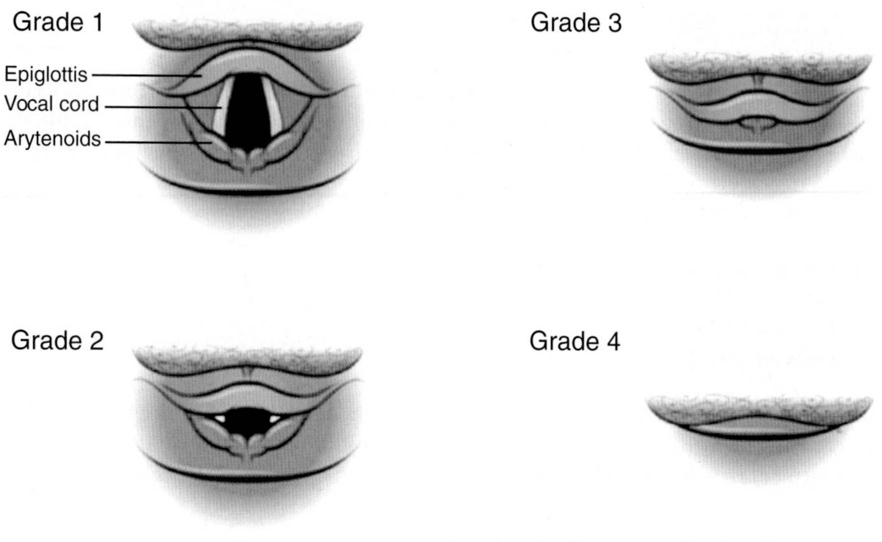


● **FIGURE 2-2.** C–L Laryngeal view grade system.

Cormack and Lehane introduced the most widely used system of categorizing the degree of visualization of the larynx during laryngoscopy, in which an ideal laryngoscopic view is designated grade 1 and the worst possible view, grade 4 (**Fig. 2-2**). Cormack–Lehane (C–L) view grade 3 (only the epiglottis is visible) and grade 4 (no glottic structures are visible) are highly correlated with difficult or failed intubation. C–L grade 1 (visualization of virtually the entire glottic aperture) and grade 2 (visualization of the posterior portion of the cords or the arytenoids) are not typically associated with difficult intubation. The C–L grading system does not differentiate precisely the degree to which the laryngeal aperture is visible during laryngoscopy: A grade 2 view may reveal little of the vocal cords, or none at all if only the arytenoids are visible. This led to adoption of a grade 2a/2b system, wherein a 2a shows any portion of the cords and a 2b shows only the arytenoids. Grade 2a airways perform comparably to those scored as grade 1, whereas grade 2b airways behave more like grade 3 airways. Grade 2b accounts for only about 20% of grade 2 views. However, when a grade 2b view occurs, two-thirds of patients are difficult to intubate, whereas only about 4% of patients with grade 2a views are characterized as difficult intubations. A grade 1 view reveals virtually the entire glottis and is associated with nearly universal intubation success.

Despite scores of clinical studies, no evidence to date has identified a full-proof set of patient attributes that, when absent, always predicts successful laryngoscopy and, when present, indicates certain intubation failure. In the absence of a proven and validated system that is capable of predicting intubation difficulty with 100% sensitivity and specificity, it is important to develop an approach that will enable a clinician to quickly and simply identify those patients who *might* be difficult to intubate so an appropriate plan can be made using the difficult airway algorithm. In other words, when asking the question, "Does this patient's airway warrant using the difficult airway algorithm, or is it appropriate and safe to proceed directly to RSI?," we value sensitivity (i.e., identifying all those who might be difficult) more than specificity (i.e., always being correct when identifying a patient as difficult).

The mnemonic LEMON is a useful guide to identify as many of the risks as possible as quickly and reliably as possible to meet the demands of an emergency situation. The elements of the mnemonic are assembled from an analysis of the difficult airway prediction instruments in the anesthesia, emergency medicine, and critical care literature. The mnemonic, which we developed for The Difficult Airway Course and the first edition of this book, has been externally validated in ED patients. The modified LEMON (all aspects of LEMON except the Mallampati score and thyromental distance) has undergone additional external validation and been found to have very high negative predictive value for both conventional and video laryngoscopy. LEMON has now been adopted as a recommended airway assessment tool in Advanced Trauma Life Support (ATLS). The mnemonic is as follows:

L—*Look externally:* Although a gestalt of difficult intubation is not particularly sensitive (meaning that many difficult airways are not readily apparent externally), it is quite specific, meaning that if the airway looks difficult, it probably is. Most of the litany of physical features associated with difficult laryngoscopy and intubation (e.g., small mandible, large tongue, large teeth, and short neck) are accounted for by the remaining elements of LEMON and so do not need to be specifically recalled or sought, which can be a difficult memory challenge in a critical situation. The external look specified here is for the "feeling" that the airway will be difficult. This feeling may be driven by a specific finding, such as external evidence of lower facial disruption and bleeding that might make intubation difficult, or it might be the ill-defined composite impression of the patient, such as the obese, agitated patient with a short neck and small mouth, whose airway appears formidable even before any formal evaluation (the rest of the LEMON attributes) is undertaken. This "gestalt" of the patient is influenced by patient attributes, the setting, and clinician expertise and experience, and likely is as valid for VL as for DL.

E—*Evaluate 3-3-2:* This step is an amalgamation of the much-studied geometric considerations that relate mouth opening and the size of the mandible to the position of the larynx in the neck in terms of likelihood of successful visualization of the glottis by DL. This concept originally was identified with "thyromental distance," but has become more sophisticated over time. The thyromental distance is the hypotenuse of a right triangle, the two legs being the anteroposterior dimension of the mandibular space, and the interval between the chin–neck junction (roughly the position of the hyoid bone indicating the posterior limit of the tongue) and the top of the larynx, indicated by the thyroid notch. The 3-3-2 evaluation is derived from studies of the geometrical requirements for successful DL, that is, the ability of the operator to create a direct line of sight from outside the mouth to the glottis. It is not known whether it has any value in predicting difficult VL, for which no straight line of sight is required. The premises of the 3-3-2 evaluation are as follows:

- The mouth must open adequately to permit visualization past the tongue when both the laryngoscope blade and the endotracheal tube are within the oral cavity.
- The mandible must be of sufficient size (length) to allow the tongue to be displaced fully into the submandibular space during DL.
- The glottis must be located a sufficient distance caudad to the base of the tongue that a direct line of sight can be created from outside the mouth to the vocal cords as the tongue is displaced inferiorly into the submandibular space.

The first "3," therefore, assesses mouth opening. A normal patient can open his or her mouth sufficiently to accommodate three of his or her own fingers between the upper and lower incisors (**Fig. 2-3A**). In reality, this is an approximate measurement as it would be unusual to ask an acutely ill or injured patient to stick three fingers in his or her mouth. If a patient is able to comply, ask if he or she can open the mouth as wide as possible. This will give a meaningful sense of whether the patient is able to open fully, partially, or not at all. The second "3" evaluates the length of the mandibular space by ensuring the patient's ability to accommodate three of his or her own fingers between the tip of the mentum and chin–neck junction (hyoid bone) (**Fig. 2-3B**). The "2" assesses the position of the glottis in relation to the base of the tongue. The space between the chin–neck junction (hyoid bone) and the thyroid notch should accommodate two of the patient's fingers (**Fig. 2-3C**). Thus, in the 3-3-2 rule, the first 3 assesses the adequacy of oral access, and the second 3 addresses the dimensions of the mandibular space to accommodate the tongue on DL. The ability to accommodate significantly more than or less than three fingers is associated with greater degrees of difficulty in visualizing the larynx at laryngoscopy: The former because the length of the oral axis is elongated, and the latter because the mandibular space may be too small to accommodate the tongue, requiring it to remain in the oral cavity or move posteriorly, obscuring the view of the glottis. Encroachment on the submandibular space by infiltrative conditions (e.g., Ludwig angina) is identified during this evaluation. The final 2 identifies the location of the larynx in relation to the base of the tongue. If significantly more than

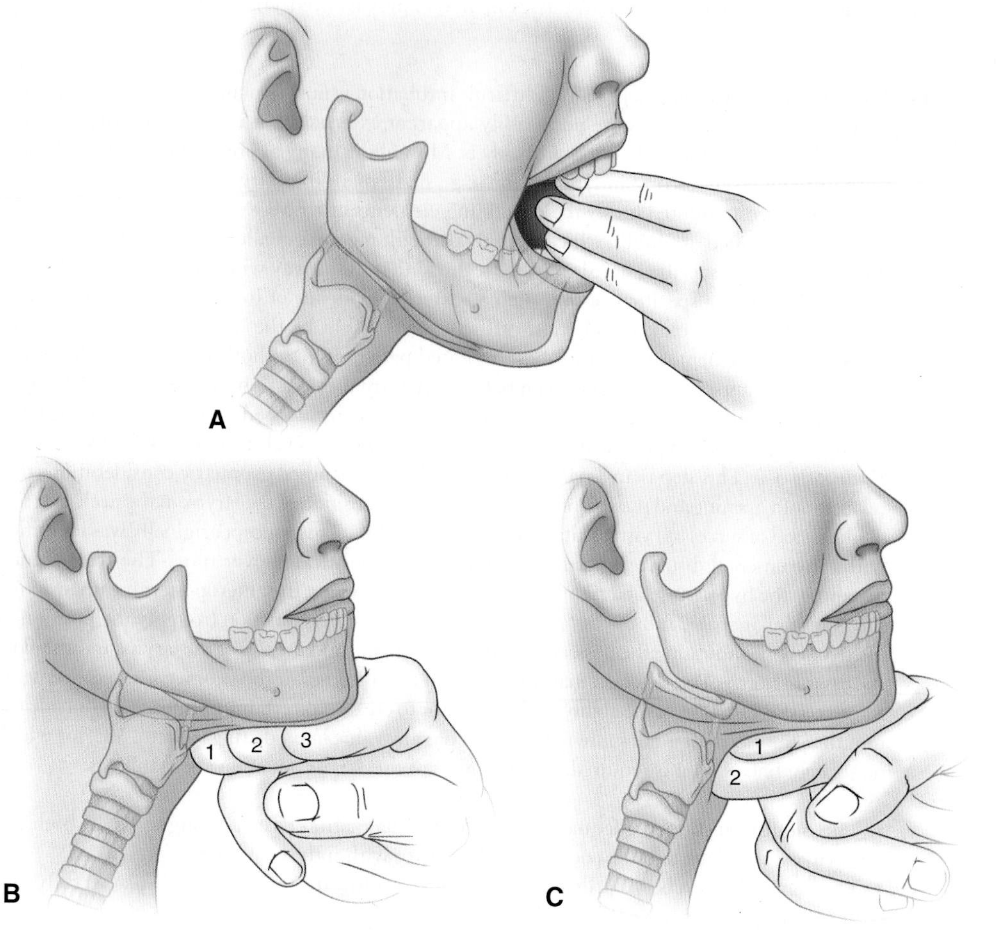


● **FIGURE 2-3.** **A:** The first 3 of the 3-3-2 rule. **B:** The second 3 of the 3-3-2 rule. **C:** The 2 of the 3-3-2 rule.

two fingers are accommodated, meaning the larynx is distant from the base of the tongue, it may be difficult to reach or visualize the glottis on DL, particularly if a smaller blade size is used initially. Fewer than two fingers may mean that the larynx is tucked up under the base of the tongue and may be difficult to expose. This condition is often imprecisely called an "anterior larynx."

M—*Mallampati score:* Mallampati determined that the degree to which the posterior oropharyngeal structures are visible when the mouth is fully open and the tongue is extruded reflects the relationships among mouth opening, the size of the tongue, and the size of the oral pharynx, which defines access through the oral cavity for intubation, and that these relationships are associated with intubation difficulty. Mallampati's classic assessment requires that the patient sit upright, open the mouth as widely as possible, and protrude the tongue as far as possible without phonating. **Figure 2-4** depicts how the scale is constructed. Class I and class II patients have low intubation failure rates; so the importance with respect to the decision whether to use neuromuscular blockade rests with those in classes III and IV, particularly class IV, where intubation failure rates may exceed 10%. By itself, the scale is neither sensitive nor specific; however, when used in conjunction with the other difficult airway assessments, it provides valuable information about access to the glottis through the oral cavity. In the emergency situation, it frequently is not possible to have the patient sit up or to follow instructions. Therefore, often only a crude

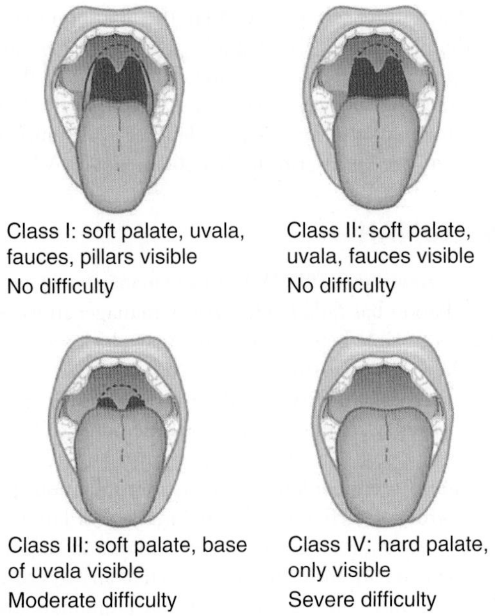


● **FIGURE 2-4. The Mallampati Scale.** In class I, the oropharynx, tonsillar pillars, and entire uvula are visible. In class II, the pillars are not visible. In class III, only a minimal portion of the oropharyngeal wall is visible, and in class IV, the tongue is pressed against the hard palate.

Mallampati measure is possible, obtained by examining the supine, obtunded patient's mouth with a tongue blade and light, or by using a lighted laryngoscope blade as a tongue depressor on the anterior half of the tongue to gain an appreciation of how much mouth opening is present (at least in the preparalyzed state) and the relationship between the size of the tongue and that of the oral cavity. Although not validated in the supine position using this approach, there is no reason to expect that the assessment would be significantly less reliable than the original method with the patient sitting and performing the maneuver actively. The laryngoscope or tongue blade should not be inserted too deeply because this may incite a gag reflex and can place a supine and compromised patient at risk for vomiting and aspiration.

O—*Obstruction/Obesity:* Upper airway obstruction is a marker for difficult laryngoscopy. The four cardinal signs of upper airway obstruction are muffled voice (hot potato voice), difficulty swallowing secretions (because of either pain or obstruction), stridor, and a sensation of dyspnea. The first two signs do not ordinarily herald imminent total upper airway obstruction in adults, but critical obstruction is much more imminent when the sensation of dyspnea occurs. Stridor is a particularly ominous sign. The presence of stridor is generally considered to indicate that the airway has been reduced to <50% of its normal caliber, or to a diameter of 4.5 mm or less. The management of patients with upper airway obstruction is discussed in Chapter 36. Although it is controversial whether obesity per se is an independent marker for difficult laryngoscopy or whether obesity simply is associated with various difficult airway attributes, such as high Mallampati score or failure of the 3-3-2 rule, obese patients frequently have poor glottic views by DL or VL, and obesity, in itself, should be considered to portend difficult laryngoscopy.

N—*Neck mobility:* The ability to position the head and neck is one of the key factors in achieving the best possible view of the larynx by DL. Cervical spine immobilization for trauma, by itself, may not create a degree of difficulty that ultimately leads one to avoid RSI after applying the thought processes of the difficult airway algorithm. However, cervical spine immobilization will make intubation more difficult and will compound the effects of other identified difficult airway markers. In addition, intrinsic cervical spine immobility, as in cases of ankylosing spondylitis or rheumatoid arthritis, can make intubation by DL extremely difficult or impossible and should be considered a much more serious issue than the ubiquitous cervical collar (which mandates inline manual immobilization). VL requires much less (or no) head extension, depending on blade shape, and provides a glottic view superior to that by DL when head extension or neck flexion is restricted. Other devices, such as the Airtraq or the Shikani optical stylet, discussed elsewhere in this manual, also may require less cervical spine movement than DL although image size and clarity are far inferior to that obtained with VL.

## Difficult BMV: ROMAN

Chapter 9 highlights the importance of BMV in airway management, particularly as a rescue maneuver when orotracheal intubation has failed. The airway manager must be confident that oxygenation with a BMV or EGD is feasible before neuromuscular blockers are administered whether or not laryngoscopy is thought to be successful.

The validated indicators of difficult BMV from various clinical studies can be easily recalled for rapid use in the emergency setting by using the mnemonic ROMAN.

**R**—*Radiation/Restriction:* Recent evidence suggests that radiation treatment to the neck is one of the strongest predictors of difficult and failed mask ventilation. Restriction refers to patients whose lungs and thoraces are resistant to ventilation and require high-ventilation pressures. These patients are primarily suffering from reactive airways disease with medium and small airways obstruction (asthma and chronic obstructive pulmonary disease [COPD]) and those with pulmonary edema, acute respiratory distress syndrome (ARDS), advanced pneumonia, or any other condition that reduces pulmonary compliance or increases airway resistance to BMV.

**O**—*Obesity/Obstruction/Obstructive sleep apnea:* We often refer to this as the "triple O" because all three attributes are important, and they are often linked (e.g., obesity with obstructive sleep apnea [OSA]). Patients who are obese (body mass index [BMI] >26 kg per $m^2$) are often difficult to ventilate adequately by bag and mask. Women in third-trimester gestation are also a prototype for this problem because of their increased body mass and the resistance to diaphragmatic excursion caused by the gravid uterus. Pregnant or obese patients also desaturate more quickly, making the bag ventilation difficulty of even greater import (see Chapters 37 and 40). Difficulty bagging the obese patient is not caused solely by the weight of the chest and abdominal walls but also the resistance by the abdominal contents to diaphragmatic excursion. Obese patients also have redundant tissues, creating resistance to airflow in the upper airway. This explains the recent association with OSA and difficult mask ventilation. Similarly, obstruction caused by angioedema, Ludwig angina, upper airway abscesses, epiglottitis, and other similar conditions will make BMV more difficult. In general, soft tissue lesions (e.g., angioedema, croup, and epiglottis) are amenable to bag-and-mask rescue if obstruction occurs, but not with 100% certainty. Similarly, laryngospasm can usually be overcome with good bag-and-mask technique. In contrast, firm, immobile lesions such as hematomas, cancers, and foreign bodies are less amenable to rescue by BMV, which is unlikely to provide adequate ventilation or oxygenation if total obstruction arises in this context.

**M**—*Mask Seal/Mallampati/Male sex*: Bushy beards, blood or debris on the face, or a disruption of lower facial continuity are the most common examples of conditions that may make an adequate mask seal difficult. Some experts recommend smearing a substance, such as KY jelly, on the beard as a remedy to this problem, although this action may simply make a bad situation worse in that the entire face may become too slippery to hold the mask in place. Both male sex and a Mallampati class 3 or 4 (see earlier) airway also appear to be independent predictors of difficult BMV.

**A**—*Age:* Age older than 55 years is associated with a higher risk of difficult BMV, perhaps because of a loss of muscle and tissue tone in the upper airway. The age is not a precise cutoff, and some judgment can be applied with respect to whether the patient has relatively elastic (young) or inelastic (aged) tissue.

**N**—*No teeth:* An adequate mask seal may be difficult in the edentulous patient because the face may not adequately support the mask. An option is to leave dentures (if available) in situ for BMV and remove them for intubation. Alternatively, gauze dressings may be inserted into the cheek areas through the mouth to puff them out in an attempt to improve the seal. Another technique for limiting mask leak involves rolling the lower lip down toward the chin and using the inner mucosal surface as a contact point for the bottom of the mask (See Chapter 9).

## Difficult EGD: RODS

In the emergency setting, extraglottic airway devices have emerged as credible first-line devices for ventilation and oxygenation, instead of the traditional bag and mask; as alternatives to tracheal intubation in some patient circumstances (especially out of hospital); and as valuable rescue devices.

Studies have identified factors that predict difficulty in placing an EGD and providing adequate gas exchange. These can be assessed using the mnemonic RODS.

**R**—*Restriction:* The restriction referred to here is similar to that for the ROMAN mnemonic, that is, "restricted" lung capacity with intrinsic resistance to ventilation from primary lung or tracheal/bronchial pathology. Ventilation with an EGD may be difficult or impossible in the face of substantial increases in airway resistance (e.g., asthma) or decreases in pulmonary compliance (e.g., pulmonary edema), although often the EGD is more effective at ventilation than is a bag and mask. In addition, restricted mouth opening will affect EGD insertion or make it impossible. Adequate mouth opening is required for insertion of the EGD. This requirement varies, depending on the particular EGD to be used. Recent operating room (OR) data have also identified restricted cervical spine mobility as a risk for difficult EGD use, likely because placement can be more challenging in these patients.

**O**—*Obstruction/Obesity:* If there is upper airway obstruction in the pharynx, at the level of the larynx or glottis, or below the vocal cords, an EGD may be impossible to insert or seat properly in order to achieve ventilation and oxygenation. In some circumstances, it will not bypass the obstruction at all. Obesity creates two challenges to oxygenation using an EGD. First, redundant tissues in the pharynx may make placement and seating of the device more difficult. Usually, this is not a significant problem. More importantly, obese patients require higher ventilation pressures, largely because of the weight of the chest wall and abdominal contents. The former causes resistance to ventilation by increasing the pressures required to expand the chest, and the latter causes resistance to ventilation by increasing the pressures required to cause the diaphragm to descend. Depending on the EGD chosen and positioning of the patient (it is better to attempt ventilation with the patient 30° head up or in reverse Trendelenberg position), ventilation resistance may exceed the ability of the EGD to seal and deliver the necessary pressures. More information on leak pressures for the variety of EGDs in circulation can be found in Chapters 10, 11, and 29.

**D**—*Disrupted or Distorted airway:* The key question here is "If I insert this EGD into the pharynx of this patient, will the device be able to seat itself and seal properly within relatively normal anatomy?" For example, fixed flexion deformity of the spine, penetrating neck injury with hematoma, epiglottitis, and pharyngeal abscess each may distort the anatomy sufficiently to prevent proper positioning of the device.

**S**—*Short thyromental distance:* A small mandibular space, as assessed by the patient's thyromental distance, may indicate that the tongue resides less in the mandibular fossa and more in the oral cavity. This can obstruct and complicate EGD insertion and has been strongly associated with difficult EGD use.

## Difficult Cricothyrotomy: SMART

There are no absolute contraindications to performing an emergency cricothyrotomy in adults (see Chapter 19). However, some conditions may make it difficult or impossible to perform the procedure, making it important to identify those conditions in advance and allow consideration of alternatives rather than assuming or hoping that cricothyrotomy, if necessary, will be successful as a rescue technique. The mnemonic SMART is used to quickly assess the patient for features that may indicate that a cricothyrotomy might be difficult. A part of patient assessment using this mnemonic, which occurs during the "A" step, is to perform a physical examination of the neck, identifying the landmarks and any barriers to the procedure. The SMART mnemonic is applied as follows:

**S**—*Surgery (recent or remote):* The anatomy may be subtly or obviously distorted, making the airway landmarks difficult to identify. Scarring may fuse tissue planes and make the procedure more difficult. Recent surgery may have associated edema or bleeding, complicating performance of the procedure.

**M**—*Mass:* A hematoma (postoperative or traumatic), abscess, or any other mass in the pathway of the cricothyrotomy may make the procedure technically difficult, and requires the operator to meticulously locate the landmarks, which may be out of the midline, or obscured.

**A**—*Access/Anatomy:* Obesity makes surgical access challenging, as it is often difficult to identify landmarks. Similar challenges are presented by subcutaneous emphysema, soft tissue infection, or edema. A patient with a short neck or overlying mandibular pannus presents challenges with both identification of landmarks and access to perform the procedure. Extraneous devices, such as a cervical immobilization collar, or a halothoracic brace also may impede access.

**R**—*Radiation (and other deformity or scarring):* Past radiation therapy may distort and scar tissues, making the procedure difficult and often causing tissues that are normally discrete to bond together, distorting tissue planes and relationships.

**T**—*Tumor:* Tumor, either inside the airway (beware of the chronically hoarse patient) or encroaching on the airway, may present difficulty, both from access and bleeding perspectives.

## SUMMARY

- When intubation is indicated, the most important question is "Is this airway difficult?" The decision to perform RSI, for example, is based on a thorough assessment for difficulty (LEMON, ROMAN, RODS, and SMART) and appropriate use of the main or difficult airway algorithms. Because most emergency department patients will have some degree of difficulty after a bedside assessment, the decision to use neuromuscular blocking agents (NMBAs) is a complex one that takes into account the degree of difficulty, the urgency for tube placement, available difficult airway tools, especially VL, and one's own skill and experience. Basically, to use NMBA, the operator must be confident that oxygenation can be maintained, and that intubation is likely to be successful, using the planned approach. See Chapter 3 for further details.
- If LEMON and ROMAN are assessed first, in order, then each component of RODS also has been assessed, with the exception of the D: distorted anatomy. In other words, if LEMON and ROMAN have identified no difficulties, then all that remains for RODS is the question: "If I insert this EGD into the pharynx of this patient, will the device be able to seat itself and seal properly within relatively normal anatomy?"
- The ability to oxygenate a patient with a bag and mask or an EGD turns a potential "can't intubate, can't oxygenate" situation requiring urgent cricothyrotomy into a "can't intubate, *can* oxygenate" situation, in which many rescue options can be considered. The ability to prospectively identify situations in which oxygenation using an EGD or a bag and mask will be difficult or impossible is critical to the decision whether to use NMBAs.
- No single indicator, combination of indicators, or even weighted scoring system of indicators can be relied on to guarantee success or predict inevitable failure for oral intubation. Application of a systematic method to identify the difficult airway and then analysis of the situation to identify the best approach, given the anticipated degree of difficulty and the skill, experience, and judgment of the individual performing the intubation, will lead to the best decisions regarding how to manage the particular clinical situation. In general, it is better to err by identifying an airway as potentially difficult, only to subsequently find this not to be the case, than the other way around.

## EVIDENCE

- **What is the incidence of difficult and failed airway?** A poor glottic view is associated with low intubation success. A meta-analysis of elective anesthesia studies found an incidence of difficult DL ranging from 6% to 27% among nine studies totaling >14,000 patients.[1] For obese patients, the incidence of difficult intubation certainly is higher, but how much of this is caused by obesity alone, and how much is a product of the presence of various difficult airway markers, such as a poor Mallampati score, is not clear. The Intubation Difficulty Score (IDS) considers the numbers of operators, devices, attempts, the C–L score, vocal cord position (abducted or not), and whether excessive lifting force or external manipulation is required.[2] In one study of 129 lean and 134 obese patients, using an IDS of five or greater as the definition of difficult intubation (a relatively high bar), investigators identified difficult intubation in 2.2% of lean patients and 15.5% of obese patients.[3] Only 1% of 663 patients in one British study had grade III glottic views, but 6.5% had grade IIb views (only arytenoids visible), and 2/3 of these were difficult to intubate.[4] In Reed's validation study of the LEMON mnemonic, 11/156 (7%) of patients had C–L grade III glottic views, and only 2/156 had grade IV views.[5] The largest emergency department series is from the National Emergency Airway Registry (NEAR) project. Glottic view is highly dependent on the type of laryngoscope chosen. Multiple ED studies have shown that glottic view is better with both the C-MAC and GlideScope compared to DL.[6–8] In an analysis of 198 video macintosh intubations (V-MAC), a grade I or II glottic view was obtained in 97% of encounters when the video screen was used, but in only 78% of encounters when the V-MAC was used as a direct laryngoscope.[7] In a single-center prospective evaluation of 750 ED intubations over a 2-year period, during which 255 intubations were performed with a C-MAC and the rest with a conventional laryngoscope, the C-MAC yielded grade I/II views in 94% of cases compared with 83% for DL.[8] In the multicenter NEAR II study, reporting on 8,937 intubations from 1997 to 2002, the first chosen method ultimately was not successful in approximately 5% of intubations. Overall airway management success was >99%, and surgical airways were performed on 1.7% of trauma patients and approximately 1% of all cases.[9] In a subset of almost 8,000 of the NEAR II patients, approximately 50% of rescues from failed attempts involved use of RSI after failure of intubation attempts without neuromuscular blockade.[10] In NEAR III, an analysis of 17,583 adult intubations from 2002 to 2012 showed that 17% of all encounters required more than one attempt before successful intubation. Ultimate intubation success was 99.5%. Rescue cricothyrotomy, a surgical airway performed after at least one intubation attempt, was lower than previously reported, occurring in 0.3% of cases and was performed twice as often in trauma patients.[11]
- **What is the evidence basis of LEMON?** There is only one published external validation of the LEMON mnemonic and one for the modified LEMON.[5,12] The American College of Surgeons adopted the LEMON mnemonic for ATLS in 2008, but mistakenly attributed it to Reed. In a recent multicenter prospective intubation registry in Japan, 3,313 patients, for whom a difficult airway assessment was performed and who were intubated using DL, the modified LEMON had a sensitivity of 86% and a negative predictive value of 98% for difficult laryngoscopy. Difficult intubation was defined as any encounter requiring two or more attempts. In other words, the LEMON assessment is most helpful when completely normal and indicates that nearly all patients would be candidates for RSI if truly LEMON-negative. Individual elements, taken in isolation, are less helpful and should never constitute the basis of a difficulty airway assessment. The gestalt of difficulty provided by the patient obviously is an intuitive notion and will vary greatly with the skills and experience of the intubator. There are no studies, of which we are aware, that assess the sensitivity or specificity of this first, quick look. We are not aware of the true origin of the 3-3-2 rule. It probably originated from a group of Canadian difficult airway experts, led by Edward Crosby, MD, but, to our knowledge, it was not published before we included it in the first edition of our book in

2000. The 3-3-2 rule has three components. The first is mouth opening, a long-identified and intuitively obvious marker of difficult DL. The second and third pertain to mandibular size and the distance from the floor of the mandible to the thyroid notch. Many studies suggest identifying decreased (and, to a lesser extent, increased) thyromental distance as a predictor of difficult DL. One study identified that it is relative, but not absolute, thyromental distance that matters; in other words, the relevant thyromental distance that predicts difficulty depends on the size of the patient.[13] This reinforces the notion of using the patient's own fingers as a size guide for thyromental distance, but also for the other two dimensions of the 3-3-2 rule. Hyomental distance has also been used, but seems less reliable, causing researchers to explore the value of repeated measurements and ratios involving different head and neck positions.[14] The eponymous Mallampati evaluation has been validated multiple times. The modified Mallampati score, the four-category method that is most familiar, was found highly reliable in a comprehensive meta-analysis of 42 studies, but the authors emphasize, as do we, that the test is important, but not sufficient in evaluating the difficult airway.[1] One study suggested that the Mallampati evaluation gains specificity (from 70% to 80%) without loss of sensitivity if it is performed with the head in extension, but this study involved only 60 patients, and performing the Mallampati, even in the neutral position, is challenging enough before emergency intubation, so we do not recommend head extension.[15] Interference with DL by upper airway obstruction is self-evident. Obesity is uniformly identified as a difficult airway marker, but, remarkably, controversy persists regarding whether obesity, per se, indicates difficult laryngoscopy, or whether obese patients simply have a greater incidence of having other difficult airway markers, such as higher Mallampati scores.[16] An opposing view suggests that, although a higher Mallampati score is associated with difficult intubation in obese patients, other traditional predictors of difficult intubation do not account for the high incidence and degree of difficulty in obese patients.[3] The only two studies to compare obese and lean patients head to head found a similar fivefold increase in intubation difficulty for obese patients (about 15% vs. about 3% of lean patients), but one study concluded that BMI was important, whereas the other concluded the opposite.[17]

- **What is the evidence basis of ROMAN?** Much of the clinical information about difficult BMV came from case reports and limited case series, and so were subject to bias and misinterpretation. The first well-designed study of difficult BMV was that of Langeron et al.,[18] where a 5% incidence of difficult BMV occurred in 1,502 patients. They identified five independent predictors of difficult BMV: presence of a beard, high BMI, age > 55 years, edentulousness, and a history of snoring. Subsequent studies by other investigators were much larger. Kheterpal et al. used a graded definition of difficult BMV in their study of >22,000 patients. They divided difficult BMV into four classes, ranging from routine and easy (class I) to impossible (class IV). Class III difficulty was defined as inadequate, "unstable," or requiring two providers. They identified class III (difficult) BMV in 313/22,600 (1.4%) and class IV (impossible) in 37 (0.16%) patients. Multivariate analysis was used to identify independent predictors of difficult BMV: presence of a beard, high BMI, age > 57 years, Mallampati class III or IV, limited jaw protrusion, and snoring. Snoring and thyromental distance < 6 cm were independent predictors of impossible BMV.[19] Subsequently, the same researchers studied 53,041 patients over a 4-year period. Independent predictors of impossible BMV included the following: presence of a beard, male sex, neck radiation changes, Mallampati class III or IV, and sleep apnea, with neck radiation having the strongest association of failed mask ventilation.[20] These studies, combined with others, and with our collective experience, are the foundation for the ROMAN mnemonic. Interestingly, Mallampati class did not fare well as a predictor of difficult BMV in Lee's meta-analysis of 42 studies with >34,000 patients, although it did quite well for difficult intubation.[1] Nevertheless, we believe that Mallampati is a worthy consideration with respect to difficult BMV, as it helps the operator to understand the extent to which the tongue might impede ventilation. Conditions that create resistance to ventilation, such as reactive airways disease and COPD, and those associated with a decrease in pulmonary compliance, such as ARDS or pulmonary edema, understandably make ventilation with a bag and mask more difficult. Why were these attributes not identified in the elegant studies of predictors of difficult BMV? Likely, patients with these conditions were too ill to be included in any such studies. Nonetheless, we are confident in including this concept in the "R" of ROMAN.

- **What is the evidence basis of RODS?** Most EGDs have not been systematically studied for predictors of difficulty. Previous information came from case reports or small case series. A recent OR-based registry of 14,480 adult patients managed with either a LMA or an iGel showed that successful oxygenation and ventilation occurred in nearly all (99.8%) cases. Multivariable analysis identified four factors predictive of difficulty: short thyromental distance, male sex, limited neck movement, and age, with short thyromental distance having the highest odds of difficulty (4.4). Interestingly, obesity was not predictive. We hesitate to remove obesity from the RODS mnemonic, however, because this study had very few difficult cases and because it has been shown previously to affect rescue mask ventilation.[21] As such, this mnemonic really represents our expert consensus rather than an assessment of high-quality evidence. The requirement for minimal mouth opening sufficient to insert the device is self-evident. Obesity and obstruction will interfere with EGD use in similar fashion to their interference with BMV. Devices vary in their utility in various patients, however, and some may be better suited for obese patients than others. One study compared 50 morbidly obese patients with 50 lean patients and identified no increase in difficulty for either ventilation or intubation with the intubating LMA.[22] Distorted anatomy is our own concept, based on the fact that each of these devices is designed to "seat" into normal human anatomy, given that the right size of device is selected.
- **How reliable are the factors we evaluate in predicting difficult intubation?** Performing a preintubation assessment confers substantial protection against unexpectedly encountering a difficult intubation. As previously mentioned, when a LEMON assessment fails to show a problem, difficult intubation may occur only in as few as 2% of patients.[12] In one study of prehospital intubations, difficult airway predictors such as obesity and cervical immobility were present in 13% and 50% of failed airways, respectively.[23] In anesthesia practice, using a definition of difficult intubation as two failed attempts despite optimal laryngeal manipulation, one study found only 0.9% unexpected difficult intubations among >11,000 patients.[24] Investigators did not report C–L scores, however. In elective anesthesia practice, difficult airway patients often are "selected out" and managed by modified anesthetic technique, such as awake flexible endoscopic intubation. The safety of performing preintubation assessment is reinforced by this practice, however, as difficult and failed BMV and intubation in this population generally are unexpected because of the prescreening, and so probably reasonably predict unexpected (i.e., not detected by preintubation assessment of difficulty) similar events during emergency intubation. In one study of almost 23,000 patients, only about 1.6% had difficult BMV, and only 0.37% or 1/300 had a combination of difficult BMV and difficult intubation.[19]
- **Does LEMON apply to** VL **also?** The short answer is no, or, at least, we do not know. Much of LEMON has to do with the need to see past the tongue, to the glottis, using a straight line of sight. VL does not involve a straight line of sight, so, for example, we do not have any reason to believe that the 3-3-2 rule applies, particularly with hyper-curved video laryngoscopes. In one study comparing the C-MAC video laryngoscope with DL in ED intubations, the aggregate effect of multiple difficult airway markers had a significant impact on first past success with DL but not with VL. Comparing first attempt success between patients without difficult airway markers with those that had three or more, the first attempt success for DL decreased from 88% to 75% but decreased only by 5% for VL (99% to 93%).[8] Mallampati is not nearly as important, because the video viewer on most video laryngoscopes is positioned beyond the tongue, thus eliminating the tongue from consideration. Mallampati assesses mouth opening, also, however, as does the first "3" of the 3-3-2 rule, and mouth opening remains important for VL, although much less so. Only one study has attempted to identify attributes associated with difficult VL, in this case the GlideScope, and it is difficult to put much weight on any conclusions because 400/400 patients had C–L class I or II views.[25] The evidence for superiority of VL over conventional laryngoscopy is presented in Chapter 14.

## REFERENCES


1. Lee A, Fan LT, Gin T, et al. A systematic review (meta-analysis) of the accuracy of the Mallampati tests to predict the difficult airway. *Anesth Analg*. 2006;102(6):1867–1878.
2. Adnet F, Borron SW, Racine SX, et al. The intubation difficulty scale (IDS): proposal and evaluation of a new score characterizing the complexity of endotracheal intubation. *Anesthesiology*. 1997;87:1290–1297.
3. Juvin P, Lavaut E, Dupont H, et al. Difficult tracheal intubation is more common in obese than in lean patients. *Anesth Analg*. 2003;97(2):595–600.
4. Yentis SM, Lee DJ. Evaluation of an improved scoring system for the grading of direct laryngoscopy. *Anaesthesia*. 1998;53(11):1041–1044.
5. Reed MJ, Dunn MJ, McKeown DW. Can an airway assessment score predict difficulty at intubation in the emergency department? *Emerg Med J*. 2005;22(2):99–102.
6. Sakles JC, Mosier JM, Chiu S, et al. Tracheal intubation in the emergency department: a comparison of GlideScope(R) video laryngoscopy to direct laryngoscopy in 822 intubations. *J Emerg Med*. 2012;42(4):400–405.
7. Brown CA 3rd, Bair AE, Pallin DJ, et al; National Emergency Airway Registry (NEAR) Investigators. Improved glottic exposure with the Video Macintosh Laryngoscope in adult emergency department tracheal intubations. *Ann Emerg Med*. 2010;56(2):83–88.
8. Sakles JC, Mosier J, Chiu C, et al. A comparison of the C-MAC video laryngoscope to the Macintosh direct laryngoscope for intubation in the emergency department. *Ann Emerg Med*. 2012;60:739–748.
9. Walls RM, Brown CA III, Bair AE, et al. Emergency airway management: a multi-center report of 8937 emergency department intubations. *J Emerg Med*. 2011;41(4):347–354.
10. Bair AE, Filbin MR, Kulkarni RG, et al. The failed intubation attempt in the emergency department: analysis of prevalence, rescue techniques, and personnel. *J Emerg Med*. 2002;23(2):131–140.
11. Brown CA 3rd, Bair AE, Pallin DJ, et al; NEAR III Investigators. Techniques, success, and adverse events of emergency department adult intubations. *Ann Emerg Med*. 2015;65(4):363–370.
12. Hagiwara Y, Watase H, Okamoto H, et al. Prospective validation of the modified LEMON criteria to predict difficult intubation in the ED. *Am J Emerg Med*. 2015;33(10):1492–1496.
13. Krobbuaban B, Diregpoke S, Kumkeaw S, et al. The predictive value of the height ratio and thyromental distance: four predictive tests for difficult laryngoscopy. *Anesth Analg*. 2005;101(5):1542–1545.
14. Huh J, Shin HY, Kim SH, et al. Diagnostic predictor of difficult laryngoscopy: the hyomental distance ratio. *Anesth Analg*. 2009;108:544–548.
15. Mashour GA, Sandberg WS. Craniocervical extension improves the specificity and predictive value of the Mallampati airway evaluation. *Anesth Analg*. 2006;103:1256–1259.
16. Brodsky JB, Lemmens HJ, Brock-Utne JG, et al. Morbid obesity and tracheal intubation. *Anesth Analg*. 2002;94(3):732–736.
17. Gonzalez H, Minville V, Delanoue K, et al. The importance of increased neck circumference to intubation difficulties in obese patients. *Anesth Analg*. 2008;106:1132–1136.
18. Langeron O, Masso E, Huraux C, et al. Prediction of difficult mask ventilation. *Anesthesiology*. 2000;92(5):1229–1236.
19. Kheterpal S, Han R, Tremper KK, et al. Incidence and predictors of difficult and impossible mask ventilation. *Anesthesiology*. 2006;105(5):885–891.
20. Kheterpal S, Martin L, Shanks AM, et al. Prediction and outcomes of impossible mask ventilation: a review of 50,000 anesthetics. *Anesthesiology*. 2009;110(4):891–897.
21. Saito T, Liu W, Chew ST, et al. Incidence of and risk factors for difficult ventilation via a supraglottic airway device in a population of 14,480 patients from SE Asia. *Anaesthesia*. 2015;70(9):1079–1083.

22. Combes X, Sauvat S, Leroux B, et al. Intubating laryngeal mask airway in morbidly obese and lean patients: a comparative study. *Anesthesiology*. 2005;102(6):1106–1109.
23. GaitherJB, Spaite DW, Stolz U, et al. Prevalence of difficult airway predictors in cases of failed prehospital endotracheal intubation. *J Emerg Med*. 2014;47(3):294–300.
24. Combes X, Le Roux B, Suen P, et al. Unanticipated difficult airway in anesthetized patients: prospective validation of a management algorithm. *Anesthesiology*. 2004;100(5):1146–1150.
25. Tremblay MH, Williams S, Robitaille A, et al. Poor visualization during direct laryngoscopy and high upper lip bite test score are predictors of difficult intubation with the GlideScope videolaryngoscope. *Anesth Analg*. 2008;106(5):1495–1500.

Chapter 3

# The Emergency Airway Algorithms

Calvin A. Brown III and Ron M. Walls

## APPROACH TO THE AIRWAY

This chapter presents and discusses the emergency airway algorithms, which we have used, taught, and refined for nearly 20 years. These algorithms are intended to reduce error and improve the pace and quality of decision making for an event that is uncommonly encountered by most practitioners, and often disrupts attempts at sound and orderly clinical management.

When we first set out to try to codify the cognitive aspects of emergency airway management, we were both liberated and impaired by the complete lack of any such algorithms to guide us. In developing The Difficult Airway Course: Emergency, The Difficult Airway Course: Anesthesia, The Difficult Airway Course: Critical Care, and The Difficult Airway Course: EMS, and in applying successively each iteration of the emergency airway algorithms to tens of thousands of real and simulated cases involving thousands of providers, we felt guided by both our continuous learning about optimal airway management and the empirical application of these principles. They are based on both the best evidence available and the opinions of the most reputable experts in the field of emergency airway management. These algorithms, or adaptations of them, now appear in many of the major emergency medicine textbooks and online references. They are used in airway courses, for residency training, and in didactic teaching sessions, both for in-hospital and out-of-hospital providers. They have stood the test of time and have benefited from constant updates.

The revolution in video laryngoscopy has caused us to rethink concepts related to the definition and management of the "difficult airway" (see Chapter 2). This fifth iteration includes the foundational concepts of our proven algorithmic approach to airway management augmented by the integration of flexible endoscopic methods, video laryngoscopy, and a focus, especially during rapid sequence intubation (RSI), on "preintubation optimization," a step designed to maximize patient physiology and, by doing so, create safer intubating conditions. Although we describe this as a new discreet step during RSI (see Chapter 20), hemodynamic optimization should occur, if time and resources allow, during *all* emergency intubations. Extraglottic devices (EGDs) continue to be refined and are now easier to use, and many offer the options of blind intubation and gastric decompression. Surgical airway management, although still an essential skill, moves from uncommon to rare as the sophistication of first-line devices, rescue tools, and safe intubation practices increases.

Together, as before, these algorithms comprise a fundamental, *reproducible* approach to the emergency airway. The purpose is not to provide a "cookbook," which one could universally and mindlessly apply, but rather to describe a reproducible set of decisions and actions to enhance performance and maximize the opportunities for success, even in difficult or challenging cases.

The specialized algorithms all build from concepts found in the universal emergency airway algorithm, which describes the priority of the key decisions: determining whether the patient represents a crash airway, a difficult airway, or a failed airway. In addition, we recommend achieving physiologic optimization as an essential step in all airway management, taking into account the patient's condition and the time and resources available. The decision to intubate is discussed in Chapter 1, and the entry point for the emergency airway algorithm is immediately after the decision to intubate has been made.

Introduced in the previous edition, we have maintained the "forced to act" option for this update. There are clinical circumstances in which it is essential to use neuromuscular blocking agents (NMBAs) even in the face of an identified difficult airway, simply because there is not sufficient time to plan any other approach. The operator who is *forced to act* uses an induction agent and an NMBA to create the best possible circumstances for intubation—in other words, to take the one best chance to secure the airway and for successful rescue should the primary method fail. An example of this might be the morbidly obese difficult airway patient who prematurely self-extubates in the ICU and is immediately agitated, hypoxic, and deteriorating. Although the patient's habitus and airway characteristics normally would argue against the use of RSI, the need to secure the airway within just a few minutes and the patient's critical deterioration mandate immediate action. By giving an NMBA and induction agent, the operator can optimize conditions for video or direct laryngoscopy, with a plan to either insert a laryngeal mask airway (LMA) or perform a surgical airway if unsuccessful. In some cases, the primary method may be a surgical airway.

The algorithms are intended as guidelines for management of the emergency airway, regardless of the locus of care (emergency department [ED], inpatient unit, operating room, ICU, and out-of-hospital). The goal is to simplify some of the complexities of emergency airway management by defining distinct categories of airway problems. For example, we single out those patients who are essentially dead or near death (i.e., unresponsive, agonal) and manage them using a distinct pathway, the crash airway algorithm. Similarly, a patient with an anatomically difficult airway must be identified and managed according to sound principles. Serious problems can ensue if an NMBA is given to a patient with a difficult airway, unless the difficulty was identified and planned for and the NMBA is part of that planned approach.

In human factors analysis, failure to recognize a pattern is often a precursor to medical error. The algorithms aid in pattern recognition by guiding the provider to ask specific questions, such as "Is this a crash airway?" and "Is this a can't-intubate-and-can't-oxygenate failed airway?" The answers to these questions group patients with certain characteristics together and each group has a defined series of actions. For example, in the case of a difficult airway, the difficult airway algorithm facilitates formulation of a distinct, but reproducible plan, which is individualized for that particular patient, yet lies within the overall approach that is predefined for all patients in this class, that is, those with difficult airways.

Algorithms are best thought of as a series of *key questions* and *critical actions*, with the answer to each question guiding the next critical action. The answers are always binary: "yes" or "no" to simplify and speed cognitive factor analysis. **Figures 3-1** and **3-2** provide an overview of the algorithms, and how they work together.

When a patient requires intubation, the first question is "Is this a crash airway?" (i.e., is the patient unconscious, near death, with agonal or no respirations, expected to be unresponsive to the stimulation of laryngoscopy?). If the answer is "yes," the patient is managed as a crash airway using the crash airway algorithm (**Fig. 3-3**). If the answer is "no," the next question is "Is this a difficult airway?" (see Chapter 2). If the answer is "yes," the patient is managed as a difficult airway (**Fig. 3-4**). If the answer is "no," then neither a crash airway nor a difficult airway is present, and RSI is recommended, as described on the main algorithm (**Fig. 3-2**). Regardless of the algorithm used initially (main, crash, or difficult), if airway failure occurs, the failed airway algorithm (**Fig. 3-5**) is immediately invoked. The working definition of the failed airway is crucial and is explained in much more detail in the following sections. It has been our experience that airway management errors occur both because the provider does not recognize the situation (e.g., failed airway), and because, although recognizing the situation, he or she does not know what actions to take.

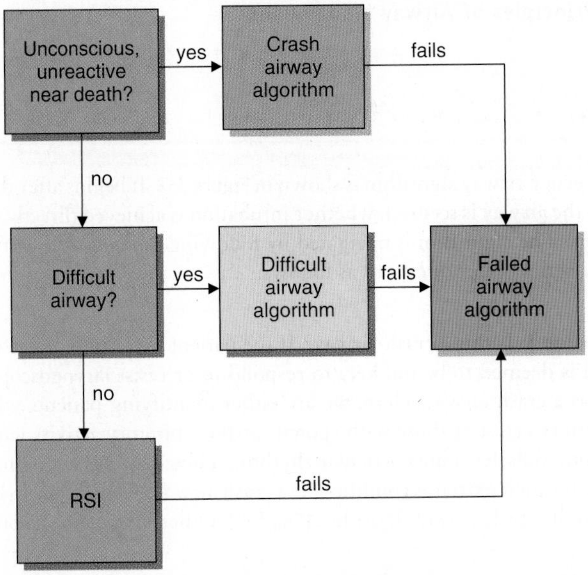


**FIGURE 3-1. Universal Emergency Airway Algorithm.** This algorithm demonstrates how the emergency airway algorithms work together. For all algorithms, green represents the main algorithm, yellow is the difficult airway algorithm, blue is the crash airway algorithm, red is the failed airway algorithm, and orange represents an end point. (© 2017 The Difficult Airway Course: Emergency.)

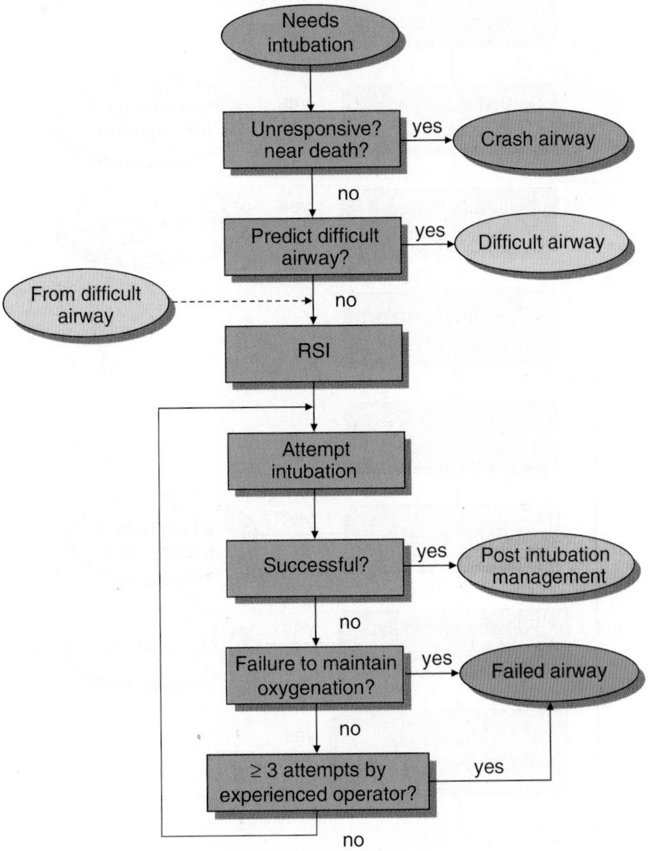


**FIGURE 3-2.** Main Emergency Airway Management Algorithm. See text for details. (© 2017 The Difficult Airway Course: Emergency.)

## THE MAIN AIRWAY ALGORITHM

The main emergency airway algorithm is shown in **Figure 3-2**. It begins after the decision to intubate and ends when the airway is secured, whether intubation is achieved directly or through one of the other algorithms. The algorithm is navigated by following defined steps with decisions driven by the answers to a series of key questions as follows:

- **Key question 1: Is this a crash airway?** If the patient presents in an essentially unresponsive state and is deemed to be unlikely to respond to or resist laryngoscopy, then the patient is defined as a crash airway. Here, we are either identifying patients who are in full cardiac or respiratory arrest or those with agonal cardiorespiratory activity (e.g., agonal, ineffective respirations, pulseless idioventricular rhythm). These patients are managed in a manner appropriate for their extremis condition. If a crash airway is identified, exit this main algorithm and begin the crash airway algorithm (**Fig. 3-3**). Otherwise, continue on the main algorithm.

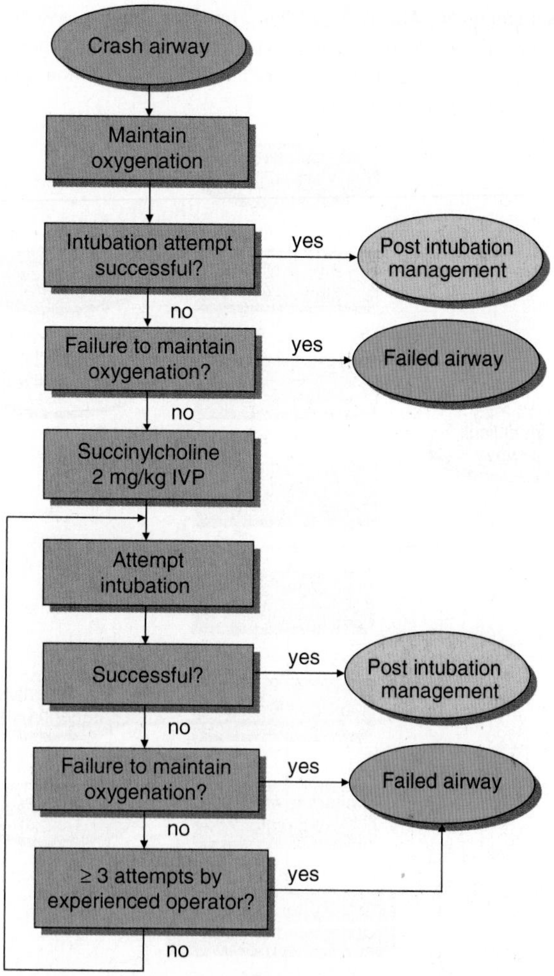


● **FIGURE 3-3. Crash Airway Algorithm.** See text for details. The portion at the bottom is essentially identical to the corresponding portion of the main emergency airway algorithm. IVP, intravenous push. (© 2017 The Difficult Airway Course: Emergency.)

- **Key question 2: Is this a difficult airway?** If the airway is not identified as a crash airway, the next task is to determine whether it is a difficult airway, which encompasses difficult direct laryngoscopy and intubation, difficult bag-mask ventilation (BMV), difficult cricothyrotomy, and difficult EGD use. Chapter 2 outlines the assessment of the patient for a potentially difficult airway using the various mnemonics (LEMON, ROMAN, RODS, and SMART) corresponding to these dimensions of difficulty. Difficult video laryngoscopy is rare as long as there is enough mouth opening to admit the device. Although some predictive parameters have started to become identified, a validated set of patient characteristics has yet to be defined. This is discussed further in Chapter 2. It is understood that virtually all emergency intubations are difficult to some extent. However, the evaluation of the patient for attributes that predict difficult airway management is extremely important. If the patient represents a particularly difficult airway situation, then he or she is managed as a difficult airway patient, using the difficult airway algorithm (**Fig. 3-4**), and one would exit the main algorithm. The LEMON assessment for difficult laryngoscopy and intubation and the ROMAN assessment for difficult rescue BMV are the main drivers of predictable airway challenges; however, an evaluation for the other difficulties (cricothyrotomy and EGD) are critical at this point as well. If the airway is not identified as particularly difficult, continue on the main algorithm to the next step, which is to perform RSI.
- **Critical action: Perform RSI.** In the absence of an identified crash or difficult airway, RSI is the method of choice for managing the emergency airway. RSI is described in detail in Chapter 20 and affords the best opportunity for success with the least likelihood of adverse outcome of any possible airway management method, when *applied to appropriately selected patients*. This step

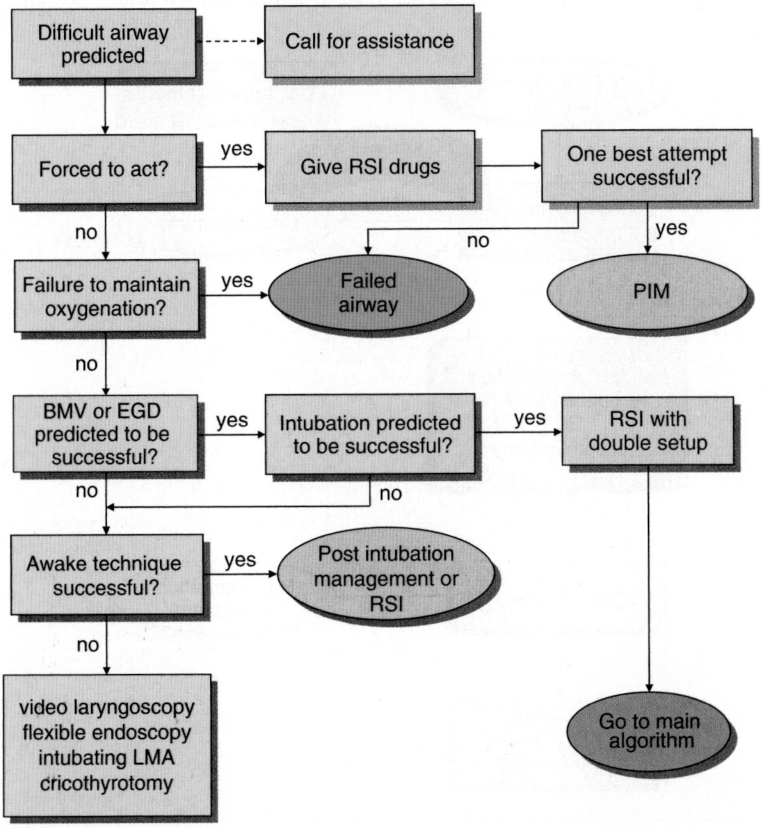


● **FIGURE 3-4. Difficult Airway Algorithm.** See text for details. BMV, bag-mask ventilation. EGD, extraglottic device. PIM, post intubation management. RSI, rapid sequence intubation. (© 2017 The Difficult Airway Course: Emergency.)

assumes that the appropriate sequence of RSI (the seven Ps) will be followed. In particular, if the patient is hemodynamically unstable and the need for intubation is *not* immediate, an effort to optimize patient physiology should occur as plans for intubation are finalized and drugs are drawn up. During RSI, intubation is attempted. According to the standard nomenclature of the National Emergency Airway Registry (NEAR), a multicenter study of emergency intubations, *an attempt is defined as activities occurring during a single continuous laryngoscopy maneuver, beginning when the laryngoscope is inserted into the patient's mouth, and ending when the laryngoscope is removed, regardless of whether an endotracheal tube is actually inserted into the patient.* In other words, if several attempts are made to pass an endotracheal tube (ETT) through the glottis during the course of a single laryngoscopy, these aggregate efforts count as one attempt. If the glottis is not visualized and no attempt is made to insert a tube, the laryngoscopy is still counted as one attempt. These distinctions are important because of the definition of the failed airway that follows.

- **Key question 3: Was intubation successful?** If the first oral intubation attempt is successful, the patient is intubated, postintubation management (PIM) is initiated, and the algorithm terminates. If the intubation attempt is not successful, continue on the main pathway.
- **Key question 4: Can the patient's oxygenation be maintained?** When the first attempt at intubation is unsuccessful, it often is possible and appropriate to attempt a second laryngoscopy without interposed BMV, since oxygen saturations often remain acceptable for an extended period of time following proper preoxygenation. Desaturation can be delayed even further by continuous supplemental oxygen by nasal cannula. In general, supplemental oxygenation with a bag and mask is not necessary until the oxygen saturation falls below 93%. Since peripheral oxygen saturation readings often lag behind actual oxy-hemoglobin levels and the rate at which hemoglobin releases its oxygen stores accelerates at this point, it is appropriate to abort laryngoscopic attempts when oxygen saturations fall below 93% and begin rescue

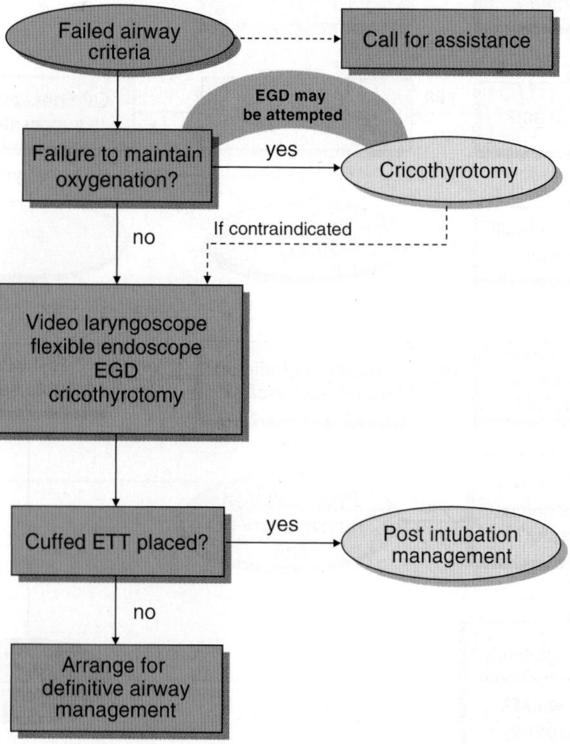


● **FIGURE 3-5. Failed Airway Algorithm.** See text for details. ETT, endotracheal tube. (© 2017 The Difficult Airway Course: Emergency.)

mask ventilation. This approach underscores the importance of assessing the likelihood of successful BMV (ROMAN, see Chapter 2) before beginning the intubation sequence. In the vast majority of cases, especially when neuromuscular blockade has been used, BMV will provide adequate ventilation and oxygenation for the patient. If BMV is not capable of maintaining the oxygen saturation at or above 93%, a better technique including oral and nasal airways, use of two-person two-handed technique with a thenar grip, and optimal patient positioning, will usually result in effective ventilation (see Chapter 9). If BMV fails and oxygen saturations keep dropping despite optimal technique, the airway is considered a failed airway, and one must exit the main algorithm immediately and initiate the failed airway algorithm (**Fig. 3-5**). Recognition of the failed airway is crucial because delays caused by persistent, futile attempts at intubation will waste critical seconds or minutes and may sharply reduce the time remaining for a rescue technique to be successful before brain injury ensues.

- **Key question 5: Have three attempts at orotracheal intubation been made by an experienced operator?** There are two essential definitions of the failed airway: (1) "can't intubate, can't oxygenate" (CICO) (described previously); and (2) "three failed attempts by an experienced operator." If three separate attempts at orotracheal intubation by an experienced operator using the best available device have been unsuccessful, then the airway is again defined as a failed airway, despite the ability to adequately oxygenate the patient using a bag and mask. If an experienced operator has used a particular method of laryngoscopy, such as video laryngoscopy or direct laryngoscopy, for three attempts without success, success with a subsequent attempt is unlikely. The operator must recognize the failed airway and manage it as such using the failed airway algorithm. If there have been fewer than three unsuccessful attempts at intubation, but BMV is successful, then it is appropriate to attempt orotracheal intubation again, provided the oxygen saturation is maintained and the operator can identify an element of the laryngoscopy that can be improved and likely to lead to success (e.g., patient positioning or different instrument). Similarly, if the initial attempts were made by an inexperienced operator, such as a trainee, and the patient is adequately oxygenated, then it is appropriate to reattempt oral intubation until three attempts by an *experienced* operator have been unsuccessful. If available, at least one of those attempts should be made with a video laryngoscope, and if the initial one or two attempts have failed using conventional laryngoscopy, we recommend switching to a video laryngoscope for the remaining attempt(s). Rarely, even a fourth attempt at laryngoscopy may be appropriate before declaring a failed airway. This most often occurs when the operator identifies a particular strategy for success (e.g., better control of the epiglottis by using a larger laryngoscope blade, switching to a video laryngoscope) during the third unsuccessful attempt. Similarly, it is possible that an *experienced* operator will recognize on the *very first attempt* that further attempts at orotracheal intubation will not be successful. In such cases, provided that the patient has been optimally positioned for intubation, good relaxation has been achieved, and it is the operator's judgment that further attempts at laryngoscopy would be futile, the airway should be immediately regarded as a failed airway, and the failed airway algorithm initiated. Thus, it is not essential to make three laryngoscopic attempts before labeling an airway as failed, but three failed attempts by an experienced operator with optimal adjuncts should always be considered a failed airway, unless the laryngoscopist identifies a particular problem and potential solution, justifying one more attempt.

## THE CRASH AIRWAY ALGORITHM

Entering the crash airway algorithm (**Fig. 3-3**) indicates that one has identified an unconscious, unresponsive, or coding patient with an immediate need for airway management. It is assumed that BMV or some other method of oxygenation is occurring throughout.

- **Key question 1: Is the patient pulseless?** If yes, then based on recent advanced cardiac life support (ACLS) recommendations, there should be immediate attempts to perform rescue ventilation with either a bag-and-mask apparatus or an EGD; however, in the initial moments of a full cardiac arrest, definitive airway placement is not required. If the patient survives his code, then plans for definitive airway management can take place.

- **Critical action: If not pulseless, intubate immediately:** The next action in the crash algorithm is to attempt oral intubation immediately by direct or video laryngoscopy without pharmacologic assistance. In these patient circumstances, direct oral intubation has success rates comparable to RSI, presumably because the patients have flaccid musculature and are unresponsive in a manner similar to that achieved by RSI. When managing crash airways, there is generally no time to consider patient optimization because the need for airway management is immediate.
- **Key question 2: Was intubation successful?** If yes, carry on with PIM and general resuscitation. If intubation was not successful, resume BMV or oxygenation using an EGD and proceed to the next step.
- **Key question 3: Is oxygenation adequate?** If oxygenation is adequate using a bag and mask or an EGD, then further attempts at oral intubation are possible. Adequacy of oxygenation with a crash airway usually is not determined by pulse oximetry but by assessment of patient color, chest rise, and the feel of the bag (reflecting patency of the airway, delivered tidal volume, airway resistance, and pulmonary compliance). *If oxygenation is unsuccessful in the context of a single failed oral intubation attempt with a crash airway, then a failed airway is present.* One further attempt at intubation may be rapidly tried, but no more than one, because intubation has failed, and the failure of oxygenation places the patient in serious and immediate jeopardy. This is a CICO-failed airway, analogous to that described previously. Exit here, and proceed directly to the failed airway algorithm (**Fig. 3-5**).
- **Critical action: Administer succinylcholine 2 mg per kg intravenous push:** If intubation is not successful, it is reasonable to assume that the patient has residual muscle tone and is not optimally relaxed. The dose of succinylcholine is increased here because these patients often have severe circulatory compromise, impairing the distribution and rapidity of the onset of succinylcholine. Bag ventilation is continued for 60 to 90 seconds to allow the succinylcholine to distribute. Remember, it is oxygen the patient requires most, not the ETT. From this point onward, the crash airway algorithm is virtually identical to the corresponding portion of the main airway algorithm, with the exception that the patient has not been adequately preoxygenated, and pulse oximetry is generally incapable of accurately reflecting the state of oxygenation in the crash airway patient. The sequence and rationale, however, are identical from this point on.
- **Critical action: Attempt intubation:** After allowing time for the succinylcholine to circulate, another attempt is made at oral intubation.
- **Key question 4: Was the intubation successful?** If intubation is achieved, then proceed to PIM. If not, another attempt is indicated if oxygenation is maintained.
- **Key question 5: Is oxygenation adequate?** If oxygenation cannot be maintained at any time, the airway becomes a CICO-failed airway, requiring implementation of the failed airway algorithm.
- **Key question 6: Have there been three or more attempts at intubation by an experienced operator?** This situation is exactly analogous to that described earlier in the RSI portion of the main airway algorithm (**Fig. 3-2**). If succinylcholine is administered to a crash patient, count the subsequent intubation attempt as attempt number one.

## THE DIFFICULT AIRWAY ALGORITHM

Identification of the difficult airway is discussed in detail in Chapter 2. This algorithm (**Fig. 3-4**) represents the clinical approach that should be used in the event of an identified potential difficult airway.

- **Critical action: Call for assistance.** The "call for assistance" box is linked as a dotted line because this is an optional step, dependent on the particular clinical circumstances, skill of the airway manager, available equipment and resources, and availability of additional personnel. Assistance might include personnel, special airway equipment, or both.

- **Key question 1: Is the operator forced to act?** In some circumstances, although the airway is identified to be difficult, patient conditions force the operator to act immediately, before there is rapid deterioration of the patient into respiratory arrest. An example of this situation is given earlier in this chapter. Another example is a patient with rapidly progressive anaphylaxis from a contrast reaction while getting an abdominal CT scan. The patient is anxious, agitated, and in severe distress. In such cases, there may not be time to obtain and administer epinephrine or antihistamines and reassess for improvement before total airway obstruction occurs. In such circumstances, a prompt decision to give RSI drugs and create circumstances for a *best single attempt* at tracheal intubation, whether by laryngoscopy or surgical airway, often is preferable to medical management alone and hoping for immediate reversal as the patient progresses to complete airway obstruction, respiratory arrest, and death. Administration of RSI drugs might permit the operator to intubate, perform a surgical airway, place an EGD, or use a bag and mask to oxygenate the patient. The key is for the operator to make the *one* best attempt that, in the operator's judgment, is most likely to succeed. If the attempt, for example, intubation using video laryngoscopy, is successful, then the operator proceeds to PIM. If that one attempt is not successful, a failed airway is present, and the operator proceeds to the failed airway algorithm.
- **Key question 2: Is there adequate time?** In the context of the difficult airway, *oxygen is time*. If ventilation and oxygenation are adequate and oxygen saturation can be maintained over 92%, then a careful assessment and a methodical, planned approach can be undertaken, even if significant preparation time is required. However, if oxygenation is inadequate, then additional oxygenation, bi-level positive airway pressure (Bi-PAP), or BMV is initiated. If oxygenation fails or saturations keep dropping despite escalating methods, immediately move to the failed airway algorithm. This situation is equivalent to a "can't intubate (the identified difficult airway is a surrogate for can't intubate), can't oxygenate (adequate oxygenation saturation cannot be achieved)" failed airway. Certain difficult airway patients will have chronic pulmonary disease, for example, and may not be able to reach an oxygen saturation of 93%, but can be kept stable and viable at, say, 88%. In addition, a patient may have been considered difficult because of a cervical collar placed by EMS after an isolated head injury, but the suspicion for cervical spine injury is low and there are no other markers of airway difficulty. In this example, an experienced airway manager, armed with a video laryngoscope, may not consider this situation analogous to a "can't intubate" scenario. In other words, whether to call these cases failed airways is a matter of judgment considering both the degree of oxygen debt and severity of predicted difficulty. If a decision is made to proceed down the difficult airway algorithm rather than switching to the failed airway algorithm, it is essential to be aware that in cases such as this, desaturation will occur rapidly during intubation attempts and to increase vigilance with respect to hypoxemia.
- **Key question 3: Should I use an NMBA on this patient? In other words, is rescue oxygenation using a bag and mask or EGD predicted to be successful? Is laryngoscopy predicted to be successful?** Having a patient in the difficult airway algorithm does not obviate RSI in all cases. It is possible that despite the presence of airway difficulty, RSI remains the best approach. This decision hinges on two key factors combined into one composite "yes or no" question.

  The first, and most important, factor is whether one predicts with confidence that gas exchange can be maintained by BMV or the use of an EGD if RSI drugs are administered rendering the patient paralyzed and apneic. This answer may already be known whether BMV has been required to maintain the patient's oxygenation or whether the difficult airway evaluation (see Chapter 2) did not identify difficulty for oxygenation using BMV or an EGD. Anticipating successful oxygenation using BMV or an EGD is an essential prerequisite for RSI, except in the "forced to act" situation described earlier. In some cases, it may be desirable to attempt a trial of BMV, but this approach does not reliably predict the ability to bag-mask ventilate the patient after paralysis.

  Second, if BMV or EGD is anticipated to be successful, then the next consideration is whether intubation is likely to be successful, despite the difficult airway attributes. In reality, many patients with identified difficult airways undergo successful emergency intubation employing RSI, particularly when a video laryngoscope is used. So if there is a reasonable likelihood of success with oral intubation, *despite predicting a difficult airway*, RSI may be undertaken. Remember, this is predicated on the fact that one has already judged that gas exchange (BMV or EGD) will be successful following neuromuscular blockade. In these cases, RSI is performed using a "double setup," in which the rescue plan (often cricothyrotomy) is clearly established, and the operator is prepared to move promptly to the rescue technique if intubation using RSI is not successful (failed airway). In most cases, however, when RSI is undertaken despite identification of difficult airway attributes, appropriate care during the technique and planning related to the particular difficulties present will result in success.

To reiterate these two fundamental principles, if gas exchange employing BMV or EGD is not confidently assured of success in the context of difficult intubation, *or* if the chance of successful oral intubation is felt to be poor, then RSI is not recommended, except in the "forced to act" scenario.

- **Critical action: Perform "awake" laryngoscopy:** Just as RSI is an essential technique of emergency airway management, "awake" laryngoscopy is the cornerstone of difficult airway management. The goal of this maneuver is to gain a high degree of confidence that the airway will be secured if RSI is performed. Alternatively, the airway can be secured during the "awake look." This technique usually requires liberally applied topical anesthesia and the judicious use of sedation in order to permit laryngoscopy without fully inducing and paralyzing the patient (see Chapter 23). The principle here is that the patient is awake enough to maintain protective airway reflexes and effective spontaneous ventilation, but is sufficiently obtunded to tolerate an awake evaluation of the airway. Thus, strictly speaking, "awake" is somewhat of a misnomer. The laryngoscopy can be done with a standard laryngoscope, flexible endoscope, video laryngoscope, or a semirigid fiberoptic or video intubating stylet. Awake video laryngoscopy has become a popular approach because the depth of blade insertion and force required to get an adequate view of the glottic inlet is less than what is required with a conventional laryngoscope. These devices are discussed in detail in Chapters 13 to 17. Two outcomes are possible from this awake examination. First, the glottis may be adequately visualized, informing the operator that oral intubation using that device is highly likely to succeed. If the difficult airway is static (i.e., chronic, such as with ankylosing spondylitis), then the best approach might be to proceed with RSI, now that it is known that the glottis can be visualized, using that same device. If, however, the difficult airway is dynamic (i.e., acute, as in smoke inhalation or angioedema), then it is likely better to proceed directly with intubation during this awake laryngoscopy, rather than to back out and perform RSI. This decision is predicated on the possibility that the airway might deteriorate further in the intervening time, arguing in favor of immediate intubation during the awake examination, rather than assuming that the glottis will be visualized with equal ease a few minutes later during RSI. Intervening deterioration, possibly contributed to by the laryngoscopy itself, might make a subsequent laryngoscopy more difficult or even impossible (see Chapter 34). The second possible outcome during the awake laryngoscopic examination is that the glottis is not adequately visualized to permit intubation. In this case, the examination has confirmed the suspected difficult intubation and reinforced the decision to avoid neuromuscular paralysis. A failed airway has been avoided, and several options remain. Oxygenation should be maintained as necessary at this point.

  Although the awake look is the crucial step in management of the difficult airway, it is not infallible. In rare cases, an awake look may provide a better view of the glottic structures than is visible after the administration of a neuromuscular blocking drug. Thus, although the likelihood that the glottis will be less well seen after paralysis than during the awake look is remote, it is not zero, and the airway manager must always be prepared for this rare eventuality.
- **Critical action: Select an alternative airway approach:** At this point, we have clarified that we have a patient with difficult airway attributes, who has proven to be a poor candidate for laryngoscopy, and therefore is inappropriate for RSI. There are a number of options available here. If the awake laryngoscopy was done using a direct laryngoscope, a video laryngoscope or flexible endoscope likely will provide a superior view of the glottis. Given the visualization advantage offered by video laryngoscopy, it should be considered a first-line device for awake laryngoscopy. The main fallback method for the difficult airway is cricothyrotomy (open or Seldinger technique), although the airway may be amenable to an EGD that facilitates intubation, that is, one of the intubating LMAs (I-LMAs). In highly select cases, blind nasotracheal

intubation may be possible but requires an anatomically intact and normal upper airway. In general, blind nasotracheal intubation is used only when flexible endoscopy is not available or is rendered impossible by excessive bleeding in the airway. The choice of technique will depend on the operator's experience, available equipment, the particular difficult airway attributes the patient possesses, and the urgency of the intubation. Whichever technique is used, the goal is to place a cuffed ETT in the trachea.

## THE FAILED AIRWAY ALGORITHM

At several points in the preceding algorithms, it may be determined that airway management has failed. The definition of the failed airway (see previous discussion in this chapter and in Chapter 2) is based on one of three criteria being satisfied: (1) a failure of an intubation attempt in a patient for whom oxygenation cannot be adequately maintained with a bag and mask, (2) three unsuccessful intubation attempts by an experienced operator but with adequate oxygenation, and (3) failed intubation using the one *best attempt* in the "forced to act" situation (this is analogous to the "CICO" situation, but oxygenation by bag and mask, or by EGD, may be possible). Unlike the difficult airway, where the standard of care dictates the placement of a cuffed ETT in the trachea providing a definitive, protected airway, the failed airway calls for action to provide emergency oxygenation sufficient to prevent patient morbidity (especially hypoxic brain injury) by whatever means possible, until a definitive airway can be secured (**Fig. 3-5**). Thus, the devices considered for the failed airway are somewhat different from, but inclusive of, the devices used for the difficult airway (see Chapter 2). When a failed airway has been determined to occur, the response is guided by whether oxygenation is possible.

- **Critical action: Call for assistance.** As is the case with the difficult airway, it is best to call for any available and necessary assistance as soon as a failed airway is identified. Again, this action may be a stat consult to emergency medicine, anesthesia, or surgery, or it may be a call for special equipment. In the prehospital setting, a second paramedic or a medical control physician might provide assistance.
- **Key question 1: Is oxygenation adequate?** As is the case for the difficult airway, this question addresses the time available for a rescue airway. If the patient is a failed airway because of three failed attempts by an experienced operator, in most cases, oxygen saturation will be adequate, and there is time to consider various approaches. If, however, the failed airway is because of a CICO situation, then there is little time left before cerebral hypoxia ensues, and immediate action is indicated. Many, or most, CICO patients will require surgical airway management, and preparation for a surgical airway should be undertaken. It is reasonable, as the first rescue step, to make a single attempt to insert a rapidly placed extraglottic airway device, *simultaneously with the preparation for a cricothyrotomy.* Placement or even use of an EGD does not preclude a surgical airway should that device fail, yet successful oxygenation using the EGD converts the CICO situation into a *can't* intubate, *can* oxygenate situation, allowing time for consideration of a number of different approaches to securing the airway.
- **Critical action:** Achieve an airway using flexible endoscopy, video laryngoscopy, an EGD, a semirigid intubating stylet, or cricothyrotomy. In the can't intubate, *can* oxygenate situation, various devices are available to provide an airway, and most also provide some degree of airway protection. Intubation by flexible endoscopy or video laryngoscopy will establish a cuffed endotracheal in the trachea. Of the EGDs, the ILMAs are preferable because they have a high likelihood of providing effective ventilation and usually permit intubation through the device (see Chapter 10). Cricothyrotomy always remains the final common pathway if other measures are not successful, or if the patient's oxygenation becomes compromised.
- **Key question 2: Does the device used result in a definitive airway?** If the device used results in a definitive airway (i.e., a cuffed ETT in the trachea), then one can move on to PIM. If an EGD has been used, or intubation was not successful through the ILMA, arrangements must

be made to provide a definitive airway. A definitive airway may be provided in the operating room, ICU, or ED, once the necessary personnel and equipment are available. Until then, constant surveillance is required to ensure that the airway, as placed, continues to provide adequate oxygenation, with cricothyrotomy always available as a backup.

## CONCLUSION

These algorithms represent our most current thinking regarding a recommended approach to emergency airway management. The algorithms are intended as guidelines only. Individual decision making, clinical circumstances, skill of the operator, and available resources will determine the final, best approach to airway management in any individual case. Understanding the fundamental concepts of the difficult and failed airway; identification, in advance, of the difficult airway; recognition of the crash airway; and the use of RSI, after physiologic optimization, as the airway management method of choice for most emergency intubations, will foster successful airway management while minimizing preventable morbidity.

## EVIDENCE

- **Evidence for the algorithms.** Unfortunately, there are no systematized data supporting the algorithmic approach presented in this chapter. The algorithms are the result of careful review of the American Society of Anesthesiologists difficult airway algorithm, the algorithms of the Difficult Airway Society of the United Kingdom, and composite knowledge and experience of the editors and faculty of The Difficult Airway Courses, who function as an expert panel in this regard.[1,2] There has not been, and likely never will be, a study comparing, for example, the outcomes of cricothyrotomy versus alternate airway devices in the CICO situation. Clearly, randomization of such patients is not ethical. Thus, the algorithms are derived from a rational body of knowledge (described previously) and represent a recommended approach, but cannot be considered to be scientifically proven as the only or even necessarily the best way to approach any one clinical problem or patient. Rather, they are designed to help guide a consistent approach to both common and uncommon airway management situations. The evidence for the superiority of RSI over other methods not involving neuromuscular blockade and the performance characteristics of video vs. direct laryngoscopy can be found in Chapters 20 and 14, respectively.

## REFERENCES

1. Apfelbaum JL, Hagberg CA, Caplan RA, et al. Practice guidelines for management of the difficult airway: an updated report by the American Society of Anesthesiologists Task Force on Management of the Difficult Airway. *Anesthesiology*. 2013;118(2):251–270.
2. Frerk C, Mitchell VS, McNary AF, et al. Difficult Airway Society 2015 guidelines for management of unanticipated difficult intubations in adults. *Br J Anaesthesia*. 2015;115(6):827–848.

Chapter 4

# Applied Functional Anatomy of the Airway

Michael F. Murphy

## INTRODUCTION

There are many salient features of the anatomy and physiology of the airway to consider with respect to airway management maneuvers. This chapter discusses the anatomical structures most involved in airway management and the innervation of the upper airway. Chapter 23 builds on these anatomical and functional relationships to describe anesthesia techniques for the airway. Chapter 24 addresses developmental and pediatric anatomical features of the airway.

This chapter describes anatomical structures in the order in which they appear as we enter the airway: the nose, the mouth, the pharynx, the larynx, and the trachea (**Fig. 4-1**).

## THE NOSE

The external nose consists of a bony vault, a cartilaginous vault, and a lobule. The bony vault comprises the nasal bones, the frontal processes of the maxillae, and the nasal spine of the frontal bone. The nasal bones are buttressed in the midline by the perpendicular plate of the ethmoid bone that forms part of the bony septum. The cartilaginous vault is formed by the upper lateral cartilages that meet the cartilaginous portion of the septum in the midline. The nasal lobule consists of the tip of the nose, the lower lateral cartilages, the fibrofatty alae that form the lateral margins of the nostril, and the columella. The cavities of each nostril are continuous with the nasopharynx posteriorly.

### Important Anatomical Considerations

- Kiesselbach's plexus (Little's area) is a very vascular area located on the anterior aspect of the septum in each nostril. Epistaxis most often originates from this area. During the act of inserting a nasal trumpet or a nasotracheal tube (NTT), it is generally recommended that the device be inserted in the nostril such that the leading edge of the bevel (the pointed tip) is away from the septum. The goal is to minimize the chances of trauma and bleeding from this very vascular area. This means that the device is inserted "upside down" in the left nostril and rotated 180° after the tip has proceeded beyond the cartilaginous septum. Although some

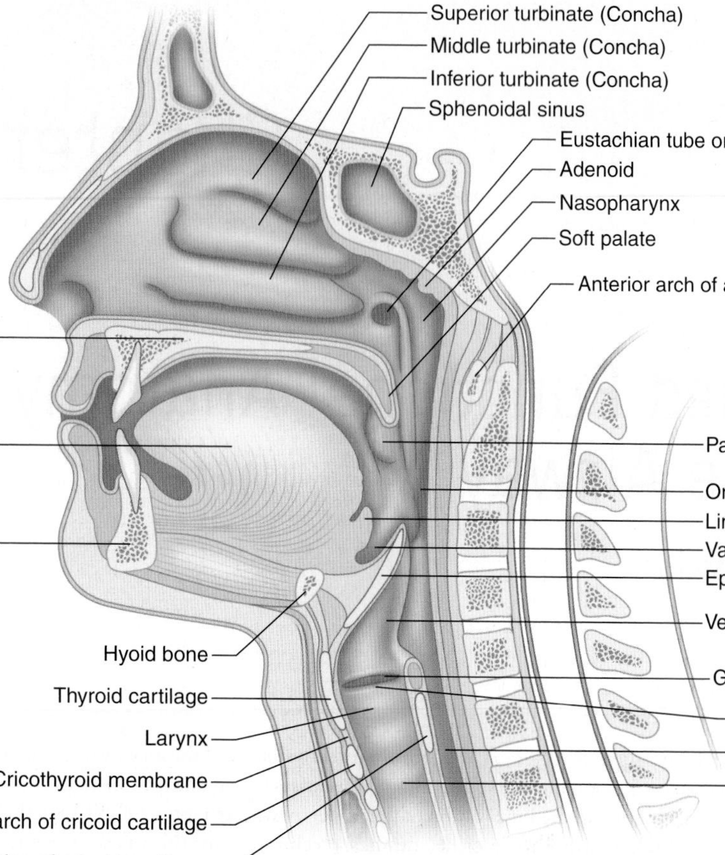


● **FIGURE 4-1. Sagittal View of the Upper Airway.** Note the subtle inferior tilt of the floor of the nose from front to back, the location of the adenoid, the location of the vallecula between the base of the tongue and the epiglottis, and the location of the hyoid bone in relation to the posterior limit of the tongue.

authors have recommended the opposite (i.e., that the bevel tip approximate the nasal septum to minimize the risk of damage and bleeding from the turbinates), the bevel away from the septum approach makes more sense and is the recommended method.

- The major nasal airway is between the laterally placed inferior turbinate, the septum, and the floor of the nose. The floor of the nose is tilted slightly downward front to back, approximately 10° to 15°. Thus, when a nasal tube, trumpet, or fiberscope is inserted through the nose, it should not be directed upward or even straight back. Instead, it should be directed slightly inferiorly to follow this major channel. Before nasal intubation of an unconscious adult patient, this author recommends gently but *fully* inserting one's gloved and lubricated little finger into the nostril to ensure patency and to maximally dilate this channel before the insertion of the nasal tube. In addition, placing the endotracheal tube (ETT; preferably an Endotrol tube) in a warm bottle of saline or water softens the tube and attenuates its damaging properties.
- The nasal mucosa is exquisitely sensitive to topically applied vasoconstricting medications such as phenylephrine, epinephrine, oxymetazoline, or cocaine. Cocaine has the added advantage of providing profound topical anesthesia and is the only local anesthetic agent that produces vasoconstriction; the others cause vasodilatation. Shrinking the nasal mucosa with a vasoconstricting agent can increase the caliber of the nasal airway by as much as 50% to 75% and may reduce epistaxis incited by nasotracheal intubation, although there is little evidence

to support this claim. Cocaine has been implicated in coronary vasoconstriction when applied to the nasal mucosa; so it should be used with caution in patients with coronary artery disease. Evidence suggests that topical vasoconstrictor and local anesthetic agents are not necessary to perform flexible nasoendoscopy.

- The nasal cavities are bounded posteriorly by the nasopharynx. The adenoids are located posteriorly in the nasopharynx just above the nasal surface of the soft palate and partially surround a depression in the mucosal membrane where the eustachian tube enters the nasopharynx. During insertion, the NTT often enters this depression, and resistance is encountered. Continued aggressive insertion can cause the NTT to penetrate the mucosa and pass submucosally deep to the naso- and oropharyngeal mucous membranes (**Fig. 4-2**). Although it is alarming when one recognizes that this has occurred, no specific treatment is indicated, except withdrawing the tube and trying the opposite nostril should nasal intubation be deemed appropriate. Despite the theoretical risk of infection, there is no literature to suggest that this occurs. Documentation of the complication and communication to the accepting team on admission is important.
- The soft palate rests on the base of the tongue during quiet nasal respiration, sealing the oral cavity anteriorly.
- The contiguity of the paranasal sinuses with the nasal cavity is believed to be responsible for the infections of the paranasal sinuses that may be associated with prolonged nasotracheal intubation. Although this fact has led some physicians to condemn nasotracheal intubation, fear of infection should not deter the emergency physician from performing nasotracheal intubation when required. Securing the airway in an emergency takes precedence over possible later infective complications, and in any case, the intubation can always be changed to an oral tube or tracheostomy, if necessary.
- A nasotracheal intubation is relatively contraindicated in patients with basal skull fractures (i.e., when the maxilla is fractured away from its attachment to the base of the skull) because of the risk of penetration into the cranial vault (usually through the cribriform plate) with the ETT. Careful technique avoids this complication: The cribriform plate is located cephalad of the nares, and tube insertion should be directed slightly caudad (see previous discussion). Maxillary fractures (e.g., LeFort fractures) may disrupt the continuity of the nasal cavities and are a relative contraindication to blind nasal intubation. Again, cautious insertion, especially if guided by a fiberscope, can mitigate the risk.

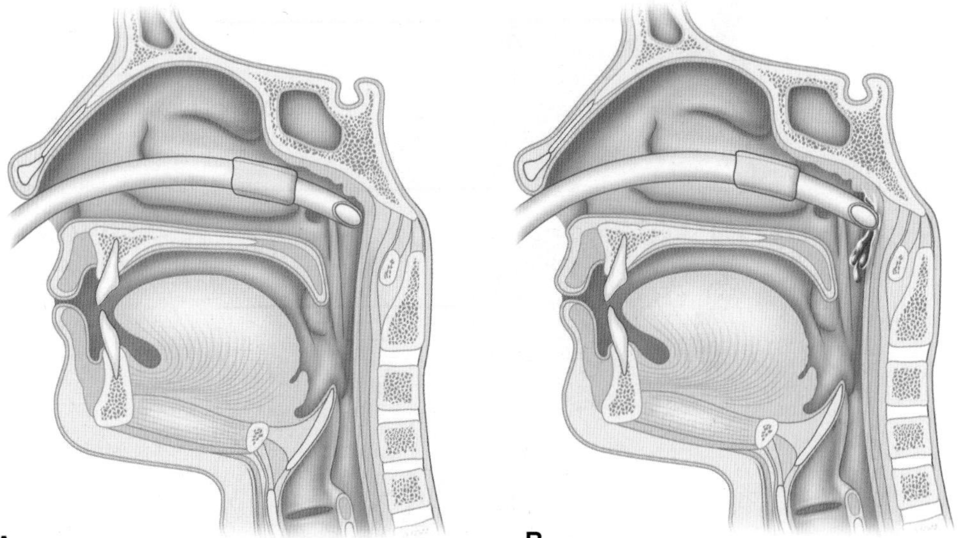

A B

● **FIGURE 4-2. Mechanism of Nasopharyngeal Perforation and Submucosal Tunneling of the NTT. A:** The NTT entering the pit of the adenoid where the eustachian tube enters the nasopharynx. **B:** The tube perforating the mucous membrane; NTT, Nasotracheal tube.

## THE MOUTH

The mouth, or oral cavity, is bounded externally by the lips and is contiguous with the oropharynx posteriorly (**Fig. 4-3**).

- The tongue is attached to the symphysis of the mandible anteriorly and anterolaterally and the stylohyoid process and hyoid bone posterolaterally and posteriorly, respectively. The hyoid is connected to the epiglottis by the hyoepiglottic ligament. The clinical relevance of this relationship explains why a jaw thrust pulls the epiglottis anteriorly exposing the laryngeal inlet. The posterior limit of the tongue corresponds to the position of the hyoid bone (**Fig. 4-1**).
- The potential spaces in the hollow of the mandible are collectively called the mandibular space, which is subdivided into three potential spaces on either side of the midline sublingual raphe: the submental, submandibular, and sublingual spaces. The tongue is a fluid-filled noncompressible structure. During direct laryngoscopy, the tongue is ordinarily displaced to the left and into the mandibular space, permitting one to expose the larynx for intubation under direct vision. If the mandibular space is small relative to the size of the tongue (e.g., hypoplastic mandible, lingual edema in angioedema, and lingual hematoma), the ability to visualize the larynx may be compromised. Infiltration of the mandibular space by infection (e.g., Ludwig angina), hematoma, or other lesions may limit the ability to displace the tongue into this space and render orotracheal intubation difficult or impossible.
- Subtle geometric distortions of the oral cavity that limit one's working and viewing space, such as a high-arched palate with a narrow oral cavity or buckteeth with an elongated oral cavity, may render orotracheal intubation difficult. Chapter 13 elaborates on these issues.
- Salivary glands continuously secrete saliva. This can hinder attempts at achieving sufficient topical anesthesia of the airway to undertake awake laryngoscopy or other active airway intervention maneuvers in the awake or lightly sedated patient—for example, laryngeal mask airway insertion.

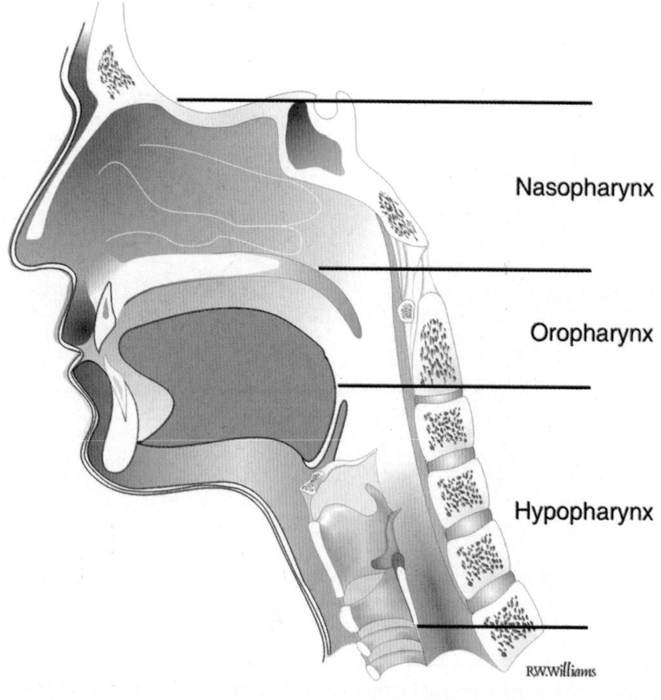


**FIGURE 4-3.** Pharynx divided into three segments: nasopharynx, oropharynx, and hypopharynx.

- The condyles of the mandible articulate within the temporomandibular joint (TMJ) for the first 30° of mouth opening. Beyond 30°, the condyles *translate* out of the TMJ anteriorly onto the zygomatic arches. After translation has occurred, it is possible to use a jaw thrust maneuver to pull the mandible and tongue forward. This is the most effective method of opening the airway to alleviate obstruction or permit bag-mask ventilation. A jaw thrust to open the airway may not be possible unless this translation has occurred (see Chapter 9).

## THE PHARYNX

The pharynx is a U-shaped fibromuscular tube extending from the base of the skull to the lower border of the cricoid cartilage where, at the level of the sixth cervical vertebra, it is continuous with the esophagus. Posteriorly, it rests against the fascia covering the prevertebral muscles and the cervical spine. Anteriorly, it opens into the nasal cavity (the nasopharynx), the mouth (the oropharynx), and the larynx (the laryngo- or hypopharynx).

- The oropharyngeal musculature has a normal tone, like any other skeletal musculature, and this tone serves to keep the upper airway open during quiet respiration. Respiratory distress is associated with voluntary pharyngeal muscular activity that attempts to open the airway further. Benzodiazepines and other sedative hypnotic agents may attenuate some of this tone. This explains why even small doses of sedative hypnotic medications (e.g., midazolam) may precipitate total airway obstruction in patients presenting with partial airway obstruction.
- An "awake look" employing direct laryngoscopy to see the epiglottis or posterior glottic structures using topical anesthesia and sedation may reassure one that at least this much, and probably more, of the airway will be visualized during a direct laryngoscopy and intubation following the administration of a neuromuscular blocking drug. In practice, the glottic view is usually improved following neuromuscular blockade. Rarely, however, the loss of pharyngeal muscle tone caused by the neuromuscular blocking agent leads to the cephalad and anterior migration of the larynx, worsening the view at direct laryngoscopy. Although uncommon, this tends to occur more often in morbidly obese or late-term pregnancy patients, in whom there may be submucosal edema.
- The glossopharyngeal nerve supplies sensation to the posterior one-third of the tongue, the valleculae, the superior surface of the epiglottis, and most of the posterior pharynx. It mediates the gag reflex. This nerve is accessible to blockade (topically or by injection) because it runs just deep into the inferior portion of the palatopharyngeus muscle (the posterior tonsillar pillar) (**Fig. 4-4**).

## THE LARYNX

The larynx extends from its oblique entrance formed by the aryepiglottic folds, the tip of the epiglottis, and the posterior commissure between the arytenoid cartilages (interarytenoid folds) through the vocal cords to the cricoid ring (**Fig. 4-5**).

- The superior laryngeal branch of the vagus nerve supplies sensation to the undersurface of the epiglottis, all of the larynx to the level of the false vocal cords, and the piriform recesses posterolateral to either side of the larynx (**Fig. 4-5**). The nerve enters the region by passing through the thyrohyoid membrane just below the inferior cornu of the hyoid bone (**Fig. 4-6**). It then divides into a superior and an inferior branch: the superior branch passes submucosally through the vallecula, where it is visible to the naked eye, on its way to the larynx; and the inferior branch runs along the medial aspects of the piriform recesses where it is also sufficiently superficial to be visible to the naked eye.

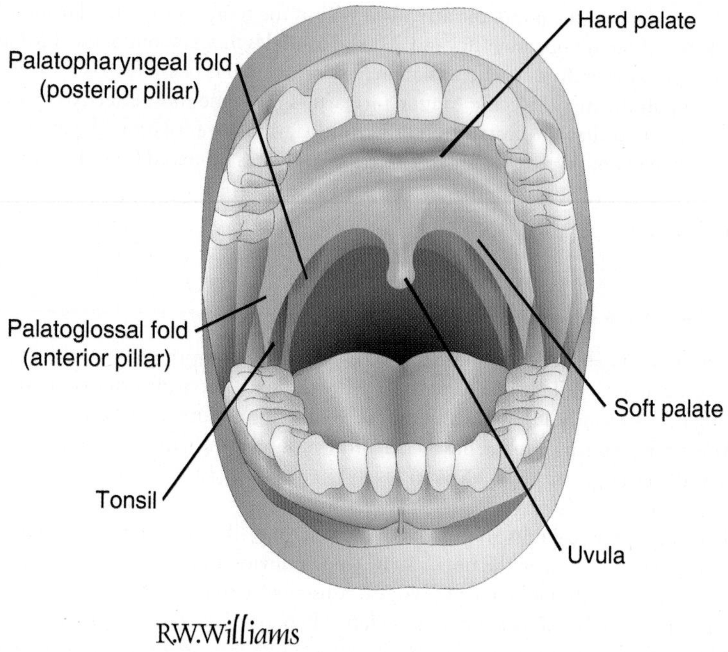


● **FIGURE 4-4. The Oral Cavity.** Note the position of the posterior tonsillar pillar. The glossopharyngeal nerve runs at the base of this structure.

- The larynx is the most heavily innervated sensory structure in the body, followed closely by the carina. Stimulation of the unanesthetized larynx during intubation causes reflex glottis closure (mediated by the vagus) and reflex sympathetic activation. BP and heart rate may as much as double as a result. This may lead to the elevation of intracranial pressure, particularly in patients with imperfect autoregulation; aggravate or incite myocardial ischemia in patients with underlying coronary artery disease; or incite or aggravate large vessel dissection or rupture (e.g., penetrating injury to a carotid, thoracic aortic dissection, or rupture of an aneurysmal abdominal aorta).
- The pyramidal arytenoid cartilages sit on the posterior aspect of the larynx (**Fig. 4-5**). The intrinsic laryngeal muscles cause them to swivel, thereby opening and closing the vocal cords. An ETT that is too large may, over time, compress these structures, causing mucosal and cartilaginous ischemia and resultant permanent laryngeal damage. A traumatic intubation may dislocate these cartilages posteriorly (more often a traumatic curved blade–related complication) or anteriorly (more often a straight blade traumatic complication), which, unless diagnosed early and relocated, may lead to permanent hoarseness.
- The larynx bulges posteriorly into the hypopharynx, leaving deep recesses on either side called the piriform recesses or sinuses. Foreign bodies (e.g., fish bones) occasionally become lodged there. During active swallowing, the larynx is elevated and moves anteriorly, the epiglottis folds down over the glottis to prevent aspiration, and the bolus of food passes midline into the esophagus. When not actively swallowing (e.g., the unconscious patient), the larynx rests against the posterior hypopharynx such that a nasogastric (NG) tube must traverse the piriform recess to gain access to the esophagus and stomach. Ordinarily, an NG tube introduced through the right nostril passes to the left at the level of the hypopharynx and enters the esophagus through the left piriform recess. Similarly, with a left nostril insertion, the NG tube gains access to the esophagus through the right piriform recess.
- The cricothyroid membrane (CTM) extends between the upper anterior surface of the cricoid cartilage to the inferior anterior border of the thyroid cartilage. Its height tends to be about

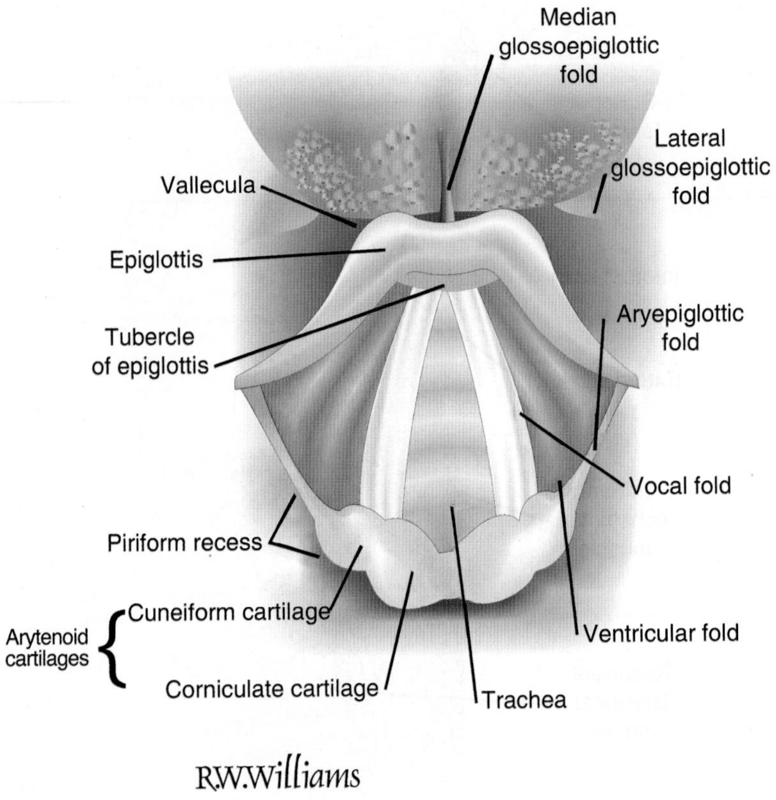


● **FIGURE 4-5. Larynx Visualized from the Oropharynx.** Note the median glossoepiglottic fold covering the hyoepiglottic ligament in the center of the vallecula. It is pressure on this structure by the tip of a curved blade that flips the epiglottis forward, exposing the glottis during laryngoscopy. Note that the valleculae and the piriform recesses are different structures, a fact often confused in the anesthesia literature. The cuneiform and corniculate cartilages are called the arytenoid cartilages. The ridge of tissue between them posteriorly is called the posterior commissure.

the size of the tip of the index finger externally in both male and female adults. Locating the cricoid cartilage and the CTM quickly in an airway emergency is crucial. It is usually easily done in men because of the obvious laryngeal prominence (Adam's apple). Locate the laryngeal prominence, and then note the anterior surface of the thyroid cartilage immediately caudad, usually about one index finger's breadth in height. There is an obvious soft indentation caudad to this anterior surface with a very hard ridge immediately caudad to it. The soft indentation is the CTM, and the ridge is the cricoid cartilage. Because of the lack of a distinct laryngeal prominence in women, locating the membrane can be much more difficult. In women, place your index finger in the sternal notch. Then drag it cephalad in the midline until the first, and ordinarily the biggest, transverse ridge is felt. This is the cricoid ring. Superior to the cricoid cartilage is the CTM, and superior to that, the anterior surface of the thyroid cartilage, and then the thyrohyoid space and thyroid cartilage. The CTM is higher in the neck in women than it is in men because women's thyroid cartilage is relatively smaller than that of men. Localization of the CTM can also be performed using the linear probe on a bedside ultrasound and may be helpful when landmarks are indistinct.

- The CTM measures 6 to 8 mm from top to bottom. The proximity of the CTM to the vocal cords is also the driving factor in using small tracheal hooks during surgical cricothyrotomy to minimize any risk to the cords (see Chapter 19).

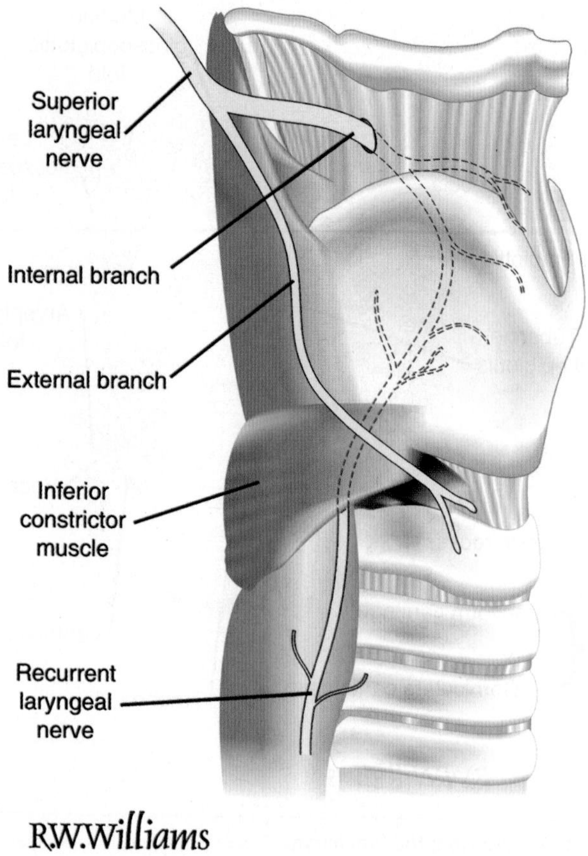


● **FIGURE 4-6. Oblique View of the Larynx.** Note how the internal branch of the superior laryngeal nerve pierces the thyrohyoid membrane midway between the hyoid bone and the superior border of the thyroid cartilage.

## TRACHEA

The trachea begins at the inferior border of the cricoid ring. The sensory supply to the tracheal mucosa is derived from the recurrent laryngeal branch of the vagus nerve. The trachea is between 9 and 15 mm in diameter in the adult and is 12 to 15 cm long. It may be somewhat larger in the elderly. The adult male trachea will generally easily accept an 8.5-mm inner diameter (ID) ETT; a 7.5-mm ID ETT is preferable in women. If the patient being intubated requires bronchoscopic pulmonary toilette after admission (e.g., chronic obstructive pulmonary disease and airway burns), consider increasing to a 9.0-mm ID tube for men and an 8.0-mm ID tube for women.

## SUMMARY

Functional anatomy is important for expert airway management. Attention to the nuances and subtleties of anatomy in relation to technique will often mean the difference between success and failure in managing airways, particularly difficult airways. A clear understanding of the relevant anatomical structures, their blood supply, and their innervation will guide the choice of intubation and anesthesia techniques and will enhance understanding regarding the best approach to each patient. It also provides a basis for understanding how complications are best avoided, or if they occur, how they may be detected.

## EVIDENCE

- **What anatomical nasal structures put a patient at risk of bleeding during nasal intubations, and how can it be mitigated?** Kiesselbach's plexus (Little's area) is a very vascular area located on the anterior aspect of the septum in each nostril. Vasoconstrictors may help limit epistaxis and have the added benefit of increasing the caliber of the nasal chamber. Many vasoconstrictors exist including topical cocaine, oxymetazoline, and neosynephrine. Cocaine should be used with caution in patients with coronary artery disease as vasospasm has been reported.[1] Although there is no solid evidence that preparatory vasoconstriction is required prior to nasal intubation, it is common practice and may be helpful in some cases.[2]
- **What anatomical structure is susceptible to trauma during nasal intubation?** Although many structures can be damaged during nasal intubations, there exists a mucosal depression at the entrance of the eustachian tube in the posterior nasopharynx that can snag the tip of the ETT and precipitate mucosal trauma or dissection. Highest-risk patients include those with chronic debilitating conditions. If this injury is suspected, antibiotics may be required to prevent infection or mediastinitis.[3–5]
- **What structural factors can complicate nasotracheal intubation?** Two other factors related to anatomy tend to be important when considering a nasotracheal intubation. First, the paranasal sinuses open into the nasal canal and may be at risk for infection with prolonged nasotracheal intubation.[6] Second, the nasal passage is bound superiorly by the cribriform plate, and with suspected or known basilar skull fractures, damage to the cribriform plate may result in migration of nasal foreign bodies into the cranial vault.[7]
- **How are men and women different with regard to CTM anatomy?** Subtle but important differences exist between the CTM in men versus women. First, the CTM is often higher, or more cephalad, in location as a result of a narrower thyroid shield. Second, the point of the upper thyroid cartilage is less prominent. As a result, anatomic localization can be more challenging.[8–10]

## REFERENCES

1. Lange RA, Hillis LD. Cardiovascular complications of cocaine use. *N Engl J Med.* 2001;345:351–358.
2. Sukaranemi VS, Jones SE. Topical anaesthetic or vasoconstrictor preparations for flexible fibre-optic nasal pharyngoscopy and laryngoscopy. *Cochrane Database Syst Rev.* 2011;(3):CD005606.
3. Tintinalli JE, Claffey J. Complications of nasotracheal intubation. *Ann Emerg Med.* 1981;10:142–144.
4. Patow CA, Pruet CW, Fetter TW, et al. Nasogastric tube perforation of the nasopharynx. *South Med J.* 1985;78:1362–1365.
5. Ronen O, Uri N. A case of nasogastric tube perforation of the nasopharynx causing a fatal mediastinal complication. *Ear Nose Throat J.* 2009;88:E17–E18.
6. Grindlinger GA, Niehoff J, Hughes SL, et al. Acute paranasal sinusitis related to nasotracheal intubation of head injured patients. *Crit Care Med.* 1987;15:214–217.
7. Marlow TJ, Goltra DD, Schabel SI. Intracranial placement of a nasotracheal tube after facial fracture: a rare complication. *J Emerg Med.* 1997;15:187–191.
8. Elliott DS, Baker PA, Scott MR, et al. Accuracy of surface landmark identification for cannula cricothyrotomy. *Anaesthesia.* 2010;65:889–894.
9. Aslani A, Ng SC, Hurley M, et al. Accuracy of identification of the cricothyroid membrane in female subjects using palpation: an observational study. *Anesth Analg.* 2012;114:987–992.
10. Lamb A, Zhang J, Hung O, et al. Accuracy of identifying the cricothyroid membrane by anesthesia trainees and staff in a Canadian Institution. *Can J Anesth.* 2015;62:495–503.

# Section II

# Oxygen Delivery and Mechanical Ventilation

Chapter 5

# Principles of Preparatory Oxygenation

Robert F. Reardon, Brian E. Driver, and Steven C. Carleton

## INTRODUCTION

Hypoxemia during emergency airway management is a feared complication and associated with dysrhythmias, hypoxic brain injury, and cardiac arrest. Critical hypoxemia often occurs when providers are focused primarily on laryngoscopy and tube placement rather than gas exchange and oxygenation. Hypoxemia could be avoided in many cases by optimal preparatory oxygenation, but the principles of preparatory oxygenation are often poorly understood and applied.

It is crucial for emergency airway providers to understand that robust preparatory oxygenation as well as the ability to reoxygenate patients with bag-mask ventilation (BMV) (Chapter 9) are the most important aspects of safe emergency airway management. The main goal of airway management is gas exchange, and although this can be accomplished through laryngoscopy and successful placement of an endotracheal tube, preventing hypoxia while this takes place is of critical importance.

Rapid sequence intubation (RSI) (Chapter 20) is the most common method for emergency airway management. Optimal preparatory oxygenation improves patient safety and reduces operator stress after neuromuscular blocking agents have been administered by prolonging the safe apnea time. "Safe apnea time" begins at the onset of paralysis and continues until the patient desaturates below 90%. Safe apnea time varies from several minutes to several seconds, depending on the patient's body habitus, comorbidities, acuity of illness, oxygen consumption, and oxygen reservoir created through the preoxygenation efforts (**Fig. 5-1**). A longer safe apnea time allows for unrushed and methodical laryngoscopy and endotracheal tube placement, while attempts at intubation can feel rushed and frantic when oxygenation levels start to fall. The stress of placing the tube correctly before critical hypoxemia ensues can transform what might have been a routine intubation into one complicated by uncertainty and poor technique, even in the hands of skilled and experienced providers.

The goal of preparatory oxygenation is to maximize this period of safe apnea, and facilitate calm and confident intubation success without hypoxemia. In this chapter, we will describe best-practice preparatory oxygenation techniques focusing on oxygen delivery, patient positioning, noninvasive positive pressure ventilation, and apneic oxygenation. We will also discuss when to abandon less aggressive techniques and take control of ventilation and oxygenation with active BMV.

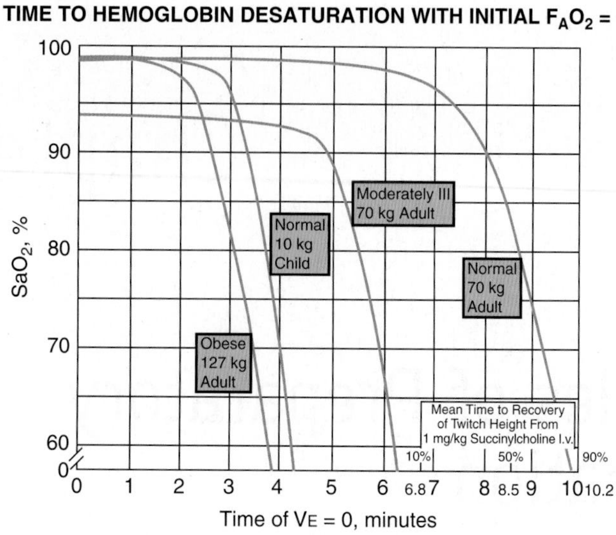


● **FIGURE 5-1.** Time to desaturation is affected by many factors, including underlying medical condition, age, body habitus, and how well preoxygenation is performed. All patients requiring emergency intubation should be assumed to be at risk for rapid desaturation, and should have maximal preoxygenation. (From Benumof JL, Dagg R, Benumof R. Critical hemoglobin desaturation will occur before return to an unparalyzed state following 1 mg/kg intravenous succinylcholine. *Anesthesiology*. 1997;87(4):979–982.)

## PREOXYGENATION

The goal of preoxygenation is to establish a reservoir of oxygen within the lungs by replacing mixed alveolar gases (mostly nitrogen) with oxygen. The volume available for this "oxygen reserve" is defined by the patient's functional residual capacity (FRC), which is approximately 30 mL per kg in adult patients. This provides a source of oxygen that the pulmonary circulation can draw from even after the patient is rendered apneic. Ideally, complete pulmonary denitrogenation is achieved, and, if measured, the fraction of expired oxygen ($Feo_2$) would be near or above 90%. In patients with healthy lungs, preoxygenation can be maximized by having the patient tidally breathe the highest fraction of inspired oxygen ($Fio_2$) as possible, ideally an $Fio_2$ of 100%, for 3 to 5 minutes. Alternatively, cooperative patients with healthy lungs can be preoxygenated by having them perform eight maximal volume deep breaths or vital capacity breaths while taking in 100% oxygen. It is imperative that emergency providers understand the differences in $Fio_2$ provided by the variety of oxygen delivery systems common to the emergency department. Preoxygenation is best accomplished with patients in the sitting or head-up position. Patients with lung pathology and decreased functional reserve capacity may require positive end-expiratory pressure (PEEP) for maximal preoxygenation. The details and rationale for these techniques are described in the following section.

### High-Concentration Oxygen versus Traditional Supplemental Oxygen

There are widespread misconceptions about the fraction of inspired oxygen ($Fio_2$) supplied by common oxygen delivery devices. Optimal preoxygenation requires delivery of high-concentration oxygen (100% $Fio_2$), but common ED oxygen delivery methods do *not* provide 100% $Fio_2$ (**Table 5-1**). The primary limitation with traditional oxygen delivery is the low oxygen flow rate used (≤15 L per minute) and the presence of significant mask leaks.

For spontaneously breathing patients, a bag-valve mask (BVM) and non-rebreather mask (NRM) can both theoretically provide 100% $Fio_2$ with a low source oxygen flow rate (15 L per

TABLE 5-1 Low $FIO_2$ Oxygen Delivery Systems

| System | Source $O_2$ Flow Rate (L/min) | $FIO_2$ (approximate) (%) |
|---|---|---|
| Nasal cannula | 2–4 | 30–35 |
| | 6 | 40 |
| Simple face mask | 6 | 45 |
| | 10 | 55 |
| Venturi mask | 15 | 50 |
| Non-rebreather mask | 15 | 70 |
| Bag-valve mask (BVM) with mask leak or without one-way valve | 15 | <50 |
| BVM without mask leak and with one-way valve | 15 | 90–100 |

minute) if they incorporate a reservoir bag, a one-way exhalation valve, and a *perfect* mask seal. This is hard to accomplish in ED patients, and attempts at oxygenation can be impeded by large volumes of room air entrainment. In low flow systems with an imperfect mask seal, $FIO_2$ decreases as the patient's minute ventilation and inspiratory flow increase, because the ventilatory demands of the patient are higher than the oxygen delivery provided by the device, and room air makes up the difference.

By altering standard flow rates, accomplished by opening a standard meter to the "flush" rate (>40 L per minute), it is possible to approach an $FIO_2$ of 100%. **Table 5-2** lists systems and accompanying flow rates that are able to deliver high $FIO_2$ regardless of the patient's minute ventilation, inspiratory flow, or mask seal. The key is to deliver 100% oxygen at a flow rate well above the patient's inspiratory needs, so that room air volume is not required to satisfy the patient's inspiratory effort.

The oxygen flow rate is likely more important than the oxygen delivery device. Although high flow rates are noisy and somewhat uncomfortable for patients, it allows delivery of high-concentration oxygen using a standard face mask or nasal cannula. In addition, very high oxygen flow rates create a small amount of PEEP, which can improve alveolar recruitment and preoxygenation efforts.

TABLE 5-2 High $FIO_2$ Oxygen Delivery Systems

| System | Source $O_2$ Flow Rate (L/min) | Approximate $FIO_2$ (%) |
|---|---|---|
| Anesthesia machine (flush valve open)[a] | 30–35 | 100 |
| Resuscitation bag (one-way valve, no mask leak) | 15 | 100 |
| NPPV machine | (wall $O_2$, ≥50 L/min) | 100 |
| High-flow nasal cannula | 40–60 | 100 |
| Non-rebreather mask | ≥40 | 100 |
| Simple mask[b] | ≥40 | 70–90 |

[a]High-flow flush compensates for a mask leak.
[b]$FIO_2$ is less predictable with simple masks because of room air entrainment and turbulent flow.

## *Nasal Cannula*

Low-flow nasal cannula is often the first-line of oxygen supplementation and is appropriate in patients with mild oxygen debt. Common initial flow rates are 2 to 4 L per minute. The traditional teaching was that the maximal effective flow rate for nasal cannula oxygen is 6 L per minute, which delivers a maximal $F_{IO_2}$ of 35% to 40%. In the last several years, oxygen delivery by high-flow nasal cannula (HFNC) has become common. Commercial HFNC systems (Optiflow, Vapotherm, Comfort Flo) provide nearly 100% $F_{IO_2}$ by using flow rates of 40 to 70 L per minute through larger caliber tubing. They also heat and humidify the oxygen, making the high flow rate more tolerable for the patient. HFNC systems have been successfully used to support patients in hypoxemic respiratory failure, although its role in preoxygenation prior to intubation is yet to be defined. The positive benefits of HFNC are washout of upper airway dead space, reduction in work of breathing by providing adequate flow, and modest amounts of PEEP. There is no literature describing the effectiveness of high-flow oxygen through standard nasal cannula tubing, but it is possible that it is more effective at preoxygenating and tolerable for short-term use.

## *Simple Face Mask*

A simple face mask is a non-form-fitting plastic mask that covers the entirety of the nose and mouth. It does not have an external bag reservoir; so the volume of oxygen available for each breath at low oxygen flow rates is only the volume contained within the mask (~100 to 150 mL). Traditionally, a simple face mask was used with flow rates between 4 and 10 L per minute. At these low flow rates, the $F_{IO_2}$ is highly variable and is dictated by the patient's respiratory pattern and the volume of room air drawn in around the mask. The traditional teaching was that the maximal $F_{IO_2}$ that could be delivered by a simple face mask is approximately 50% (with an oxygen flow rate of 15 L per minute). However, there is good evidence that high-concentration oxygen ($F_{IO_2} > 90\%$) can be delivered by a simple face mask when the source oxygen flow rate is set to a higher level (≥40 L per minute). In addition, high-flow face mask oxygen should theoretically provide the same benefits as a HFNC—washout of upper airway dead space, reduction in work of breathing by providing adequate flow, and mild PEEP. For all of these reasons, some experts believe that a simple face mask with a high flow rate (≥40 L per minute) is a reasonable way to provide maximal preoxygenation prior to emergency RSI (see the Evidence section). However, it is more prudent to use a NRM for two reasons. First, the most commonly used simple mask (Hudson DCI) has small holes adjacent to where the oxygen tubing connects to the mask; with very high oxygen flow rates, the Venturi effect will draw room air into the mask next to the oxygen stream and dilute the $F_{IO_2}$ (**Fig. 5-2A**). Second, very high flow rates (≥50 L per minute) of the oxygen flow in a simple mask can be turbulent, thereby providing less $F_{IO_2}$ than at lower flow rates. Most NRMs do not have these limitations.

## *Nonrebreather Mask*

A NRM is a simple face mask with a 500 to 1,000 mL reservoir bag from which the patient can draw 100% oxygen during inspiration. NRMs also contain one or two crude one-way valves on the side of the mask, which are supposed to open during expiration and close during inspiration, limiting entrainment of room air into the system. In order to achieve a high $F_{IO_2}$ with a NRM at low flow rates, there must be a decent mask seal, the one-way valves must be present and functioning properly, and all inspired air must come from the reservoir bag. In practice, there is a poor mask seal, inconsistent function of the one-way valves, and entrainment of room air with inspiration from around the mask, which limits its efficacy (**Fig. 5-2B**). Multiple studies show that a NRM with an oxygen flow rate of 15 L per minute delivers a maximal $F_{IO_2}$ of 70%. As with a simple mask, using a NRM with a very high source oxygen flow rate ("flush" rate ≥ 40 L per minute) delivers an $F_{IO_2}$ of nearly 100% (see Evidence section). This is an excellent system for providing high-concentration oxygen for preoxygenation prior to emergency RSI. Although the reservoir

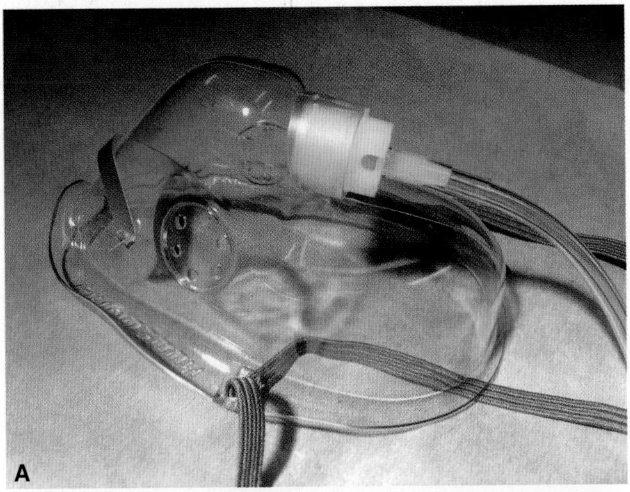

A

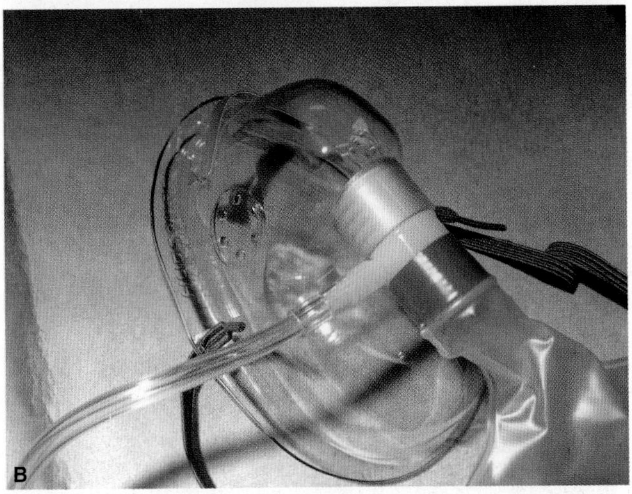

B

● **FIGURE 5-2.** **A:** Simple (Hudson) face mask. This mask delivers an $F_{IO_2}$ of about 50% with an oxygen flow rate of 15 L per minute and about 70% with an oxygen flow rate ≥40 L per minute. Note the open-side ports and the small hole in the white plastic adjacent to where the oxygen tubing connects, which likely entrains room air into the system via the Venturi effect. Also, turbulent flow likely occurs at flow rates >50 L per minute, which also entrains room air. **B:** Non-rebreather mask. This mask delivers an $F_{IO_2}$ of about 70% with a standard oxygen flow rate (15 L per minute), but can provide an $F_{IO_2}$ of 100% with a "flush" flow rate (≥40 L per minute).

bag is probably not helpful in most patients, it has a theoretical benefit in patients with extremely high minute ventilation.

## How to Deliver High-Flow Oxygen with Standard Flowmeters

Standard wall-mounted oxygen flowmeters (with gradations up to 15 L per minute) typically mark a maximum flow rate, also known as the "flush" flow rate, which is approximately 40 L per minute or more (**Fig. 5-3A**). To achieve the "flush" flow rate, simply turn the oxygen flowmeter knob until it does not turn further; the high flow of oxygen will be easily audible. This will enable delivery of nearly 100% $F_{IO_2}$ with a NRM. Alternatively, there are commercially available oxygen flowmeters that allow flow rates up to 70 L per minute (**Fig. 5-3B**).

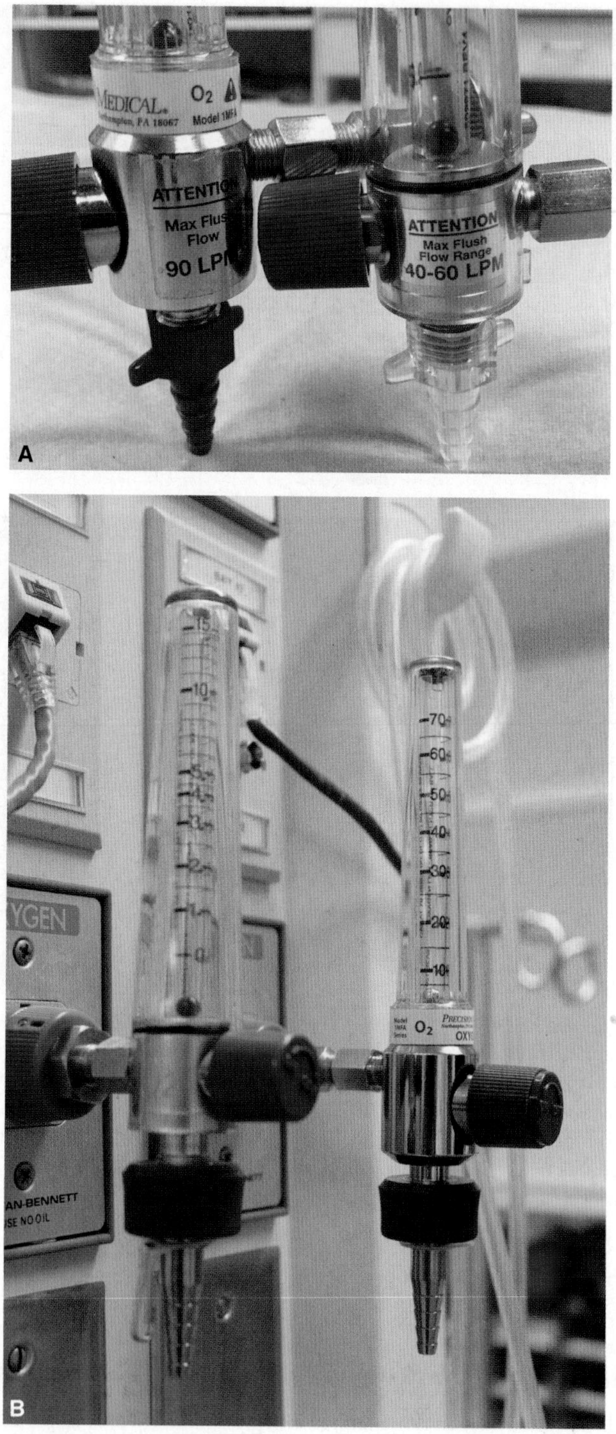


● **FIGURE 5-3. A:** Flush rate labels on standard oxygen flowmeters. The maximum flow rate for oxygen flowmeters, known as the "flush" rate, is typically marked on the side of the device. Standard flowmeters that show a maximum gradation of 15 L per minute at the top of the clear cylinder are usually able to deliver oxygen at >40 L per minute. **B:** Standard and high-flow oxygen flow meters. On the left is a standard flow meter (0 to 15 L per minute, with a "flush rate" of 40 to 60 L per minute). On the right is a high-flow meter (0 to 70 L per minute, with a flush rate of 90 L per minute).

## *Venturi Mask*

Venturi masks are traditionally referred to as "high flow" supplemental oxygen devices, but they should not be confused with high-concentration oxygen delivery devices. They are designed to be used with source oxygen flow rates of 12 to 15 L per minute and can deliver a maximal $FIO_2$ of 50%. The principle benefit of Venturi masks is their ability to provide consistent $FIO_2$ by fixing the degree of room air entrainment and should be considered "precision control" oxygen delivery devices rather than high-flow devices. They are commonly used in the ICU setting rather than the ED and are most helpful when titratable amounts of oxygen supplementation are important or when there is concern about excessive oxygen administration, as in patients with chronic obstructive pulmonary disease. They can deliver between 24% and 50% $FIO_2$.

## *Bag-Valve Mask*

BVM devices provide 100% $FIO_2$ during active positive pressure ventilation in patients with apnea. For spontaneously breathing patients, BVMs may provide an $FIO_2$ of more than 90% as long as a robust mask seal is maintained and room air admixture is minimal. If the mask seal is compromised, the patient will draw in room air around the mask during inspiration and significantly lower the $FIO_2$. In spontaneously breathing patients, preoxygenation with a BVM and a good mask seal is better than a NRM at standard flow rates. Using high flow rates ($\geq$40 L per minute) with a BVM device has not been studied, but this may be reasonable if there is a poor mask seal.

Providers should be acutely aware that not all BVM devices are the same. BVM devices without a one-way exhalation valve allow entrainment of significant room air (**Fig. 5-4**) and deliver an $FIO_2 < 50\%$ in spontaneously breathing patients. BVMs with a one-way valve on the exhalation port prohibit entrainment of room air during inspiration, and can provide an $FIO_2$ of nearly 100% if there is a perfect mask seal. Adding a PEEP valve to the BVM device during preoxygenation of spontaneously breathing patients is theoretically helpful but has not been well studied and may be counterproductive (see Evidence section).

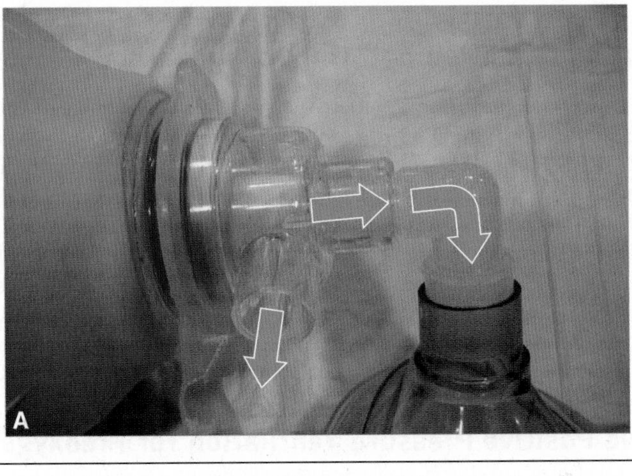


● **FIGURE 5-4. A:** Resuscitation bag used with positive pressure (when bag is being squeezed) and no active breathing by the patient. Whether or not a one-way exhalation valve is present, the patient receives 100% oxygen from the bag reservoir, as long as the mask seal is effective. **B:** Resuscitation bag during spontaneous breathing (when bag is not being squeezed). Note that there is no one-way exhalation valve. The exhalation port is open to the room air. When the patient inhales, a large amount of room air ($FIO_2$ 21%) is entrained, resulting in an $FIO_2$ as low as 30%. **C:** Resuscitation bag during spontaneous breathing with one-way exhalation valve (bag is not being squeezed). Room air cannot enter via the exhalation port, so the $FIO_2$ approaches 100%.

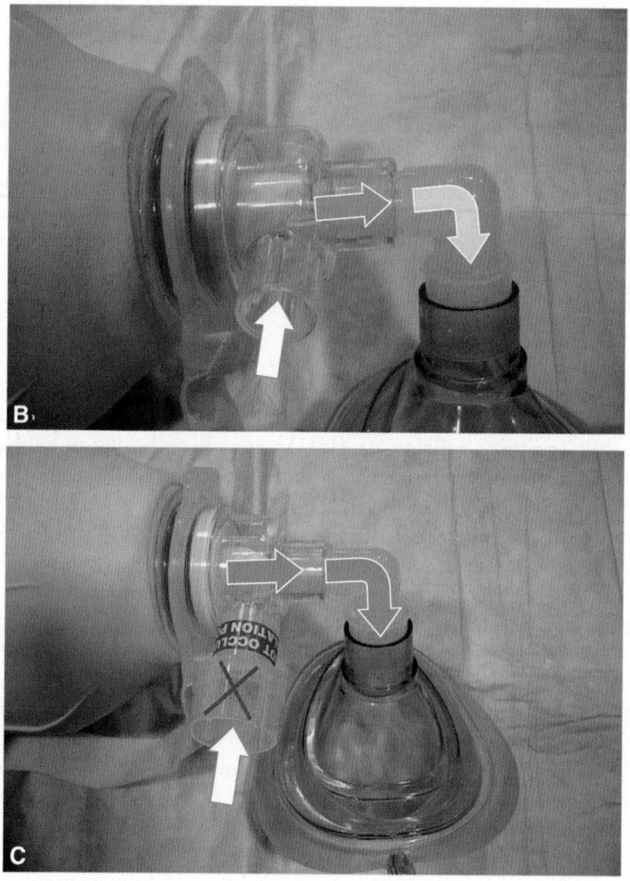

● **FIGURE 5-4.** *(continued)*

## Optimal Patient Positioning for Preoxygenation

Position has been shown to influence the effectiveness of preoxygenation and safe apnea time. The oxygen storage capacity of the lungs is greatest when patients are in the upright position and lowest in the supine position. Multiple studies have shown that preoxygenation is significantly more effective in an upright position by allowing full utilization of a patient's FRC. The FRC is a potential space, rarely used during normal tidal breathing, but recruited during preoxygenation efforts to store high-concentration oxygen that can then be drawn from by the pulmonary circulation to maintain oxygenation during RSI. Those who cannot tolerate the upright position (e.g., those with spinal precautions) should be preoxygenated in a reverse Trendelenberg position. Upright or head-up positioning during preoxygenation is especially important in obese patients, who are prone to rapid desaturation during RSI, and in patients whose abdominal mass further restricts use of the FRC (**Fig. 5-1**).

## Noninvasive Positive Pressure Ventilation for Preoxygenation

Patients with underlying lung pathology, such as pulmonary edema, severe pneumonia, and acute respiratory distress syndrome, and those who are morbidly obese, cannot achieve maximal preoxygenation without PEEP. These patients have alveoli that are perfused but not ventilated, or high intrinsic airway pressures that confound preoxygenation efforts. They need increased airway pressure to open these alveoli for maximal nitrogen washout, oxygen storage, and gas exchange. Therefore, patients who are morbidly obese or relatively hypoxemic (oxygen saturation < 95%) despite administration of high-concentration oxygen should be preoxygenated upright with non-invasive positive pressure ventilation (NPPV) whenever possible.

When using NPPV, it is best to provide both inspiratory and expiratory pressure support. This can be accomplished using the bilevel positive airway pressure (BiPAP) mode on a noninvasive machine or a standard ventilator with pressure support mode plus PEEP. Alternatively, positive airway pressure can be applied using a disposable continuous positive airway pressure (CPAP) mask setup or a PEEP valve attached to a standard BVM device. Delivery of bilevel positive pressure using a specialized NPPV machine is probably the best "go to" technique because these machines compensate for mask leaks. Delivering an end-expiratory pressure of 5 to 10 cm $H_2O$ and an inspiratory pressure of 10 to 20 cm $H_2O$ are good starting points in most cases (see Chapter 6 for more about NPPV).

### *Concept of "Delayed Sequence Intubation"*

"Delayed sequence intubation" is not a change in how the RSI medications are delivered, as the name implies, but is a form of "procedural sedation" to facilitate patient compliance with attempts at preoxygenation. Often employed for agitated or delirious patients, the goal is to provide a low dose of an agent (like ketamine) that is unlikely to affect the patient's respiratory drive or protective airway reflexes while sedating the patient enough to accept NPPV or high-flow oxygen by face mask. This technique has been shown to be effective in the hands of highly skilled airway managers, but should be undertaken with great caution because sedation of critically ill and decompensated patients may result in respiratory depression, arrest, or inability to protect their airway. Because this technique has not been extensively studied, the rate of adverse events is not known. If this technique is to be attempted, the airway manager needs to be fully prepared for immediate definitive airway management if one of these events take place (see Chapter 20 for more detail).

## APNEIC OXYGENATION

Apneic oxygenation involves the administration of oxygen during the apneic period of RSI, usually applied via a standard nasal cannula with a flow rate of 5 to 15 L per minute. Because oxygen diffuses across the alveoli more readily than carbon dioxide and has a high affinity for hemoglobin, more oxygen leaves the alveoli than carbon dioxide enters during apnea. This creates a pressure gradient that causes oxygen to travel from the nasopharynx to the alveoli and into the bloodstream by a physiologic principle known as "aventilatory mass flow".

With the exception of a crash airway or a "forced to act" imperative during which preoxygenation is trumped by the immediacy of tube placement, apneic oxygenation should be considered for every tracheal intubation to decrease the chance of severe hypoxemia. A standard nasal cannula is placed beneath the main preoxygenation device (face mask or BVM). If the patient is awake, the flow rate should be as high as the patient can tolerate, typically between 5 and 15 L per minute, during the preoxygenation phase. If the patient is comatose or unresponsive, the nasal cannula can be set to 15 L per minute or higher when initially placed. When the preoxygenation mask is removed for intubation, the nasal cannula remains in place. During intubation attempts, the nasal cannula should be set to at least 15 L per minute. It may be beneficial to turn the oxygen flowmeter up as high as possible, because higher flow rates have been shown to provide higher $F_{IO_2}$. If there is nasal obstruction, a nasopharyngeal airway can be placed in one or both nares to facilitate oxygen delivery to the posterior nasopharynx. To optimize gas flow past the upper airway, the patient should be ideally positioned for tracheal intubation, and maneuvers to ensure upper airway patency should be performed (i.e., jaw thrust, head tilt/chin lift).

Multiple studies in the operating room setting have shown that apneic oxygenation increases safe apnea time, especially in obese patients. Although a recent randomized trial of critically ill ICU patients showed no benefit of apneic oxygenation after optimal preoxygenation, the results of this trial are not generalizable to ED patients, who are often intubated within minutes of arrival and who are not on supplemental oxygen for hours preceding intubation. In addition, a recent observational ED study on apneic oxygenation demonstrated an increase in first-pass intubation success without hypoxemia (see Evidence section). With an intervention as simple and inexpensive as nasal cannula use, we recommend routine use of apneic oxygenation.

## RESCUE OXYGENATION

RSI is a nonbagging procedure, and active BMV is not recommended during the apneic period of RSI as long as the patient maintains adequate oxygenation (≥93%) when the RSI medications are pushed. Those who cannot be adequately preoxygenated despite optimal technique are at high risk for rapid desaturation and should be actively ventilated/oxygenated with BMV during the onset and duration of apnea.

When an intubation attempt is prolonged or fails and the oxygen saturation drops below 93%, the airway manager's attention should be focused on ventilation and oxygenation rather than persisting with the intubation attempt. Optimal BMV with a well-fitting mask is the first-line technique for active ventilation and oxygenation. The goal is to increase the oxygen saturation as high as possible (ideally 100%) to allow continued safe apnea time for subsequent intubation attempts. Providers should be aware that there will be a delay of about 30 seconds between the onset of adequate BMV and an increase in oxygen saturation as measured by a pulse oximeter. This is often a time of high anxiety for the provider performing BMV as well as other team members caring for the patient. The key is to ensure that good quality BMV is being provided (see Chapter 9) and to evaluate for adequate gas exchange by looking for chest rise, listening to breath sounds, and monitoring end-tidal carbon dioxide using a continuous waveform monitor (see Chapter 8). The ability to provide high-quality BMV is an underestimated and difficult skill, and many emergency airway providers perform this in a suboptimal fashion. Practicing and optimizing BMV skills saves lives and significantly decreases the anxiety associated with emergency airway management.

Patients with difficult BMV due to head-and-neck radiation changes, poor mask seal (beard, facial trauma), obesity, or other factors may be good candidates for an extraglottic device (EGD). EGDs are easy to insert and provide adequate ventilation and oxygenation in nearly all patients regardless of the experience of the provider. In this scenario, the EGD can be used similar to a BMV: to temporarily provide ventilation and oxygenation until the oxygen saturation rises. The EGD is then removed, and further intubation attempts can proceed. Another option is to use an intubating laryngeal mask airway for ventilation and oxygenation and as a conduit for blind or flexible endoscopic intubation (see chapters 16 and 18).

## SUMMARY

Preparatory oxygenation maximizes pulmonary oxygen reserves to create an oxygen reservoir, which increases safe apnea time during RSI. Traditional methods of supplemental oxygen delivery are inadequate for preparatory oxygenation. The keys to preparatory oxygenation are understanding how to deliver high-concentration (≈100%) oxygen, using apneic oxygenation, ensuring proper head-up positioning, and knowing when to use positive pressure ventilation and rescue BMV.

## EVIDENCE

- **What is the best way to preoxygenate for RSI?** Prior to intubation, the gold standard for delivering 100% $F_{IO_2}$ is an anesthesia machine with a well-fitted mask; however, both a BVM and a NRB mask with flush rate oxygen have been shown to be equivalent to an anesthesia machine.[1,2] A recent study by Groombridge et al.[1] compared several common preoxygenation methods to an anesthesia circuit and found that only the BVM (with a one-way exhalation valve) device was comparable. However, in that study, the flow rate used for the simple mask and NRM was only 15 L per minute. The benefit of using a simple or NRM is that they require no specialized equipment, and are "hands-off" techniques, allowing personnel to attend to other important tasks during the preintubation period. A NRM is preferred to the simple mask because of concerns with room air entrainment via the Venturi effect and turbulent flow. A recent study showed that the fraction of expired oxygen ($FeO_2$) with a NRM and oxygen delivered at the "flush flow" rate of >40 L per minute was noninferior to

BVM with 15 L per minute of oxygen flow.[3] At 15 L per minute oxygen flow, a BVM device provides higher $F_{IO_2}$ than face mask devices; however, this can only occur if the former has a functioning one-way valve on the exhalation port and a good mask seal. Many BVM devices do not have one-way valves,[2,4] and deliver close to room air with spontaneous respirations. Also, BMV is a "hands-on" technique that requires the full attention of at least one team member; furthermore, many patients who need emergency airway management do not tolerate a tight mask seal. Both BMV at 15 L per minute flow and NRM with a flush flow rate of at least 40 L per minute are good options for preoxygenation in spontaneously breathing patients.

Patients should be in the upright or head-up position during preoxygenation whenever possible. Several randomized studies of both obese and nonobese patients have shown that preoxygenation in the upright or 20° to 25° head-up position significantly increases safe apnea time.[5–9]

Patients who are hypoxemic (oxygen saturation less than 93%) despite maximal passive oxygen delivery and those who are morbidly obese need positive pressure ventilation for optimal preoxygenation. This is best accomplished with a noninvasive machine or a standard ventilator with pressure support plus PEEP.[10–16] Alternatively, positive airway pressure can be applied using a disposable CPAP mask setup. Using a BVM device with a PEEP valve has been proposed but is not well studied.[17]

HFNC is a simple method for providing both preoxygenation and apneic oxygenation. One prospective randomized trial of hypoxemic patients in an ICU setting showed that preoxygenation plus apneic oxygenation with HFNC was equivalent to preoxygenation (without apneic oxygenation) with a face mask set at 15 L per minute.[18] A before and after study of hypoxemic ICU patients showed that preoxygenation with HFNC was better than using a NRM with an $O_2$ flow rate of 15 L per minute.[19] Although these studies are interesting, they both compared HFNC to a low-flow face mask, which is known to be inadequate for maximal preoxygenation. Studies comparing preoxygenation with HFNC to a high-flow face mask (≥40 L per minute), an anesthesia machine, or a BVM device are needed. Currently, there is not enough information in ED populations to formally recommend HFNC as a preoxygenation strategy.

- **Does apneic oxygenation prolong desaturation time during RSI?** In one study of obese patients undergoing general anesthesia, those who received continuous oxygenation using nasal cannula at a 5 L per minute flow rate during apnea maintained $S_{PO_2}$ >95% for significantly longer than controls (5.3 vs. 3.5 minutes) and had a significantly higher minimum $S_{PO_2}$ (94.3% vs. 87.7%).[20] An observational study of ED RSI showed that apneic oxygenation with a standard nasal cannula was associated with a significant increase in first-pass success without hypoxemia.[21] In addition, a before and after study in the EMS setting showed that the introduction of apneic oxygenation was associated with decreased incidence of desaturation in patients undergoing RSI.[22] Although a recent prospective randomized trial of critically ill ICU patients showed no benefit of apneic oxygenation after optimal preoxygenation,[23] the results of this trial are not generalizable to ED patients, who are often intubated within minutes of arrival and who are not on supplemental oxygen for hours preceding intubation. Because there is little downside to providing apneic oxygenation, we recommend that oxygen be routinely delivered via nasal cannula at 15 L per minute during the apneic period of RSI.
- **Can a checklist help improve preparatory oxygenation and avoid hypoxemia during emergency RSI?** Yes, the use of a preprocedural checklist prior to intubation of severely injured trauma patients has been shown to be associated with a significant reduction in oxygen desaturation (<90%) due to increased utilization of maximal preoxygenation and apneic oxygenation.[24]

## REFERENCES

1. Groombridge CJ, Chin CW, Hanrahan B, et al. Assessment of common preoxygenation strategies outside of the operating room environment. *Acad Emerg Med*. 2016;23:342–346.
2. Cullen P. Self-inflating ventilation bags. *Anaesth Intensive Care*. 2001;29(2):203.
3. Driver BE, Prekker ME, Kornas RL, et al. Flush rate oxygen for emergency airway preoxygenation. *Ann Emerg Med*. 2017;69:1–6.

4. Nimmagadda U, Salem MR, Joseph NJ, et al. Efficacy of preoxygenation with tidal volume breathing. Comparison of breathing systems. *Anesthesiology*. 2000;93(3):693–698.
5. Altermatt FR, Munoz HR, Delfino AE, et al. Pre-oxygenation in the obese patient: effects of position on tolerance to apnoea. *Br J Anaesth*. 2005;95(5):706–709.
6. Baraka AS, Hanna MT, Jabbour SI, et al. Preoxygenation of pregnant and nonpregnant women in the head-up versus supine position. *Anesth Analg*. 1992;75(5):757–759.
7. Dixon BJ, Dixon JB, Carden JR, et al. Preoxygenation is more effective in the 25 degrees head-up position than in the supine position in severely obese patients: a randomized controlled study. *Anesthesiology*. 2005;102(6):1110–1115; discussion 5A.
8. Lane S, Saunders D, Schofield A, et al. A prospective, randomised controlled trial comparing the efficacy of pre-oxygenation in the 20 degrees head-up vs supine position. *Anaesthesia*. 2005;60(11):1064–1067.
9. Ramkumar V, Umesh G, Philip FA. Preoxygenation with 20 masculine head-up tilt provides longer duration of non-hypoxic apnea than conventional preoxygenation in non-obese healthy adults. *J Anesth*. 2011;25(2):189–194.
10. Baillard C, Fosse JP, Sebbane M, et al. Noninvasive ventilation improves preoxygenation before intubation of hypoxic patients. *Am J Respir Crit Care Med*. 2006;174(2):171–177.
11. Cressey DM, Berthoud MC, Reilly CS. Effectiveness of continuous positive airway pressure to enhance pre-oxygenation in morbidly obese women. *Anaesthesia*. 2001;56(7):680–684.
12. De Jong A, Futier E, Millot A, et al. How to preoxygenate in operative room: healthy subjects and situations "at risk". *Ann Fr Anesth Reanim*. 2014;33(7–8):457–461.
13. Delay JM, Sebbane M, Jung B, et al. The effectiveness of noninvasive positive pressure ventilation to enhance preoxygenation in morbidly obese patients: a randomized controlled study. *Anesth Analg*. 2008;107(5):1707–1713.
14. Futier E, Constantin JM, Pelosi P, et al. Noninvasive ventilation and alveolar recruitment maneuver improve respiratory function during and after intubation of morbidly obese patients: a randomized controlled study. *Anesthesiology*. 2011;114(6):1354–1363.
15. Gander S, Frascarolo P, Suter M, et al. Positive end-expiratory pressure during induction of general anesthesia increases duration of nonhypoxic apnea in morbidly obese patients. *Anesth Analg*. 2005;100(2):580–584.
16. Harbut P, Gozdzik W, Stjernfalt E, et al. Continuous positive airway pressure/pressure support pre-oxygenation of morbidly obese patients. *Acta Anaesthesiol Scand*. 2014;58(6):675–680.
17. Weingart SD, Levitan RM. Preoxygenation and prevention of desaturation during emergency airway management. *Ann Emerg Med*. 2012;59(3):165.e1–175.e1.
18. Vourc'h M, Asfar P, Volteau C, et al. High-flow nasal cannula oxygen during endotracheal intubation in hypoxemic patients: a randomized controlled clinical trial. *Intensive Care Med*. 2015;41(9):1538–1548.
19. Miguel-Montanes R, Hajage D, Messika J, et al. Use of high-flow nasal cannula oxygen therapy to prevent desaturation during tracheal intubation of intensive care patients with mild-to-moderate hypoxemia. *Crit Care Med*. 2015;43(3):574–583.
20. Ramachandran SK, Cosnowski A, Shanks A, et al. Apneic oxygenation during prolonged laryngoscopy in obese patients: a randomized, controlled trial of nasal oxygen administration. *J Clin Anesth*. 2010;22(3):164–168.
21. Sakles JC, Mosier JM, Patanwala AE, et al. First pass success without hypoxemia is increased with the use of apneic oxygenation during RSI in the emergency department. *Acad Emerg Med*. 2016;23:703–710.
22. Wimalasena Y, Burns B, Reid C, et al. Apneic oxygenation was associated with decreased desaturation rates during rapid sequence intubation by an Australian helicopter emergency medicine service. *Ann Emerg Med*. 2015;65(4):371–376.
23. Semler MW, Janz DR, Lentz RJ, et al. Randomized trial of apneic oxygenation during endotracheal intubation of the critically ill. *Am J Respir Crit Care Med*. 2016;193:273–280.
24. Smith KA, High K, Collins SP, et al. A preprocedural checklist improves the safety of emergency department intubation of trauma patients. *Acad Emerg Med*. 2015;22(8):989–992.

Chapter 6

# Noninvasive Mechanical Ventilation

Alan C. Heffner and Peter M.C. DeBlieux

## INTRODUCTION

Patients with severe respiratory symptoms are common in the emergency department (ED) and comprise >10% of all presentations. Over the past decade, ED presentations of asthma, pneumonia, and chest pain have increased. A thorough knowledge of mechanical ventilatory support, both invasive and noninvasive, is essential for practicing emergency medicine clinicians. This chapter discusses noninvasive positive-pressure ventilation (NPPV), while Chapter 7 focuses on mechanical ventilation after tracheal intubation. The use of NPPV has grown steadily as a result of evidence-based research, cost effectiveness, and consideration of patient comfort and complications.

The advantages of NPPV over mechanical ventilation include preservation of speech, swallowing, and physiologic airway defense mechanisms; reduced risk of airway injury; reduced risk of nosocomial infection; enhanced patient comfort; and a decreased length of stay in the ICU and hospital.

## TECHNOLOGY OF NONINVASIVE MECHANICAL VENTILATION

Noninvasive ventilators have several characteristics that are distinct from standard invasive mechanical ventilators. NPPV offers a more portable technology because of the reduced air compressor size, but because of this, noninvasive ventilators are not able to generate pressures as high as standard critical care invasive ventilators. Noninvasive ventilators have a single-limb tubing circuit that delivers oxygen to the patient and allows for exhalation. To prevent accumulation of carbon dioxide, this circuit is continuously flushed with supplemental oxygen during the expiratory phase. Exhaled gases are released through a small exhalation port near the patient's mask. During the respiratory cycle, the machine continuously monitors the degree of air leak and compensates for this loss of volume. NPPV is designed to tolerate air leak and compensates by maintaining airway pressures. This is in sharp contrast to the closed system found in invasive, critical care ventilators consisting of a dual, inspiratory and expiratory tubing system that does not tolerate air leak or compensate for lost volume. The device that makes physical contact between the patient and the ventilator is termed the interface. Interfaces for NPPV come in a variety of shapes and sizes designed to cover the individual nares, the nose only, the nose and mouth, the entire face, or fitted as a helmet. Ideally, interfaces should be comfortable and offer a good seal with minimal leak and limited dead space.

## MODES OF NONINVASIVE MECHANICAL VENTILATION

In a manner analogous to invasive mechanical ventilation, understanding the modes of NPPV is based on knowledge of three essential variables: the *trigger*, the *limit*, and the *cycle*. The *trigger* is the event that initiates inspiration: either patient effort or machine-initiated positive pressure. The *limit* refers to the airflow parameter that is regulated during inspiration: either airflow rate or airway pressure. The *cycle* terminates inspiration: either a pressure is delivered over a set time period or the patient ceases inspiratory efforts.

### Continuous Positive Airway Pressure

Continuous positive airway pressure (CPAP) is a mode for invasive and noninvasive mechanical ventilation. CPAP is not a stand-alone mode of assisted mechanical ventilation. It is equivalent to positive end-expiratory pressure (PEEP) and facilitates inhalation by reducing the pressure threshold to initiate airflow (see Chapter 7). Positive airway pressure is provided throughout the respiratory cycle with constant pressure maintained during both inhalation and exhalation. This mode should never be used in patients at risk of apnea, because of the lack of a backup respiratory rate.

### Spontaneous and Spontaneous/Timed Modes

In spontaneous mode, the airway pressure cycles between an inspiratory positive airway pressure (IPAP) and an expiratory positive airway pressure (EPAP). This is commonly referred to as bilevel or biphasic positive airway pressure (BL-PAP or BiPAP). The patient's inspiratory effort triggers the switch from EPAP to IPAP. The limit during inspiration is the set level of IPAP. The inspiratory phase cycles off, and the machine switches back to EPAP when it detects a cessation of patient effort. This is indicated by a decrease in inspiratory flow rate, or once a maximum inspiratory time is reached, which is typically set at 3 seconds. Tidal volume varies breath to breath and is determined by the degree of IPAP, patient effort, and lung compliance. Work of breathing (WOB) is primarily dictated by initiation and maintenance of inspiratory airflow, with additional WOB linked to active contraction of the expiratory muscles.

Spontaneous mode relies on patient effort to trigger inhalation. In this mode, a patient breathing at a low rate can develop a respiratory acidosis. The spontaneous/timed (ST) mode prevents this clinical consequence. The trigger in the ST mode can be the patient's effort, or an elapsed time interval that is predetermined by a set respiratory backup rate. If the patient does not initiate a breath in the prescribed interval, then IPAP is triggered. For machine-generated breaths, the ventilator cycles back to EPAP based on a set inspiratory time. For patient-initiated breaths, the ventilator cycles as it would in the spontaneous mode.

Conceptually, one can consider BiPAP as CPAP with pressure support (PS). The pressure during the inspiratory phase is termed IPAP and is analogous to PS, a pressure boost during inspiratory efforts. The pressure during the expiratory phase is termed EPAP and is analogous to CPAP, or PEEP, which maintains a set minimum positive pressure throughout the entire respiratory cycle. The IPAP is necessarily set higher than EPAP by a minimum of 5 cm $H_2O$, and the difference between the two settings is equivalent to the amount of PS provided.

Humidified high-flow nasal cannula (HFNC) has recently been utilized as a mode of NPPV with some promising results. The high flow rates of oxygen (up to 60 L per minute) are heated and humidified, able to meet high inspiratory demands without room air entrainment, and can generate low-level positive pressure in the upper airways (up to 8 cm of $H_2O$). The fraction of inspired oxygen can be adjusted by changing the fraction of oxygen in the driving gas. The high flow rates may also flush expired carbon dioxide from the upper airway, ultimately diminishing physiologic dead space and improving WOB.

The keys to successfully using NPPV on an emergency basis are patient selection and aggressive therapy to reverse the disease inciting respiratory failure.

## INDICATIONS AND CONTRAINDICATIONS

The indications for NPPV in the emergency setting are straightforward. The eligible patient must have a patent, stable airway, be conscious and cooperative, have preserved spontaneous ventilatory drive and a disease process that is likely to improve quickly with medical and ventilator management. Target patients may have hypercarbia, hypoxemia, or both. Acute exacerbation of chronic obstructive pulmonary disease (COPD), moderate to severe asthma, and acute pulmonary edema are classic patient situations to consider NPPV; however, NPPV is *contraindicated* if the patient has a threat to the airway, is unable to cooperate, or is apneic. If the patient is in extremis, with severe hypoxemia and severe or worsening ventilatory inadequacy, immediate intubation is usually indicated. In such cases, it is not appropriate to delay intubation for a trial of NPPV. This is a relative contraindication and clinical judgment is required. In some cases, NPPV can also be used to enhance preoxygenation in preparation of anticipated intubation.

The objectives of NPPV are the same as those for invasive mechanical ventilation: to improve pulmonary gas exchange, alleviate respiratory distress and WOB, alter adverse pressure/volume relationships in the lungs, permit lung healing, and avoid complications. Patients on NPPV must be monitored closely, using familiar parameters such as vital signs, oximetry, capnography, chest radiograph, bedside spirometry, and arterial blood gases (ABGs).

## INITIATING NONINVASIVE MECHANICAL VENTILATION

For CPAP or BiPAP, either a face mask or a nasal mask can be used, but a nasal mask is generally better tolerated. There are varying mask sizes and styles, and a respiratory therapist should measure the patient to ensure a good fit and seal. First, explain the process to the patient before applying the mask. Initially, supply 3 to 5 cm $H_2O$ of CPAP with supplemental oxygen. Acceptance by the patient may improve if they are allowed to hold the mask against the face. The mask is secured with straps once the patient demonstrates acceptance. Next, explain that the pressure will change, and either sequentially increase the CPAP pressure by 2 to 3 cm $H_2O$ increments every 5 to 10 minutes, or initiate BiPAP to support the patient's respiratory efforts. Recommended initial settings for BiPAP is IPAP of 8 cm $H_2O$ and EPAP of 3 cm $H_2O$, for a PS (IPAP minus EPAP) of 5 cm $H_2O$. The level of supplemental oxygen flowing into the circuit should be governed by pulse oximetry and corroborated by ABG results if necessary. It is appropriate to initiate oxygen therapy with 2 to 5 L per minute, but this amount should be adjusted with each titration of IPAP or EPAP.

The same general principles apply for the initiation of HFNC. Patient selection is critical, and special nasal cannula that permit humidified high flows of 20 L per minute to 60 L per minute are required. Initial flows of 20 L per minute should be instituted and titrated based on patient response.

### Response to Therapy

Following patient acceptance, support pressures should be titrated to optimize respiratory support. One common approach in the management of hypoxemic respiratory failure is to titrate EPAP and IPAP in tandem via 2 to 3 cm $H_2O$ steps, allowing a brief trial period (e.g., 5 minutes) at each level. If the patient is hypercapnic, it may be better to raise the IPAP in 2 cm $H_2O$ steps, with the EPAP being kept stationary or increased in a ratio to IPAP of approximately 1:2.5 (EPAP:IPAP). The intrinsic PEEP ($PEEP_i$), or auto-PEEP, cannot be measured by a noninvasive ventilator; therefore, EPAP should generally be maintained below 8 to 10 cm $H_2O$ to be certain that it does not exceed $PEEP_i$ in patients with obstructive lung disease. The IPAP must always be set higher than EPAP by at least 5 cm $H_2O$. The goals are to reduce the patient's WOB, improve comfort, meet oxygen saturation goals, improve gas exchange, foster patient compliance, and maintain a respiratory rate of $<30$ breaths per minute. If the patient is not approaching these goals after the first hour of NPPV, then strong consideration should be made for intubation and institution of invasive mechanical ventilation.

## TIPS AND PEARLS

- Patients with inadequate airway protection are poor candidates for NPPV owing to risk of aspiration.
- Patients with both a patent airway and preserved respiratory drive—even if that drive is failing—may be candidates for NPPV.
- Patients most likely to respond to NPPV in the ED (and therein avoid intubation) are those with acutely reversible etiologies of respiratory failure, such as COPD exacerbation and acute cardiogenic pulmonary edema.
- The ventilatory management of patients in frank or impending respiratory failure with NPPV is a *minute-to-minute*, ongoing strategic decision. Virtually, every modern ventilator is capable of delivering noninvasive ventilation (NIV) (BiPAP, CPAP) and should be readily accessible to the ED or other critical care areas in the hospital. Physicians, nurses, and respiratory care personnel must be comfortable with NPPV use and knowledgeable of its limitations.
- Patient selection must consider the overall condition of the patient, tolerance of the NPPV interface, and the anticipated reversibility of the underlying insult.
- NPPV should be accompanied by aggressive medical therapy of the underlying condition (e.g., vasodilators and diuretics for pulmonary edema, β-adrenergic agonist, and anticholinergic aerosols and corticosteroids for reactive airways disease).
- Be prepared for prompt intubation (i.e., difficult airway assessment completed along with drugs, equipment, and plan established) in case NPPV fails.
- Patients should be carefully monitored for progress of therapy, tolerance of NPPV, and any signs of clinical deterioration that indicate a need for intubation and mechanical ventilation.
- NPPV response is typically recognized within 20 to 30 minutes of initiation. Early intubation should be considered for patients who fail to improve quickly in order to avoid complicated emergency intubation in the midst of deterioration on NPPV.
- Patients treated with NPPV may require judicious sedation for anxiety in order to tolerate the mask. Careful dosing is required to preserve respiratory drive and avoid precipitating deterioration.

## EVIDENCE

- **When is NPPV most helpful in managing ED patients?** Most studies compare NPPV to standard medical care with favorable outcome measures of endotracheal intubation and ICU and hospital length of stay. Mortality benefit has not been substantiated. In some series, ED patients successfully supported with NPPV and avoided ICU admission, thereby incurring a significant health care cost savings. The strongest level of evidence supports NPPV use for COPD exacerbations and acute cardiogenic pulmonary edema. Uncontrolled studies suggest that NPPV may be successful in a larger variety of patients.[1,2]
- **What is the role for HFNC?** Studies to date confirm that HFNC is feasible and provides a safe alternative for effective and titratable oxygen therapy in acute hypoxemic respiratory failure.[3,4] Patient tolerance is a recognized benefit compared to traditional oxygen devices, including NPPV. Initial studies also suggest improved outcome, but more comparative evidence is required before a firm assessment can be made. HFNC appears to be a natural adjunct to improve preoxygenation during emergency rapid sequence intubation. Limited studies to date in ICU populations have shown conflicting results in HFNC's ability to abort desaturation during emergency airway management.[5,6]

## REFERENCES

1. Schnell D, Timsit JF, Darmon M, et al. Noninvasive mechanical ventilation in acute respiratory failure: trends in use and outcomes. *Intensive Care Med*. 2014;40:582–591.
2. Ozyilmaz, E, Ozsancak U, Nava S. Timing of noninvasive ventilation failure: causes, risk factors, and potential remedies. *BMC Pulm Med*. 2014;14:19.
3. Stephan F, Barrucand B, Petit P, et al; BiPOP Study Group. High-flow nasal oxygen vs noninvasive positive airway pressure in hypoxemic patients after cardiothoracic surgery; a randomized clinical trial. *JAMA*. 2015;313(23):2331–2339.
4. Frat JP, Thille AW, Mercat A, et al; FLORALI Study Group; REVA Network. High-flow oxygen through nasal cannula in acute hypoxemic respiratory failure. *N Engl J Med*. 2015;372:2185–2196.
5. Miguel-Montanes R, Hajage D, Messika J, et al. Use of high-flow nasal cannula oxygen therapy to prevent desaturation during tracheal intubation of intensive care patients with mild-to-moderate hypoxemia. *Crit Care Med*. 2015;43(3):574–583.
6. Vourc'h M, Asfar P, Volteau C, et al. High-flow nasal cannula oxygen during endotracheal intubation in hypoxemic patients: a randomized controlled clinical trial. *Intensive Care Med*. 2015;41(9):1538–1548.

Chapter 7

# Mechanical Ventilation

Alan C. Heffner and Peter M.C. DeBlieux

## INTRODUCTION

Acute respiratory failure is a common acute critical condition, and initiation of mechanical ventilation is a required skill for all emergency physicians. The etiologies for respiratory failure are expansive, and the choice between invasive and noninvasive mechanical ventilation can be a challenging clinical decision. This chapter focuses on initiation of safe and effective invasive mechanical ventilation following endotracheal intubation. Chapter 6 focuses on respiratory failure requiring noninvasive mechanical ventilation.

Spontaneous ventilation draws air into the lungs under negative pressure, whereas mechanical ventilation uses positive pressure to provide airflow. In either case, the amount of negative or positive pressure required to deliver the tidal volume ($V_t$ or TV) must overcome resistance to airflow. Positive-pressure ventilation alters normal pulmonary physiology by increasing airway and intrathoracic pressure, decreasing venous return to the thorax, and altering ventilation–perfusion matching in the lung.

## TERMINOLOGY OF MECHANICAL VENTILATION

The following variables are important to best understand mechanical ventilation:

- **$V_t$ or TV** is the volume of a single breath. During mechanical ventilation, the contemporary safe goal TV is ≤7 mL per kg of ideal body weight (IBW). It is important to note that IBW is more a function of patient height rather than weight or overall size. TVs may be reduced (to 6 or lower mL per kg IBW) in certain circumstances to minimize ventilator-induced lung injury (VILI) associated with excessive airway pressure that risk overdistention of functional lung units.

  The airway conduits do not exchange gas and therefore represent anatomical dead space that accounts for a fixed volume of each tidal breath. The remaining TV participates in gas exchange and constitutes alveolar ventilation. As TV is reduced, anatomical dead space makes up a proportionally larger portion of each breath. It is important to increase minute ventilation through enhanced respiratory rate (RR) to balance the decrease in effective alveolar ventilation with TV reduction.
- **RR or frequency (*f*)** is simply the number of breaths per minute. Usual starting RR is 12 to 20 breaths per minute in adults. Higher rates are typical in neonates, infants, and small children.

  Given our attention to low-TV ventilation, even in patients without lung injury, minute ventilation is typically modified by increasing RR rather than TV. In addition to compensating for the relative proportion of dead space mentioned earlier, enhanced RR may be used to provide compensation for metabolic acidosis or enhanced carbon dioxide ($CO_2$) production (e.g., fever/hyperthermia, sepsis, and hypermetabolic conditions).

In reactive airways diseases, the concept of permissive hypercapnia refers to the use of low RR (8 to 10 breaths per minute), allowing for adequate expiratory time for complete exhalation of the former TV to avoid trapped air that leads to dynamic hyperinflation and auto-Positive end-expiratory pressure (PEEP).

- **Fractional concentration of inspired oxygen ($FIO_2$)** ranges from the concentration of oxygen in room air (0.21 or 21%) to that of pure oxygen (1.0 or 100%). When initiating mechanical ventilation, start with a $FIO_2$ of 100% and reduce the $FIO_2$ based on continuous pulse oximetry. During acute critical illness, titrating $FIO_2$ to maintain $SpO_2 \geq 95\%$ is appropriate for most conditions. The lowest $FIO_2$ required to maintain adequate oxygenation should be used.
- **Inspiratory flow rate (IFR)** is the rate at which a TV is delivered during inspiration. In an adult, this is typically set at 60 L per minute. Cases of reactive airways disease may require peak IFR to be increased to 90 to 120 L per minute in order to shorten the inspiratory time (Ti), and thus increase expiratory time and diminish dynamic hyperinflation.
- **PEEP** provides a static pressure to the airways during inspiration and expiration, and is typically set at a minimum of 5 cm $H_2O$. PEEP increases alveolar recruitment, functional residual capacity, total lung volume, and pulmonary and intrathoracic pressure. When a patient is unable to meet oxygenation goals on $FIO_2 > 50\%$, PEEP is typically increased to augment mean airway pressure to improve oxygenation. However, excessive PEEP can lead to pathologic overdistention of healthy lung tissue contributing to ineffective gas exchange and VILI. Elevated intrathoracic pressure can also compromise venous return with consequent hemodynamic deterioration.
- **Peak inspiratory pressure (PIP) and plateau pressure ($P_{plat}$)**: The PIP is the greatest pressure reached during the inspiratory cycle, and is a function of the ventilator circuitry, endotracheal tube (ETT), ventilator flow rate, and patient lung and thoracic compliance. It is useful for rapid assessment of a patient during acute changes, but does not accurately reflect lung compliance or the risk of VILI. Risk of pulmonary overdistention is better represented by the $P_{plat}$, measured at the end of inspiration (via an inspiratory pause). The inspiratory pause enables equilibration of pressure between the ventilator and lung units to measure the *static pressure* of the thoracic compartment. $P_{plat}$ correlates with the risk of VILI, and current recommendations aim to maintain safe $P_{plat} \leq 30$ cm $H_2O$ via reduction in TV when advanced lung disease is the cause for elevated $P_{plat}$.

## VENTILATION MODES

There are a variety of modes of invasive mechanical ventilation, and the key to understanding the differences between these modes centers on three variables: the trigger, the limit, and the cycle.

- The trigger is the event that initiates inspiration: either patient effort or machine-initiated positive pressure.
- The limit refers to the airflow parameter that is used to regulate inspiration: either airflow rate or airway pressure.
- The cycle terminates inspiration: via delivered set volume in volume-control ventilation (VCV), pressure delivered over a set time period in pressure-control ventilation (PCV), or by patient termination of inspiratory effort in pressure support ventilation (PSV).
- The best mode in a given circumstance depends on the needs of the patient.

Commonly used ventilation modes are as follows:

- **Control mode ventilation (CMV)** is almost exclusively relegated to the operating room in sedated and paralyzed patients, but an understanding of this mode provides appreciation of the support provided through other modes. In CMV, all breaths are triggered, limited, and cycled by the ventilator. The clinician sets the TV, RR, IFR, PEEP, and $F_{IO_2}$. The ventilator then delivers the prescribed TV (the cycle) at the set IFR (the limit). Even if the patient wanted to initiate an additional breath, the machine would not respond. In addition, if the patient has not completely exhaled before initiation of the next breath, the machine would generate the required pressure to deliver the full TV breath. For these reasons, CMV is only used in those patients who are sedated and paralyzed.

- **Assist control (AC)** is the preferred mode for patients with acute respiratory failure. The clinician sets the TV, RR, IFR, PEEP, and $F_{IO_2}$. In contrast to all other modes, the trigger that initiates inspiration can be either patient effort or an elapsed time interval. When either of these occurs, the ventilator delivers the prescribed TV. The ventilator synchronizes set RRs with patient efforts, and if the patient is breathing at or above the set RR, then all breaths are patient initiated. The work of breathing (WOB) is primarily limited to the patient's effort to trigger the ventilator and can be altered by adjusting the sensitivity threshold.
- **Synchronized intermittent mandatory ventilation (SIMV with or without PS)** is commonly misunderstood and can lead to excessive patient WOB. The physician sets the TV, RR, IFR, PEEP, and $F_{IO_2}$. Importantly, the trigger that initiates inspiration depends on the patient's RR relative to the set RR. When the patient is breathing at or below the set RR, the trigger can be patient effort or elapsed time. In these cases, the ventilator operates similar to an AC mode. If the patient is breathing above the set RR, the ventilator does not automatically assist the patient efforts, and the TV is determined by effort and resistance to airflow through the ETT and ventilator circuit. In these instances, WOB can be excessive.

  Addition of PSV to the SIMV mode provides a set inspiratory pressure that is applied during patient-initiated breaths, which exceed the set RR. Appropriate PSV balances the inherent resistance of the artificial airways and supports the patient's physiologic situation to limit undue WOB. Insufficient PSV is associated with high RR and low TV, also known as rapid, shallow breathing. Sustained tachypnea greater than 24 breaths per minute is a helpful marker to consider evaluating if the PSV level is appropriate to the patient condition. SIMV provides no clear benefit over AC mode ventilation. Although previously used as a weaning mode wherein the set rate is progressively decreased to allow the patient to assume increased WOB, the absence of additional PSV substantially increases WOB and is frequently overtaxing. Spontaneous breathing trials using minimal PSV, without SIMV, is the current standard approach to assess readiness for liberation from mechanical ventilation.
- **Continuous positive airway pressure (CPAP)** is not a true mode of invasive mechanical ventilation. It is equivalent to PEEP in that it provides a static positive airway pressure throughout the entire respiratory cycle.

  In a fashion similar to SIMV, PS can be added to CPAP to function as an assisted form of ventilation. In the CPAP-PS mode, the patient determines the RR, initiating and terminating each breath. The TV is dependent on patient effort and the degree of PS relative to the resistance of the airway circuit. This mode should never be used in patients at risk for hypoventilation or apnea, because there is no mandatory backup rate to support the patient in case of failure.

## VENTILATOR TV DELIVERY

### Volume-Control Ventilation

In this method of delivering a breath, the operator sets the TV of each breath. The pressure required to deliver this volume varies by the flow rate selected, the resistance of the airway circuit and lungs, and compliance of lungs and thorax. In adults, the initial peak flow is usually set to 60 L per minute.

VCV also allows selection of the flow characteristics of a delivered breath. The waveform may be square or decelerating (**Fig. 7-1**). A square wave delivers the TV at a constant peak flow throughout inspiration. This waveform usually generates a higher peak pressure than the decelerating waveform, but has the advantage of a shorter Ti, providing more time for expiration. A decelerating flow wave

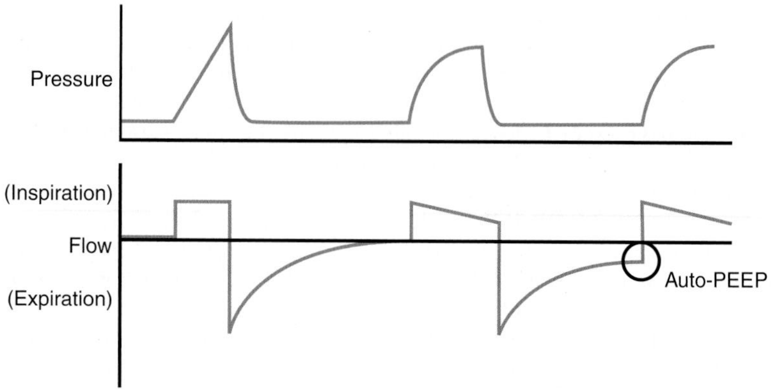


● **FIGURE 7-1. Volume-Control Ventilation (VCV).** The lower trace demonstrates a square flow waveform first followed by a decelerating waveform. Note that the peak pressure generated by the square waveform exceeds that of the decelerating waveform. The third waveform demonstrates breath initiation before expiratory flow reaches zero. This is an example of breath stacking that leads to dynamic hyperinflation and auto-PEEP.

delivers the initial TV at a selected flow that decelerates as the breath is delivered. Because resistance to flow normally increases during inspiration, the decelerating waveform generally results in lower PIP. This approach increases Ti at the expense of expiratory time, which may potentiate dynamic hyperinflation and auto-PEEP. For this reason, the IFR set for decelerating flow wave is usually higher than that used in a square wave flow pattern. When setting up the ventilator, one can try different flow patterns to determine which offers the best patient synchrony.

## Pressure-Control Ventilation

PCV should not be confused with PSV ventilation, described previously. The limit during PCV is a set airway pressure. Instead of TV, the cycle during PCV is a set Ti. Some PCV ventilator models require a set RR and inspiratory to expiratory (I:E) ratio. Ti is then calculated by the ventilator based on these settings. The clinician specifies an inspiratory pressure and an inspiratory–expiratory (I:E) ratio predicted to provide a reasonable TV and RR, based on the patient's expected resistance and compliance. TV may vary from breath to breath based on airway resistance, lung compliance, and patient effort, but it should generally meet the same ≤7 mL per kg IBW goal discussed earlier.

In this mode, the peak flow of the administered tidal breath and the flow waveform vary according to airway and lung characteristics. Early in inspiration, the ventilator generates a flow rate that is sufficiently rapid to reach the preset pressure and then automatically alters the flow rate to stay at that pressure, and cycles off at the end of the predetermined Ti. The flow waveform created by this method is a decelerating pattern (**Fig. 7-2**). A normal I:E ratio is 1:2. If the RR is 10 breaths per minute evenly distributed over a minute, each cycle of inspiration and expiration is 6 seconds. With an I:E ratio of 1:2, inspiration is 2 seconds, and expiration is 4 seconds.

The I:E ratio is usually determined by simply observing the pressure and flow waveforms on the ventilator monitor. After the inspiratory pressure is adjusted to meet the target TV, the Ti is adjusted while monitoring end-expiratory flow. Terminal end-expiratory flow should approach zero to confirm exhalation is complete, and avoid retained intrathoracic volume. Small fractions of retained TV compounded by the ventilator rate can quickly lead to dynamic hyperinflation with increased intrathoracic pressure known as auto-PEEP that affects venous return, respiratory mechanics, and can put the patient at risk for barotrauma (**Fig. 7-3**). In contrast, overly brief Ti can lead to low TVs and hypoventilation.

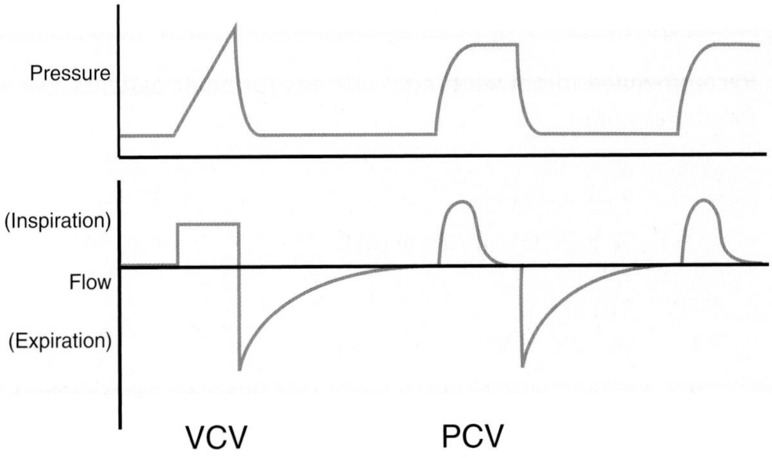


● **FIGURE 7-2. Pressure-Control Ventilation (PCV).** These waveforms demonstrate the differing waveform characteristics between volume-control (VCV) and PCV. Note that PCV generates lower peak pressures than VCV.

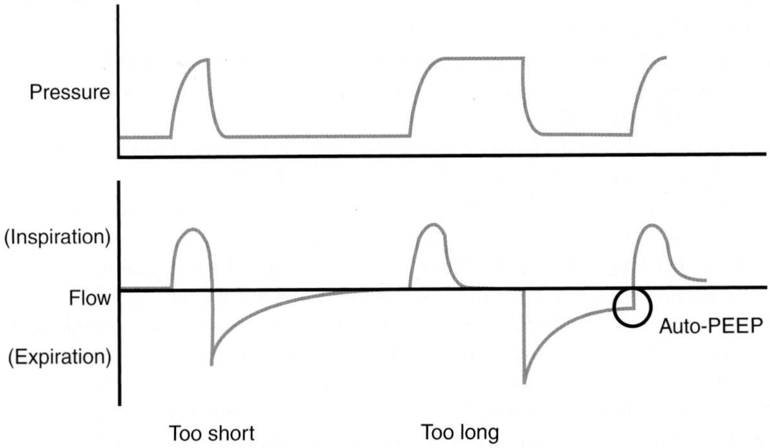


● **FIGURE 7-3. Pressure-Control Ventilation and Inspiratory-Expiratory Ratio.** The first waveform demonstrates inspiratory time that is so short that the tidal volume is likely insufficient. The second and third waveforms demonstrate how prolonged inspiratory time may contribute to breath stacking and auto-PEEP.

## INITIATING MECHANICAL VENTILATION

The patient who is spontaneously breathing possesses a complex series of physiologic feedback loops that control the volume of gas moved into and out of the lungs each minute (minute ventilation). They automatically determine the RR and the volume of each breath necessary to effect gas exchange and maintain homeostasis. Patients dependent on ventilators have no such servo control and must rely on individualized ventilator settings to meet their physiologic needs. In the past, this required frequent blood gas determinations. Now we rely more heavily on noninvasive techniques such as pulse oximetry and end-tidal $CO_2$ monitoring.

**BOX 7-1**

**Recommended initial ventilator settings for adult patients.** *See text for abbreviations.*

- Mode AC
- $V_t$ 7 mL per kg IBW
- *f* 12 to 20 breaths per minute
- $FIO_2$ 1.0
- PEEP 5.0 cm $H_2O$
- IFR 60 L per minute

A certain amount of ventilation is required (minute ventilation or minute volume) to remove the $CO_2$ produced by metabolism and delivered to the lungs by the circulatory system each minute. This minute volume approximates 100 mL per kg, under normal metabolism. Hypermetabolic and febrile patients can produce up to 25% more $CO_2$ compared with normal resting steady state. Minute ventilation would need to increase proportionally to accommodate this increased production.

Our recommended initial ventilator settings for adult patients are shown in **Box 7-1**. For the vast majority of patients, this formula produces reasonable gas exchange to provide adequate oxygenation and ventilation. The components of minute ventilation (TV and RR) are manipulated to provide adequate minute volume. If smaller TV is desired, compensatory increase in respiratory frequency may be required.

Supranormal TV and high airway pressure risk VILI during mechanical ventilation. This underlies the recommended starting TV $\leq$ 7 mL per kg IBW. For some patients, the most difficult task in optimizing mechanical ventilation is balancing TV and distending lung pressure. Plateau airway pressure correlates with the risk of VILI, and current recommendations aim to maintain $P_{plat} \leq 30$ cm $H_2O$. Because many of these patients require PEEP augmentation for oxygenation, this is often best managed by reducing TV to a range of 4 to 6 mL per kg IBW.

Positive-pressure breathing increases intrathoracic pressure that is transmitted to the great vessels and can compromise venous return. This can seriously compromise cardiovascular performance and precipitate shock or cardiac arrest (i.e., pulseless electrical activity) when unrecognized dynamic hyperinflation with auto-PEEP occurs, especially in patients with low intravascular volume.

In other situations, ventilator modifications aim to balance minute ventilation with airflow dynamics. The intubated patient with obstructive lung disease such as severe asthma is a good example. Minute volume aims to provide reasonable minute ventilation relative to $CO_2$ production, but must be balanced to complete TV exhalation and avoid retained intrathoracic volume. *Frequency has the greatest impact on expiratory time and should start as low as 8 breaths per minute in patients with obstructive lung physiology.* The inspiratory cycle can also be shortened by increasing the IFR to maximize expiratory time. Auscultation of the chest is a rapid means to clarify if initiation of the next breath occurs before complete exhalation (typically manifest as persistent wheezing). Incomplete exhalation, commonly called "breath stacking," leads to dynamic hyperinflation of the lungs. The flow-time graphic on modern ventilators is also helpful as return to zero flow is another aid to judge adequacy of exhalation.

In extreme cases, deliberate hypoventilation is performed to avoid dynamic hyperinflation and high intrathoracic pressure that can lead to barotrauma and cardiovascular compromise from limited venous return. Permissive hypercapnia (respiratory acidosis with pH $>$ 7.10) is the expected cost of this strategy. Equipment considerations may also contribute to airflow obstruction and deserves special attention (**Box 7-2**).

**BOX 7-2**

**Recommendations for mechanical ventilation for adult patients with obstructive lung physiology.** *See text for abbreviations.*

- Use as large an ETT as possible
- Cut the ETT and ventilator circuit to minimize dead space
- Set initial RR at 8 breaths per minute
- Set initial TV at 7 mL per kg IBW
- Increase IFR at 90 to 120 L per minute
- Use clinical auscultation and ventilator flow-time graphics to confirm cessation of airflow prior to the following breath

## TIPS AND PEARLS

- Have a respiratory therapist (RT) review the features and graphics of ventilators available at your particular institution. Make sure that your RTs are familiar with the ARDSnet protocol, $P_{plat}$ measurements, and the concept of permissive hypercapnia.
- When a ventilator alarms, you must know how to take a patient off the ventilator and resume bag ventilation until an RT can assist. To do this, you must be able to turn the ventilator on and off and know how to silence the alarms. These minimal steps will preserve calm until the RT can respond. Bag ventilation effectively deals with temporary ventilator malfunction and provides immediate manual feedback of airway, pulmonary, and thoracic resistance and compliance.
- Understand the typical resistance and compliance characteristics of various respiratory disorders. This information may help predict specific TV and rate settings for your patients.
- Use AC as your primary mode following initial intubation. This provides support for apneic patients and relieves the patient of the WOB.
- Disconnect the patient from the breathing circuit and provide bag ventilation support during transport, unless a small transport ventilator is used. The circuit is heavy and may drag the ETT out, especially in infants and children.

## EVIDENCE

- **What is permissive hypercapnia, and is there evidence that it is safe?** All patients are capable of trapping inspired air if the expiratory period is inadequate. Patients with obstructive lung disease are particularly vulnerable. Maximizing expiratory period through ventilator modifications (i.e., low RR and TV with rapid IFR) may require sacrificing normal physiologic minute ventilation to avoid dynamic hyperinflation. Permissive hypercapnia is the technique of providing intentional hypoventilation and allowing respiratory acidosis until airways resistance improves. Moderate to severe acidemia (pH $> 7.10$) is well tolerated. Significant sedation, and even neuromuscular paralysis, is required to suppress patient respiratory effort from triggering the ventilator in this situation.
- **What is the current ventilator management strategy to limit lung injury (VILI) in acute respiratory distress syndrome (ARDS)?** Contemporary mechanical ventilation aims to

minimize VILI induced by lung overdistention, even in patients without pulmonary disease. Low TV (≤7 mL per kg IBW) reduces mortality and ventilator days in patients with ARDS.[1] Recognizing that TV is distributed predominantly to healthy, patent alveoli, lower TV prevents overdistention injury of functional lung units. $P_{plat}$ (goal ≤ 30 cm $H_2O$) is used as the surrogate measure of lung compliance to individualize the appropriate reduction of TV. Further reduction in TV (to 4 to 6 mL per kg IBW) may be required to minimize distending pressure to meet this goal in patients with severe lung disease.

Neuromuscular blockade improves gas exchange in patients with severe lung disease, presumably via removal of patient-ventilator dysynchrony. Early continuous paralysis is also now recognized to improve mortality in patients with severe ARDS (defined by partial pressure of arterial oxygen [$Pao_2$]/$Fio_2$ < 150).[2] Attention to maintain appropriate sedation under the influence of neuromuscular blockade is essential to avoid patient awareness.

## REFERENCES

1. The Acute Respiratory Distress Syndrome Network Authors. Ventilation with lower tidal volumes as compared with traditional tidal volumes for acute lung injury and the acute respiratory distress syndrome. *N Engl J Med*. 2000;342:1301–1308.
2. Papazian L, Forem JM, Gacouin A, et al. Neuromuscular blockers in early acute respiratory distress syndrome. *N Engl J Med*. 2010;363:1107–1116.

Chapter 8

# Oxygen and Carbon Dioxide Monitoring

Robert F. Reardon and Jennifer L. Avegno

## PULSE OXIMETRY

The amount of oxygen reversibly bound to hemoglobin in arterial blood is defined as hemoglobin saturation ($Sao_2$), a critical element of systemic oxygen delivery. Unfortunately, clinical detection of hypoxemia is unreliable. Pulse oximeters enable in vivo, noninvasive, and continuous measurement of arterial oxygen saturation at the bedside. Reliable interpretation of the information provided by these devices requires appreciation of their technology and limitations.

### Principles of Measurement

Pulse oximetry relies on the principle of spectral analysis, which is the method of analyzing physiochemical properties of matter based on their unique light-absorption characteristics. For blood, absorbance of transmitted light is dependent on the concentration of hemoglobin species. Oxygenated hemoglobin absorbs more infrared light and allows more red light to pass through than deoxygenated hemoglobin.

Oximeters are made up of a light source, photodetector, and microprocessor. Light-emitting diodes (LED) emit high-frequency signals at 660 nm (red) and 940 nm (infrared) wavelengths. When positioned to traverse or reflect from a cutaneous vascular bed, the opposed photodetector measures the light intensity of each transmitted signal. Signal processing exploits the pulsatile nature of arterial blood to isolate arterial saturation. The microprocessor averages these data over several pulse cycles and compares the measured absorption to a reference standard curve to determine hemoglobin saturation, which is displayed as percentage of oxyhemoglobin ($Spo_2$). $Spo_2$ and $Sao_2$ correlation vary with manufacturer but exhibit high accuracy ($\pm 2\%$) within normal physiologic range and circumstances.

Anatomical locations with high vascular density are preferred for probe placement, and two oximetry techniques are used in clinical practice. Transmission oximetry deploys the LED and photodetector on opposite sides of a tissue bed (e.g., digit, nose, or ear lobe) such that the signal must traverse tissue. Reflectance oximeters position the LED and photodetector side by side on a single surface and can be placed in anatomical locations without an interposed vascular bed (e.g., forehead). This facilitates more proximal sensor placement with improved response time relative to core body $Sao_2$.

## Indications

Pulse oximetry provides important, real-time physiologic data and is the standard noninvasive measure of arterial saturation. It is now widely considered one of the standard measurements in patient vital signs. Continuous monitoring is indicated for any patient at risk or in the midst of acute cardiopulmonary decompensation. Reliable continuous oximetry is mandatory for patients requiring airway management and should be a component of each preintubation checklist. If placed on an extremity, the probe is preferably placed on the opposite side of the blood pressure cuff to avoid interruptions in $Sa_{O_2}$ readings during cuff inflation.

## Limitations and Precautions

Pulse oximeters have a number of important physiologic and technical limitations that influence bedside use and interpretation (Table 8-1).

## Signal Reliability

Proper pulse oximetry requires pulse detection to distinguish light absorption from arterial blood relative to the background of other tissues. Abnormal peripheral circulation as a consequence of shock, vasoconstriction, or hypothermia may prevent pulsatile flow detection. Heart rate and plethysmographic waveform display verify arterial sensing, and $Sp_{O_2}$ should be considered inaccurate unless corroborated by these markers. Varying pulse amplitude is easily recognized on the monitor

TABLE 8-1 **Etiology and Examples of Unreliable Pulse Oximetry**

| Etiology | Examples |
|---|---|
| Sensor location | Critical illness (forehead probe is best) |
| | Extraneous light exposure |
| Motion artifact | Exercise |
| | Cardiopulmonary resuscitation (CPR) |
| | Seizure |
| | Shivering/tremor |
| | Prehospital transport |
| Signal degradation | Hypothermia |
| | Hypotension/shock |
| | Hypoperfusion |
| | Vasoconstriction |
| | Nail polish/synthetic nails |
| Physiologic range | Increasingly inaccurate when systolic BP < 80 mm Hg |
| | Increasingly inaccurate when $Sa_{O_2} < 75\%$ |
| | Severe anemia |
| | Sickle cell anemia |
| Dyshemoglobinemia | CO-Hgb (overestimates $Sp_{O_2}$) |
| | Met-Hgb (variable response) |
| Intravenous dye | Methylene blue |
| | Indocyanine green |

and represents the measure of arterial pulsatility at the sampled vascular bed. Quantification in the form of perfusion index is being incorporated into some software to verify signal reliability and gauge microvascular flow.

Even with verified signal detection, measurement bias limits $Spo_2$ reliability during physiologic extremes. Reliability deteriorates with progressive hypotension below systolic BP of 80 mm Hg, and in these patients, readings generally underestimate true $Sao_2$. Severe hypoxemia with $Sao_2 <$ 75% is also associated with increased measurement error as comparisons to reference standards are limited below this value. However, patients with this severity of hypoxemia are typically receiving maximized intervention, and closer discrimination in this range rarely imparts new information that alters management.

A number of physical factors affect pulse oximetry accuracy. Signal reliability is influenced by sensor exposure to extraneous light, excessive movement, synthetic fingernails, nail polish, intravenous dyes, severe anemia, and abnormal hemoglobin species. Diligent probe placement and shielding the probe from extraneous light should be routine. Surface extremity warming may improve local perfusion to enable arterial pulse sensing, but $Spo_2$ accuracy using this technique is not confirmed.

Dyshemoglobinemias such as carboxyhemoglobin (CO-Hgb) and methemoglobin (Met-Hgb) absorb light at different wavelengths and may affect the accuracy of oximetry readings. Co-oximeters (and some new generation pulse oximeters) use four wavelengths of light stimulus to selectively discriminate these species. However, CO-Hgb absorbance is close to oxyhemoglobin such that most conventional pulse oximeters sum up their measurement and give artifactually high $Spo_2$ readings. Met-Hgb produces variable error, depending on the true oxy- and Met-Hgb levels. $Spo_2$ classically approximates 85% in severe toxicity.

## Response Time

Pulse oximetry readings lag the patient's physiologic state; signal averaging of 4 to 20 seconds is typical of most monitors. Delay because of sensor anatomical location and abnormal cardiac performance compound the lag relative to central $Sao_2$. Forehead and ear probes are closer to the heart and respond more quickly than distal extremity probes. Response difference compared to central $Sao_2$ is also compounded by hypoxemia (i.e., starting on the steep portion of the oxyhemoglobin dissociation curve) and slower peripheral circulation such as low cardiac output states. As such, forehead reflectance probes are often preferred in critically ill patients. All of these response delays become more clinically important during rapid desaturation such as that which may occur during airway management and is the basis for our general recommendation to abort most intubation attempts when the $Spo_2$ falls below 93%.

## Physiologic Insight and Limitations

Hemoglobin saturation is just one part of the assessment of systemic oxygenation. Although monitoring is continuous, $Spo_2$ provides momentary information on arterial saturation without true insight into systemic oxygenation and respiratory reserve. The physiologic context of oximetry is critical for appropriate interpretation and assists estimation of a patient's cardiopulmonary reserve for planning and execution of an airway management plan.

Oximetry measures arterial hemoglobin saturation but not the arterial oxygen tension or oxygen content of blood. The oxyhemoglobin dissociation curve (see Chapters 5 and 20) describes the relationship of oxygen partial pressure ($Pao_2$) and saturation ($Sao_2$). Its sigmoidal shape hinges on varying hemoglobin affinity with successive oxygen binding. It is important to note that $Spo_2$ provides poor correlation with $Pao_2$ in the normal range. Normal $Sao_2$ is associated with a wide range of $Pao_2$ (80 to 400 mm Hg), which includes two extremes of oxygen reserve. Similarly, oximetry is insensitive at detecting progressive hypoxemia in patients with high-baseline $Pao_2$. Correlation is established in the hypoxemic range at and below the upper inflection point of the oxyhemoglobin curve ($Pao_2 <$ 60 mm Hg approximating $Sao_2$ 90% at normal pH) where desaturation is rapid with declining $Pao_2$.

Hemoglobin saturation must also be interpreted in the context of inspired oxygen fraction ($Fio_2$) to provide insight into gas exchange and physiologic reserve. Simple observation at the bedside provides qualitative assessment. More formal calculation of the $Spo_2/Fio_2$ (SF) ratio is advocated. For the same reasons discussed earlier, SF ratio correlates with $Pao_2/Fio_2$ (PF) ratio in the hypoxemic range ($Spo_2 < 90\%$) but not in the normal range. As such, observation of the patient's condition before supplemental oxygen escalation or preoxygenation provides more insight into the physiologic state. Correct interpretation of $Spo_2$ relative to $Fio_2$ is also important in assessing for failure of noninvasive ventilation. Hypoxemia and/or requirement of oxygen escalation above $Fio_2 > 70\%$ leaves a thin margin of physiologic reserve for preoxygenation and execution of safe, uncomplicated endotracheal intubation.

Although $Pao_2$ (with or without conscious calculation of PF ratio) is a traditional and reliable gauge of pulmonary gas exchange and reserve, measurement of $Pao_2$ through arterial blood gas sampling before airway management is not generally helpful. The aim to maximize preoxygenation in all patients supersedes this strategy. However, knowledge of these principles and relationships provides insight into physiologic events and the fallibility of current technology during the management of critical illness.

The context of cardiac performance is also vital to interpretation of oximetry data. Although saturated hemoglobin accounts for the majority of blood oxygen content, systemic oxygen delivery is largely regulated (and limited) by cardiac performance. Pertinent to airway management, rapid desaturation and delayed response to pulmonary oxygenation should be anticipated in the setting of low cardiac output.

Finally, oxygen saturation is an unreliable gauge of ventilation, $Paco_2$ level, or acid–base status. Normal arterial saturation does not ensure appropriate ventilation. Oxygenation often is adequate with minimal volume of gas exchange, whereas carbon dioxide ($CO_2$) removal relies on pulmonary ventilation. Arterial blood gas analysis is the traditional means to measure $Paco_2$, but alternative noninvasive $CO_2$ monitoring provides additional insight.

## END-TIDAL $CO_2$ MONITORING

$CO_2$ is a normal byproduct of systemic metabolism. The quantity of expired $CO_2$ is dependent on three factors: metabolic production, venous return and pulmonary circulation to deliver $CO_2$ to the lungs, and alveolar ventilation. Capnography, therefore, provides insight into each of these factors. The corollary is that interpretation of exhaled $CO_2$ is not always straightforward as a consequence of its dependence on these three functions.

### Basics of $CO_2$ Monitoring

$CO_2$ monitors measure the partial pressure of $CO_2$ (in millimeters of mercury) in expired gas. A variety of methods and devices are available. Qualitative (or semiquantitative) colorimetric monitors simply detect expired $CO_2$ above a threshold concentration. Quantitative devices include nonwaveform capnometers and waveform capnographers, which display the partial pressure of $CO_2$ in each breath. When measured at the end of expiration, this is referred to as end-tidal $CO_2$ ($ETCO_2$), which approximates alveolar $CO_2$. Waveform capnographers display a continuous waveform, representing exhaled $CO_2$ concentration over time and therein provide the most comprehensive data on ventilation, metabolism, and perfusion.

### Colorimetric $CO_2$ Detectors

Colorimetric $CO_2$ detectors use pH-sensitive filter paper impregnated with metacresol purple, which changes color from purple (<4 mm Hg $CO_2$) to tan (4 to 15 mm Hg $CO_2$) to yellow (>20 mm Hg $CO_2$), depending on the concentration of exhaled $CO_2$. The indicator, housed in a plastic casing, is typically interposed between the endotracheal tube (ETT) and ventilator bag. Qualitative colorimetric detectors are inexpensive and easy to use, making them an excellent choice for ETT confirmation. One important limitation of qualitative colorimetric detectors is that they have a 25% false-negative

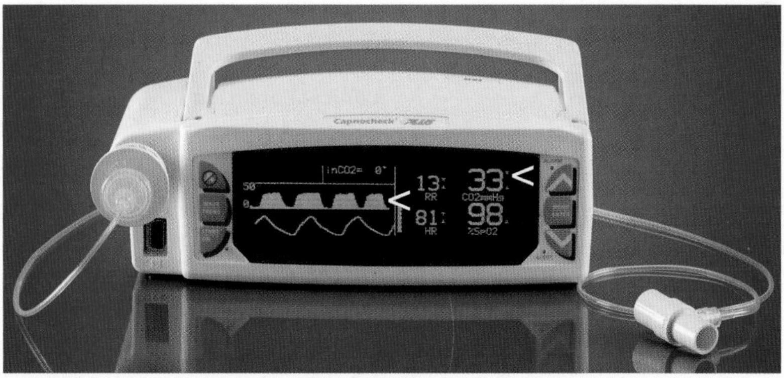


● **FIGURE 8-1. Waveform Capnographer.** Display showing the $ETCO_2$ value (<) with each breath and a waveform (<) representing exhaled $CO_2$ concentration over time.

rate (no color change with correct intubation) in the setting of (usually prolonged) cardiac arrest resulting from the absence of circulatory distribution of $CO_2$ to the lungs.

## Quantitative $CO_2$ Monitors

Quantitative monitors include nonwaveform capnometers, which display $ETCO_2$ of each breath, and waveform capnographers, which display $ETCO_2$ and a continuous waveform representing exhaled $CO_2$ over time (**Fig. 8-1**). Most of these devices use an infrared sensor, which measures the amount of infrared light absorbed by $CO_2$ in the exhaled gases.

There are two types of capnographers: sidestream monitors withdraw gas samples from the airway with a thin tube, and mainstream monitors sample gas with an in-line sensor. Both types can be used for intubated patients. Nonintubated patients undergoing sedation are usually monitored with a sidestream capnographer through a nasal cannula. Capnography face masks that use both sidestream and mainstream technology are also available for monitoring nonintubated patients.

## Capnography Interpretation

In healthy patients, a close correlation exists between $ETCO_2$ and arterial $CO_2$ ($Paco_2$) such that $ETCO_2$ is approximately 2 to 5 mm Hg less than $Paco_2$ (normal $ETCO_2$ is 35 to 45 mm Hg). Unfortunately, changes in ventilation and perfusion alter the alveolar to arterial gradient such that absolute $Paco_2$ can be difficult to predict based on capnography. This does not detract from the utility of capnographic waveform and trend analysis (**Table 8-2**).

Capnography monitors can display at a high-recording rate, which allows assessment of individual waveforms, or a low-recording rate, which allows a better assessment of trends (**Figs. 8-2** and **8-3**). A normal waveform has a characteristic rectangular shape and should start from 0 mm Hg and return to 0 mm Hg. Elevation of the baseline above zero implies $CO_2$ rebreathing or hypoventilation. The upstroke should be rapid and almost vertical. A slurred upstroke occurs with expiratory obstruction caused by bronchospasm, chronic lung disease, or a kinked ETT. The plateau tends to slope gently upward to the end of expiration where the $ETCO_2$ value is measured. Beginning with inspiration, there is a rapid vertical drop back to the baseline.

## Clinical Utility of Quantitative Capnometry and Capnography

### *Confirmation of ETT Placement and Detection of Accidental Extubation*

Continuous waveform capnography and nonwaveform capnometry are the most accurate methods for confirming ETT placement. Esophageal intubation results in an absent or abnormal $ETCO_2$

TABLE 8-2 Abnormal $ETCO_2$ Values

| $ETCO_2$ | Physiology | Clinical Condition |
|---|---|---|
| Increased | Decreased $CO_2$ clearance | Classic hypoventilation |
| | Increased circulation | Return of spontaneous circulation in cardiac arrest |
| | Increased $CO_2$ production | Increased metabolism (fever and seizure) |
| Decreased | Increased $CO_2$ clearance | Hyperventilation |
| | Lack of $CO_2$ in gas | Hypopneic hypoventilation |
| | Sample decreased circulation | Low cardiac output |
| | Decreased $CO_2$ production | Pulmonary embolism |
| | | Decreased metabolism (hypothermia) |
| Zero | No ventilation | Esophageal intubation |
| | | Accidental extubation |
| | | Apnea |
| | No circulation | Cardiac arrest |

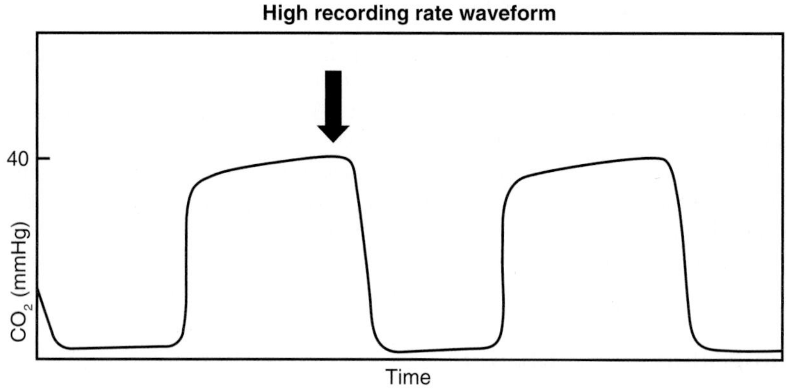


● **FIGURE 8-2.** Normal capnography waveform at a high-recording rate (12.5 mm per second) with a characteristic rectangular shape. The upstroke and downstroke are nearly vertical, the plateau rises slightly throughout expiration, and the $ETCO_2$ value (about 40 mm Hg) is measured at the end of expiration (*arrow*).

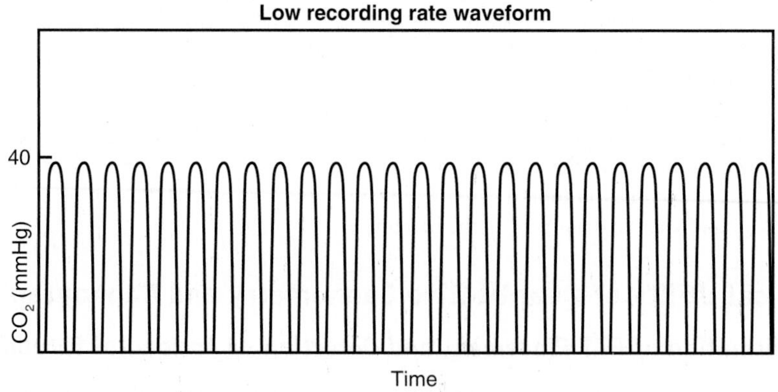


● **FIGURE 8-3.** Normal capnography waveform at a low-recording rate (25 mm per minute). The low-recording rate is useful for monitoring $ETCO_2$ trends, not waveform shape.

value or waveform after the first few breaths (**Fig. 8-4**). Correct ETT placement results in a reasonable $ETCO_2$ value and a characteristic rectangular waveform. The $ETCO_2$ value and waveform can be continuously monitored during prehospital and intrahospital transport. Sudden waveform loss is the earliest sign of accidental extubation and may precede oxygen desaturation by minutes.

## *Capnography during Cardiopulmonary Resuscitation*

Capnography is a sensitive indicator of cardiovascular status. Exhaled $CO_2$ is dependent on pulmonary circulation, which is absent during untreated cardiac arrest. The 2015 American Heart Association (AHA) guidelines encourage the use of continuous waveform capnography to optimize chest compressions during CPR. Effective chest compressions lead to an immediate rise in $ETCO_2$ as a result of effective pulmonary circulation (**Fig. 8-5**). $ETCO_2 < 10$ mm Hg signals ineffective circulation despite CPR or a prolonged arrest with poor prognosis. Return of spontaneous circulation (ROSC) is unlikely if $ETCO_2$ persists $<10$ mm Hg after correct ETT placement and optimal CPR. An abrupt increase in $ETCO_2$ to normal values ($>30$ mm Hg) during CPR is an early indicator of ROSC and often precedes other clinical signs. Be aware that intravenous bicarbonate administration liberates $CO_2$ and causes a transient rise in $ETCO_2$, which should not be misinterpreted as optimized CPR or ROSC.

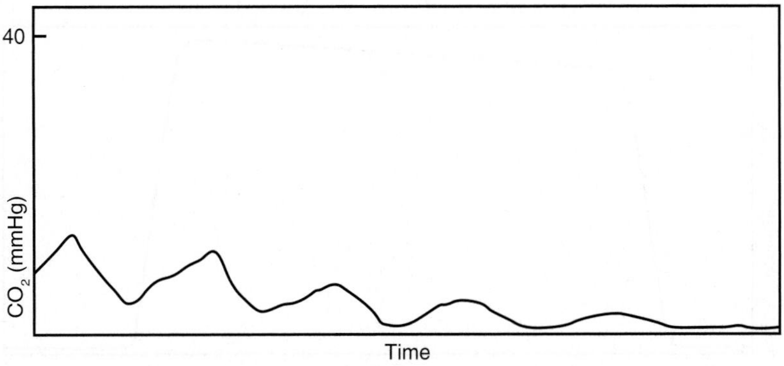


● **FIGURE 8-4. Esophageal Intubation.** Note that there is a minimal abnormal waveform that disappears within five to six breaths.

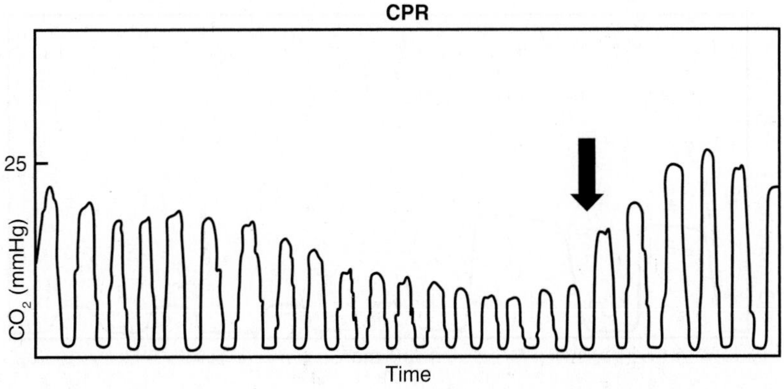


● **FIGURE 8-5.** Capnography waveform during CPR displayed at a low-recording speed for trend analysis. $ETCO_2$ values during CPR are closely correlated with circulation. This trend waveform shows an increase in $ETCO_2$ with improved chest compressions (*arrow*). ROSC also results in an abrupt rise in $ETCO_2$.

### *Monitoring Ventilation during Procedural Sedation*

In the setting of procedural sedation, capnography is the most sensitive indicator of hypoventilation and apnea. Several studies show that patients undergoing procedural sedation have a high rate of acute respiratory events including hypoventilation and apnea, and clinical assessment of chest rise is not sensitive for detecting these events. Oxygen desaturation is a late finding in hypoventilation, especially in patients receiving supplemental oxygen. Addition of capnography to standard monitoring provides advanced warning and reduces hypoxic events.

When using capnography to assess for respiratory depression, it is important to understand that hypoventilation can result in an increase or decrease in $ETCO_2$. Capnographic evidence of respiratory depression includes $ETCO_2 > 50$ mm Hg, a change of $ETCO_2$ of 10% from baseline (or absolute change of 10 mm Hg), or loss of waveform. Bradypneic (classic) hypoventilation results in a waveform of increased amplitude and width (**Fig. 8-6**). Hypopneic hypoventilation (shallow ineffective breathing) results in a low-amplitude waveform, despite rising alveolar $CO_2$ (**Fig. 8-7**). In this case, the measured $ETCO_2$ value will decline because of the relative decrease in the volume of exhaled gas relative to the fixed volume of dead-space gas, thus diluting the $CO_2$ in the sample as indicated.

Analogous to its use in procedural sedation, capnography can be used to gauge adequacy of spontaneous ventilation whenever there is a concern for respiratory depression, similar to that in patients with depressed mental status caused by disease, trauma, or pharmacologic agents.

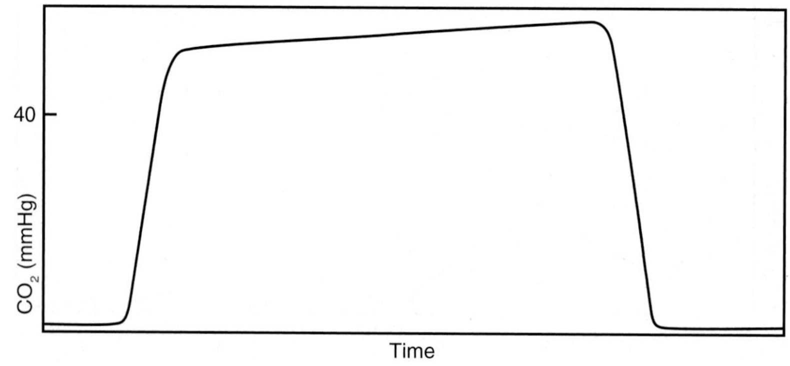


● **FIGURE 8-6. Bradypneic (Classic) Hypoventilation.** Note that the waveform is wide and has increased amplitude, with an $ETCO_2 > 50$ mm Hg.

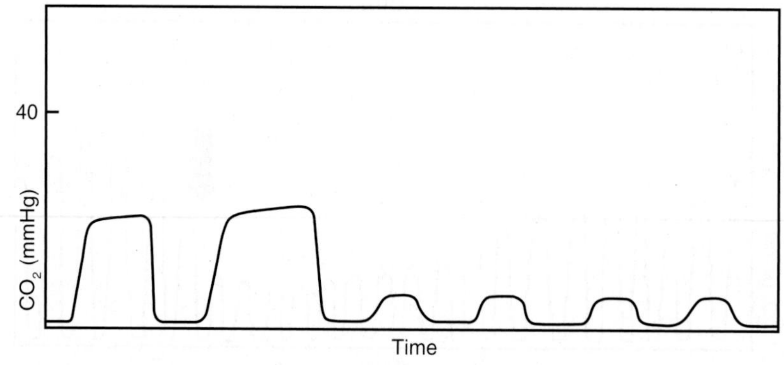


● **FIGURE 8-7. Hypopneic Hypoventilation.** Very shallow breathing results in a low-amplitude waveform and a low $ETCO_2$, despite a rising alveolar $CO_2$.

### Surveillance and Monitoring of Mechanically Ventilated Patients

Capnography is useful for determining adequacy of ventilation in mechanically ventilated patients. Although $ETCO_2$ can be an unreliable gauge of $Paco_2$ because of variation in alveolar-arterial gradient, $ETCO_2$ can be incorporated as a surrogate for $Paco_2$ to minimize routine blood gas analysis. An initial arterial blood gas sample allows comparison of $Paco_2$ and $ETCO_2$ and establishes calibration so that $ETCO_2$ monitoring provides a continuous gauge of $Paco_2$, assuming no major clinical change in patient condition. This is especially helpful for maintaining normocapnia in intubated patients who may be harmed by hypercapnea or hyperventilation, such as those with intracranial hypertension or brain injury.

### Assessment and Monitoring of Patients in Respiratory Distress

Capnography can be useful for monitoring patients presenting with respiratory distress. A large pulmonary embolism can cause a decrease in $ETCO_2$ because of a lack of pulmonary perfusion, but most patients with severe respiratory distress are hypercapnic. Chronic obstructive lung disease and bronchospasm display a characteristic waveform with a slurred upstroke. The waveform shape may normalize with treatment of the underlying disease. Increasing $ETCO_2$ usually indicates worsening of respiratory distress, and decreasing $ETCO_2$ usually indicates improvement of respiratory distress. $ETCO_2$ values and waveform trends may help guide management decisions, such as endotracheal intubation or intensive care observation, in patients with respiratory distress from any etiology.

## EVIDENCE

- **What key points of pulse oximetry monitoring are particularly pertinent during emergency airway management?** Rapid change in arterial saturation is common during airway management. Although pulse oximetry is continuous, there is a delay in peripheral cutaneous oximetry relative to central $Sao_2$. Monitor averaging, probe location, circulatory and oxygenation status, and rate of desaturation all contribute to the degree of correlation. Sensor anatomical location is an easily modifiable factor: Forehead probes are closer to the heart and respond more quickly than distal extremity probes. Although most sensors lose reliability during hypotension, hypoperfusion, and hypothermia, forehead reflectance probes maintain reliability during these conditions in most patients.[1–3] As such, they are often preferred in the management of critically ill patients.[4,5]
- **Is there evidence for the use of capnography in emergency settings?** The 2015 AHA ACLS guidelines recommend the use of capnography for confirmation of correct ETT placement, monitoring CPR quality, and indicating ROSC. Continuous waveform capnography is recommended, in addition to clinical assessment, as the most reliable method of confirming and monitoring correct placement of an ETT.[6] If continuous waveform capnometry is not available, a nonwaveform $CO_2$ detector is a reasonable alternative.[6] Colorimetric detectors are less accurate for confirming correct ETT placement during cardiac arrest. However, colorimetric and nonwaveform capnometers are nearly 100% accurate for confirming correct ETT placement in patients with circulation.[7] AHA guidelines also recommend waveform capnography to optimize CPR performance.[6] ROSC is unlikely when $ETCO_2$ values are persistently less than 10 mm Hg in intubated patients receiving good quality CPR.[8] A sudden increase in $ETCO_2$ to normal values (>30 mm Hg) during CPR is an early indication of ROSC.[9] The use of waveform capnography during procedural sedation is well accepted and recommended as a standard for the safe practice of anesthesia worldwide.[10] Although it is not used in some emergency departments (EDs), there is good evidence that waveform capnography is the most sensitive early indicator of hypoventilation and apnea, and its use has been shown to decrease the incidence of hypoxia during ED procedural sedation.[11–14]

## REFERENCES

1. Chan ED, Chan MM, Chan MM. Pulse oximetry: understanding its basic principles facilitates appreciation of its limitations. *Respir Med*. 2013;107(6):789–799.
2. Jubran A. Pulse oximetry. *Crit Care*. 2015;19:272.
3. Schallom L, Sona C, McSweeney M, et al. Comparison of forehead and digit oximetry in surgical/trauma patients at risk for decreased peripheral perfusion. *Heart Lung*. 2007;36(3):188–194.
4. Branson RD, Mannheimer PD. Forehead oximetry in critically ill patients: the case for a new monitoring site. *Respir Care Clin N Am*. 2004;10(3):359–367, vi–vii.
5. Nesseler N, Frenel JV, Launey Y, et al. Pulse oximetry and high-dose vasopressors: a comparison between forehead reflectance and finger transmission sensors. *Intensive Care Med*. 2012;38(10):1718–1722.
6. Link MS, Berkow LC, Kudenchuk PJ, et al. Part 7: Adult Advanced Cardiovascular Life Support: 2015 American Heart Association Guidelines Update for cardiopulmonary resuscitation and emergency cardiovascular care. *Circulation*. 2015;132(18, suppl 2):S444–S464.
7. Ornato JP, Shipley JB, Racht EM, et al. Multicenter study of a portable, hand-size, colorimetric end-tidal carbon dioxide detection device. *Ann Emerg Med*. 1992;21(5):518–523.
8. Levine RL, Wayne MA, Miller CC. End-tidal carbon dioxide and outcome of out-of-hospital cardiac arrest. *N Engl J Med*. 1997;337(5):301–306.
9. Falk JL, Rackow EC, Weil MH. End-tidal carbon dioxide concentration during cardiopulmonary resuscitation. *N Engl J Med*. 1988;318(10):607–611.
10. Merry AF, Cooper JB, Soyannwo O, et al. International standards for a safe practice of anesthesia 2010. *Can J Anaesth*. 2010;57(11):1027–1034.
11. Deitch K, Miner J, Chudnofsky CR, et al. Does end tidal CO2 monitoring during emergency department procedural sedation and analgesia with propofol decrease the incidence of hypoxic events? A randomized, controlled trial. *Ann Emerg Med*. 2010;55(3):258–264.
12. Krauss B, Hess DR. Capnography for procedural sedation and analgesia in the emergency department. *Ann Emerg Med*. 2007;50(2):172–181.
13. Mohr NM, Wessman B. Continuous capnography should be used for every emergency department procedural sedation. *Ann Emerg Med*. 2013;61(6):697–698.
14. Waugh JB, Epps CA, Khodneva YA. Capnography enhances surveillance of respiratory events during procedural sedation: a meta-analysis. *J Clin Anesth*. 2011;23(3):189–196.

# Section III

# Basic Airway Management

Chapter 9

# Bag-Mask Ventilation

Steven C. Carleton, Robert F. Reardon, and Calvin A. Brown III

## INTRODUCTION

Bag-mask ventilation (BMV) is a foundational skill in airway management and a consideration in every airway intervention. Evaluation for potential difficulty in bagging is a fundamental component of every airway assessment. Effective BMV reduces both the urgency to intubate and the anxiety that accompanies challenging laryngoscopy and intubation, buying time as one works through potential solutions for a difficult or failed airway. The confident application of BMV is particularly critical when muscle relaxants are used to facilitate intubation; confidence with BMV should be considered a prerequisite to using paralytic agents. The ability to oxygenate and ventilate a patient with a bag and mask effectively eliminates the "can't oxygenate" portion of the can't intubate, can't oxygenate scenario (see Chapter 2), leaving three unsuccessful attempts at intubation, or a failed best attempt in the "forced to act" scenario, as the only pathways to a failed airway.

In spite of its importance, there is a paucity of literature that adequately describes effective BMV. Most health care providers mistakenly think that they are proficient at it, and it is given less attention in training for airway management than more glamorous, but less frequently applied, airway techniques. Nonetheless, BMV is among the most difficult airway skills to master, requiring a clear understanding of functional airway obstruction, familiarity with the required equipment, mechanical skill, teamwork, and an organized approach when initial efforts are suboptimal.

Successful BMV depends on three factors: (1) a patent airway, (2) an adequate mask seal, and (3) proper ventilation. A patent airway permits the delivery of appropriate tidal volumes with the least possible positive pressure. Basic methods for opening the airway include patient positioning, and the chin lift and jaw thrust maneuvers. Creating an adequate mask seal requires an understanding of the design features of the mask, the anatomy of the patient's face, and the interrelationship between the two. Proper ventilation involves delivering an appropriate volume at a rate and force that minimize gastric insufflation and the potential for breath stacking and barotrauma.

The specific type of bag used is critically important. Self-inflating bags are the most useful in the emergency situation because of their low cost, simplicity, and broad availability. Resuscitation bags vary in volume depending on their intended use, with adult bags typically having a volume of 1,500 mL, whereas those for children and infants have volumes of 500 and 250 mL, respectively. Bags that minimize dead space, incorporate unidirectional inspiratory and expiratory airflow valves, and have an oxygen reservoir are essential to optimize oxygenation during BMV (see Chapter 5). Bags with a pop-off pressure valve minimize the potential for barotrauma; most with this feature allow the valve to be manually disabled when high ventilation pressures are required.

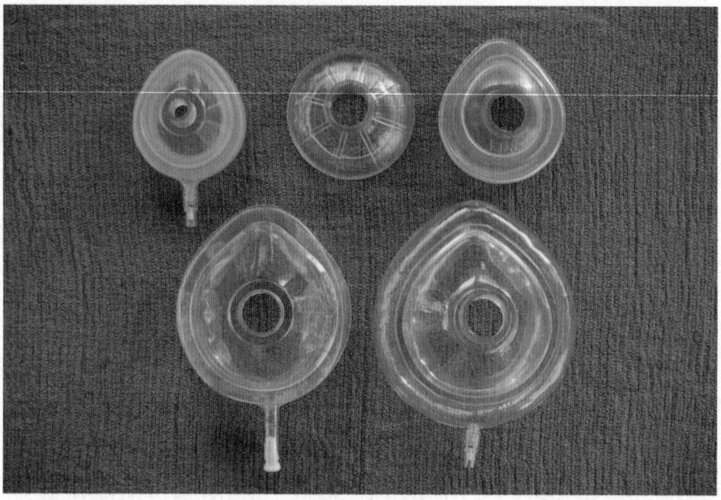

● **FIGURE 9-1.** Face masks of various types in sizes from infant to large adult.

Face masks for BMV in the emergency department and prehospital setting are usually disposable, plastic models. Three sizes (small, medium, and large) are sufficient to accommodate most adults and school-aged children. Choice of size is empiric. Smaller masks are available for use in toddlers, infants, and newborns. A selection of face masks is shown in **Figure 9-1**. Note that it is generally easier to establish an adequate mask seal if the mask is too large than if it is too small because the mask must cover both the mouth and nose. A typical mask consists of three components:

- A round orifice that fits over the standard 22-mm outside diameter connector on the bag assembly
- A hard shell or body; this is often clear, to allow continuous monitoring of the patient's mouth and nose for regurgitation
- A circumferential cushion or inflatable cuff to evenly distribute downward pressure onto the patient's face, filling irregular contours and promoting an effective seal

Although newer, ergonomically designed face masks may be more effective in reducing mask leaks than standard, disposable masks; such masks are not widely available and have yet to be evaluated in the emergency setting.

## OPENING THE AIRWAY

The airway should be opened *before* placing the mask on the face. Functional occlusion of the airway is common in supine, obtunded patients, particularly when neuromuscular blocking agents have been given. Occlusion results from posterior displacement of the tongue onto the posterior oropharynx wall as the genioglossus, geniohyoid, and hyoglossus muscles relax. Airway closure also may result from occlusion of the hypopharynx by the epiglottis, or by circumferential collapse of the hypopharynx when airway tone is lost. Airway collapse is exacerbated by flexion of the head on the neck and by widely opening the mouth. Maneuvers to open the airway are directed at counteracting these conditions by anterior distraction of the mandible and hyoid. The head tilt/chin lift is an initial maneuver that may be used in any patient in whom cervical spine injury is not a concern. In this technique, the clinician applies downward pressure to the patient's forehead with one hand while the index and middle fingers of the second hand lift the mandible at the chin, pulling the tongue from the posterior pharynx, and slightly extending the head on the neck. Airway caliber may be augmented by coupling atlanto-occipital extension with slight flexion of the lower cervical spine (i.e., the "sniffing position") similar to optimal positioning for direct laryngoscopy (see Chapter 13). Although chin lift may be sufficient

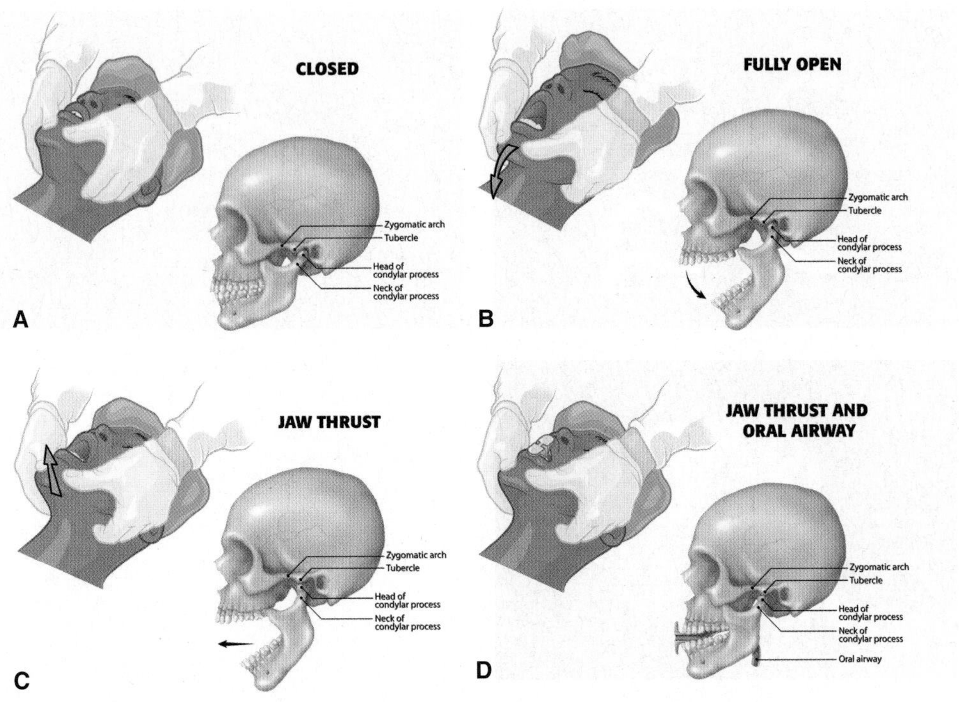


● **FIGURE 9-2.** Relieving upper airway obstruction by "creating an underbite" with the jaw thrust maneuver. This is the most important technique for opening and maintaining the airway. **A:** From the head of the bed, the closed mandible is grasped between the thumbs and fingers of both hands. **B:** The mandible is widely opened. **C:** The open mandible is displaced anteriorly out of the temporomandibular joint. **D:** The mandible is closed on the bite block of an OPA to maintain the jaw thrust with the lower teeth in front of the upper teeth.

in some patients, the jaw thrust maneuver is more effective in displacing the mandible, hyoid, and tongue anteriorly. The jaw thrust is achieved by forcibly and fully opening the mouth to translate the condyles of the mandible out of the temporomandibular joints, then pulling the mandible forward (**Fig. 9-2A–D**). This is most easily accomplished from the head of the bed, by placing the fingers of both hands on the body, angle, and ramus of the mandible with the thumbs on the mental processes. The forward position of the mandible can be maintained, and anterior traction on the hyoid and tongue can be increased, by closing the mandible on an oropharyngeal airway (OPA). It is useful to think of the jaw thrust maneuver as "creating an underbite" with the bottom incisors placed anterior to the upper incisors. The fingers maintain this position while the mask is applied to the face. The jaw thrust is the safest first approach to opening the airway of a patient with a potential cervical spine injury; if properly performed, it can be accomplished without moving the head or neck.

## ORAL AND NASAL PHARYNGEAL AIRWAYS

Once an open airway has been established, it must be maintained. OPAs and nasopharyngeal airways (NPAs) are necessary adjuncts in achieving this goal. Rescue bag-and-mask ventilation in a supine, unresponsive patient is ineffective without either an OPA or a NPA. Both prevent the tongue from falling back and occluding the airway and provide an open conduit for ventilation. OPAs are available in a variety of lengths, measured in centimeters (**Fig. 9-3A**). They are intended to extend from the central incisors to just short of the epiglottis and posterior pharyngeal wall. The appropriate size can be estimated by choosing an OPA that extends from the lips to just beyond the angle of the mandible when held alongside the face. Sizes from 8 to 10 cm suffice for the majority of adults. Two methods of

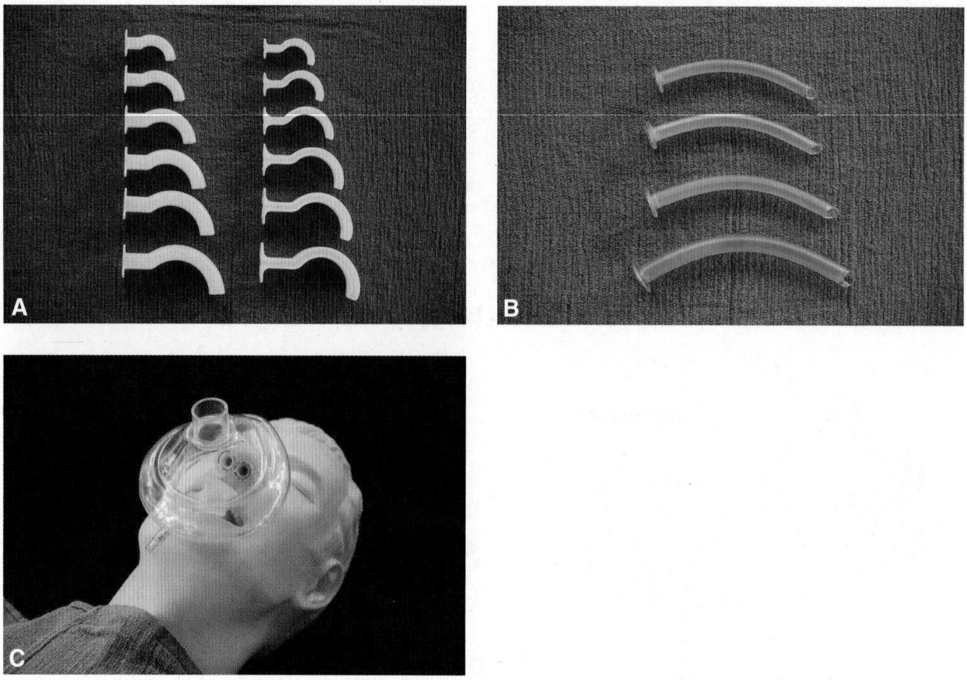

● **FIGURE 9-3. A:** Guedel **(left)** and Berman **(right)** OPAs. **B:** NPAs. **C:** OPA and two NPAs in place within the body of the mask to optimize airway maintenance.

insertion are in common use. In one, the OPA is inserted into the open mouth in an inverted position with its tip sliding along the palate. As the insertion is completed, the OPA is rotated 180° into its final position with the flange resting against the lips. This method is designed to minimize the likelihood of the OPA impinging the tongue and displacing it posteriorly. In the second method, the tongue is pulled forward manually, and the OPA is inserted with its curve paralleling that of the airway until the flange rests against the lips. The latter technique has less potential for causing trauma to oropharyngeal structures. NPAs are available in various sizes based on internal luminal diameter (**Fig. 9-3B**). Sizes from 6 to 8 mm accommodate most adult patients. The appropriate size is commonly stated as the diameter of the patient's small finger, or 0.5 to 1.0 mm smaller than the endotracheal tube size for the patient, but neither method of estimation has been validated. For the purpose of augmenting BMV while minimizing the potential for nasal trauma, the smallest effective tube should be used; generally, this is 6 mm in adult females and 7 mm in adult males. When time permits, the larger nostril should be chosen based on inspection and decongested with oxymetazoline or neosynephrine spray. Topical anesthetics such as 4% aqueous lidocaine or 2% lidocaine jelly also can be applied. A generously lubricated NPA is then inserted through the inferior nasal meatus parallel to the palate until the flange rests at the nostril. When introducing a NPA, the recommended position is with the point of the nasal trumpet away from the anterior nasal septum (bevel side facing medially) in order to reduce injury to Kiesselbach's plexus and reduce the risk of epistaxis. A slight rotatory motion during insertion may facilitate passage. If resistance is met, the tube should either be downsized, or insertion should be attempted through the contralateral nostril. An NPA should never be forced when resistance is encountered, because bleeding will inevitably result. Relative contraindications to NPA insertion should be observed, including bleeding diathesis and suspected basilar skull fracture.

OPAs generally facilitate airway maintenance more reliably than NPAs, but OPAs are tolerated poorly in patients with intact gag and cough reflexes. Use of an NPA, particularly when time permits topical anesthesia of the nose, may be tolerated in this circumstance. When airway patency during BMV is difficult to maintain with an OPA alone, it can be supplemented by one or two NPAs (**Fig. 9-3C**). The following cannot be stated strongly enough: an adjunctive airway should *always* be used to maintain airway patency when bagging a patient for his or her life.

## POSITIONING AND HOLDING THE MASK

Once the airway is opened, the mask is placed to obtain a seal on the face. This should be accomplished with the mask *detached* from the bag to permit optimal positioning free from the unbalanced weight and bulk of the complete assembly. The cuff on the mask is intended to seat on the bridge of the nose, the malar eminences of the maxillae, the maxillary and mandibular teeth, the anterior body of the mandible, and the groove between the chin and alveolar ridge of the mandible. This ensures that the mouth and nose will be covered entirely and that the cuff will be supported by bony structures. In general, the seal between the mask and face is least secure laterally over the cheeks. This is particularly true in edentulous patients where the unsupported soft tissue of the cheeks may incompletely contact the cuff. In this circumstance, adequate facial support for the cuff can be maintained by leaving dentures in place during BMV, or restored by packing gauze rolls into the cheeks. Medial compression of the soft tissue of the face against the outside margins of the cuff can also mitigate leakage. Shifting the mask such that the caudal edge of the cuff rests inside the lower lip may improve the seal between the mask and face in edentulous patients (**Fig. 9-4**).

Optimal placement of the mask is facilitated by grasping its body between the thumbs of both hands and then spreading the cuff with the fingers (**Fig. 9-5**). Initially, the nasal part of the mask is placed on the bridge of the nose, and the mask is adjusted superiorly or inferiorly to optimize coverage. The body of the mask is then lowered onto the patient's face, and the cuff is released once in firm contact with the skin. This effectively pulls the soft tissue of the face into the body of the

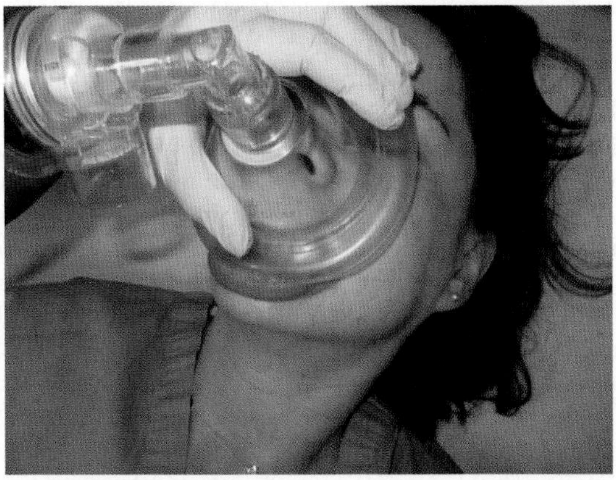

● **FIGURE 9-4.** Lower-lip positioning of the mask. This position may improve the mask seal in edentulous patients. (Photograph courtesy of Tobias D. Barker, MD.)

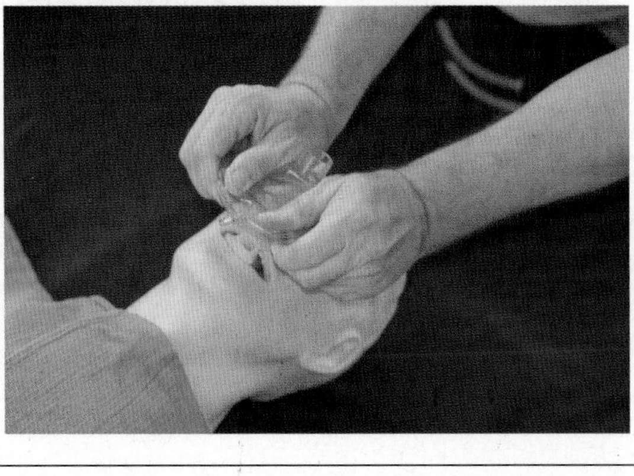

● **FIGURE 9-5.** Spreading the cuff of the mask before seating it on the face to improve the mask seal.

mask, improving the mask seal. In masks with inflatable cuffs, the cuff volume can be adjusted with a syringe to further augment the seal if leakage is encountered. Once the mask is in full contact with the face, the fingers can be released and used to pull the lower face upward into the mask as the grip on the mask is maintained with the thumbs. The bag is then attached, and ventilation is initiated. The tendency to rest the hands or the cuff on the orbits should be avoided during BMV. Compression of the eyes may cause injury or a vagal response.

With proper technique, the mask is not pushed down onto the patient's face during BMV. Rather, the patient's face is pulled upward into the mask. This has significant implications on the most effective method of holding the mask after the initial seal is obtained. As discussed in the following section, whenever possible, a two-handed and two-person technique employing a thenar mask grip should be used.

## Single-Handed Mask Hold

Securing the mask to the face using one hand may be necessary when personnel are limited, but this should be a very rare scenario. Single-handed BMV can be successful in selected, unchallenging patients, particularly when the operator's hands are large and strong enough to maintain a robust seal for extended periods of time. However, when it is difficult to achieve or maintain a good mask seal, two-person, two-handed technique is used. In the one-handed technique, the operator's dominant hand is used to hold and compress the bag, while the nondominant hand is placed on the mask with the thumb and the index finger partially encircling the mask connector, as if making an "OK" sign. This grip is also referred to as the "EC grip," because the third through fifth fingers form the letter "E" and the thumb and index finger form the letter "C" while grasping the mask. The grasping hand and mask are then rocked from side to side to achieve the best seal. The ring finger and little finger are typically used to pull the body of the mandible upward toward the mask (**Fig. 9-6A**) while the tip of the long finger is placed beneath the point of the chin to maintain the chin lift. When the operator's hands are of sufficient size, the pad of the little finger can be placed posterior to the angle of the mandible to augment chin lift with a degree of jaw thrust. Fingers grasping the mandible should contact only its bony margin to avoid pressure on the submandibular and submental soft tissues, which may occlude the airway. When holding the mask with one hand, it may be necessary to gather the cheek with the ulnar aspect of the grasping hand and compress it against the mask cuff to establish a more effective seal. One-handed bagging can be extremely fatiguing. A common tendency, especially during difficult bagging or with operator fatigue, is to deform the body of the mask by squeezing it between the thumb and index finger. This may create or worsen a mask leak.

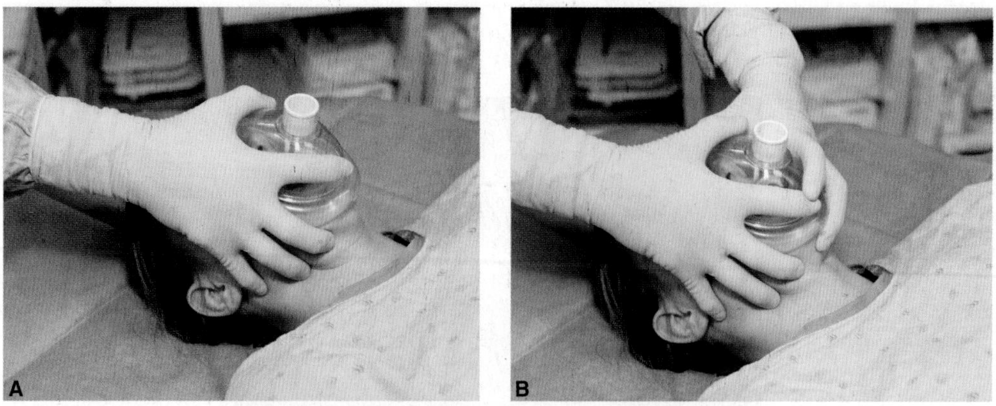


● **FIGURE 9-6. A:** Single-handed mask hold with the "OK" or "EC" grip. **B:** Two-handed mask hold with the conventional, double "OK" grip.

## Two-Handed Mask Hold

The two-handed mask hold is the most effective method of opening the airway while achieving and maintaining an adequate mask seal. It is the method of choice in the emergency situation, whenever two operators are available. The two-handed, two-person technique mandates that one operator's sole responsibility is to ensure proper placement of the mask, an effective mask seal, and a patent airway. Usually, the more experienced member should handle the mask. The other member provides bag ventilation.

The operator's hands may be placed on the mask in one of two ways. The traditional method involves placing the index fingers and thumbs of each hand on the body of the mask in an identical fashion to that of one-hand, "OK" mask grip (**Fig. 9-6B**). The tips of the remaining three fingers of each hand are used to capture the mandible and perform a chin lift and a partial jaw thrust, opening the airway, pulling the face upward into the mask, and creating a mask seal. This method provides a more effective seal than the one-handed technique but is still subject to hand fatigue if bagging is difficult or prolonged. In the second method, both thenar eminences are positioned on the body of the mask, parallel to one another, with the thumbs pointing caudally. The cuff of the mask is placed on the bridge of the nose, and the remainder of the mask is lowered onto the face (**Fig. 9-7A**). The index, long, ring, and small fingers of each hand grasp the body, angle, and ramus of the mandible and pull the mandible forward into the mask to produce a seal. The jaw thrust maneuver produced in this manner is much more effective than that produced with the conventional two-handed grip, and the mask seal is more robust than in either alternative technique described. Recent evidence has shown that the thenar grip results in fewer ventilation failures and larger ventilation volumes than other mask holds. In addition, the two-handed, thenar mask hold is also more comfortable and less tiring compared with the other methods. When extremely difficult BMV is encountered, a more aggressive version of the thenar grasp may be useful. Here, the operator stands on a stool, or has the bed lowered until the arms are straight, with the second to fifth fingers pointing straight toward the floor as the thenar grip on the mask is maintained. The fingers of each hand are shifted posteriorly to grasp the mandible by the angle and ramus to perform a more robust jaw thrust.

If clinical circumstances require that the operator perform BMV from a position facing the patient, the thenar mask grip, reversed so that the thumbs point cephalad, is the best method. This grip can also be applied successfully in seated patients (**Fig. 9-7B**). In circumstances where there is a lone rescuer and difficulty is encountered in obtaining a mask seal, the care provider can free both hands for the two-hand, thenar mask grip and still provide ventilation by compressing the bag

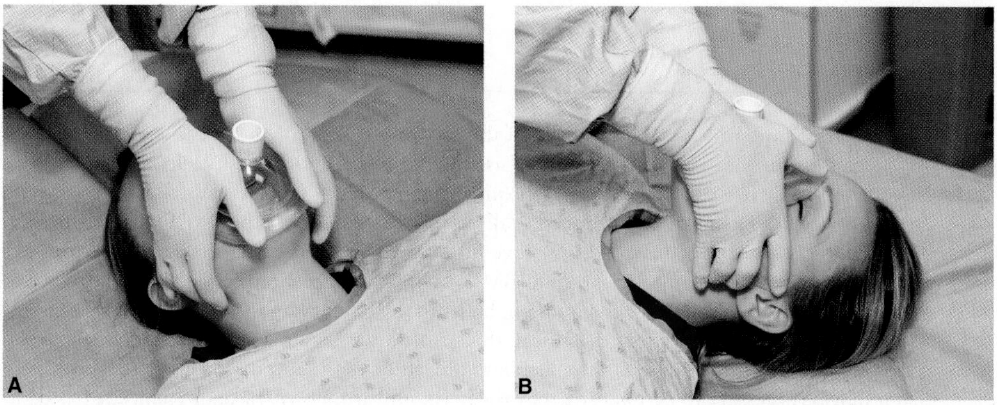


● **FIGURE 9-7. A:** Two-handed, thenar mask grip. This grip provides a superior face seal, better airway maintenance, and is less fatiguing than the alternative methods. **B:** The two-handed, thenar mask grip applied from the side in a semi-seated patient.

between their elbow and lateral torso if standing, or between their knees if kneeling on the floor. When the prospective assessment for difficult bagging is highly unfavorable, or a single rescuer anticipates insurmountable difficulty performing one-person technique, consideration should be given to bypassing BMV in favor of placing an extraglottic device as the initial means of ventilation (see Chapters 10 and 11).

## VENTILATING THE PATIENT

Once the airway is opened and an optimal mask seal is obtained, the bag is connected to the mask, and ventilation is initiated. The entire volume of the self-inflating resuscitation bag cannot, and should not, be delivered. Overzealous volume delivery may exceed the opening pressures of the upper and lower esophageal sphincters (approximately 20 to 25 cm $H_2O$ pressure), insufflating gas into the stomach and increasing the risks of regurgitation and aspiration. It also may result in breath stacking leading to pulmonary barotrauma, and loss of functional residual capacity as the abdomen distends and compresses the diaphragms. The goal for effective oxygenation and ventilation without excessive inspiratory pressure is to deliver 10 to 12 reduced tidal volume breaths (5 to 7 mL per kg; approximately 500 mL in an average adult) per minute over 1 to 2 seconds each. Factors that increase peak inspiratory pressures include shorter inspiratory times, larger tidal volumes, incomplete airway opening, increased airway resistance, and decreased lung or chest compliance. Several of these factors are controllable, and attention should be paid by the clinician to maintenance of airway patency, delivery of inspiration over a 1- to 2-second period, and limiting tidal volume to that sufficient to produce visible chest rise.

## SELLICK MANEUVER

During BMV, studies demonstrate that application of Sellick maneuver (see Chapter 20) may reduce gastric insufflation. If resources permit, we recommend applying Sellick maneuver during bag ventilation of an unresponsive patient. Sellick maneuver involves pressing the cricoid cartilage posteriorly, attempting to occlude the cervical esophagus against the anterior vertebral bodies. Two errors are commonly committed. The first is to apply pressure to the thyroid cartilage instead of the cricoid cartilage, failing to compress the esophagus and potentially occluding the airway. The second is to press too hard resulting in distortion of the airway and more difficult ventilation.

## SUMMARY

BMV is a dynamic process. The patency of the airway, position of the mask, and adequacy of gas exchange must be assessed continually. Listening and feeling for mask leaks, monitoring the compliance of the bag during delivery of breaths, and observing the rise and fall of the chest are crucial to success. The most important role falls to the person holding the mask, but coordination of the efforts of this individual, the person ventilating with the bag, and the person performing Sellick maneuver are essential to optimal BMV. Two-handed technique with the thenar mask grip is the preferred method for maintaining both airway patency and the mask seal. In addition to optimizing the jaw thrust and mask seal, this grip allows a lateral mask leak to be felt by the provider's hands. Compression of the cheek into the lateral mask cuff may occlude the leak. Note that it may be necessary to periodically rock the mask upward, downward, or from side to side to reacquire the best seal. It also may be necessary to reapply the jaw thrust maneuver to reestablish airway patency because of the tendency of the mandible to fall back into the temporomandibular joints. When delivering tidal volumes with the bag, the operator should simultaneously feel for the resistance of the bag to compression, and observe the patient's chest for rise and fall during ventilation. This feedback can provide clues about the patient's lung and chest wall compliance and can influence bagging technique in response. Other important signs of satisfactory ventilation are maintenance of adequate oxygen saturation and the appearance of an appropriate waveform on end-tidal $CO_2$ capnography.

Occasionally after a breath is delivered, passive expiration fails to occur. This generally indicates closure of the airway because of an inadequate jaw thrust. Removal of the mask from the face and reapplication of a vigorous jaw thrust will generally relieve the blockage and permit expiration.

Whenever BMV fails to establish or maintain adequate oxygen saturation, the bag-and-mask technique must be adjusted to compensate. Simply stated, when bagging fails, bag better. Bagging better requires a systematic reappraisal of the adequacy of airway opening, the mask seal, and the mechanics of ventilation with the bag. If a single-handed mask hold is being used by a lone provider, the mask grip should immediately shift to two-handed thenar technique, and the bag should be compressed by one of the alternative methods described earlier. If two providers are available, two-person, two-handed thenar technique should be used, and the providers should focus on the following questions:

1. Does the jaw thrust maneuver need to be redone to more effectively open the airway? Optimal jaw thrust is facilitated by positioning the person holding the mask at the head of the bead, with the bed at a height that allows the provider to shift the fingers posteriorly to grasp the angle and ramus of the mandible, and comfortably maintain the upward pull required to open the airway. Jaw thrust is easier when performed by an individual with large hands; if an experienced operator with large hands is available, they must be recruited for this task.
2. Is the mask seal optimal? If not, the seal may be improved by applying an occlusive plastic membrane to a beard, by reinserting dentures or packing fluffed gauze inside the cheeks of an edentulous patient, by gathering and compressing both cheeks inside the body of the mask, by ensuring that the entire mouth and nose are within the body of the mask, by rocking the mask to reestablish cuff contact with the face, or by considering lower-lip mask positioning in the edentulous patient. Positioning a morbidly obese patient in a semi-seated position during BMV may improve pulmonary dynamics and ease difficult bagging. This may require the person holding the mask to use a stool or to move to a position facing the patient, and adjust their mask grip accordingly.
3. Are airway adjuncts being used? A common error in BMV is failure to use OPAs and NPAs. A minimum of one of these adjuncts should *always* be used during BMV of an unresponsive patient. An OPA and two NPAs should be used in cases where persistent difficulty is encountered in delivering adequate ventilation and oxygenation.
4. Does a more experienced person need to be recruited to optimize efforts at BMV? The learning curve for proficiency with BMV is long. Novice providers may fail to achieve the most effective possible ventilation and should be replaced by the most experienced available operator when difficult bagging fails to respond to simple countermeasures.

## EVIDENCE

- **What is the best method for maintaining a mask seal during BMV?** Simulation studies suggest that two-handed mask techniques facilitate delivery of greater tidal volumes and peak airway pressures than the one-handed technique in both child and adult manikin models.[1,2] The traditional two-handed and two-handed thenar mask grips yielded similar results in the adult study, but fatigue with prolonged bagging was not evaluated. A clinical trial comparing the two-handed grip where the mask was grasped with the thumbs and standard one-handed technique clearly document the superiority of the two-handed thenar grip in delivering greater tidal volumes in apneic patients.[3] In another trial, the thenar grip was also found to be more effective than the two-handed "E-C grip" when performed by novice practitioners.[4] Mask seal in edentulous patients may be improved by modifying placement of the caudal margin of the mask cuff to a position inside of the lower lip, bearing on the alveolar ridge.[5] Further, in edentulous patients with dentures, ventilation and gas flow during BMV are facilitated by leaving the dentures in place during bagging.[6] Newer, ergonomically designed masks improve the mask seal with the face in comparison to standard, disposable masks with inflatable cuffs during simulated BMV.[7]

- **What is the optimal technique to ventilate the patient during BMV?** The primary goal is oxygenation without gastric inflation. This is best accomplished by avoiding high airway pressures during BMV (e.g., longer inspiratory times, smaller tidal volume, and optimal airway opening).[8,9] The recommended adult tidal volume of approximately 500 mL is best achieved by squeezing the bag with the hands, rather than compressing it between the arm and torso.[10]
- **Should Sellick maneuver be performed during BMV?** If the necessary personnel are available, it may be helpful to use this technique during prolonged BMV. Proper application of cricoid pressure does appear to reduce the volume of air entering the stomach when BMV is performed with low to moderate inspiratory pressures.[11] Other cross-sectional radiology studies indicate that this technique may not reliably occlude the esophagus or may impair ventilation by partially obstructing the airway.[12,13] Furthermore, there is evidence to suggest that Sellick maneuver may either improve or worsen laryngoscopic view of the glottis.[14–16]
- **How easily can competence in BMV be achieved?** An evaluation of the number of repetitions required for novice physicians to achieve a success rate of 80% for BMV found that 25 training runs were necessary.[17] It should be noted that an 80% success rate is an insufficiently rigorous goal for a frequently applied, life-sustaining procedure, highlighting the necessity for frequent, scrupulous training in BMV.

## REFERENCES

1. Davidovic L, LaCovey D, Pitetti RD. Comparison of 1—versus 2-person bag-valve-mask techniques for manikin ventilation of infants and children. *Ann Emerg Med*. 2005;46:37–42.
2. Reardon R, Ward C, Hart D, et al. Assessment of face-mask ventilation using an airway simulation model. *Ann Emerg Med*. 2008;52(4):S114.
3. Joffe AM, Hetzel S, Liew EC. A two-handed jaw-thrust technique is superior to the one-handed "EC-clamp" technique for mask ventilation in the apneic, unconscious person. *Anesthesiology*. 2010;113:873–875.
4. Gerstein NS, Carey MC, Braude DA, et al. Efficacy of facemask ventilation techniques in novice providers. *J Clin Anesth*. 2013;24:193–197.
5. Racine SX, Solis A, Hamou NA, et al. Face mask ventilation in edentulous patients. A comparison of mandibular groove and lower lip placement. *Anesthesiology*. 2010;112:1190–1193.
6. Conlon NP, Sullivan RP, Herbison PG, et al. The effect of leaving dentures in place on bag-mask ventilation at induction of general anesthesia. *Anesth Analg*. 2007;105:370–373.
7. Bauman EB, Joffe AM, Lenz L, et al. An evaluation of bag-valve-mask ventilation using an ergonomically designed facemask among novice users: a simulation-based pilot study. *Resuscitation*. 2010;81:1161–1165.
8. American Heart Association. 2005 American Heart Association guidelines for cardiopulmonary resuscitation and emergency cardiovascular care. *Circulation*. 2005;112(suppl I):IV1–IV203.
9. Uzun L, Ugur MB, Altunkaya H, et al. Effectiveness of the jaw-thrust maneuver in opening the airway: a flexible fiberoptic endoscopic study. *ORL J Otorhinolaryngol Relat Spec*. 2005;67:39–44.
10. Wolcke B, Schneider T, Mauer D, et al. Ventilation volumes with different self-inflating bags with reference to the ERC guidelines for airway management: comparison of two compression techniques. *Resuscitation*. 2000;47:175–178.
11. Petito SP, Russell WJ. The prevention of gastric inflation—a neglected benefit of cricoid pressure. *Anaesth Intensive Care*. 1988;16:139.

12. Smith KJ, Dobranowski JD, Yip G, et al. Cricoid pressure displaces the esophagus: an observational study using magnetic resonance imaging. *Anesthesiology*. 2003;99:60–64.

13. Hartsilver EL, Vanner RG. Airway obstruction with cricoid pressure. *Anaesthesia*. 2000;55:208–211.

14. Levitan RM, Kinkle WC, Levin WJ, et al. Laryngeal view during laryngoscopy: a randomized trial comparing cricoid pressure, backward-upward-rightward pressure, and bimanual laryngoscopy. *Ann Emerg Med*. 2006;47:548–555.

15. Snider DD, Clarke D, Finucane BT. The "BURP" maneuver worsens the glottic view when applied in combination with cricoid pressure. *Can J Anaesth*. 2005;52:100–104.

16. Harris J, Ellis DY, Foster L. Cricoid pressure and laryngeal manipulation in 402 pre-hospital emergency anaesthetics: essential safety measure or a hindrance to rapid safe intubation? *Resuscitation*. 2010;81:810–816.

17. Komatsu R, Kayasu Y, Yogo H, et al. Learning curves for bag-and-mask ventilation and orotracheal intubation: an application of the cumulative sum method. *Anesthesiology*. 2010;112:1525–1531.

# Chapter 10

# Extraglottic Devices: Supraglottic Type

Michael F. Murphy and Jennifer L. Avegno

## INTRODUCTION AND TERMINOLOGY

The terminology related to airway management devices that are inserted into the hypopharynx and upper esophagus is not standardized. We will employ the term *extraglottic devices* (EGDs) to refer to this collection of devices. Those that sit on top of the larynx are *supraglottic* devices (SGDs), and those that are blindly inserted into the upper esophagus are *retroglottic* devices (RGDs). This latter group might also be referred to as an infraglottic devices (IGDs). RGDs such as the Combitube, King LT airway, and EasyTube are covered in the following chapter. Most EGDs are single-use, but some are available in reusable variants.

EGDs differ from face mask gas delivery apparatus in that they are inserted through the mouth to a position where they provide a direct conduit for air to flow through the glottis and into the lungs. They vary in size and shape, and most have balloons or cuffs that, when inflated, provide a reasonably tight seal in the upper airway to permit positive-pressure ventilation with variable limits of peak airway pressure. This chapter deals with SGDs such as the LMA family of devices, Cook ILA and Air Q, Ambu Aura family, and the i-gel.

The SGD Class is further divided into first generation (no gastric drainage lumen) and second generation (possessing a gastric drainage tube).

## INDICATIONS FOR USE

Although bag-mask ventilation (BMV) is relatively simple in concept, it is difficult or impossible to perform in selected patients (see Chapter 9), even in the hands of experts. Use of an EGD is a more easily acquired skill than BMV for the nonexpert airway practitioner. Similarly, tracheal intubation is the "gold standard" for effective ventilation and airway protection from aspiration, but the skill is not easily mastered or maintained. EGDs are a viable alternative to tracheal intubation in many emergency settings, particularly in prehospital care.

Finally, airway management difficulty and failure are associated with significant morbidity and mortality. EGDs have a potential role in managing or rescuing both the difficult and failed airway (see Chapters 2 and 3).

The indications for these devices have expanded over the past three decades and include potential for use as:

- An airway rescue device when BMV is difficult and intubation has failed;
- A "single attempt" rescue device performed simultaneously with preparation for cricothyrotomy in the "*can't* intubate, *can't* oxygenate" (CICO) failed airway (see Chapter 3);
- An easier and more effective alternative to BMV in the hands of basic life support providers or nonmedical rescue personnel;
- An alternative to endotracheal intubation by advanced life support providers;
- An alternative to endotracheal intubation for elective airway management in the operating room (OR) for appropriately selected patients; and
- A conduit to facilitate endotracheal intubation (certain types of intubating SGDs).

## SUPRAGLOTTIC DEVICES

The Laryngeal Mask Company developed the original SGD, the LMA Classic (**Fig. 10-1**), which serves as the prototype for much of the supraglottic class, although other designs exist. The company also makes several other versions of the LMA, including both reusable and nonreusable (disposable) devices as follows:

- LMA Unique (disposable variant of the LMA Classic)
- LMA Flexible (reinforced tube variant of the LMA Classic)
- LMA ProSeal (reusable) (**Fig. 10-2**)
- LMA Supreme (disposable) (**Fig. 10-3**)
- Fastrach or intubating LMA (ILMA) (reusable and disposable) (**Fig. 10-4**)

Other companies also make SGDs, both LMA type and non-LMA type, including

- A variety of disposable LMA Classic type designs (e.g., Portex and Solus);
- Ambu LMA (ALMA) family of devices (AuraOnce, Aura Straight, Aura-i; disposable and reusable) (**Fig. 10-5**);
- Cookgas ILA (reusable) and Air Q (disposable) (**Fig. 10-6A** and **B**); and
- i-gel (**Fig. 10-7**).

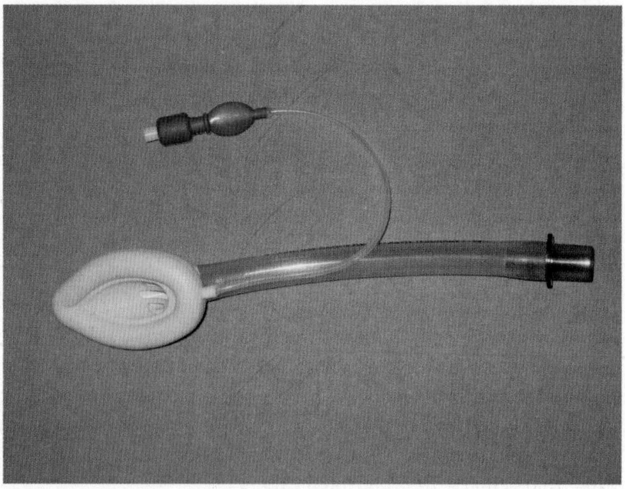

● **FIGURE 10-1. LMA Classic.** Note the aperture bars at the end of the plastic tube intended to limit the ability of the epiglottis to herniate into this opening.

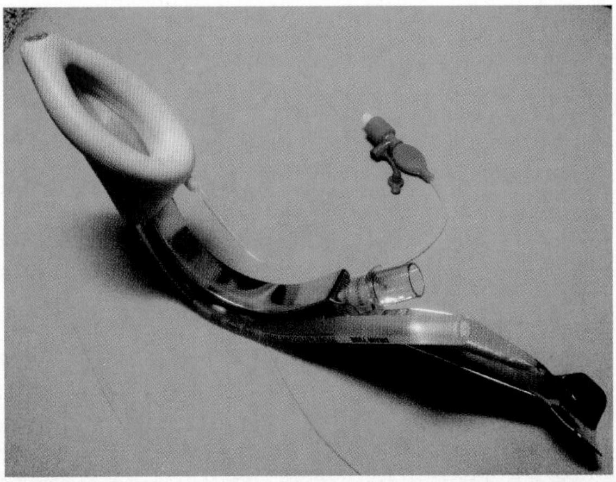

● **FIGURE 10-2. LMA ProSeal.** Note the drain tube and distal orifice to permit gastric tube passage and drainage.

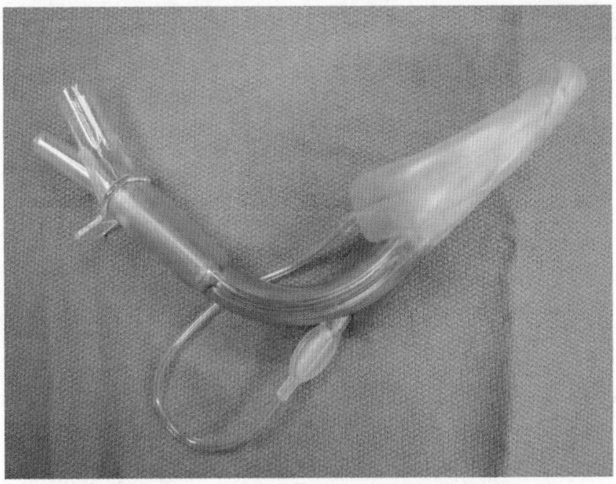

● **FIGURE 10-3. LMA Supreme.** The rigid construction of the tube and the curvature of the device enhance insertion characteristics and the immediacy of the seal obtained once inflated.

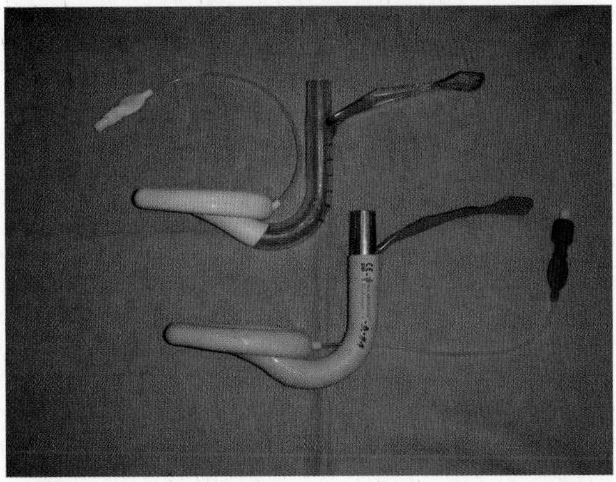

● **FIGURE 10-4. LMA Fastrach or ILMA.** Both the reusable **(bottom)** and disposable **(top)** variants are pictured. The most unique feature of this device that confers a particular advantage is the handle to permit positioning in the hypopharynx to improve airway seal and the capacity for adequate gas exchange. This factor may be crucial in rescuing a failed airway.

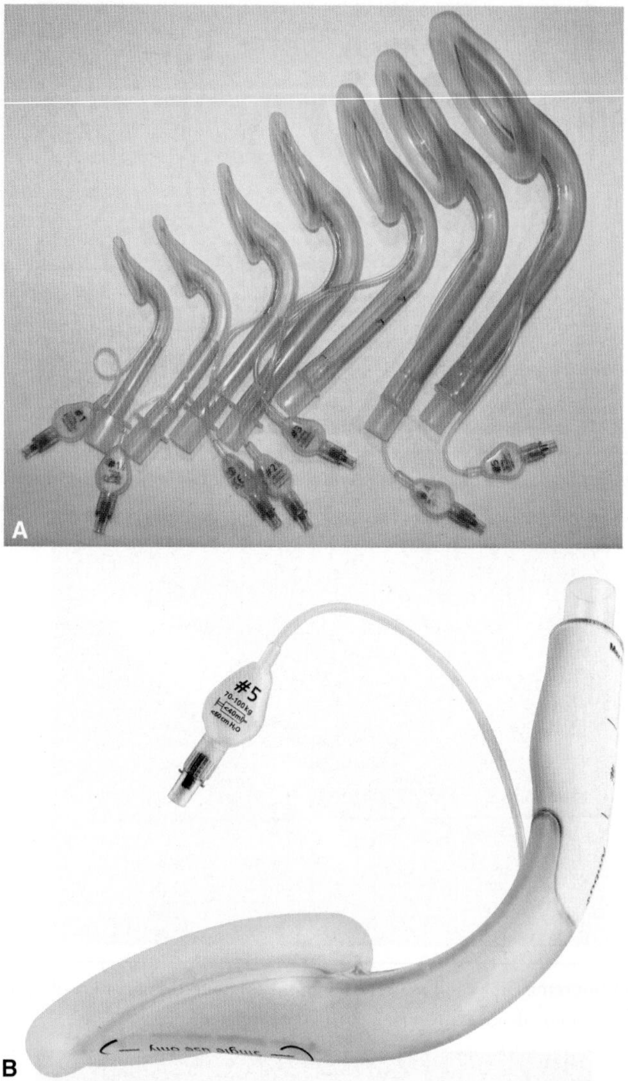


● **FIGURE 10-5.** **A:** Range of sizes of the Ambu AuraOnce LMA. **B:** Ambu Aura-i LMA, specifically designed to be used with the Ambu A Scope for endoscopic intubation.

The LMA Company (now owned by Teleflex) has recently introduced two new single-use devices that have novel features: The LMA Protector (**Fig. 10-8**) is a second-generation silicone single-use device that is available with both a gastric drainage tube and a vent (second-generation SGA) that incorporates Cuff Pilot technology, a pilot balloon pressure indicator. The device bears similarity to the LMA Supreme, but is easier to intubate through. It is also similar in feel and shape to the Fastrach LMA, although it lacks the handle and endotracheal tube ramp.

The single-use Unique EVO (**Fig. 10-9**) is a successor to the LMA Unique, with a couple of design modifications: a more robust cuff design meant to produce better seal characteristics and Cuff Pilot technology.

These devices are easy to use, generally well tolerated, produce little in the way of adverse hemodynamic responses on insertion, and play a significant role in rescue emergency airway management. Ventilation success rates near 100% have been reported in OR series, although patients with difficult

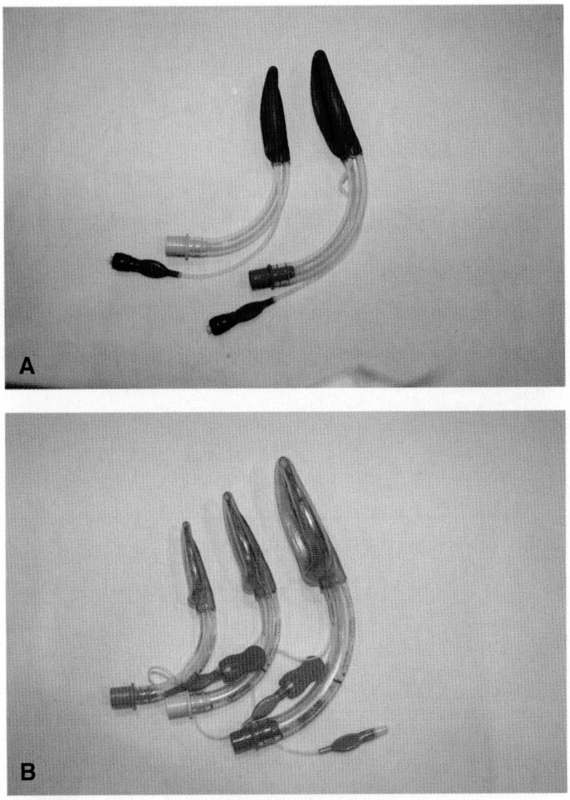


● **FIGURE 10-6. A:** The reusable Cookgas ILA. **B:** The disposable Air Q variant.

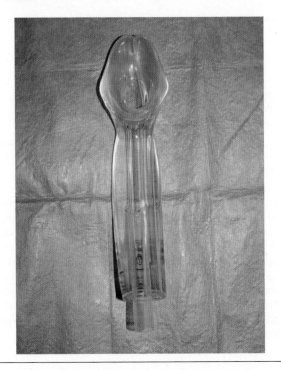

● **FIGURE 10-7. The i-gel Device**. Note the esophageal drainage tube.

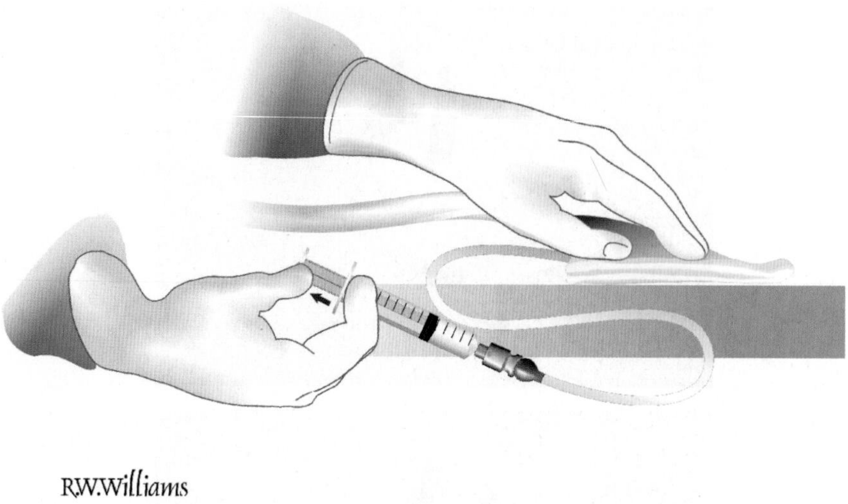


● **FIGURE 10-8.** Correct method of deflating the LMA Cuff.

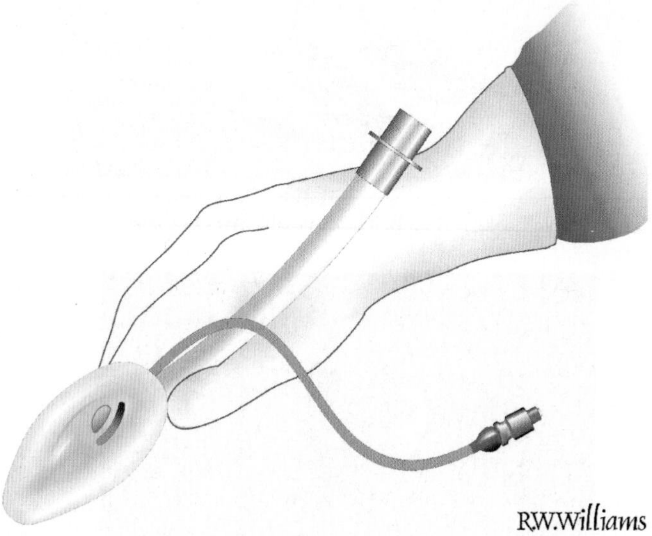


● **FIGURE 10-9.** Correct position of the fingers for LMA Insertion.

airways were excluded. It is likely that emergency airway ventilation success rates are somewhat lower. Intubation success rates through the ILMA are as high as 95% after three attempts, comparable to success rates with flexible endoscopic intubation and significantly better than through the standard LMA (See evidence section). However, an LMA does not constitute *definitive airway management*, defined as a protected airway (i.e., a cuffed endotracheal tube [ETT] in the trachea). Although they do not reliably prevent the gastric insufflation or the regurgitation and aspiration of gastric contents, LMAs confer some protection of the airway from aspiration of blood and saliva from the mouth and pharynx.

Maximal success is only achievable when the patient has effective topical airway anesthesia (see Chapter 23) or is significantly obtunded (e.g., by rapid sequence intubation medications) to tolerate insertion of these devices.

## LARYNGEAL MASK COMPANY DEVICES

### Standard, Non-ILMAs

The original LMA, now called the LMA Classic, was introduced into clinical practice in 1981 and looks like an ETT equipped with an inflatable, elliptical, silicone rubber collar (laryngeal mask) at the distal end (**Fig. 10-1**). The laryngeal mask component is designed to surround and cover the supraglottic area, providing upper airway continuity. Two rubber bars cross the tube opening at the mask end to prevent herniation of the epiglottis into the tube portion of the LMA.

The LMA Classic is a multiuse (reusable) device. The disposable and much less expensive variety of this device is called the LMA Unique. A similar product, the LMA Flexible, incorporates wire reinforcement in the tube portion of the device to prevent kinking as the tube warms. We do not recommend the LMA Flexible for management of the emergency airway.

The reusable LMA ProSeal incorporates an additional lumen through which one can pass a suction catheter into the esophagus or stomach. In addition to the standard perilaryngeal cuff, it also has a "directional sealing cuff" dorsally. This design modification results in higher sealing pressure capacity than the LMA Classic (28 vs. 24 cm $H_2O$), theoretically conferring an advantage for ventilating patients requiring higher airway pressures, although the difference may not be clinically significant. Because of its expense, relative difficulty with insertion characteristics, and marginal benefit in the emergency situation, the LMA ProSeal does not currently have a place in emergency airway management.

A disposable device similar to the LMA Classic called the LMA Supreme has compelling design characteristics that may make it a good rescue device for emergency airway management. It is easy to insert, seals readily, has higher leak pressures than do earlier LMA iterations, has a built-in bite block, and contains a channel through which a gastric tube can be passed. This device can be considered as a replacement for BMV in the hands of nonexpert airway managers or when rescue BMV is expected to be prolonged. It is the preferred device for emergency airway management if a nonintubating style of LMA is desired.

### Intubating LMAs

The LMA Fastrach, also called the ILMA, is the most important version of the LMA for emergency airway management because it combines the high insertion and ventilation success rate of the other LMAs with specially designed features to facilitate blind intubation. It has an epiglottic elevating bar and a rigid guide channel that directs an ETT in a superior direction into the larynx, enhancing the success rate when passed blindly. The LMA Fastrach device is a substantial advancement in airway management, particularly as a rapidly inserted rescue device in the CICO situation while preparations for cricothyrotomy are underway. It is supplied in both reusable and disposable forms.

### Indications and Contraindications

The LMA and LMA Fastrach have two principal roles in rescue emergency airway management: (1) as a rescue device in a "*can't* intubate, *can* oxygenate" situation, and (2) as a single attempt to effect gas exchange in the CICO failed airway as one concurrently prepares to perform a cricothyrotomy (see Chapter 3). The success rate of LMA-facilitated ventilation in the difficult airway may be eroded if multiple preceding intubation attempts have traumatized the upper airway.

The handle of the LMA Fastrach enhances its insertion characteristics and allows for manipulation to achieve optimum seal once the cuff is inflated. The LMA Fastrach can be used as a rescue device for a CICO airway when upper airway anatomy is believed to be normal, thus allowing for a proper "seat." LMAs have been used successfully in pediatrics, by novice intubators, during cardiopulmonary resuscitation (CPR), and in emergency medical services (EMS).

## Technique: LMA Classic, LMA Unique, and LMA Supreme

The LMA Classic, Unique, and Supreme can all be rapidly inserted as primary airway management devices, but most often will be used in emergency airway management to rescue a failed airway. First, the appropriate size of LMA should be selected based on patient characteristics. The LMA Classic and Unique come in sizes 1 to 6 (ranging from neonates < 5 kg to adults > 100 kg); the Supreme sizes range from 1 to 5. For adults, the simplest sizing formula is weight-based, regardless of patient size: size 3, 30 to 50 kg; size 4, 50 to 70 kg; and size 5, >70 kg. For patients on the borderline between one mask size and another, it is generally advisable to select the larger mask because it provides a better seal.

1. Place the device such that the collar is on a flat surface, and then inflate; then deflate the mask by aspirating the pilot balloon (**Fig. 10-8**). Completely deflate the cuff and ensure that it is not folded. Inflating the mask and then deflating it while pressing the ventral surface of the inflatable collar firmly against a flat surface produces a smoother and "flipped-back" leading edge, enhancing insertion characteristics. The collar is designed to flip backward so that the epiglottis is not trapped between the collar and the glottic opening and to minimize "tip roll." Curling of the mask tip can also be mitigated by adding 5 mL of air into the cuff, creating enough "body" within the mask to prevent this phenomenon. Lubricate both sides of the LMA with water-soluble lubricant to facilitate insertion.
2. Open the airway by using a head tilt as one would in basic airway management, if possible. Some, including the device inventor, recommend that a jaw lift be performed with the nondevice insertion hand to aid insertion.
3. Insert the LMA into the mouth with the laryngeal surface directed caudally and the tip of your index or long finger resting against the cuff-tube junction (**Fig. 10-9**). Press the device onto the hard palate (**Fig. 10-10**), and advance it over the back of the tongue as far as the length of your index or long finger will allow (**Fig. 10-11**). Then use your other hand to push the device to its final seated position (**Fig. 10-12**), allowing the natural curve of the device to follow the natural curve of the oro- and hypopharynx to facilitate its falling into position over the larynx. The dimensions and design of the device allow it to wedge into the esophagus with gentle caudad pressure and to stop in the appropriate position over the larynx.
4. Inflate the collar with air—20 mL, no. 3; 30 mL, no. 4; and 40 mL, no. 5—or until there is no leak with bag ventilation (**Fig. 10-13**). If a leak persists, ensure that the tube of the LMA emerges from the mouth in the midline, ensure that the head and neck are in anatomical alignment (i.e., neither flexed nor extended), withdraw the device approximately 6 cm with the cuff inflated, readvance it (the "up–down" maneuver, intended to free a folded or trapped epiglottis), reinsert the device, or go to the next larger size.

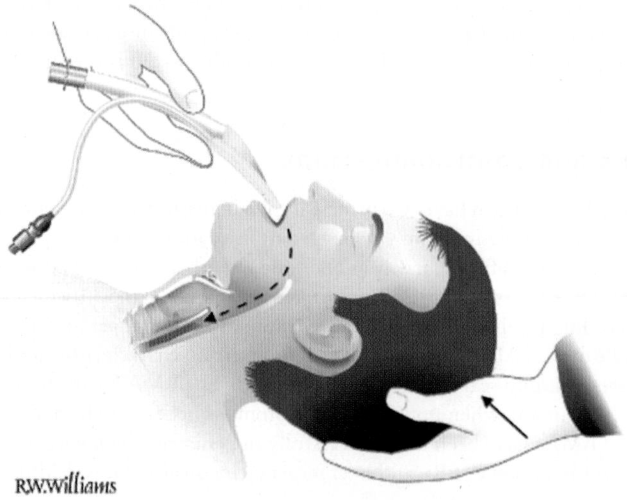


● **FIGURE 10-10.** Starting insertion position for the LMA Classic and LMA Unique.

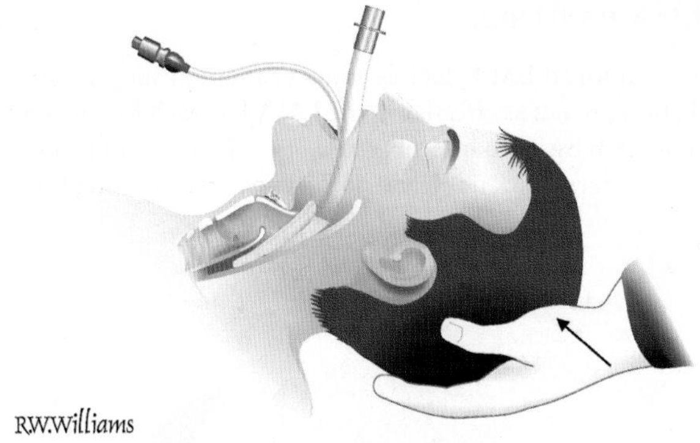


● **FIGURE 10-11.** Insert the LMA to the limit of your finger length.

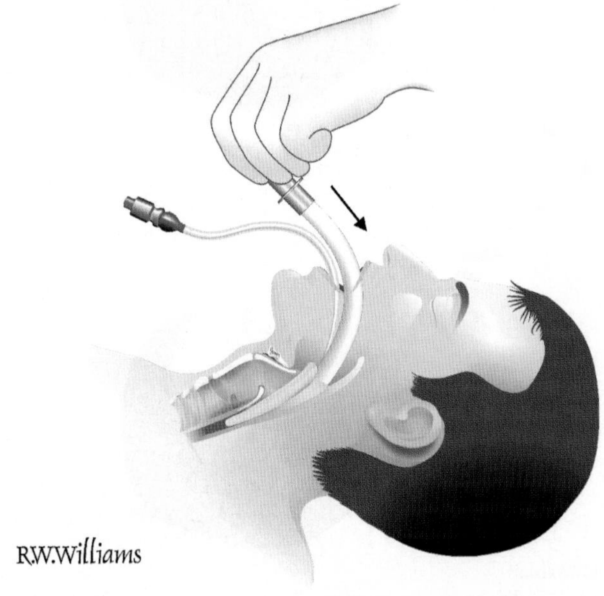


● **FIGURE 10-12.** Complete the insertion by pushing the LMA in the remainder of the way with your other hand.

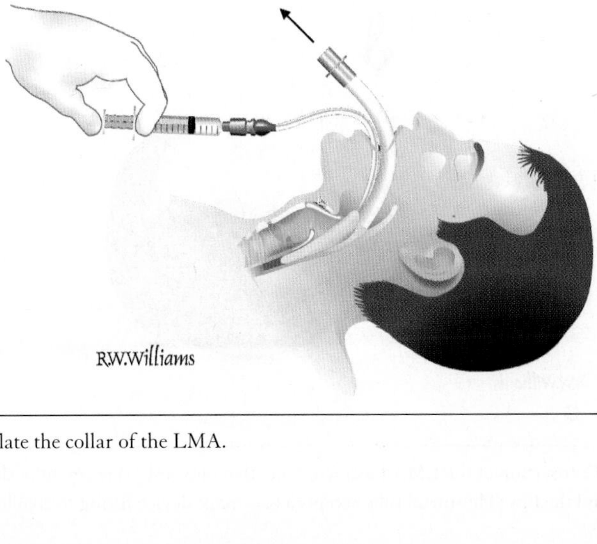


● **FIGURE 10-13.** Inflate the collar of the LMA.

## Technique: LMA Fastrach

Although the aforementioned LMA devices enjoy ventilation success rates comparable to that of the LMA Fastrach, they are not as effective as the LMA Fastrach for facilitating intubation. In fact, the LMA Fastrach is often easier to insert because of the handle and metal tube design. The LMA Fastrach comes in three sizes: no. 3, no. 4, and no. 5, with corresponding ETT sizes of 6.0 to 8.0. The

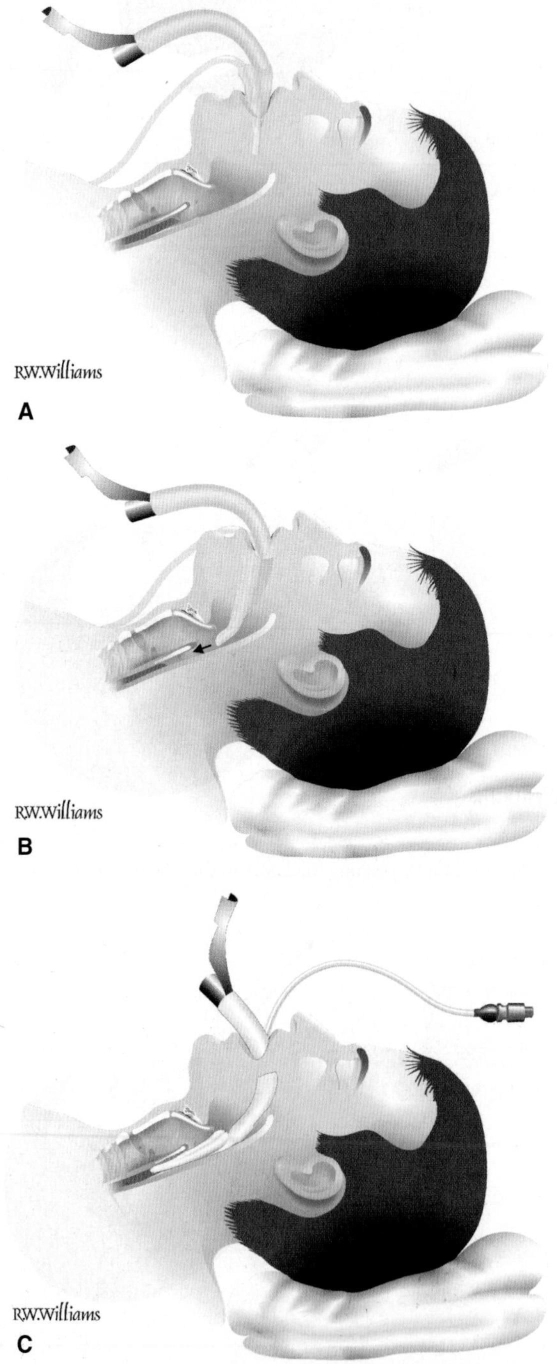


● **FIGURE 10-14.** A–C: Insertion of the LMA Fastrach. Note that only a short segment of the tubular portion of the device extends beyond the lips. This metal tube accepts a bag-mask device fitting to enable BMV.

no. 3 will fit a normal-size 10- to 12-year-old child and small adults, and sizing is as recommended earlier. There are no neonatal, infant, or toddler ILMA sizes.

The intention is to rescue a patent airway initially and recover the oxygen saturations by ventilating through the LMA Fastrach device. Once the saturations are adequate, the operator intubates through the device using the manufacturer-supplied silicone-tipped ETT (although conventional ETTs can be used as well). Intubation can be done blindly or by using a flexible endoscope.

1. Select the appropriate-sized LMA Fastrach. Deflate the cuff of the mask (**Fig. 10-8**), and apply a water-soluble lubricant to the anterior and posterior surfaces and the greater curvature of the bend of the rigid "stem." Hold the device in the dominant hand by the metal handle, and open the airway. Insert the collar in the mouth, ensuring that the curved tube portion of the device is in contact with the chin and the mask tip is flat against the palate before rotation (**Fig. 10-14A**).
2. Rotate the mask into place with a circular motion, maintaining firm pressure against the palate and posterior pharynx (**Fig. 10-14B** and **C**). Insert the device until resistance is felt and only the proximal end of the tube protrudes from the airway.
3. Inflate the cuff of the LMA Fastrach, and hold the metal handle firmly in the dominant hand, using a "frying pan" grip. Ventilate the patient through the device. While ventilating, manipulate the mask with the dominant hand by a lifting motion in a direction similar to that used for direct laryngoscopy (i.e., toward the ceiling over the patient's feet, **Fig. 10-15**). This may enhance mask seal and intubation success. Best mask positioning will be identified by essentially noiseless ventilation, almost as if the patient is being ventilated through a cuffed ETT.
4. Visually inspect and test the cuff of the silicone-tipped ETT that is supplied with the LMA Fastrach. *Fully deflate* the cuff (important), lubricate the length of the ETT liberally, and pass it through the LMA Fastrach. With the black vertical line on the ETT facing the operator (indicates that the leading edge of the bevel will advance through the cords in an A–P orientation), insert the ETT to the 15-cm-deep marker, which corresponds to the transverse black line on the silicone-tipped ETT. This indicates that the silicone tip of the tube is about to emerge from the LMA Fastrach, pushing the epiglottic elevating bar up to lift the epiglottis. Use the handle to gently lift the LMA Fastrach as the ETT is advanced (**Fig. 10-16**). Carefully advance the ETT until intubation is complete. Do not use force of the ETT. Inflate the ETT cuff, and confirm intubation. Then deflate the cuff on the LMA Fastrach.

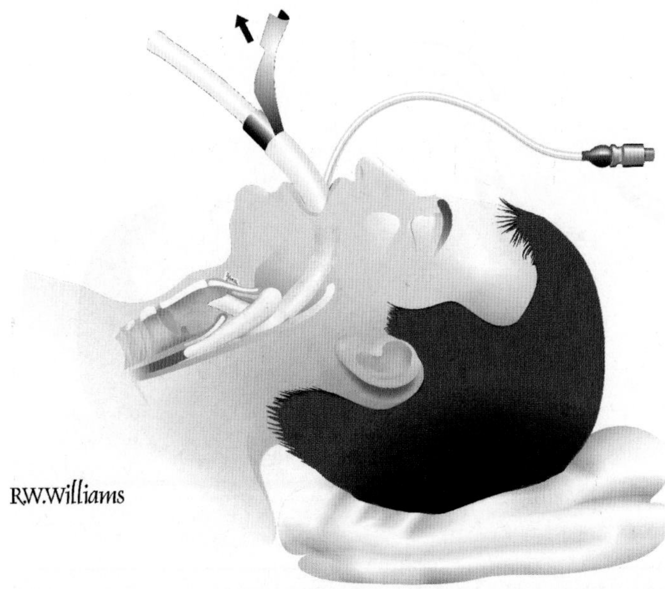


● **FIGURE 10-15.** Lift the handle of the LMA Fastrach as the ETT is about to pass into the larynx to improve the success rate of intubation. **This** is called the Chandy maneuver, after Dr. Archie Brain's associate Dr. Chandy Vergese.

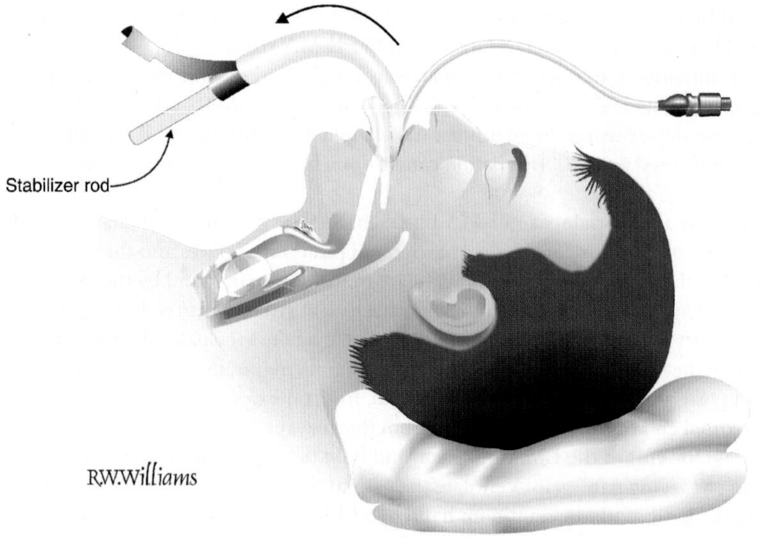


● **FIGURE 10-16.** Use of the stabilizer rod to ensure the ETT is not inadvertently dragged out of the trachea as the LMA Fastrach is removed.

5. After intubation, the LMA Fastrach can be removed fairly easily, leaving just the ETT in place. The key to successful removal of the mask is to remember that one is attempting to keep the ETT precisely in place and to remove the mask over it. First remove the 15-mm connector from the ETT. Then immobilize the ETT with one hand, and gently ease the deflated LMA Fastrach out over the ETT with a rotating motion until the proximal end of the mask channel reaches the proximal end of the ETT. Use the stabilizer rod provided with the device to hold the ETT in position as the LMA Fastrach is withdrawn over the tube (**Fig. 10-17**). Remove the stabilizer rod from the LMA Fastrach, and grasp the ETT at the level of the incisors (**Fig. 10-17**). *The stabilizer bar must be removed to allow the pilot balloon of the ETT to pass through the LMA Fastrach* (**Fig. 10-18**). Failure to do so may result in the pilot balloon being avulsed from the ETT, rendering the balloon incompetent and necessitating reintubation, preferably over an ETT changer.

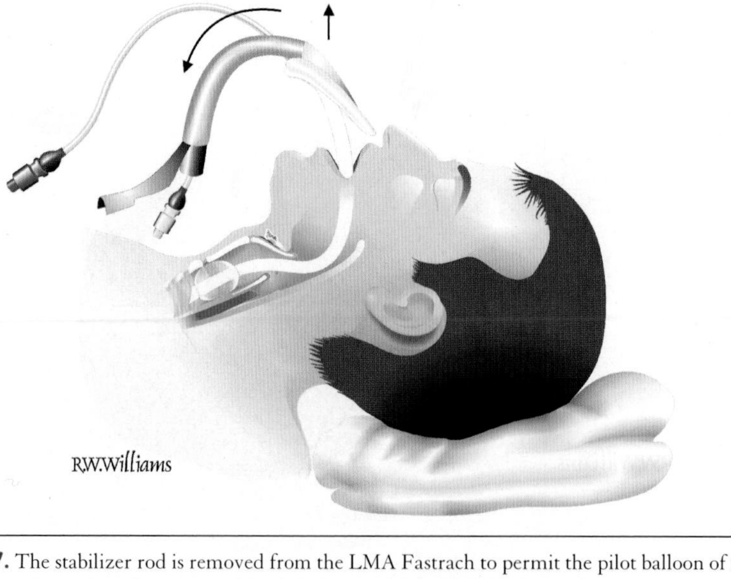


● **FIGURE 10-17.** The stabilizer rod is removed from the LMA Fastrach to permit the pilot balloon of the ETT to go through the LMA Fastrach and prevent it from being avulsed from the ETT.

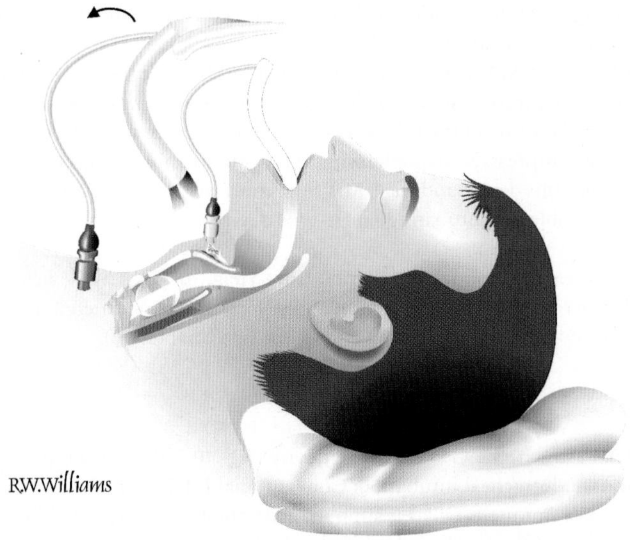


● **FIGURE 10-18.** The pilot balloon of the ETT emerges from the end of the LMA Fastrach intact.

### Complications and Limitations

Unfortunately, the distal collar tip of the Laryngeal Mask Company Limited devices can "roll up" on insertion, creating a partial "insertion block" hindering optimal placement. This feature also likely contributes to pharyngeal abrasion and bleeding that is sometimes seen with these devices. Some authorities recommend partial inflation of the cuff to minimize tip roll, although there is little evidence that this helps; others suggest the up/down maneuver (see above). Insertion of the LMA Classic and LMA Unique "upside down," and rotating into place once in the hypopharynx, has also been described and is preferred by some. Our preferred method is as described earlier.

Achieving a seal sufficient to enable positive-pressure ventilation with an LMA may be difficult. Keeping the tube portion of the device in the midline and altering the position of the head and neck from flexion (more usual) to neutral or extension may be of help. Overall, ventilation success rates are very high with all LMA-type devices. Optimal positioning improves ventilatory effectiveness and, in the case of the LMA Fastrach, facilitates intubation.

It is not known to what extent the LMA protects the airway against the aspiration of gastric contents; so the device is considered a temporizing measure only. This limits its usefulness in pre-hospital and emergency airway care, except when the LMA Fastrach is used to achieve intubation.

## OTHER SUPRAGLOTTIC DEVICES

### Disposable LMA-Type Designs

Several manufacturers produce disposable devices that appear almost identical to the LMA Classic. Although they do not incorporate the vertical bars intended to prevent epiglottic intrusion as are present in the LMA Classic and LMA Unique, the effect of this absence is not clear. These devices have the same indications, contraindications, insertion techniques, and complications as similar Laryngeal Mask Company Limited devices.

The Ambu LMA (**Fig. 10-5A**) devices have several unique design features that may confer particular insertion and seal advantages:

- The device is semi-inflated in the package. This feature provides an "immediate seal" once inserted, minimizing the inflation step and speeding the time to ventilation.

- The leading tip of the inflatable collar is reinforced and "spatulated" to minimize tip roll and improve insertion characteristics.
- The AuraOnce LMA incorporates a tube that is flexible at the curved portion and more rigid proximally to improve insertion characteristics. In a recent design modification, the plastic in the curved portion of the tube was softened in response to concerns that this portion of the tube might compress the hypopharyngeal mucous membrane and lead to ischemia. Evidence suggests that this device and the LMA Supreme are the most easily inserted and rapid to seal of the disposable nonintubating LMA-type devices.

Ambu has recently introduced the Ambu Aura-i (**Fig. 10-5B**). This device is single-use, virtually identical in design to the Ambu AuraOnce, and is specifically modified to be used with the Ambu A Scope System, a disposable intubating endoscope (see Chapter 16).

### Cookgas ILA and Air Q

Like the LMA Fastrach, the Cookgas ILA device (**Fig. 10-6A**) is a supraglottic ventilatory device that also permits endotracheal intubation. Conventional ETTs (size 5.0 to 8.5) are used for intubation as opposed to a unique ETT as is supplied with the LMA Fastrach. The Air Q (**Fig. 10-6B**) is a disposable version of the Cookgas ILA. Like the Fastrach, the Cookgas device may be removed over the ETT (once ETT placement is confirmed) with use of a special stabilizing rod.

### I-Gel Airways

The i-gel family of devices (**Fig. 10-8**) all contain preshaped, noninflatable masks made of a soft, gel-like substance that theoretically reduces insertion trauma. They include an integral bite block and gastric channel, and are available in a range of sizes from small infant to large adult. Advantages include ease of insertion without a cuff inflation step and decreased minor adverse effects; however, the preformed sizes may make an exact fit more difficult than other SGDs. It has been used with success in emergency medicine and EMS.

## EVIDENCE–SGDS

- **Is the LMA effective in emergency, difficult, and failed airway management?** There is ample evidence that LMAs are useful in emergency airway management, both for the management of the difficult airway and rescue of the failed airway.[1–5] SGAs that optimize first-pass success, high seal pressure, and an ability to permit ETI are generally preferred. Furthermore, numerous studies have demonstrated that the LMA is at least as effective as other methods of airway management for patients requiring CPR.[6–8]
- **What success rates have been achieved intubating through the ILMAs (Fastrach and Cookgas)?** Success rates for blind intubation through these devices range from 70% to 99%.[1,9,10] Techniques that employ a fiberscope to aid in ETI through devices have success rates routinely over 90%.[11,12]
- **Is the LMA effective in the pediatric population?** There is ample evidence that the traditional LMA are appropriate and widely accepted as rescue devices in children.[13,14] Some authors have described guidelines for selecting the appropriate size in children, and the manufacturer provides a pocket card to guide clinicians. There is also evidence to support the use of ILMAs in both routine and difficult pediatric airway management.[15]
- **How easy is it for nonexperts to successfully use these LMA devices?** A variety of authors have described successful insertion and use of both classic and newer devices by minimally trained rescuer nonmedical personnel, prehospital care providers, nurses, and respiratory therapists and naive airway managers.[16,17] Some of the EMS literature has questioned the ease of use of the device as a primary method of airway management in EMS,[9] although analysis has shown that training is key to its successful use.[18]

- **What complications with short-term use of the LMA might I expect?** The incidence of difficult ventilation or major airway adverse events with an LMA is quite low and is thought to be significantly less than standard tracheal intubation or Bag Mask Ventilation.[19] The LMA may fail to provide a seal sufficient to permit adequate ventilation, often attributed to the sensitivity of the seal to head and neck position.[20,21] Insufflation of the stomach may occur. Although SGDs may not offer total protection from the aspiration of regurgitated gastric contents, they protect the aspiration of material produced above the device with varying degrees of success.[22] Cricoid pressure may or may not interfere with proper functioning of an LMA, although in practice each case is evaluated individually.[23] Negative-pressure pulmonary edema (mentioned previously) is caused by a patient sucking hard to inspire against an obstruction, where fluid is sucked into the alveolar spaces. This complication has been reported with patients biting down on the LMA and can be prevented by placing folded gauze flats between the molar teeth on either side.[24]
- **How do the preformed cuffless devices compare to more traditional cuffed LMAs?** The I-Gel has compared favorably in most aspects to other LMA products. Compared to the LMA Classic/Unique, physiologic response to insertion is equivalent or improved, and there is less gastric insufflation and increased leak pressures in both children and adults.[1,25,26] Evidence is mixed regarding ease of insertion and first-pass success, and the I-Gel seal adequacy has been found to be nonsuperior compared with some of the LMA devices.[27,28]
- **How do the ILMA devices compare to one another?** Both the Cookgas and LMA Fastrach devices have been shown to have excellent insertion success rates and ventilatory function as an SGD; however, the blind endotracheal intubation rates are consistently >90% for the Fastrach only.[1,29]

## REFERENCES


1. Kapoor S, Jethava DD, Gupta P, et al. Comparison of supraglottic devices i-gel(®) and LMA® Fastrach(®) as conduit for endotracheal intubation. *Indian J Anaesth*. 2014;58:397–402.
2. Wong DT, Yang JJ, Jagannathan N. Brief review: The LMA Supreme™ supraglottic airway. *Can J Anaesth*. 2012;59:483–493.
3. Frerk C, Mitchell VS, McNarry AF, et al; Difficult Airway Society Intubation Guidelines Working Group. Difficult Airway Society 2015 guidelines for management of unanticipated difficult intubation in adults. *Br J Anaesth.* 2015;115(6):827–848.
4. Parmet JL, Colonna-Romano P, Horrow JC, et al. The laryngeal mask airway reliably provides rescue ventilation in cases of unanticipated difficult tracheal intubation along with difficult mask ventilation. *Anesth Analg*. 1998;87:661–665.
5. Wetsch WA, Schneider A, Schier R, et al. In a difficult access scenario, supraglottic airway devices improve success and time to ventilation. *Eur J Emerg Med*. 2015;22(5):374–376.
6. Grayling M, Wilson IH, Thomas B. The use of the laryngeal mask airway and Combitube in cardiopulmonary resuscitation: a national survey. *Resuscitation*. 2002;52:183–186.
7. Kurz MC, Prince DK, Christenson J, et al. Association of advanced airway device with chest compression fraction during out-of-hospital cardiopulmonary arrest. *Resuscitation*. 2016;98:35–40.
8. Benoit JL, Gerecht RB, Steuerwald MT, et al. Endotracheal intubation versus supraglottic airway placement in out-of-hospital cardiac arrest: a meta-analysis. *Resuscitation*. 2015;93:20–26.
9. Fukutome T, Amaha K, Nakazawa K, et al. Tracheal intubation through the intubating laryngeal mask airway (LMA®-Fastrach) in patients with difficult airways. *Anaesth Intensive Care*. 1998;26:387–391.
10. Karim YM, Swanson DE. Comparison of blind tracheal intubation through the intubating laryngeal mask airway (LMA® Fastrach) and the Air-Q. *Anaesthesia*. 2011;66:185–190.
11. Moore A, Gregoire-Bertrand F, Massicotte N, et al. I-gel™ versus LMA-Fastrach™ supraglottic airway for flexible bronchoscope-guided tracheal intubation using a Parker (GlideRite™) endotracheal tube: a randomized controlled trial. *Anesth Analg*. 2015;121(2):430–436.

12. Kannan S, Chestnutt N, McBride G. Intubating LMA® guided awake fibreoptic intubation in severe maxillo-facial injury. *Can J Anaesth*. 2000;47:989–991.
13. Greif R, Theiler L. The use of supraglottic airway devices in pediatric laparoscopic surgery. *Minerva Anestesiol*. 2010;76:575–576.
14. Sanket B, Ramavakoda CY, Nishtala MR, et al. Comparison of second-generation supraglottic airway devices (i-gel versus LMA ProSeal) during elective surgery in children. *AANA J*. 2015;83(4):275–280.
15. Jagannathan N, Roth AG, Sohn LE, et al. The new air-Q intubating laryngeal airway for tracheal intubation in children with anticipated difficult airway: a case series. *Paediatr Anaesth*. 2009;19:618–622.
16. Braun P, Wenzel V, Paal P. Anesthesia in prehospital emergencies and in the emergency department. *Curr Opin Anaesthesiol*. 2010;23:500–506.
17. Stroumpoulis K, Isaia C, Bassiakou E, et al. A comparison of the i-gel and classic LMA insertion in manikins by experienced and novice physicians. *Eur J Emerg Med*. 2012;19(1):24–27.
18. Ruetzler K, Roessler B, Potura L, et al. Performance and skill retention of intubation by paramedics using seven different airway devices—a manikin study. *Resuscitation*. 2011;82(5):593–597.
19. Cook TM, Woodall N, Ferk C; on behalf of the Fourth National Audit Project. Major complications of airway management in the UK: results of the Fourth National Audit Project of the Royal College of Anaesthetists and the Difficult Airway Society. Part I: anesthesia. *Br J Anaesth*. 2011;106:617–631.
20. Bercker S, Schmidbauer W, Volk T, et al. A comparison of seal in seven supraglottic airway devices using a cadaver model of elevated esophageal pressure. *Anesth Analg*. 2008:445–448.
21. Park SH, Han SH, Do SH, et al. The influence of head and neck position on the oropharyngeal leak pressure and cuff position of three supraglottic airway devices. *Anesth Analg*. 2009;108(1):112–117.
22. Schmidbauer W, Bercker S, Volk T, et al. Oesophageal seal of the novel supralaryngeal airway device I-Gel™ in comparison with the laryngeal mask airways Classic™ and ProSeal™ using a cadaver model. *Br J Anaesth*. 2009;102(1):135–139.
23. Li CW, Xue FS, Xu YC, et al. Cricoid pressure impedes insertion of, and ventilation through, the ProSeal laryngeal mask airway in anesthetized, paralyzed patients. *Anesth Analg*. 2007;104(5):1195–1198.
24. Vandse R, Kothari DS, Tripathi RS, et al. Negative pressure pulmonary edema with laryngeal mask airway use: recognition, pathophysiology and treatment modalities. *Int J Crit Illn Inj Sci*. 2012;2(2):98–103.
25. Ismail SA, Bisher NA, Kandil HW, et al. Intraocular pressure and haemodynamic responses to insertion of the i-gel, laryngeal mask airway or endotracheal tube. *Eur J Anaesthesiol*. 2011;28:443–448.
26. Maitra S, Baidya DK, Bhattacharjee S, et al. Evaluation of i-gel™ airway in children: a meta-analysis. *Pediatr Anaesth*. 2014;24(10):1072–1079.
27. Beleña JM, Núñez M, Vidal A, et al. Randomized comparison of the i-gel(TM) with the LMA Supreme(TM) in anesthetized adult patients. *Anaesthesist*. 2015;64(4):271–276.
28. Middleton PM, Simpson PM, Thomas RE, et al. Higher insertion success with the i-gel® supraglottic airway in out-of-hospital cardiac arrest: a randomised controlled trial. *Resuscitation*. 2014;85(7):893–897.
29. Liu EH, Goy RW, Lim Y, et al. Success of tracheal intubation with intubating laryngeal mask airways. *Anesthesiology*. 2008;108(4):621–626.

# Chapter 11

# Extraglottic Devices: Retroglottic Type

Erik G. Laurin, Leslie V. Simon, Darren A. Braude, and Michael F. Murphy

## INTRODUCTION

The term *extraglottic device* (EGD) is divided into two main subclasses: supraglottic devices and retroglottic devices. Supraglottic devices are defined and discussed in Chapter 10, along with general indications and contraindications. This chapter focuses on the retroglottic EGDs (rEGD). Since these devices sit posterior to the glottis in the proximal esophagus, they are contraindicated in patients with known esophageal disease such as strictures and presumed esophageal disease as in caustic ingestions; otherwise, they share the same indications and contraindications as the supraglottic EGDs.

Retroglottic devices such as the Esophageal Obturator Airway and the Esophageal Gastric Tube Airway were among the first extraglottic airways to be put into practice, back in the 1970s, but no longer have a role in emergency airway management. Modern rEGDs represent a dramatic improvement over these early devices and have demonstrated their effectiveness and safety in rapidly establishing oxygenation and ventilation in a variety of emergency situations.

## RETROGLOTTIC DEVICES

To many practitioners, the most familiar and prototypical EGD is the Esophageal-Tracheal Combitube (ETC) (**Fig. 11-1**) (Tyco-Healthcare-Kendall-Sheridan, Mansfield, MA). It has been in use since 1987 and has substantial evidence and experience supporting its use. It is generally easier to use and more effective for novices than is BMV and easier to place than an endotracheal tube (ETT). The success of the ETC has spawned the development of devices based on the same principles, attempting to replicate or improve on its safety, ease of use, and ability to facilitate oxygenation and ventilation. These most common of these devices, and the two examples discussed in this chapter, include the Rusch EasyTube (**Fig. 11-2**) and the King Laryngeal Tube (King LT) (Ambu Inc. USA Columbia, MD) variants (**Fig. 11-3**).

All of these devices share the design feature of two high-volume, low-pressure balloons. The proximal balloon seals the oropharynx, whereas the distal balloon seals the esophagus, with gas exiting and entering the device and the laryngeal inlet between the two. The ETC and the EasyTube use two separate inflation ports to enable independent balloon inflation; the King LT has a single

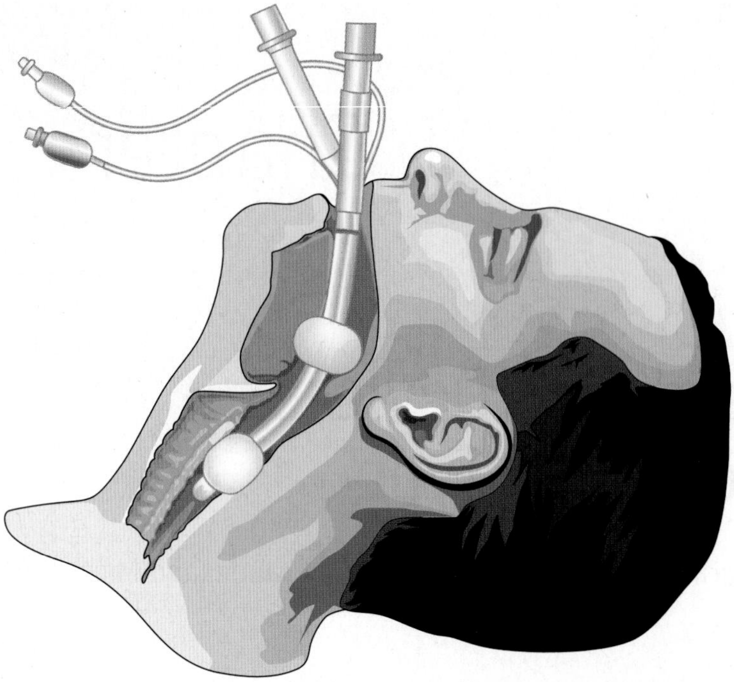

● **FIGURE 11-1. The Combitube Inserted and Seated.** Note how the laryngeal aperture is trapped between the two balloons.

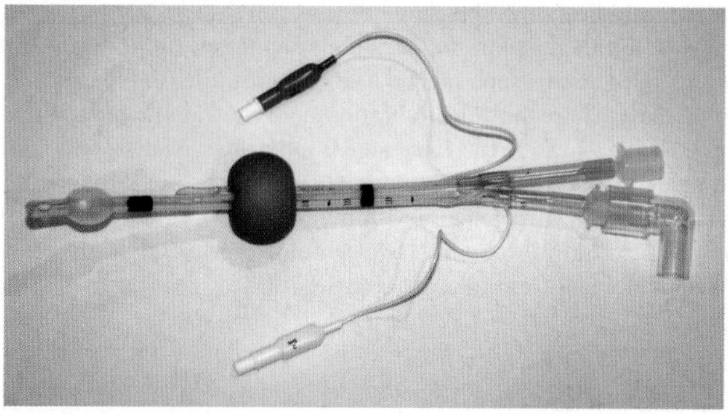

● **FIGURE 11-2. Rusch EasyTube.**

inflation port that inflates both the upper and lower portions of the balloon with a single bolus of air. The advantage of the latter is simplicity, but during tube device exchange it is beneficial to be able to maintain esophageal occlusion while deflating the upper balloon for laryngoscopy. The ETC and EasyTube both have dual lumens that allow for ventilation whether the device ends up in the proximal esophagus as intended or in the trachea; the King LT has a single lumen based on the reality that placement of these devices almost always results in esophageal positioning.

In common practice these devices are all inserted blindly, but there is a strong literature base supporting direct visualization for placement of the ETC when the equipment and expertise exists, which can be extrapolated to the EasyTube and possibly even the King LT. Such placement technique may mitigate some of the common issues encountered with these devices during insertion, particularly trauma to the posterior pharynx.

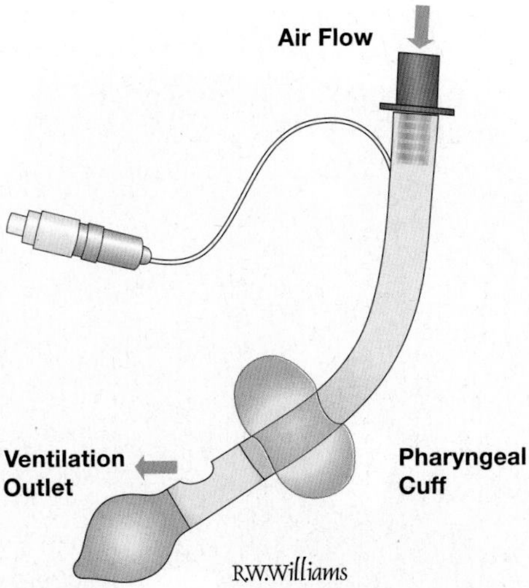


● **FIGURE 11-3. The King LT Airway.** Note that there is only one inflation port to inflate both balloons.

When compared with SGDs, retroglottic EGDs typically have a tighter seal, resulting in higher cuff leak pressures (up to 35 to 40 cm $H_2O$ compared with 25 to 30 cm $H_2O$), which may be advantageous in patients with intrinsic high airway resistance requiring high peak airway pressures (asthma and obesity) or if glottic anatomy is distorted from hematoma, infection, or mass, requiring increased inflation pressure. These devices may also provide some tamponade effect for upper airway bleeding. There is some concern that these devices exert more pressure on the carotid vessels than do SGDs. This might increase vagal tone and impede resuscitation efforts, leading some to advocate for SGDs over rEGDs as the airway device of choice during cardiac arrest. This concern arose largely from animal (swine) study and has been countered in a small human case series.

## Combitube

The ETC (**Fig. 11-1**) has been in clinical use for a much longer period of time than any of the other EGDs and therefore it has accumulated the largest body of evidence describing its indications, contraindications, benefits, and risks. As discussed above, the ETC is a dual-lumen, dual-cuff, disposable rEGD intended to be inserted into the esophagus, although it may rarely enter the trachea on insertion (generally <5% of insertions) and is designed to function adequately in either position. The ETC is supplied in two sizes: 37F catheter SA (small adult) and 41F catheter Regular, which, according to the package insert, are to be used for patients 4 ft (1.22 m) to 5 ft 6 in (1.67 m) tall and more than 5 ft 6 in tall, respectively. However, postmarketing research has demonstrated that the small adult size should be used all the way up to 6 ft tall. There is no ETC suitable for use in children or patients <4 ft tall. Due to its large robust balloons, the ETC can generate some of the highest peak ventilation pressures before leak occurs (up to 40 cm $H_2O$) and may be the EGD of choice when ventilation is predicted to be challenging.

The Combitube has been shown to be an easy and effective primary airway, particularly in the prehospital setting, and rescue airway in the event of a failed intubation. Like any EGD, it does not provide optimum protection against aspiration, although the protection provided is substantial and reports of aspiration are infrequent. The relative merit of the ETC compared with all the available newer retroglottic and supraglottic devices is not well established.

### *Insertion Technique*

Insertion of the Combitube is typically a blind technique intended for providers that do not have training in laryngoscopy; however, a laryngoscope can and should be used when available to lift the

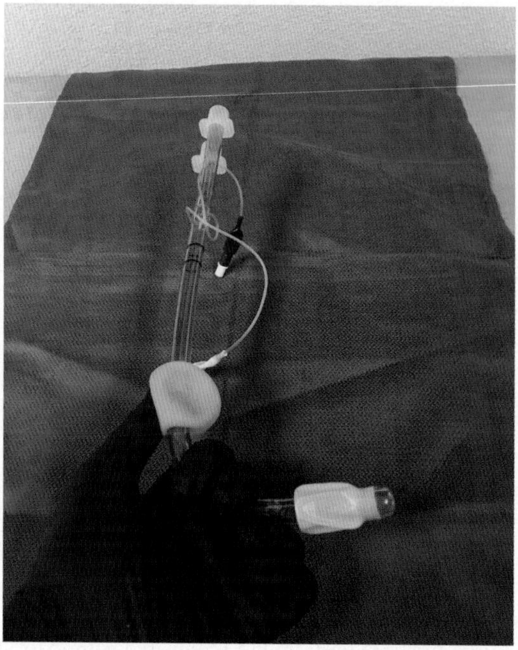

● **FIGURE 11-4. Lipp maneuver.**

tongue and permit direct visualization of esophageal placement, as was done in all the preliminary trials in the operative setting. Although the Combitube has been inserted in almost every conceivable patient position, the technique described here assumes the patient is in the supine position and the provider does not have a laryngoscope available or cannot perform laryngoscopy within their scope of practice.

1. First perform a Lipp maneuver to gently preshape the device to pass easily around the tongue (**Fig. 11-4**).
2. With the patient supine and the head and neck in a neutral position, lift the tongue and jaw upward (jaw lift) with the nondominant hand.
3. Insert the preshaped device in the midline, allowing the curve of the device to follow the natural curve of the airway around the tongue, and advance the device until the upper incisors (or alveolar ridge if the patient is edentulous) lie between the imprinted black circular bands on the device. Minimal force is required to enable the device to pass through the pharyngeal constrictor muscles into the esophagus; resistance should prompt the operator to withdraw, reassess patient positioning and device shape, consider use of a laryngoscope, and gently readvance. Using the syringe provided, inflate the proximal large oropharyngeal balloon with 100 mL of air (Regular) or 85 mL of air (SA) through the blue pilot balloon port labeled no. 1.
4. Inflate the distal small balloon with 15 mL of air (Regular) or 12 mL of air (SA) through the white pilot balloon port labeled no. 2. This presumes the device is sitting in the distensible upper esophageal tissues.
5. Begin ventilation using the longer blue connecting tube (labeled no. 1), which will deliver air out the ventilation holes on the side of the device between the proximal and distal balloons. The presence of air entry into the lung, the detection of end-tidal carbon dioxide, and the absence of gastric insufflation by auscultation all indicate that the Combitube is situated in the esophagus, which occurs with nearly every insertion. With the Combitube in this position, aspiration and continuous suctioning of gastric contents is possible by passing the provided suction catheter or any 12F catheter or smaller catheter through the clear connecting tube (labeled no. 2) into the stomach.

6. If ventilation using the longer blue tube no. 1 does not result in breath sounds and end-tidal carbon dioxide detection, then the Combitube may have ended up in the trachea and ventilation should be attempted through the shorter clear connection tube no. 2. In this case, air should be withdrawn carefully from the distal balloon until an air leak is just heard and then just enough added back to overcome the leak to avoid pressure injury in the trachea. In this tracheal position, gastric decompression through the device is not possible.
7. The absence of end-tidal $CO_2$ and any sounds on auscultation while ventilating both ports may indicate severe patient pathology, incorrect sizing, or that the device has been inserted too far and should be withdrawn carefully.

### *Complications*

Complications are rare, but occasionally very serious and likely underreported, with most related to upper airway and esophageal trauma from overly aggressive insertion or balloon overinflation. These include hematomas, mucosal lacerations, pyriform sinus perforation, and perforation of the esophagus. Most complications can be overcome with proper training and technique. Other issues are related to potential mucosal ischemic injury and possible impairment of carotid blood flow as discussed above. Finally, it should be noted that the pharyngeal balloon on the Combitube (as opposed to the Rusch EasyTube or the King LT airway) is made of latex and should be avoided in patients with this allergy.

## Rusch EasyTube

The Rusch EasyTube (**Fig. 11-2**) is a dual-lumen tube designed for difficult or emergency airway intubation and ventilation. Like the Combitube, the EasyTube can be placed either in the trachea or in the esophagus and creates a viable airway in either position. When placed in the esophagus, the EasyTube allows the passage of a flexible endoscope, a suction catheter, or a tracheal tube introducer through the proximally terminating ventilation lumen. This distinguishes it from the Combitube, which does not permit passage of a tube exchanger to potentially establish a definitive airway through the device. If placed in the trachea, the size and shape of the distal tip are similar to a standard ETT. It is suggested by the manufacturer that the risk of tracheal trauma relative to the Combitube is reduced because of the smaller diameter of EasyTube device at the distal tip.

The EasyTube is latex free and supplied in two sizes, 28F catheter and 41F catheter. As for the Combitube, the manufacturer claims that the smaller size can be used in older children. There is minimal evidence from human studies to demonstrate the relative success rate of the EasyTube versus the LMA, Combitube, or King LT, although initial data appear promising. Multiple manikin studies show that it is similar to a Combitube in speed of insertion, successful ventilations, and skill retention. More data are needed to determine its role in emergency airway management.

## The Laryngeal Tube Airway

The Laryngeal Tube airway (known as King Airway or King LT in North America) (**Fig. 11-3**) is a newer latex-free silicon single-lumen retroglottic device that is built on the presumption that blind insertion will virtually always result in esophageal placement. The two balloons are inflated simultaneously via a single port. It is supplied in blind distal tip (King LT, LT-D) and open distal tip (King LTS, LTS-D) variants, the latter to permit gastric decompression. Approximate interdental distance of 20 mm is required for insertion, comparable to the ETC. Sizing of the Laryngeal Tube is primarily height based, like the ETC, though there are weight-based sizing guidelines provided as well for children. A full size range from newborn to adult is available in some parts of the world; the smallest size in North America is currently a size #2 to be used for patients down to 12 kg. A new iLT-D version to facilitate intubation and gastric access for adults recently became available in parts of the world and should be available soon in the United States. There is not sufficient data available yet to evaluate this product.

The King LT is inserted through the pharynx and blindly into the esophagus in a similar fashion as the ETC except there is less reported experience using a laryngoscope and the Lipp maneuver is not recommended. There have been rare published reports of unanticipated tracheal placements with this technique. The King LT is advanced until the 15/22-mm bag connector flange touches the incisors, unless resistance is encountered. The balloons should be inflated through the single port with the recommended amount of air. Ventilation is then attempted *while* the device is slowly withdrawn, monitoring carefully until unrestricted ventilation and chest rise is noted along with capnography and equal lung sounds. It is common for providers to stop withdrawal when the very first sign of ventilation is noted, which may leave the distal ventilation outlets too deep such that they may be delivering air to the stomach and not the lungs. We suggest withdrawing about 1 or 2 cm (less for smaller pediatric sizes and more for large adult sizes) *past* the point when ventilation first occurs and halting when ventilation becomes most prominent and easy to accomplish. This ensures all ventilation is directed to the lungs.

If a properly sized device is unable to ventilate, it is most commonly overinserted. Once correctly positioned, the King LT works in a fashion that is very similar to that of the ETC with similar ventilation and oxygenation capabilities and aspiration protection. Although there have not been extensive reports of complications, airway trauma has been reported. Clinically significant tongue swelling has also been reported, in one case occurring as early as 45 minutes post insertion, but such cases seem rare. Still, prolonged insertion of any rEGD is not recommended and exchange for an ETT is encouraged within 2-4 hours when it can be done safely. Because of concerns about possible effects on the cerebral perfusion, it is advisable to use a manometer to check balloon pressures, when possible, instead of relying on suggested volumes.

## EVIDENCE

- **What is the role of the Combitube as a rescue airway device?** The Combitube has been identified as a rescue airway device for the failed airway by authoritative bodies in the United States and Canada.[1,2] Its use is well described in the anesthesia, resuscitation, emergency medicine, and emergency medical services (EMS) literature both as a first-line device and as a device to be used in the face of a difficult or failed airway.[3–9] Several authors have identified the Combitube as a valuable adjunct in cardiopulmonary resuscitation,[10–12] performing as well as or better than the LMA and bag-mask ventilation.
- **What kind of airway management success rates have been reported with the Combitube?** Success rates of 98% to 100% are regularly reported in these studies. The ease of insertion[13–17] and adequacy of ventilation by physicians and nonphysician providers is well established.[18–20]
- **Has the Combitube been successful in the management of the difficult or failed airway?** The device is useful in the management of the difficult airway[21] and in rescuing a failed airway[22–24] while one prepares to undertake a cricothyrotomy.
- **Has the Combitube been used in any unusual situations?** It has been demonstrated to protect the airway, control bleeding, and permit ventilation in a case of craniofacial trauma associated with oropharyngeal severe bleeding[25] and to secure an airway in a case of severe facial burns preventing intubation.[26]
- **What precautions should I be aware of with this device?** It is unclear whether the Combitube provides protection against the aspiration of gastric contents.[27] The downside of the Combitube includes reports of potentially serious complications related to its use, particularly pyriform sinus perforation[28–32] and esophageal perforation.[33–37] Mucosal pressures exerted by the inflated balloons may exceed mucosal perfusion pressure, leading to mucosal ischemia, and the degree of balloon inflation should be deliberate and closely monitored.[38]
- **Has the King LT airway been demonstrated to be similarly effective in nonemergency airway management as the LMA and Combitube?** Simple handling, possible aspiration protection, and availability in newborn to adult sizes are considered to be advantages of this airway device.[39–42]

- **Does the King LT have a place in EMS as an airway management device?** There is some evidence that this device is easily learned by EMS personnel and provides more effective ventilation than bag-mask devices.[43–45]
- **Is the King LT airway useful as an emergency airway adjunct?** The evidence that the King LT is useful as a rescue airway or in patients where intubation has failed is limited and for the most part is based on case reports.[46–48] However, a recent publication provides compelling evidence that this device may well be of use in the difficult and failed airway.[49]
- **Are there potential problems that I ought to be aware of with this device?** As with the Combitube, mucosal compression by the inflated balloons may lead to mucosal ischemic injury.[38,50]
- **Is the King LT useful in pediatric patients?** Manikin studies suggest that the pediatric Kings LT can be placed more rapidly and with a greater degree of success compared with endotracheal intubation by prehospital providers.[51,52] The very low rate of advanced airway management in pediatric patients in the prehospital setting limits meaningful data on pediatric use.[53]
- **The EasyTube looks as though it would be easier to insert in an emergency than the Combitube. Is there evidence to that effect?** Perhaps, but at this point, the available evidence is relatively thin.[38,54–68] Much of the published information is from simulated patients or manikins,[54,55,62,65] an operating theater,[58,60,64] or is based on opinion.[57,60] However, there is sufficient evidence to suggest that this device is at least competitive with the Combitube and King LT to be a consideration for prehospital airway management.
- **Is there evidence to support the use of the iLTS-D?** A preliminary study on the iLTS-D suggests a high rate of success for both initial placement and subsequent intubation under direct visualization using flexible bronchoscopy on 30 ENT patients with apparently normal airways.[68] A manikin-based study suggests similar timing and intubation success rates between the iLTS-D and the LMA-Fastrach.[69] Further studies are needed before this device can be recommended for routine use.

## REFERENCES


1. Crosby ET, Cooper RM, Douglas MJ, et al. The unanticipated difficult airway with recommendations for management. *Can J Anaesth*. 1998;45:757–776.
2. American Society of Anesthesiologists Task Force on Management of the Difficult Airway. Practice guidelines for management of the difficult airway. An updated report by the American Society of Anesthesiologists Task Force on Management of the Difficult Airway. *Anesthesiology*. 2003;98:1269–1277.
3. Mercer M. The role of the Combitube in airway management. *Anaesthesia*. 2000;55:394–395.
4. Gaitini LA, Vaida SJ, Agro F. The esophageal-tracheal Combitube. *Anesthesiol Clin North Am*. 2002;20:893–906.
5. Idris AH, Gabrielli A. Advances in airway management. *Emerg Med Clin North Am*. 2002;20:843–857.
6. Agro F, Frass M, Benumof JL, et al. Current status of the Combitube: a review of the literature. *J Clin Anesth*. 2002;14:307–314.
7. Keller C, Brimacombe J, Boehler M, et al. The influence of cuff volume and anatomic location on pharyngeal, esophageal, and tracheal mucosal pressures with the esophageal tracheal Combitube. *Anesthesiology*. 2002;96:1074–1077.
8. Shuster M, Nolan J, Barnes TA. Airway and ventilation management. *Cardiol Clin*. 2002;20:23–35.
9. Agro F, Frass M, Benumof J, et al. The esophageal tracheal Combitube as a non-invasive alternative to endotracheal intubation: a review. *Minerva Anesthesiol*. 2001;67:863–874.
10. Grayling M, Wilson IH, Thomas B. The use of the laryngeal mask airway and Combitube in cardiopulmonary resuscitation: a national survey. *Resuscitation*. 2002;52:183–186.
11. Gabrielli A, Layon AJ, Wenzel V, et al. Alternative ventilation strategies in cardiopulmonary resuscitation. *Curr Opin Crit Care*. 2002;8:199–211.

12. Frass M, Staudinger T, Losert H, et al. Airway management during cardiopulmonary resuscitation—a comparative study of bag-valve-mask, laryngeal mask airway and Combitube in a bench model. *Resuscitation*. 1999;43:80–81.
13. Levitan RM, Kush S, Hollander JE. Devices for difficult airway management in academic emergency departments: results of a national survey. *Ann Emerg Med*. 1999;33:694–698.
14. Lefrancois DP, Dufour DG. Use of the esophageal tracheal Combitube by basic emergency medical technicians. *Resuscitation*. 2002;52:77–83.
15. Ochs M, Vilke GM, Chan TC, et al. Successful prehospital airway management by EMT-Ds using the Combitube. *Prehosp Emerg Care*. 2000;4:333–337.
16. Tanigawa K, Shigematsu A. Choice of airway devices for 12,020 cases of nontraumatic cardiac arrest in Japan. *Prehosp Emerg Care*. 1998;2:96–100.
17. Rumball CJ, MacDonald D. The PTL, Combitube, laryngeal mask, and oral airway: a randomized prehospital comparative study of ventilatory device effectiveness and cost-effectiveness in 470 cases of cardiorespiratory arrest. *Prehosp Emerg Care*. 1997;1:1–10.
18. Calkins MD, Robinson TD. Combat trauma airway management: endotracheal intubation versus laryngeal mask airway versus Combitube use by Navy SEAL and Reconnaissance Combat Corpsmen. *J Trauma*. 1999;46:927–932.
19. Yardy N, Hancox D, Strang T. A comparison of two airway aids for emergency use by unskilled personnel: the Combitube and laryngeal mask. *Anaesthesia*. 1999;54:181–183.
20. Dorges V, Ocker H, Wenzel V, et al. Emergency airway management by non-anaesthesia house officers—a comparison of three strategies. *Emerg Med J*. 2001;18:90–94.
21. Staudinger T, Tesinsky P, Klappacher G, et al. Emergency intubation with the Combitube in two cases of difficult airway management. *Eur J Anaesthesiol*. 1995;12:189–193.
22. Blostein PA, Koestner AJ, Hoak S. Failed rapid sequence intubation in trauma patients: esophageal tracheal Combitube is a useful adjunct. *J Trauma*. 1998;44:534–537.
23. Enlund M, Miregard M, Wennmalm K. The Combitube for failed intubation—instructions for use. *Acta Anaesthesiol Scand*. 2001;45:127–128.
24. Della Puppa A, Pittoni G, Frass M. Tracheal esophageal Combitube: a useful airway for morbidly obese patients who cannot intubate or ventilate. *Acta Anaesthesiol Scand*. 2002;46:911–913.
25. Morimoto F, Yoshioka T, Ikeuchi H, et al. Use of esophageal tracheal Combitube to control severe oronasal bleeding associated with craniofacial injury: case report. *J Trauma*. 2001;51:168–169.
26. Wagner A, Roeggla M, Roeggla G, et al. Emergency intubation with the Combitube in a case of severe facial burn. *Am J Emerg Med*. 1995;13:681–683.
27. Mercer MH. An assessment of protection of the airway from aspiration of oropharyngeal contents using the Combitube airway. *Resuscitation*. 2001;51:135–138.
28. Urtubia RM, Gazmuri RR. Is the Combitube traumatic? *Anesthesiology*. 2003;98:1021–1022.
29. Urtubia RM, Carcamo CR, Montes JM. Complications following the use of the Combitube, tracheal tube and laryngeal mask airway. *Anaesthesia*. 2000;55:597–599.
30. Oczenski W, Krenn H, Dahaba AA, et al. Complications following the use of the Combitube, tracheal tube and laryngeal mask airway. *Anaesthesia*. 1999;54:1161–1165.
31. Moser MS. Piriform sinus perforation during esophageal-tracheal Combitube placement. *J Emerg Med*. 1999;17:129.
32. Richards CF. Piriform sinus perforation during esophageal-tracheal Combitube placement. *J Emerg Med*. 1998;16:37–39.
33. Krafft P, Nikolic A, Frass M. Esophageal rupture associated with the use of the Combitube. *Anesth Analg*. 1998;87:1457.
34. Krafft P, Frass M, Reed AP. Complications with the Combitube. *Can J Anaesth*. 1998;45:823–824.

35. Walz R, Bund M, Meier PN, et al. Esophageal rupture associated with the use of the Combitube. *Anesth Analg*. 1998;87:228.

36. Vezina D, Lessard MR, Bussieres J, et al. Complications associated with the use of the esophageal-tracheal Combitube. *Can J Anaesth*. 1998;45:76–80.

37. Klein H, Williamson M, Sue-Ling HM, et al. Esophageal rupture associated with the use of the Combitube. *Anesth Analg*. 1997;85:937–939.

38. Ulrich-Pur H, Hrska F, Krafft P, et al. Comparison of mucosal pressures induced by cuffs of different airway devices. *Anesthesiology*. 2006;104(5):933–938.

39. Dorges V, Ocker H, Wenzel V, et al. The laryngeal tube S: a modified simple airway device. *Anesth Analg*. 2003;96:618–621.

40. Genzwuerker HV, Hilker T, Hohner E, et al. The laryngeal tube: a new adjunct for airway management. *Prehosp Emerg Care*. 2000;4:168–172.

41. Dorges V, Ocker H, Wenzel V, et al. The laryngeal tube: a new simple airway device. *Anesth Analg*. 2000;90:1220–1222.

42. Agro F, Cataldo R, Alfano A, et al. A new prototype for airway management in an emergency: the laryngeal tube. *Resuscitation*. 1999;41:284–286.

43. Kette F, Reffo I, Giordani G, et al. The use of laryngeal tube by nurses in out-of-hospital emergencies: preliminary experience. *Resuscitation*. 2005;66:21–25.

44. Kurola J, Harve H, Kettunen T, et al. Airway management in cardiac arrest—comparison of the laryngeal tube, tracheal intubation and bag-mask-ventilation in emergency medical training. *Resuscitation*. 2004;61:149–153.

45. Asai T, Hidaka I, Kawachi S. Efficacy of the laryngeal tube by inexperienced personnel. *Resuscitation*. 2002;55:171–175.

46. Asai T. Use of the laryngeal tube for difficult fiberoptic tracheal intubation. *Anaesthesia*. 2005;60:826.

47. Matioc A, Olson J. Use of the laryngeal tube in two unexpected difficult airway situations: lingual tonsillar hyperplasia and morbid obesity. *Can J Anaesth*. 2004;51:1018–1021.

48. Genzwuerker H, Dhonau S, Ellinger K. Use of the laryngeal tube for out-of-hospital resuscitation. *Resuscitation*. 2002;52:221–224.

49. Winterhalter M, Kirchhoff K, Groschel W, et al. The laryngeal tube for difficult airway management: a prospective investigation in patients with pharyngeal and laryngeal tumours. *Eur J Anaesthesiol*. 2005;22:678–682.

50. Keller C, Brimacombe J, Kleinsasser A, et al. Pharyngeal mucosal pressures with the laryngeal tube airway versus ProSeal laryngeal mask airway. *Anasthesiol Intensivmed Notfallmed Schmerzther*. 2003;38:393–396.

51. Ritter SC, Guyette FX. Prehospital pediatric King LT-D use: a pilot study. *Prehosp Emerg Care*. 2011:15(3):401–404.

52. Byars DV, Brodsky RA, Evans D, et al. Comparison of direct laryngoscopy to Pediatric King LT-D in simulated airways. *Pediatr Emerg Care*. 2012;28(8):750–752.

53. Hansen M, Lambert W, Guise JM, et al. Out-of-hospital pediatric airway management in the United States. *Resuscitation*. 2015;90:104–110.

54. Ruetzler K, Gruber C, Nabecker S, et al. Hands-off time during insertion of six airway devices during cardiopulmonary resuscitation: a randomised manikin trial. *Resuscitation*. 2011;82:1060–1063.

55. Ruetzler K, Roessler B, Potura L, et al. Performance and skill retention of intubation by paramedics using seven different airway devices—a manikin study. *Resuscitation*. 2011;82:593–597.

56. Chenaitia H, Soulleihet V, Massa H, et al. The Easytube for airway management in prehospital emergency medicine. *Resuscitation*. 2010;81:1516–1520.

57. Bollig G. The EasyTube and users' preferences: implications for prehospital medicine and research. *Eur J Anaesthesiol*. 2010;27:843–844.

58. Lorenz V, Rich JM, Schebesta K, et al. Comparison of the EasyTube and endotracheal tube during general anesthesia in fasted adult patients. *J Clin Anesth*. 2009;21:341–347.

59. Cavus E, Deitmer W, Francksen H, et al. Laryngeal tube S II, ProSeal laryngeal mask, and EasyTube during elective surgery: a randomized controlled comparison with the endotracheal tube in nontrained professionals. *Eur J Anaesthesiol*. 2009;26:730–735.

60. Bollig G. Combitube and Easytube should be included in the Scandinavian guidelines for pre-hospital airway management. *Acta Anaesthesiol Scand*. 2009;53:139–140.

61. Trabold B, Schmidt C, Schneider B, et al. Application of three airway devices during emergency medical training by health care providers—a manikin study. *Am J Emerg Med*. 2008;26:783–788.

62. Bercker S, Schmidbauer W, Volk T, et al. A comparison of seal in seven supraglottic airway devices using a cadaver model of elevated esophageal pressure. *Anesth Analg*. 2008;106:445–448.

63. Urtubia RM, Leyton P. Successful use of the EasyTube for facial surgery in a patient with glottic and subglottic stenosis. *J Clin Anesth*. 2007;19:77–78.

64. Bollig G, Lovhaug SW, Sagen O, et al. Airway management by paramedics using endotracheal intubation with a laryngoscope versus the oesophageal tracheal Combitube and EasyTube on manikins: a randomized experimental trial. *Resuscitation*. 2006;71:107–111.

65. Thierbach AR, Werner C. Infraglottic airway devices and techniques. *Best Pract Res Clin Anaesthesiol*. 2005;19:595–609.

66. Thierbach AR, Piepho T, Maybauer M. The EasyTube for airway management in emergencies. *Prehosp Emerg Care*. 2005;9:445–448.

67. Thierbach AR, Piepho T, Maybauer MO. A new device for emergency airway management: the EasyTube. *Resuscitation*. 2004;60:347.

68. Bergold MN, Kahle S, Schulzik T. Intubating laryngeal tube suction disposable: initial clinical experiences with a novel device for endotracheal intubation [in German]. *Anaesthesist*. 2016;65:30–35.

69. Ott T, Fischer M, Limbach T. The novel intubation laryngeal tube (iLTS-D) is comparable to the intubations laryngeal mask (Fastrach)—a prospective randomized manikin study. *Scand J Trauma Resusc Emerg Med*. 2015;23:44.

# Chapter 12

# Managing the Patient with an Extraglottic Device in Place

Darren A. Braude, Michael T. Steuerwald, and Eli Torgeson

## INTRODUCTION

Extraglottic devices (EGDs) are being used increasingly often in emergency settings, especially in the prehospital environment, as many emergency medical service (EMS) companies are promoting them as the principal mode of airway management. Because most EGDs need to be converted to a definitive airway, providers must be comfortable assessing and managing a patient once an EGD is in place, whether placed in the emergency department (ED) or before arrival. An EGD may have been used as a primary airway without prior attempts at intubation or secondarily in the event of a failed intubation, which can have important clinical implications. Hospital-based providers should become familiar with devices used within their agency/institution and by EMS agencies in their catchment area. This should include hands-on practice whenever possible. Intensive care units (ICUs), EDs, and critical care transport agencies should consider keeping samples of devices on hand for rapid reference. In-depth knowledge of the various EGDs in use will improve patient care and facilitate further management.

## MANAGING A PATIENT WITH AN EGD IN PLACE

Although EGDs are not definitive airways—they are not cuffed tubes that exist within the tracheal lumen—they are reliable conduits for oxygenation and ventilation and offer variable degrees of aspiration protection. Therefore, the provider's initial thought process should focus on confirming and optimizing gas exchange rather than on immediate exchange for an endotracheal tube (ETT). Most critically ill or injured patients with an EGD in situ have other competing priorities; if further airway interventions can be safely deferred for even a few minutes, it will allow the provider to address these other issues. We provide **Figure 12-1** to help think through the process.

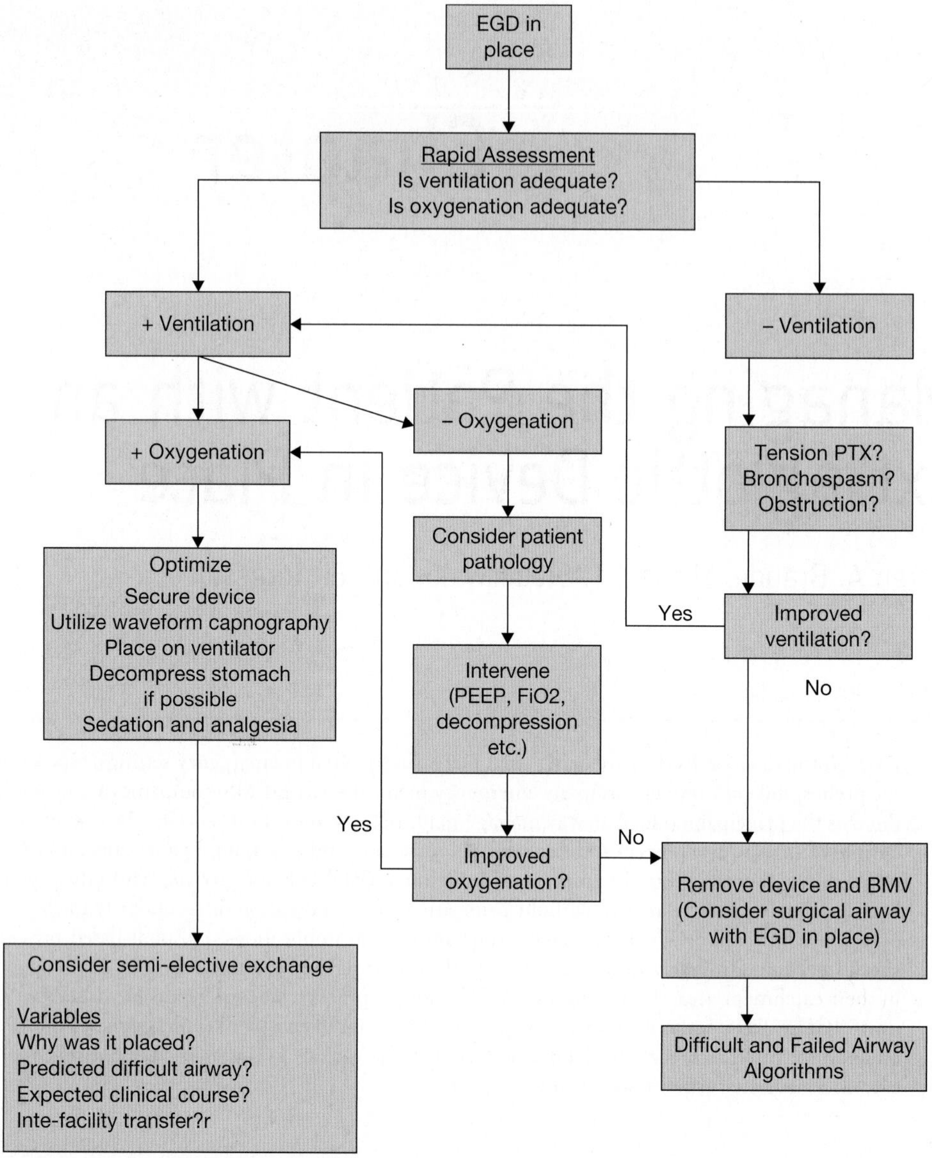


● **FIGURE 12-1. Management Algorithm for an in situ EGD.**

## Assessment

Rapid assessment of gas exchange (both ventilation and oxygenation) should be the first step. Adequate gas exchange is confirmed in the same way as for an ETT. Clinical observations such as breath sounds, chest rise, and gastric distension are important, but waveform capnography is paramount (**Fig. 12-2**). If the provider concludes that ventilation is taking place, then oxygenation should next be considered. Simultaneously, the provider should visually assess whether or not the device appears to be sized correctly and is sitting in a grossly appropriate position, whether or not the pilot balloon pressures seem appropriate (if present), and whether or not a substantial air leak is present. Any correctable issues should be rapidly addressed, such as repositioning the device or adding/removing air from inflatable cuffs. If any major issues that cannot be quickly corrected are present, the device should be removed and rescue bag mask ventilation (BMV) initiated (Chapter 9).

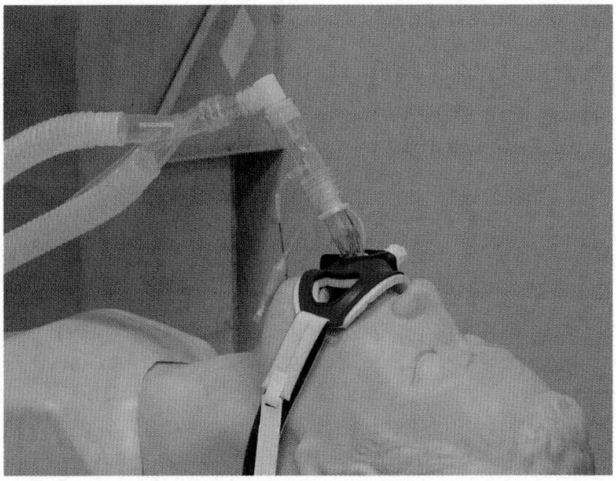

● **FIGURE 12-2.** Ventilator tubing as well as waveform capnography equipment attached to an EGD, specifically the King LTS-D (seated in mannequin). The device has been secured with a commercially available tube holder.

### Optimization

Once general function has been assessed and assured, the provider can focus on optimizing the situation. Ventilators may be employed just as if the patient were intubated. A ventilator will free up hands and assure consistent, lung protective ventilation as appropriate for the patient's condition; tens of thousands of patients are managed in this fashion in the operating room every day. Reassessment for air leak should take place after any changes in ventilator parameters. Patients should receive appropriate analgesia and sedation, and occasionally neuromuscular blockade, just as if they were intubated with an ETT. Patients should be routinely monitored for common complications of any positive pressure ventilation, such as pneumothorax. If not already present, a gastric tube should be inserted if a conduit exists. All "second-generation" EGDs facilitate gastric tube placement, but not all EMS providers that place these devices are allowed to perform gastric decompression or stock the appropriate-sized gastric tubes, especially in pediatrics. Bite blocks should be used for spontaneously breathing patients if the EGD does not have one built-in.

## TROUBLESHOOTING

If ventilation is adequate but oxygenation is poor, hypoxemia is more likely on account of patient pathology than device failure. The provider should seek to intervene by increasing positive end expiratory pressure if not contraindicated, increasing the $FiO_2$, adding sedation and analgesia and possibly neuromuscular blockade, and treating pneumothorax if present. If such maneuvers are successful, semielective exchange can be considered. If such maneuvers are unsuccessful, then the provider should err on the side of rapid exchange to ensure that the device was not contributing to oxygenation failure. An option for this type of exchange is rapid sequence intubation (RSI) with a "double setup" for surgical airway. After induction and neuromuscular blockade, the EGD can be pulled and one best attempt at laryngoscopy made before moving to a cricothyrotomy because rescue with another EGD is assumed to be unreliable. Another option in this situation is to continue ventilating via the EGD to oxygenate as well as possible while performing a surgical airway with the EGD in situ.

If ventilation is inadequate in the setting of a well-sized and positioned EGD, the next task is to determine whether the problem is intrinsic to the patient or the device. Patient issues that can be rapidly corrected include tension pneumothorax, mucus plugging, and bronchospasm. Device issues that may be rapidly addressed include obstructing secretion or blood clots or herniation of the epiglottis into the outlet of the supraglottic airway; both will become apparent and possibly solved with passage of a suction catheter. If these maneuvers improve air movement, then oxygenation can be addressed as described above. If these maneuvers do not improve air movement, the device should be immediately removed, BMV commenced, and definitive airway management performed according to the Difficult and Failed Airway Algorithms (see Chapter 3).

## WHEN TO CONSIDER SEMI-ELECTIVE EXCHANGE

When a device is clearly not working and troubleshooting, as discussed earlier, is unsuccessful, the decision to remove it is easy. However, the decision to remove a functioning EGD (i.e., a semi-elective exchange) is much more challenging. Semi-elective exchange for an ETT is not without risk and is a decision that should not be taken lightly.

The reason the device was initially placed should be considered. If the EGD was placed as a matter of protocol, then a routine airway assessment should be performed using the LEMON, ROMAN, and SMART mnemonics (see Chapter 2). If the EGD was placed by an experienced provider after a failed intubation, then the airway should be considered difficult regardless of other predictors.

The expected clinical course for the patient must also be considered. If the patient requires urgent imaging or a critical procedure, these should not be delayed if the device is functioning and adequate gas exchange is taking place. If the patient has a deteriorating upper airway condition, such as a thermal inhalation injury that is anticipated to eventually preclude EGD functioning, then the EGD should be exchanged as soon as possible. If the patient is headed emergently to the operating room, then it may be reasonable to defer exchange to anesthesia providers. If, on the other hand, the patient is going to the interventional radiology suite or the cardiac catheterization lab, then the threshold to exchange for an ETT should probably be lowered. These are all decisions that should be made in consultation with the providers accepting the patient.

Finally, if the patient is being transferred between institutions, the threshold for intubation is also lowered, although it is very reasonable to transfer a patient with a well-functioning EGD in place if: (1) the exchange is predicted to be difficult; (2) the clinical condition is not likely to change over the course of transport such that the EGD would no longer be expected to provide effective oxygenation and ventilation; and (3) it is expected the device would remain in place no longer than 4 hours, after which the risk of ischemic mucosal injury (even with properly inflated devices) increases. This decision should be made in conjunction with the receiving hospital, transport team, and transport agency medical director whenever possible.

## HOW TO PERFORM A SEMI-ELECTIVE EXCHANGE FOR AN ETT

We strongly discourage rushing to remove an EGD until the airway is thoroughly assessed and device-specific plans can be made. The techniques available for exchange will vary according to the attributes of each device (Table 12-1), available equipment, expertise, and the clinical situation.

### Removal with Routine Intubation via Direct/Video Laryngoscopy

An EGD can always be deflated and removed. This approach may be utilized with any EGD when a difficult airway is not anticipated, patient physiology is favorable, and sufficient equipment for a more secure exchange is not available. It is advisable to decompress the stomach first when possible. The patient should be appropriately sedated and paralyzed as during an RSI procedure. Reinsertion of the same EGD is a consideration if intubation proves difficult or impossible, provided that it was not damaged when removed. Reinsertion does not guarantee success, however, with a number of anecdotes and case reports describing both intubation difficulty and subsequent EGD use after removal.

TABLE 12-1 Attributes of Common EGDs and Selected Exchange Techniques

| Device | Type | Blind Passage of ETT through EGD Lumen | Visualized Passage of ETT through Lumen Using Endoscope or Intubating Stylet | Use of the Aintree Catheter for Exchange |
|---|---|---|---|---|
| Combitube | Dual balloon<br>Dual lumen<br>Retroglottic | Not possible | Not possible | Not possible |
| King Larygneal Tube | Dual balloon<br>Single lumen<br>Retroglottic | Not possible | Not possible | Possible |
| King iLT-D | Dual balloon<br>Single lumen<br>Retroglottic | Possible<br>Reliability not established | Possible | Possible |
| LMA Unique | Supraglottic | Not reliable | Possible | Possible |
| LMA Supreme | Supraglottic | Not possible | Not possible | Difficult |
| LMA Fastrach | Supraglottic | Reliable | Possible (flexible endoscope only) | Possible |
| Intersurgical i-gel | Supraglottic | Not reliable | Possible | Possible |
| CookGas air-Q | Supraglottic | Not reliable | Possible | Possible |
| Ambu AuraGain | Supraglottic | Not reliable | Possible | Possible |

## Working around the Device and Performing Intubation with Direct/ Video Laryngoscopy

This approach is particularly useful in situations where a retroglottic EGD such as the Combitube or King LT is in place. In these cases, leaving the device in place effectively blocks the esophagus, limiting the potential for tube misplacement. Specifically, with the Combitube the proximal balloon may be deflated while the distal balloon is left inflated to minimize regurgitation; with the King LT both balloons must be deflated simultaneously. Because all second-generation EGDs have integrated channels for passage of an orogastric tube, gastric decompression should take place whenever possible before airway manipulation. All of these devices may be swept far to the left side of the mouth to allow for laryngoscopy and tube passage; use of an ETT introducer may be helpful here with either direct or video laryngoscopy because the working space that remains is often tight; use of video laryngoscopy and a bougie has been specifically recommended (**Figs. 12-3A** and **12-3B**). If this strategy proves challenging, the device may either be drawn back partially or removed entirely to allow for more working space or rapidly reinflated to allow for further ventilation and oxygenation.

## Blind Exchange

The only EGD that has proven to reliably and safely facilitate blind intubation without any adjuncts is the LMA Fastrach, using the techniques described in Chapter 10. It may be possible to blindly intubate through other devices such as the Cookgas air-Q, Aura-i, or King iLT-D, but the reported success rates thus far are either lower or not yet known. Another approach to blind intubation through an EGD is to pass a bougie through the device and hope it passes into the trachea. If this passage occurs, as noted by the typical tactile feedback, the EGD may be removed and an ETT railroaded over the bougie in the usual fashion. A major safety concern described in the literature is airway perforation. Therefore, we do not recommend this approach.

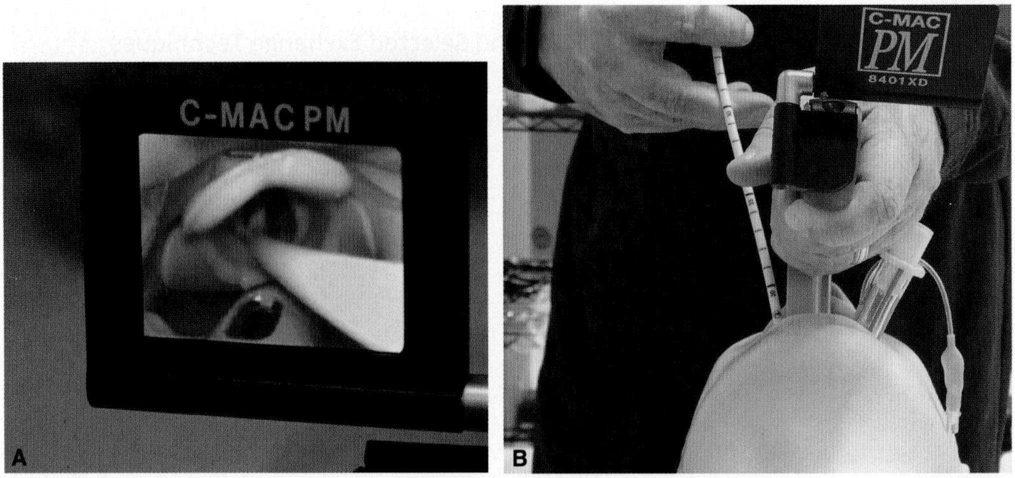


● **FIGURE 12-3. A:** A standard geometry video laryngoscope (Macintosh shape) being used to visualize the glottis while an EGD, specifically the King LTS-D, is in place. **B:** A tracheal tube introducer (e.g., bougie) has been used to access the trachea.

## Endoscopic Exchange

Endoscopic exchange is the ideal approach when the necessary equipment is available. Because such exchanges are usually undertaken only when the EGD is functioning well, the ventilation orifice is likely sitting directly in front of the glottic opening, which makes the procedure simple and highly successful.

Those EGDs that can accommodate an ETT can be simply exchanged once an endoscope or intubating stylet has been used to visualize the trachea. Most of these EGDs indicate the appropriate-sized tube to use directly on the side of the device. We recommend first loading the well-lubricated ETT into the EGD until the cuff is within the lumen, followed by inflating the balloon with just enough air to secure it there (usually about 2 to 3 mL). Ideally, an endoscopic port adapter (i.e., "bronch adapter" or "bronch elbow") will be placed on the end of the ETT during these maneuvers to allow for continuous ventilation and oxygenation while the endoscope is advanced. The lubricated endoscope is then advanced through the ETT and EGD lumen and visually guided into the trachea (**Fig. 12-4**). At this point, the cuff of the ETT can be deflated to permit its passage into the trachea. After the patient has been intubated, the endoscope may be removed. The soon to be available retroglottic "intubating King Airway," the King iLT-D, should be able to accomplish these steps as well.

For those EGDs that do not have a large enough bore to accommodate an ETT, an Aintree Catheter (**Fig. 12-5**) or other airway exchange kit such as the Arndt Airway Exchange Catheter Kit is required. The Aintree catheter is a device that resembles a hollow bougie designed to fit over a flexible pediatric endoscope yet still allowing the scope to exit the distal end and be maneuvered. After this has been done, the scope can be driven down the lumen of the EGD into the airway. After the scope and EGD are carefully removed, the Aintree remains within the trachea and can be used like a bougie to guide an ETT into position. A standard Macintosh laryngoscope should be inserted to displace the tongue forward into the mandibular fossa in order to keep pressure off the Aintree, which can cause it to bend backward in the pharynx and hinder tube passage. Of note, the catheter itself can be used to rescue oxygenate a patient if delay in passing the ETT is encountered. This is done using a custom 15 mm connector (**Fig. 12-6**) that comes with the device and can quickly be attached to its end.

Exchange kits utilize similar principles. The Arndt Airway Exchange Catheter Set works by passing a wire through the working channel of the endoscope to facilitate passage of the catheter overtop after scope removal. This technique is rarely used in the ED.

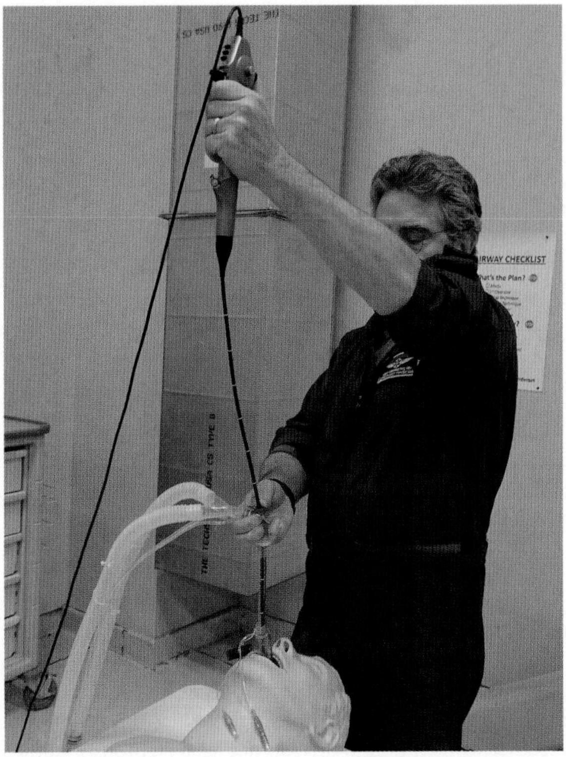

● **FIGURE 12-4.** An ETT has been preloaded into an EGD, namely the Cookgas air-Q, which has been placed in a mannequin; 2 to 3 mL of air was delivered to the ETT cuff to secure it there, and to provide a seal. An endoscopic port adapter is being used to maintain the ventilation circuit. A video endoscope scope is being driven through the port, through the ETT and EGD, and into the trachea with ease while maintaining oxygenation and ventilation. After the trachea has been accessed with the scope, the ETT can simply be advanced over it.

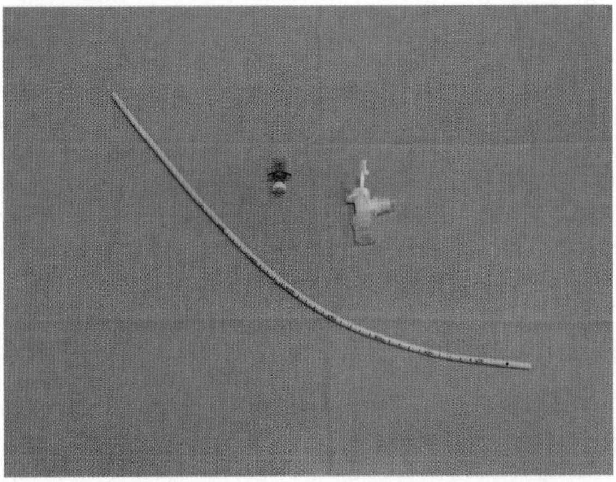

● **FIGURE 12-5. The Aintree Catheter.** Pictured are the catheter, an included endoscopic port adapter, and a specialized 15 mm connector that can be affixed to the end to provide rescue oxygenation.

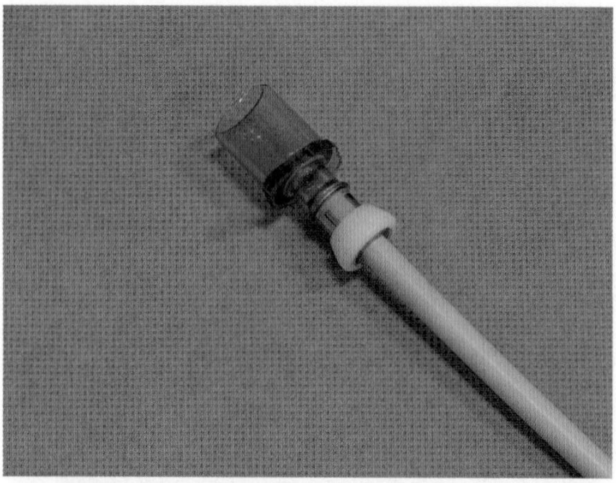

● **FIGURE 12-6. A Specialized 15 mm Connector Attached to the Aintree Catheter.** This can be attached for the provision of rescue oxygenation.

Lastly, if other options do not exist, and the provider has a disposable Ambu A-scope available but not a compatible Aintree Catheter, it is possible to use the A-scope wand "as the bougie." In other words, after the A-scope is driven into the airway under visualization, the wand may be cut from the head with trauma shears (or a large pocket knife) and used as a bougie; the wand is disposable, and there is no power running through it. Once this is done, the capability for further visualization is of course lost. Although this has not been rigorously studied, it has been successful in our experience in a limited number of cases, but challenging because we have found the wand to be short and not as stiff as most modern tracheal tube introducers.

## Removal after Intubation

Removal of an EGD after an ETT has been passed through its lumen is anxiety provoking and introduces the risk of accidentally extubating the patient. It is our prediction that this is why some providers prefer an Aintree Catheter to other methods, even though its use may require more specialized steps.

If this exchange was performed in the setting of a predicted difficult airway, it is our recommendation that any inflatable cuffs on the EGD be deflated, and the device left in place until additional resources are available, which may require transfer to the ICU, operating room, or another facility. If, for some other reason, it is deemed imperative to remove the EGD after it has been used as a conduit for intubation, the central tenet of the removal is simply to maintain the position of the ETT regardless of what other maneuvers are being made. Commercially produced tube exchange devices are available for the LMA Fastrach and the Cookgas air-Q. If a commercially available device is not available, a smaller ETT can be used to "extend" the length of the ETT already in place, making it possible to keep a hold on it (**Fig. 12-7**). Making sure that the pilot balloon of the ETT does not become pinned inside the EGD by the tube exchange device or second ETT is imperative.

## Surgical Airway

The final means of "exchange" is to perform a surgical airway while continuing to ventilate through the EGD. This is a reasonable approach when the EGD is providing some degree of oxygenation, very difficult intubating conditions are expected, and the time, equipment, and/or expertise for an endoscopic exchange is not available (or a device such as a Combitube that does not permit endoscopic passage is in situ). Although high-level evidence for this approach is lacking, it intuitively makes sense, and the authors have utilized this approach under rare circumstances and found it to be very effective.

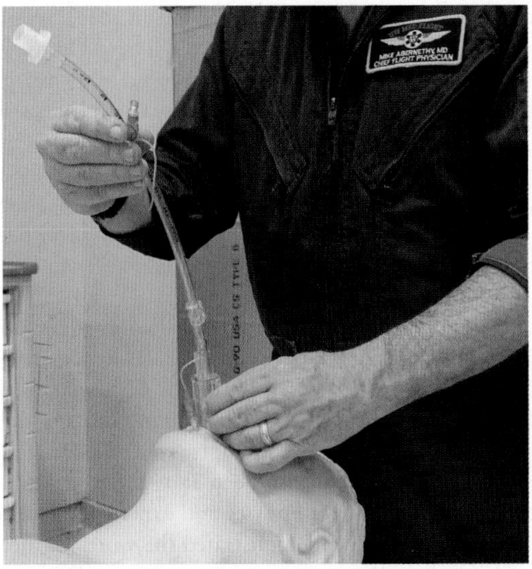


● **FIGURE 12-7.** A size 7.0 ID ETT being "extended" by a size 6.5 ID ETT.

## CAN A PATIENT BE PRONOUNCED DEAD WITH AN EGD IN PLACE?

The question often arises regarding whether or not it is permissible to pronounce a patient in cardiac arrest dead after cardiopulmonary resuscitation if the airway management strategy during the care has been done entirely with an EGD, or, alternatively, if a "gold standard" ETT must be placed first. The authors suggest that as long as the EGD is ventilating the patient, it is a very reasonable decision to not exchange the device for an ETT before terminating resuscitative efforts if they are deemed futile.

## EVIDENCE

- **Have paradigm shifts in prehospital care led to more patients presenting to EDs with EGDs in place?** There has been a prehospital airway management practice shift in many communities over the past 10 years de-emphasizing endotracheal intubation, especially for patients in cardiac arrest. Many EMS providers now place EGDs as their initial airway strategy, whereas in other communities EGDs are utilized as back-up devices, although the threshold for moving to a back-up has dropped considerably.[1,2] Thus, emergency physicians (EPs) are likely to manage patients who arrive with an EGD in place. This can pose a challenge if the EGD is not functioning appropriately or the EP is not familiar with the device itself.
- **Is the traditional role of the EGD expanding in ED patients?** The traditional role of the EGD in EMS was to "rescue" failed intubation. This traditional role was later extended to allow providers not trained in ETI to obtain a "more advanced" and "more efficacious" airway than using BMV alone. These roles have yet again been further extended in many EMS systems to include primary use in out-of-hospital cardiac arrest situations. In advanced prehospital care systems and in the ED, primary use of EGDs in medication-facilitated airway management, termed Rapid Sequence Airway (RSA), has also been advocated by some authors and is used by some EMS systems.[3] EGDs designed to facilitate intubation may be placed in the ED to manage difficult and failed airway situations, often averting surgical airway placement. The effect of video laryngoscopy on the need for EGD rescue is unclear. EGDs may also be placed to assist with preoxygenation, potentially as part of an RSA.[4,5]

- **How long can a functioning EGD safely be left in place?** Authors have reported use of the LMA-Supreme without complication for 9 hours.[3] On the other hand, complications with some other similar devices have been reported after much less time.[6] In a report by Gaither et al., massive tongue engorgement was noted after a King LTS-D was in place for 3 hours.[7] Although experience is limited, and there are likely differences in tolerability between devices, it would seem reasonable to leave most EGDs in place for no more than 4 hours if that time facilitates transfer for, or arrival of, consultants to assist with exchange in a predicted very difficult airway. This duration can likely be longer if the device is deflated after having been used as an intubation conduit, but this has not been extensively evaluated to our knowledge.
- **Is an endoscopic exchange of EGDs for ETTs superior to the blind approach when all the necessary equipment is available?** Several studies have demonstrated the viability of visualized exchange, while the only EGD that has proven to reliably and safely facilitate blind intubation is the LMA Fastrach: the first pass success rate utilizing the recommended technique is over 90%, and success within three attempts is over 97%, regardless of obesity, secretions, or cervical precautions.[8–18] It has also been shown that visualized endoscopic exchange through an EGD is a skill that both novice and expert providers can perform at an equally high level.[19] Several studies have demonstrated the worth of the Aintree Catheter in EGD exchange procedures.[20–25] The worth of the Arndt Airway Exchange Catheter Set to maintain airway control during exchange of an EGD, specifically the King LT, for an ETT has also been documented.[26] Lastly, if an endoscope is not available, authors have demonstrated that a retroglottic EGD can be "intubated around" using a standard geometry video laryngoscope and a tracheal tube introducer.[27]
- **Is blind passage of an ETT introducer, such as a bougie, through an EGD recommended?** The question of safety exists as airway perforation was noted in a cadaver study examining this procedure through a King LT. The same risk would be present with any EGD.

## REFERENCES


1. Gahan K, Studnek JR, Vandeventer S. King LT-D use by urban basic life support first responders as the primary airway device for out-of-hospital cardiac arrest. *Resuscitation*. 2011;82:1525–1528.
2. Guyette FX, Greenwood MJ, Neubecker D, et al. Alternate airways in the prehospital setting (resource document to NAEMSP position statement). *Prehosp Emerg Care*. 2007;11(1):56–61.
3. Braude D, Southard A, Bajema T, et al. Rapid sequence airway using the LMA-Supreme as a primary airway for 9 h in a multi-system trauma patient. *Resuscitation*. 2010;81(9):1217.
4. Braude D, Richards M. Rapid Sequence Airway (RSA)—a novel approach to prehospital airway management. *Prehosp Emerg Care*. 2007;11:250–252.
5. Weingart SD, Levitan RM. Preoxygenation and prevention of desaturation during emergency airway management. *Ann Emerg Med*. 2012;59:165–175.
6. Gerstein NS, Braude D, Harding JS, et al. Lingual ischemia from prolonged insertion of a fastrach laryngeal mask airway. *West J Emerg Med*. 2011;12(1):124–127.
7. Gaither JB, Matheson J, Eberhardt A, et al. Tongue engorgement associated with prolonged use of the King LT laryngeal tube device. *Ann Emerg Med*. 2010;55:367–369.
8. Jagannathan N, Roth AG, Sohn LE. The new air-Q intubating laryngeal airway for tracheal intubation in children with anticipated difficult airway: a case series. *Pediatric Anesthesia*. 2009;19:618–622.
9. Kleine-Brueggeney M, Theiler L, Urwyler M, et al. Randomized trial comparing the i-gel and Magill tracheal tube with the single-use ILMA and ILMA tracheal tube for fibreoptic-guided intubation in anaesthetized patients with a predicted difficult airway. *Br J Anaesth*. 2011;107:251–257.

10. Bakker EJ, Valkenburg M, Galvin EM. Pilot study of the air-Q intubating laryngeal airway in clinical use. *Anaesth Intensive Care*. 2010;38:346–348.
11. Joffe AM, Liew EC, Galgon RE, et al. The second-generation air-Q intubating laryngeal mask for airway maintenance during anaesthesia in adults: a report of the first 70 uses. *Anaesth Intensive Care*. 2011;39:40–45.
12. Campbell J, Michalek P, Deighan M. I-gel supraglottic airway for rescue airway management and as a conduit for tracheal intubation in a patient with acute respiratory failure. *Resuscitation*. 2009;80:963.
13. Sharma S, Scott S, Rogers R, et al. The i-gel airway for ventilation and rescue intubation. *Anaesthesia*. 2007;62:419–420.
14. Michalek P, Hodgkinson P, Donaldson W. Fiberoptic intubation through an I-gel supraglottic airway in two patients with predicted difficult airway and intellectual disability. *Anesth Analg*. 2008;106:1501–1504.
15. Gerstein NS, Braude DA, Hung O, et al. The Fastrach Intubating Laryngeal Mask Airway: an overview and update. *Can J Anaesth*. 2010;57(6):588–601.
16. Liu EH, Goy RW, Yvonne Lim Y, et al. Success of tracheal intubation with intubating laryngeal mask airways: a randomized trial of the LMA Fastrach(tm) and LMA CTrach(tm). *Anesthesiology*. 2008;108:621–626.
17. Erlacher W, Tiefenbrunner H, Kastenbauer T. CobraPLUS and Cookgas air-Q versus Fastrach for blind endotracheal intubation: a randomized controlled trial. *Eur J Anaesthesiol*. 2011;28:181–186.
18. Karim YM, Swanson DE. Comparison of blind tracheal intubation through the intubating laryngeal mask airway (LMA Fastrach) and the Air-Q. *Anesthesia*. 2011;66:185–190.
19. Hodzovic I, Janakiraman C, Sudhir G, et al. Fibreoptic intubation through the laryngeal mask airway: effect of operator experience. *Anesthesia*. 2009;64:1066–1071.
20. Zura A, Doyle DJ, Orlandi M. Use of the Aintree intubation catheter in a patient with an expected difficult airway. *Can J Anaesthesia*. 2005;52:646–649.
21. Higgs A, Clark E, Premraj K. Low-skill fibreoptic intubation: use of the Aintree catheter with the Classic LMA. *Anaesthesia*. 2005;60:915–920.
22. Cook TM, Silsby J, Simpson TP. Airway rescue in acute upper airway obstruction using a Proseal Laryngeal mask airway and an Aintree catheter: a review of the ProSeal laryngeal mask airway in the management of the difficult airway. *Anaesthesia*. 2005;60:1129–1136.
23. Cook TM, Bigwood B, Cranshaw J. Complications of transtracheal jet ventilation and use of the Aintree Intubating Catheter for airway rescue. *Anaesthesia*. 2006;61:692–697.
24. Blair EJ, Mihai R, Cook TM. Tracheal intubation via the Classic and Proseal laryngeal mask airways: a manikin study using the Aintree Intubating Catheter. *Anaesthesia*. 2007;62:385–387.
25. Galgon RE, Joffe AM, Willman K, et al. Fiberoptic, wire guided king laryngeal tube exchange in trauma patients: a case series. *JACS*. 2012; doi:10.7243/2049-9752-1-15, www.hoajonline.com (open access).
26. Klein L, Paetow G, Kornas R, et al. Technique for exchanging the king laryngeal tube for an endotracheal tube. *Acad Emerg Med*. 2016;23:e2.
27. Lutes M, Worman DJ. An unanticipated complication of a novel approach to airway management. *J Emer Med*. 2010;38(2):222–224.

# Section IV

# Tracheal Intubation

Chapter 13

# Direct Laryngoscopy

Robert F. Reardon and Steven C. Carleton

## DIRECT LARYNGOSCOPY

Although video laryngoscopy (VL) has become the device of choice for many emergency physicians, direct laryngoscopy (DL) is still a common technique for tracheal intubation in the emergency setting. In experienced hands, DL has a high success rate, and the equipment is inexpensive, reliable, and widely available. However, DL requires significant experience to gain proficiency and has inherent limitations that manifest when factors such as decreased cervical mobility, a large tongue, a receding chin, or prominent incisors are present.

## BASICS OF DIRECT LARYNGOSCOPY

The concept of DL is simple—to create a straight line of sight from the mouth to the larynx in order to visualize the vocal cords. The tongue is the greatest obstacle to laryngoscopy. The laryngoscope is used to control the tongue and displace it out of the line of sight. A laryngoscope consists of a handle, a blade, and a light source. It is used as a left-handed instrument regardless of the operator's handedness. In general, DL blades are either curved (Macintosh) or straight (Miller) (**Fig. 13-1**). Both blades come in a variety of sizes from newborn to large adult, and sizes 3 and 4 are commonly used in adults. Macintosh blades have a gentle curve, a vertical flange for displacing the tongue, and a relatively wide square tip with an obvious knob. Variations of the original Macintosh blade design, which include a smaller vertical flange and a shorter light-to-tip distance, have also been manufactured. The vertical flange height of the size 3 and 4 blades is similar, making it reasonable to start with the longer size 4 blade in all adults. Curved blades are intended to be advanced into the vallecula, and when the knob on the tip makes contact and depresses the hyoepiglottic ligament, the epiglottis elevates, exposing the vocal cords (**Fig. 13-2**).

Miller blades have a narrower and shorter flange and a slightly curved tip without a knob. The smaller flange may be advantageous when there is less mouth opening, but makes tongue control more difficult and decreases the area of displacement for visualization and tube placement. Size 3 and 4 Miller blades are nearly identical except for length, so it may be reasonable to start with the longer size 4 blade in most adults. Miller blades are intended to be passed posterior to the epiglottis, to lift it directly in order to expose the vocal cords (**Fig. 13-3**). Most operators prefer the curved Macintosh blade because it is wider and allows better control of the tongue; however, the straight

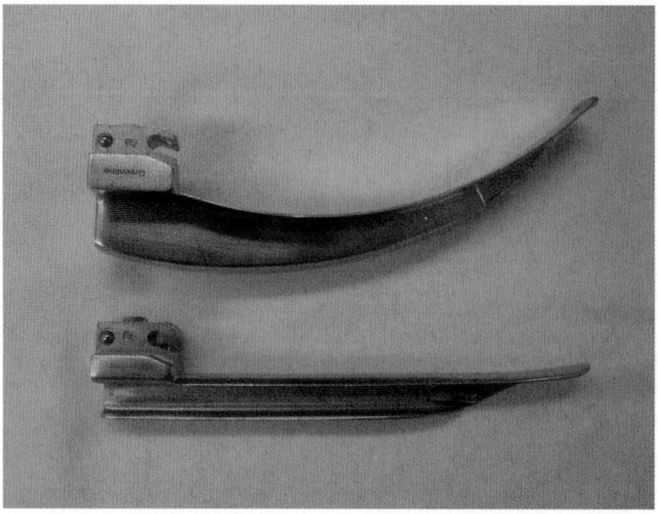

● **FIGURE 13-1. Macintosh (top) and Miller (bottom) Laryngoscope Blades.** The curved blade is a size 4 German Macintosh, which is a good blade for routine use in adults, unlike the American design, which has a taller flange height. The straight blade is a size 3 Miller, for normal sized adults. Most Miller blades have the light on the left side (as shown here), which can embed in the tongue, but better designs place the light on the right side of the blade.

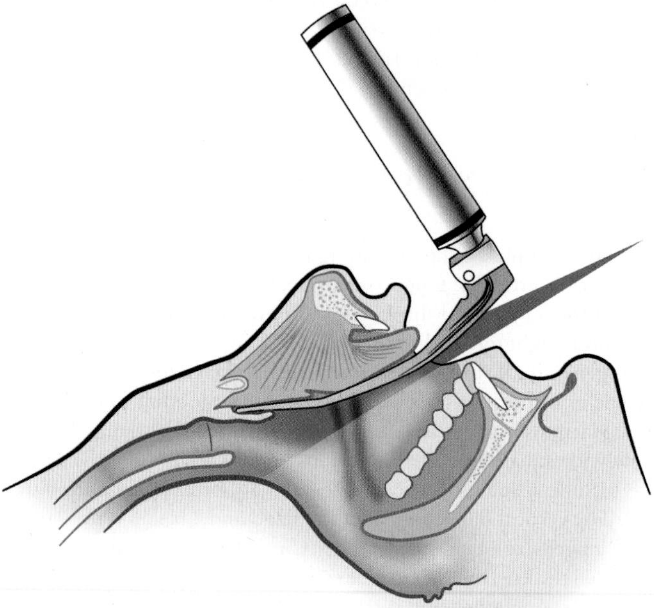

● **FIGURE 13-2. Direct Laryngoscopy with a Macintosh Blade.** Note that the tip of the blade is properly placed into the base of the vallecula and elevates the epiglottis by pushing against the hyoepiglottic ligament.

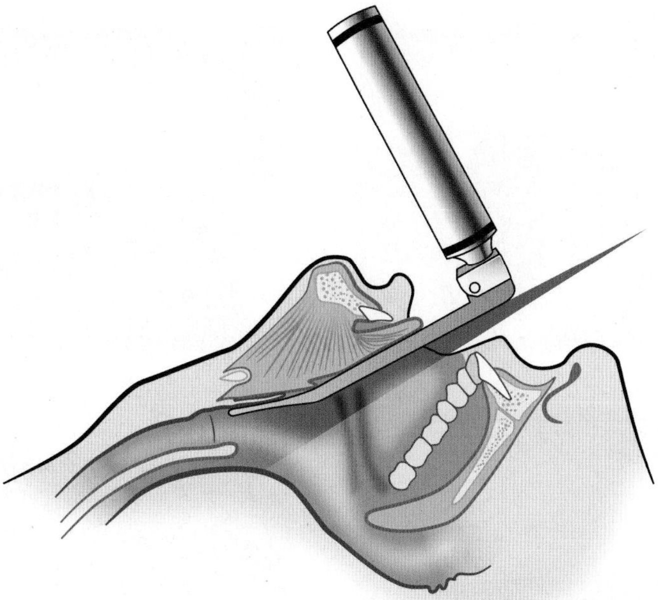

● **FIGURE 13-3. Direct Laryngoscopy with a Miller Blade.** The tip of the blade is used to lift the epiglottis directly.

Miller blade may provide better visualization of the glottis when there is limited cervical movement, prominent upper incisors, a large tongue, limited mouth opening, or a large and floppy epiglottis, so it is important to master both techniques.

## ANATOMY FOR DIRECT LARYNGOSCOPY

Recognition of anatomic landmarks is critical to DL success (see **Figs. 13-4**). For laryngoscopy, the most important laryngeal structures are the epiglottis, the posterior arytenoid cartilages, interarytenoid notch, and the vocal cords. Tracheal intubation is accomplished by passing the endotracheal tube (ETT) through the vocal cords. Success is more likely if the vocal cords are well visualized and a near certainty if a full view is obtained; however, tracheal intubation does not always require visualization of the vocal cords. If only the posterior cartilages are visible, the tube can be passed anterior to these structures in the midline and will usually enter the trachea (**Fig. 13-4B**). Furthermore, intubation can often be accomplished when the only visible structure is the epiglottis (**Fig. 13-4C**), especially if an ETT introducer (ETI or "bougie") is used. If the epiglottis cannot be identified, the likelihood of successful tracheal intubation is very low (**Fig. 13-4D**).

## PREPARATION AND ASSISTANCE

Before embarking on the intubation attempt, the airway manager must ensure that the following are available:

- Established IV and monitoring systems.
- Oxygen saturation and cardiac monitoring.
- All required equipment and medications.

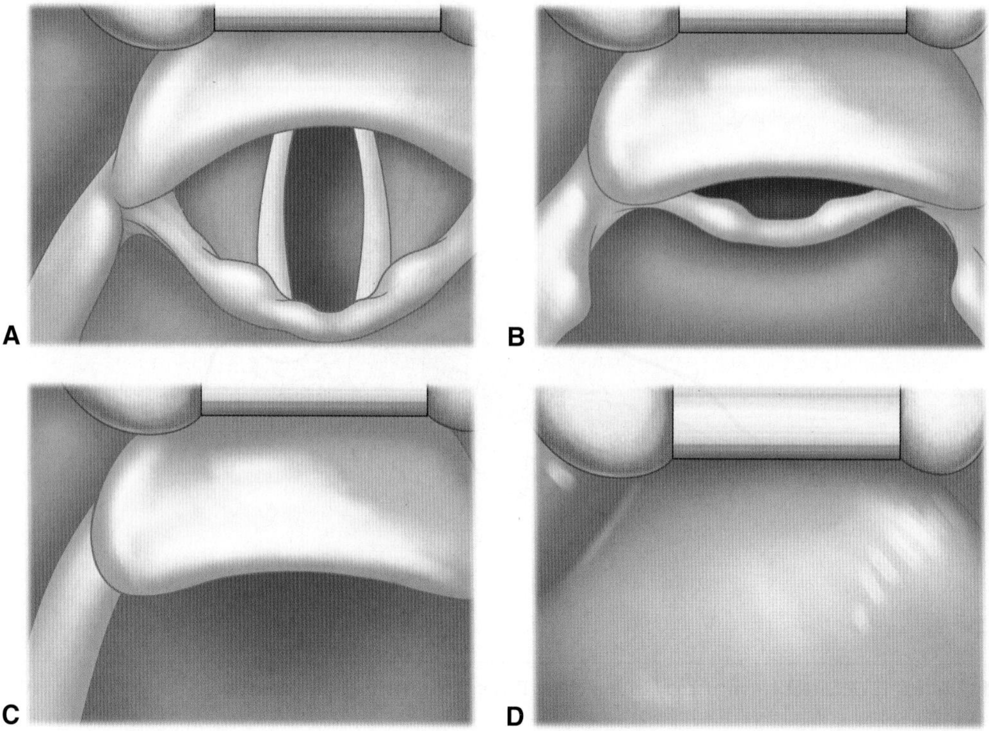


● **FIGURE 13-4. Laryngoscopic Views (Correlating with the Cormack-Lehane system).** **A:** Full view of the vocal cords (grade 1). **B:** Only the posterior glottic structures/cartilages are visible (grade 2). **C:** Only the epiglottis is visible (grade 3). **D:** Neither the epiglottis nor the glottic structures are visible, only the soft palate (grade 4).

- Laryngoscope blade and handle, ETT and backup ETT of a smaller size, 10 mL syringe, lubrication, working suction, and rapid sequence intubation drugs.
- ETI (disposable or reusable bougie, see page 150).
- Adequate suction.
- Trained assistant standing on the patient's right.

The assistant should be prepared to do the following:

- Pass equipment as needed to the airway manager.
- Hold the head in a position as stipulated.
- Perform laryngeal manipulation as instructed.
- Retract the corner of the mouth during intubation.

## PREINTUBATION ASSESSMENT AND EQUIPMENT CHOICE

Preintubation assessment of the patient's airway is essential and must, when time allows, be performed on every patient before administration of neuromuscular blockers. In the mnemonic LEMON, discussed in Chapter 2, the *M* stands for Mallampati, serving as a reminder to examine the oral cavity to assess the relative size of the tongue in relationship to the oropharynx and the mandibular space (see Chapters 2 and 4). The laryngoscope blade is the tool that controls and maneuvers the tongue. Fundamental to successful laryngoscopy is blade selection, curved or straight, that will be wide and long enough to capture the tongue during laryngoscopy, sweep it leftward and then forward into the mandibular space out of the visual field, and permit direct visualization of the airway. The larger flange of the curved Macintosh blade usually provides better tongue control than the thinner blade of the straight Miller blade. Many operators prefer a size 4 Macintosh blade for most emergency airways to assure adequate blade length. However, choice of a laryngoscope blade and the technique used to facilitate intubation is best guided by personal choice and experience. The literature suggests that straight blades improve laryngoscopic view (increased exposure of the vocal cords), whereas curved blades provide better intubating conditions (continuous visualization of the vocal cords during ETT passage). Using an ETI (bougie) improves intubation success rates with the straight-blade technique.

## HANDLING THE LARYNGOSCOPE AND POSTURE OF THE OPERATOR

The laryngoscope should be held low on the handle, so the proximal end of the blade pushes into the thenar or hypothenar eminence of the left hand. This grip will encourage lifting from the shoulder, keeping the elbow low, and keeping the wrist stiff during laryngoscopy. The operator should be in an upright position with his or her arms and hands at a comfortable working height, rather than stooping or straining to reach the patient. The patient's bed should be elevated and the operator should step back from the patient so that his or her back is relatively straight during laryngoscopy.

## PATIENT POSITIONING

Optimal head and neck positioning for DL is often described as the "sniffing position": lower cervical flexion and atlanto-occipital extension. The sniffing position attempts to align the oral, pharyngeal, and laryngeal axes of the upper airway (**Fig. 13-5**). Absent contraindications, alignment of these axes is important for optimizing the laryngoscopic view. The optimal degree of lower cervical flexion brings the external auditory meatus to the level of the sternal notch or anterior surface of the shoulder. In adult patients of normal body habitus, a 4 to 6 cm pad beneath the occiput usually suffices for this purpose. Alternatively, the operator can extend and lift the head with his or her right hand during laryngoscopy to determine the optimal position empirically. The head can then be supported by an assistant standing on the right side of the patient while the operator intubates or performs external laryngeal manipulation. In morbidly obese patients, optimal positioning will often require a ramp to be constructed from linens or pads placed beneath the upper torso, shoulders, neck, and occiput in order to align the ear canal with the sternal angle of Louis (see **Fig. 40-1**). Airway ramps are also commercially available for this purpose. In small children with a protuberant occiput, the torso may need to be raised to allow the external meatus to fall back to the desired plane (see **Fig. 25-2**). Because of individual variations in anatomy, the optimal head and neck position is often unpredictable, and may require empiric adjustment during the intubation attempt. It is critically important that some means of adjusting the patient's position be available before initiating the procedure. Understanding optimal head and neck positioning will help operators appreciate the difficulty of performing DL on trauma patients and others who must be intubated in a fixed position.

## STANDARD DIRECT LARYNGOSCOPY TECHNIQUE

This is the standard technique used with both curved and straight blades.

- Open the mouth as widely as possible.
- Insert the blade in the right lingual gutter along the inside of the mandibular molars and sweep the tongue to the left.

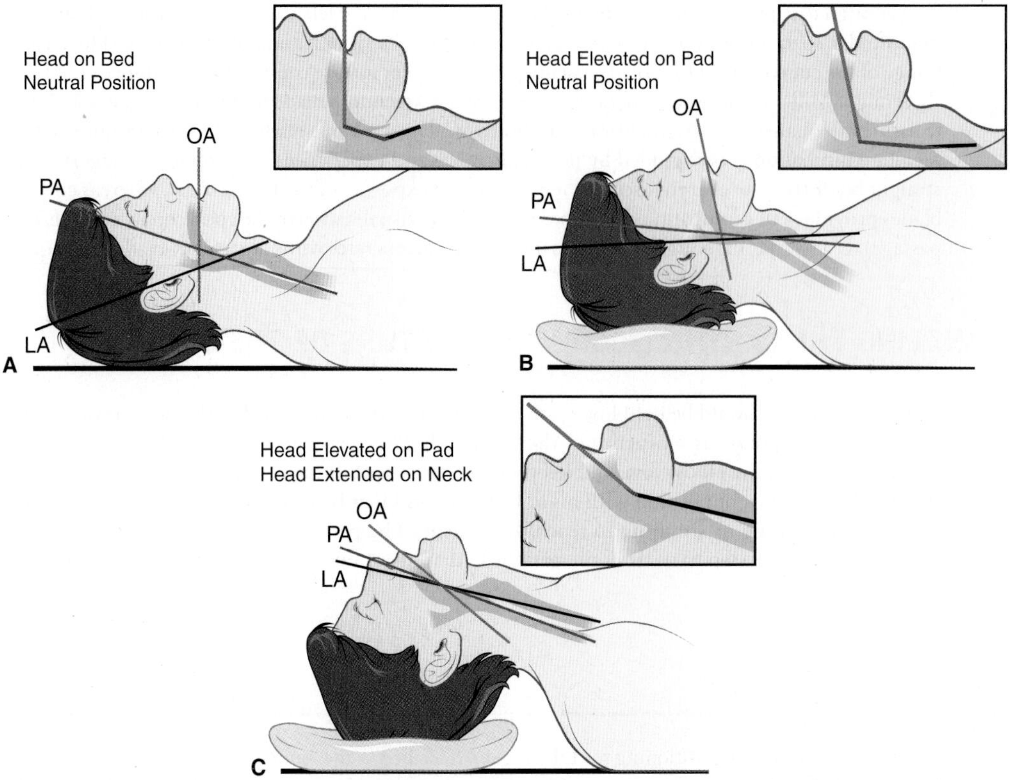


● **FIGURE 13-5.** **A:** Anatomical neutral position. The oral axis (OA), pharyngeal axis (PA), and laryngeal axis (LA) are not aligned. **B:** Head, still in neutral position, has been lifted by a pillow flexing the lower cervical spine and aligning the PA and LA. **C:** The head has been extended on the cervical spine, aligning the OA with the PA and LA, creating the optimum sniffing position for intubation.

- Use a "look as you go" approach—that is, advance the tip of the blade down the tongue in a careful step-by-step manner, lifting intermittently to ascertain the location of the tip in relation to anatomic structures, until the epiglottis is located. The epiglottis is the main anatomic landmark because the glottis can be consistently found just posterior and inferior to it.
- Lift the epiglottis. When using the curved blade, displace the epiglottis indirectly by pressing against the hyoepiglottic ligament at the base of the vallecula (**Figs. 13-2** and **13-6**). When using the straight blade, lift the epiglottis directly with the tip of the blade (**Figs. 13-3** and **13-7**).
- Identify the posterior cartilages and interarytenoid notch. These structures make up the posterior border of the glottis and separate the tracheal inlet from the esophagus. Tracheal intubation can be accomplished by passing the tube anterior to these structures, even when the vocal cords cannot be seen.
- Visualize the vocal cords, if possible.
- Pass the tube through the vocal cords and into the trachea.

## PARAGLOSSAL (RETROMOLAR) STRAIGHT-BLADE TECHNIQUE

This is an alternative technique that may be useful when standard DL is unexpectedly difficult because of prominent upper incisors, a large tongue, or limited mouth opening.

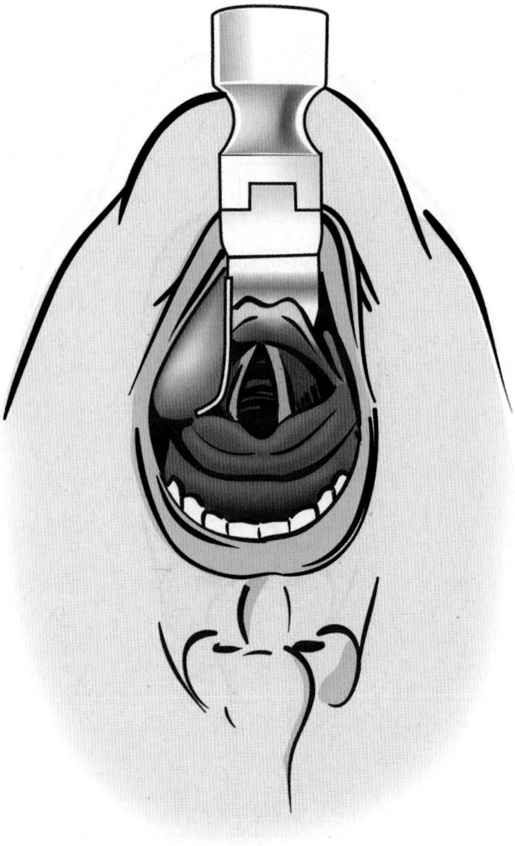

● **FIGURE 13-6. Direct Laryngoscopy with a Macintosh Blade.** The mouth is opened wide, and the tongue is well controlled and kept entirely to the left by the large flange of the Macintosh blade. The epiglottis is visualized, and the tip of the blade is pushed into the vallecula to elevate the epiglottis and expose the vocal cords. Force is applied by lifting the entire blade upward, not by tilting the butt of the blade toward the upper incisors.

- Insert the Miller blade into the right corner of the mouth.
- Pass the blade along the groove between the tongue and the tonsil.
- Sweep the tongue to the left and maintain it to the left of the blade.
- Advance the tip of the blade toward the midline, keeping the back of the blade to the right side of the mouth adjacent to the molars (**Fig. 13-8**).
- Identify the epiglottis and lift its tip to expose the vocal cords.
- Have an assistant retract the right corner of the mouth.
- Pass the tube through the vocal cords and into the trachea. Often, one needs to use an ETI (bougie) down the channel of the scope with this approach because of limited space preventing ETT advancement. The ETI was specifically designed for this purpose.

## BLIND INSERTION TECHNIQUE FOR THE STRAIGHT BLADE

This is an alternative technique often used in neonates, infants, and small children using a straight blade, or in adults when other techniques are predicted to be difficult or have failed. There are two phases to this method: (1) blind insertion of the tip of the laryngoscope blade beyond the glottic

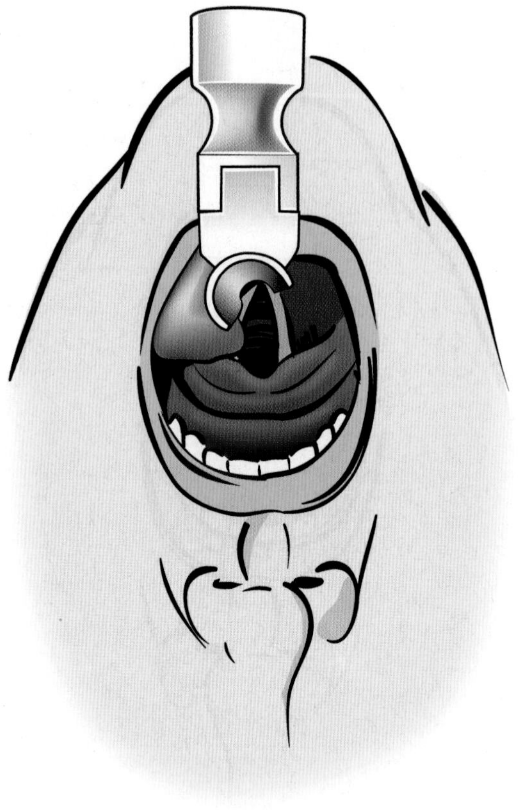

● **FIGURE 13-7. Direct Laryngoscopy with a Miller Blade.** The mouth is opened wide, and the tongue is difficult to control with the small flange of the Miller blade, but it is kept entirely to the left. The epiglottis is identified and then lifted with the tip of the blade (so it is no longer visible here) to expose the vocal cords. Force is applied by lifting the entire blade upward, not by tilting the butt of the blade toward the upper incisors.

inlet and into the esophagus, and (2) visualization of the glottis during withdrawal. The potential for esophageal and tracheal injury or regurgitation resulting from opening the upper esophageal sphincter during blind insertion of the blade has not been studied.

- Place the blade into the right side of the mouth and maintain the tongue to the left.
- Hold the laryngoscope with the fingertips and gently advance the entire length of the blade blindly toward the midline, past the base of the tongue, posterior to the glottis, and into the proximal esophagus. If there is any resistance, stop and withdraw slightly, then realign and advance completely.
- While looking into the airway, lift the blade and then slowly and deliberately withdraw until the glottis drops down into view. If the epiglottis also drops into view, lift it with the tip of the blade to expose the vocal cords.
- Pass the tube through the vocal cords and into the trachea.

## INTUBATING THE TRACHEA

If the glottis is directly visualized, it is usually easy to pass a tube into the trachea. However, even with excellent glottic exposure, it is possible to block the line of sight with the ETT during the intubation

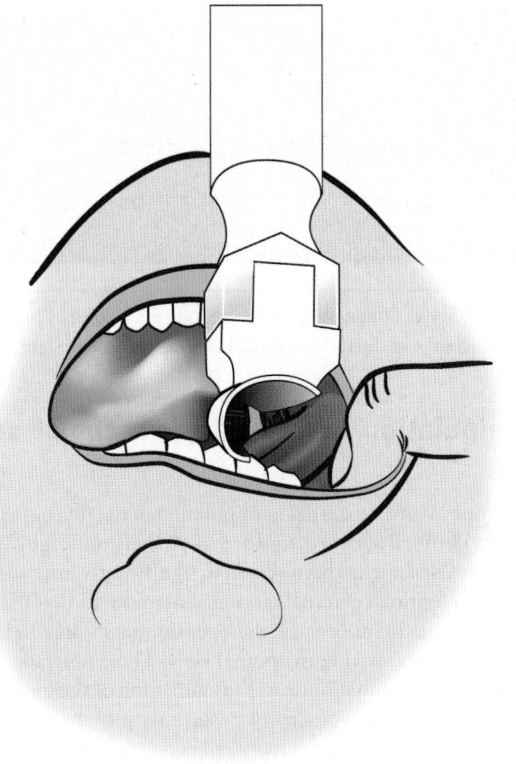

● **FIGURE 13-8. Paraglossal (Retromolar) Straight-Blade Technique.** The Miller blade enters the right corner of the mouth, and the tip advances toward the midline while the proximal blade remains in the right side of the mouth. Note that the tongue is entirely to the left of the blade. This technique may improve glottic visualization in difficult situations but does not leave much room for passage of the ETT. Have an assistant retract the lip to create more room as shown.

attempt. This possibility can be minimized by inserting the tube from the extreme right-hand corner of the mouth while an assistant retracts the lip, and by keeping the tube below the line of sight while advancing it toward the glottis, raising it over the posterior landmarks only during the terminal phase of insertion. Tube shape can also influence the ease of visualization during intubation. Using a malleable stylet to produce a straight tube with a single "hockey stick" bend of <35° just proximal to the balloon facilitates cord visualization during passage, by keeping the tube out of the line of sight until it passes the cords (**Fig. 13-9**). As the tube approaches the depth of the glottis, it is raised up over the posterior landmarks and passed through the vocal cords. A banana-shaped tube tends to cross the visual axis twice in the course of insertion and may interfere with visual guidance during placement.

## TROUBLESHOOTING DIFFICULT DIRECT LARYNGOSCOPY

### Paralysis

Neuromuscular blockade greatly facilitates DL. The reflexes and muscle tone of the upper airway are difficult to overcome in patients who are sedated but not paralyzed. Airway managers should understand the indications for, and use of, neuromuscular blocking agents (see Chapters 2, 3, and 22).

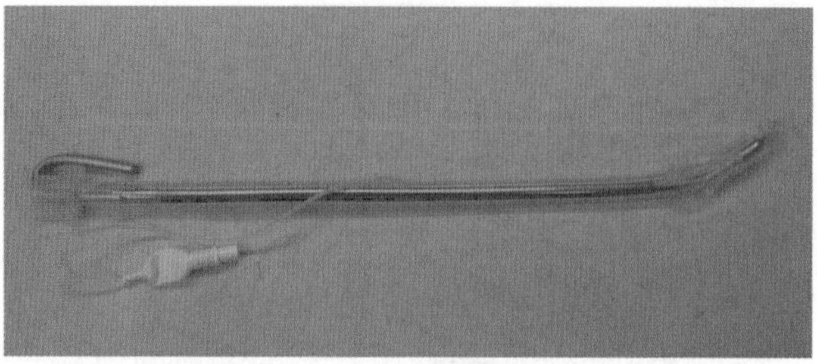

● **FIGURE 13-9. Optimal ETT/Stylet Shape.** A relatively straight ETT with a "hockey stick" shape, with a bend angle <35°. This shape allows passage of the ETT without blocking the line of sight.

## External Manipulation by the Laryngoscopist versus an Assistant or Instructor

Bimanual laryngoscopy involves external manipulation of the thyroid cartilage with the laryngoscopist's right hand (**Fig. 13-10**). Backward, upward (cephalad), and rightward pressure (BURP) on the thyroid cartilage, by an assistant, has been shown to significantly improve glottic visualization during laryngoscopy. However, optimal external laryngeal manipulation (OELM) by the laryngoscopist is better than BURP by an assistant because the operator gets immediate feedback and can quickly determine which movements provide an optimal view. These movements might include BURP, but can also involve any movement that improves visualization of the glottis. Firm downward pressure on the thyroid cartilage moves the vocal cords posteriorly into the line of sight of the laryngoscopist. Also, during curved blade laryngoscopy, downward pressure on the thyroid cartilage helps to drive the

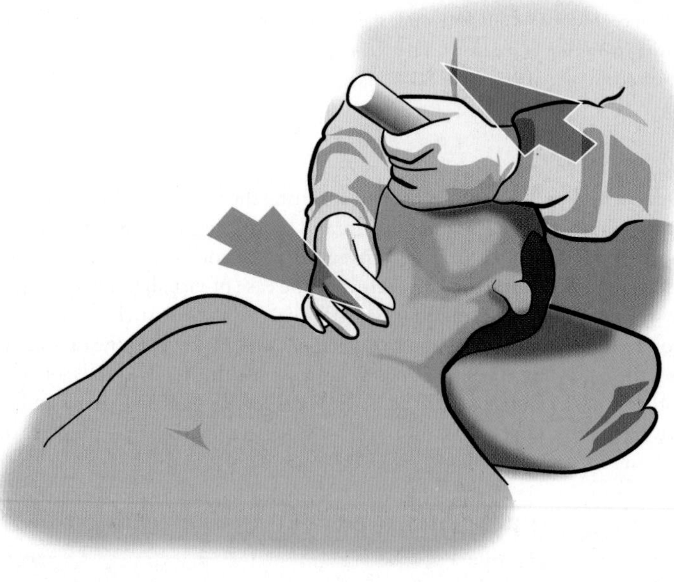

● **FIGURE 13-10. Bimanual Laryngoscopy.** The laryngoscopist uses his/her right hand to manipulate the thyroid cartilage. Optimal external manipulation often involves firm pressure on the thyroid cartilage and movement to the right (backward, upward [cephalad], and rightward pressure). The advantage of the laryngoscopist performing this maneuver (not an assistant) is that he/she gets immediate visual feedback and can quickly determine what constitutes *optimal* external manipulation.

tip of the laryngoscope into the hyoepiglottic ligament, further lifting the epiglottis out of the visual axis. When the laryngoscopist finds the best view, an assistant can hold the thyroid cartilage in the optimal position while the ETT is placed. Bimanual laryngoscopy should not be confused with cricoid pressure (Sellick's maneuver), which is performed during BMV to avoid regurgitation. In teaching situations, it may beneficial for an instructor to apply external manipulation (downward pressure on the thyroid cartilage) and/or perform a mandibular advancement (jaw thrust) maneuver to help the operator obtain the best laryngeal view during DL. Using a device that allows simultaneous DL and VL, like the C-MAC, or the GlideScope teaching blade, allows an assistant or instructor to help optimize the laryngeal view. This is especially important in teaching institutions where relatively inexperienced operators may be intubating critically ill or injured patients while still learning the finer points of DL (see Evidence section).

## Endotracheal Tube Introducer

An ETI or bougie is a simple, inexpensive adjunct that can improve intubation success when visualization of the glottis is difficult (**Fig. 13-11**). It is most helpful when the epiglottis is visualized, but the vocal cords and posterior cartilages cannot be seen. The ETI is a long (60 cm), narrow (5 mm), flexible plastic (SunMed Bougie, Largo, FL) or spun nylon (Eschmann Bougie/Guide, Smiths Medical-Portex, St. Paul, MN) device with a fixed 40° bend at the distal end (Coudé tip). Insertion is often facilitated by making a 60° anterior bend approximately 10 to 15 cm from the distal tip (**Fig. 13-11**, inset). The ETI is held with the tip pointing upward. Under visual guidance with a laryngoscope, it is passed just under the epiglottis and upward into the tracheal inlet (**Fig. 13-12**). Tracheal placement results in palpable vibrations of the introducer as the Coudé tip bumps against the tracheal rings during insertion. Alternatively, tracheal placement can be confirmed by a hard stop at about 40 cm of insertion. Placement in the esophagus provides no such hard stop. The ETT is placed over the ETI by an assistant until the proximal end of the ETI is grasped while the operator keeps the laryngoscope in place, continuing to displace the tongue into the mandibular fossa. This is a critical, and often neglected, point. The operator then passes the ETT distally. As the tip of the

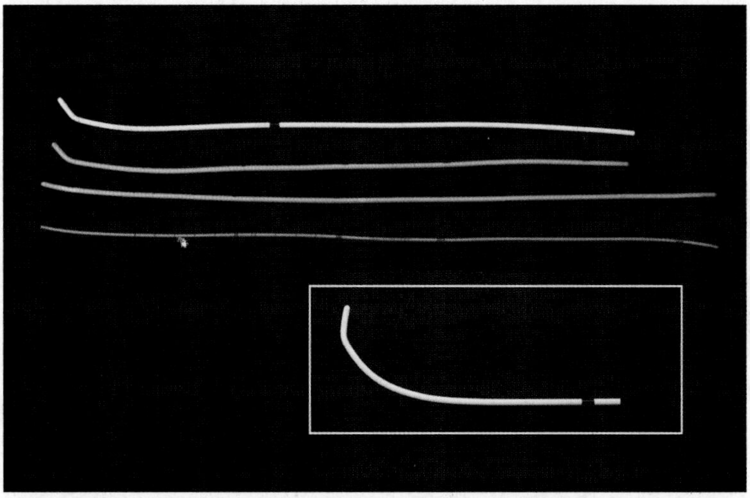

● **FIGURE 13-11. Endotracheal Tube Introducers (Bougies).** The classic gum elastic bougies (yellow) are reusable, 60 to 70 cm long, and available with straight and Coudé tip designs. A reusable (blue) polyethylene introducer is available with a Coudé tip and is 60 cm in length. Adult tracheal tube introducers are 5 mm in diameter. A thinner pediatric introducer can accommodate a 4.0-mm ETT. The lower right inset demonstrates the 60° optimal curve for attempting intubation when none of the glottic structures (only the epiglottis) can be visualized with laryngoscopy.

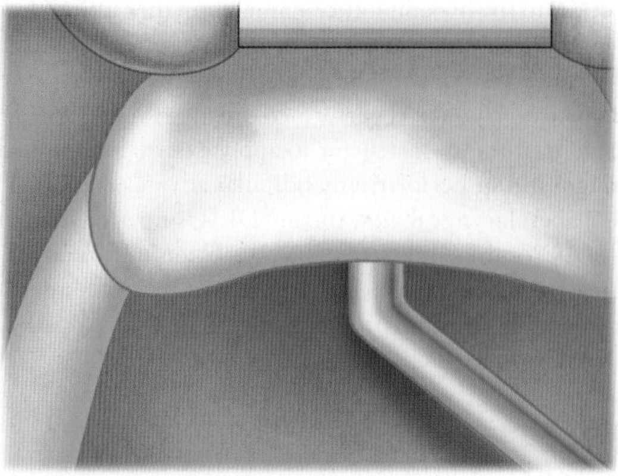

● **FIGURE 13-12.** Endotracheal tube introducer (bougie) facilitating intubation with difficult (grade 3—"epiglottis only" view) laryngoscopy. The disposable blue introducer is passed beneath the epiglottis and then anteriorly and caudally through the glottic inlet. The operator can immediately confirm tracheal placement by feeling the introducer against the tracheal rings or feeling a hard stop as the introducer enters a bronchus.

ETT passes the glottis, the laryngoscopist should rotate it counterclockwise to facilitate passage through the vocal cords (**Fig. 13-13A**–C).

## Failed Laryngoscopy and Intubation

When tracheal intubation is unsuccessful, the patient should be ventilated with BMV and high-flow oxygen if the saturations are <90%. During this reoxygenation time, the laryngoscopist should systematically analyze the likely causes of failure (**Table 13-1**). It makes no sense to attempt a second laryngoscopy without changing some aspect of the technique to improve chances for success. The following questions should be addressed:

- Is the patient in the optimum position for laryngoscopy and intubation? If the patient was placed in the sniffing position initially and the larynx still appears quite anterior, reducing

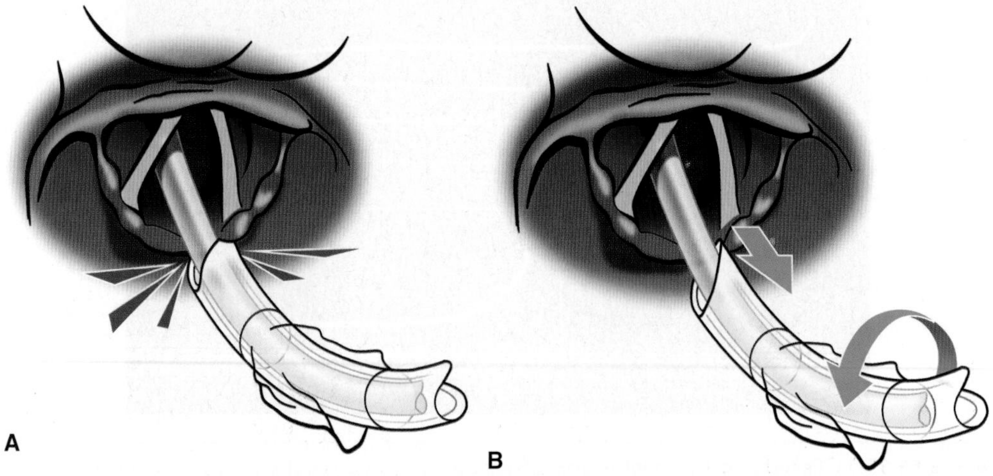


● **FIGURE 13-13.** Counterclockwise rotation of the endotracheal tube (ETT) during insertion over an introducer. **A:** The tip of the ETT is hung up on the glottis, which is common. **B:** The ETT is withdrawn 1 to 2 cm and then rotated 90° counterclockwise. **C:** With the bevel facing posteriorly, the ETT passes smoothly through the glottis.

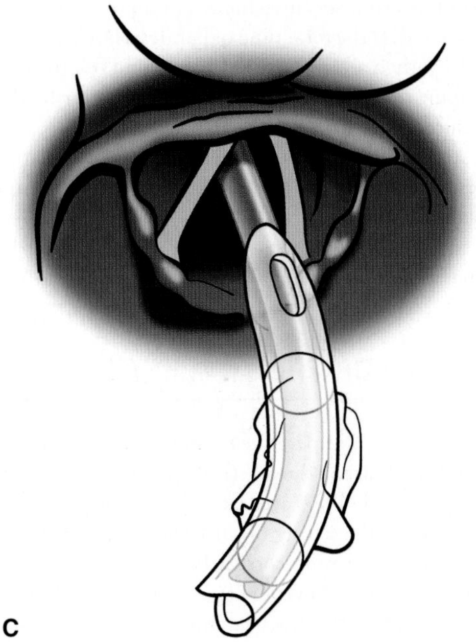

C

● **FIGURE 13-13.** (*continued*)

the degree of head extension could be helpful. It may occasionally help to elevate and flex the patient's head and neck with the laryngoscopist's free right hand while performing laryngoscopy to create a better view of a true anterior airway.

- Would a different blade provide a better view? If the initial attempt at laryngoscopy was done with a curved blade, it may be advisable to change to a straight blade, and vice versa. Alternatively, a different size blade of either type might be helpful.
- Is the patient adequately relaxed? Appropriate neuromuscular blockade can improve the view of laryngoscopy one full Cormack–Lehane grade. Laryngoscopy may have been attempted

TABLE 13-1 **Errors Associated with Failed Laryngoscopy**

| | |
|---|---|
| Rushed/frantic laryngoscopy | If the patient is rapidly desaturating, do not try to intubate hurriedly. Use BMV to improve oxygenation and then perform relaxed, methodical laryngoscopy |
| Laryngoscopy without a plan | Do not just insert the blade and hope that the vocal cords appear. This will usually result in advancing the blade too deeply, missing anatomic landmarks. Use a methodical approach with progressive visualization of anatomic structures—follow the tongue to the epiglottis and then the epiglottis to the vocal cords |
| Poor tongue control | No tongue should be visible on the right side of the blade during properly performed laryngoscopy. This will prevent good visualization of the glottis and passage of the ETT |
| Poor ergonomics | Holding the laryngoscope incorrectly, bending over in an awkward position, resting your elbow on the patient or the bed, and positioning your eyes too close to the procedure are recipes for failure |

too soon after administering succinylcholine, or an inadequate dose of succinylcholine may have been administered. If the total time of paralysis has been such that the effect of succinylcholine is dissipating, then administration of a second full paralyzing dose of succinylcholine is advisable. Atropine should be available to treat bradycardia that occasionally accompanies repeat dosing of succinylcholine.

- Would external laryngeal manipulation be helpful? Manipulation of the thyroid cartilage by the laryngoscopist or the assistant, as described above, often improves the laryngeal view by one full Cormack–Lehane grade.
- Is a more experienced laryngoscopist available? If so, a call for help may be in order.
- If DL has been maximized, is a VL available? If so, recourse to VL should be considered early.

## CONFIRMING INTUBATION OF THE TRACHEA

Once the ETT has been placed, it is imperative to confirm that it is in the trachea. The current standard is the detection of end-tidal carbon dioxide ($ETCO_2$). Both qualitative colorimetric detectors and quantitative capnography are nearly 100% accurate for confirming tracheal tube placement in patients who are not in cardiac arrest. In the setting of cardiac arrest, continuous waveform capnography is the most reliable method for confirming correct ETT placement. Colorimetric $ETCO_2$ detectors quickly change from purple ("poor") to yellow ("yes") when $ETCO_2$ is detected. This color change should occur within a few breaths after tracheal intubation, and a lack of color change indicates an esophageal intubation. Uncommonly, $CO_2$ from the stomach can create a color change to yellow, but this will revert to purple within six breaths. With proper tracheal intubation, the color should continue to change from purple to yellow with each breath. A color change to tan, rather than bright yellow, may indicate esophageal or supraglottic misplacement. In cardiac arrest, colorimetric detectors are of limited value because the $ETCO_2$ may be less than the detectable limit for color change (usually 5% $CO_2$ in exhaled gas), so capnography or suction esophageal detection devices (see below) should be used. When waveform capnography is used, tracheal intubation is confirmed by visualization of a square waveform that persists for at least six breaths. Absence of a waveform confirms esophageal placement. In cardiac arrest, the presence of a waveform confirms endotracheal intubation, whereas the lack of a waveform is indeterminate, requiring use of an alternative detection method. There are two types of suction esophageal detecting devices (EDDs): the piston syringe and the self-inflating bulb. Studies have shown that the sensitivity of the self-inflating bulb is greater than that of the piston syringe. The principle behind these devices is simple: releasing the deflated bulb or pulling back on the piston creates a negative pressure at the tip of the device. The negative pressure causes the esophagus to collapse around the tip of the device in an esophageal intubation, preventing the bulb from reinflating or the syringe plunger from being pulled back easily. The trachea does not collapse easily with negative pressure, so tracheal placement is confirmed if the bulb reinflates or the piston is easily pulled back. These devices are quite sensitive and specific, but are not perfect, so they should be used in combination with other confirmation methods, such as visualizing the ETT passing through the vocal cords. Bronchoscopic confirmation of tracheal intubation is helpful when other methods of confirmation are confusing, especially in cardiac arrest. Auscultation is important for detecting mainstem intubation and pulmonary pathology, but is unreliable for confirming tracheal tube placement. Chest x-rays should not be used to differentiate whether the ETT is in the trachea or the esophagus, but only to assess proper ETT depth and to evaluate for mainstem intubation. Fogging (condensation) of the ETT is a *completely unreliable* method of confirming tracheal intubation and should not be used.

## EVIDENCE

- **What is the safest way to teach DL in the emergency setting?** A minimum of 50 intubations are needed to become proficient at DL in the elective setting.[1] It is more difficult to teach and learn DL in the emergency setting, and the number of intubations needed to gain proficiency in difficult emergency airways is likely much higher than 50. Teaching DL with a traditional laryngoscope in the emergency setting can be challenging for both trainees and the instructors given that only one person can view the airway directly.[2] The rate of complications increases dramatically when there are multiple intubation attempts, so the goal should be first pass success.[3,4] VL has been shown to increase intubation success even in difficult airways; however, many do not recreate DL mechanics.[5–7] Despite its drawbacks, DL remains an important skill that trainees should master. Today, several VLs allow DL and VL simultaneously for both adult and pediatric patients.[8–10] There is subjective and objective evidence that these devices shorten the learning curve for DL.[8–11] In a small randomized trial of 198 patients intubated with either the C-MAC or a DL, first attempt success was higher with VL (92% vs. 86%), although the small sample size kept this from being statistically significant.[12] Eight patients (8%) failed DL intubation on the first attempt, and all were successfully intubated using VL on the second attempt. Interestingly, the residents involved in this study learned DL using the C-MAC, and this is the first ED-based study demonstrating the effectiveness of learning and performing DL with a Macintosh shaped VL.

- **How should the head and neck be best positioned for laryngoscopy?** Cormack and Lehane devised the most widely accepted system of categorizing the view of the larynx achieved with an orally placed laryngoscope.[13] The sniffing position (head extension and neck flexion) has been widely accepted as the optimum position for orotracheal intubation. However, there is conflicting evidence that increased head elevation (increased neck flexion) or just simple extension (head extension and neck extension) may be better than the sniffing position.[14,15] Although the question of optimal head positioning remains, it is likely that it will vary from patient to patient. This highlights the importance of a two-handed technique for intubation, allowing for individualized adjustments during laryngoscopy. Morbidly obese patients should be placed in a "ramped" position, with significant elevation of the shoulders, neck, and head such that a horizontal line can be drawn from the tragus of the ear to the sternal notch.[16–18]
- **What is the utility of external laryngeal manipulation during DL?** It has been clearly shown that external laryngeal manipulation, one example of which is BURP, improves laryngeal view by one full grade, on average. In addition, one recent study demonstrated the importance of operator-directed laryngeal manipulation (as opposed to assistant-directed manipulation) in maximizing visualization of the glottic structures.[19] The importance of laryngoscopy being a bimanual technique is emphasized regardless of which direction the thyroid cartilage is displaced. In addition, one OR-based study showed that mandibular elevation (a jaw thrust) in addition to BURP improved the glottic view during DL by inexperienced laryngoscopists.[20]
- **Is an ETI or bougie truly helpful?** The literature clearly supports the use of ETIs to enhance success rates of intubation, particularly with grade 3 views.[21–24] In one study, the success rate improved from 66% to 96% when an ETI was used. When using an ETI, it is important to continue laryngoscopy while the ETT is placed over the ETI and rotate the ETT counter-clockwise as it passes through the larynx. Also, it may help to release cricoid pressure as the ETT is passed over the ETI.[25]
- **Does it matter which laryngoscopic blade I use?** It is generally believed that one's choice of a laryngoscope blade and the technique used to facilitate intubation is best guided by personal choice and experience.[26,27] The literature suggests that straight blades improve laryngoscopic view (increased exposure of the vocal cords), whereas curved blades provide better intubating conditions (continuous visualization of the vocal cords during ETT passage).[26]
- **What are the best methods for confirming correct ETT placement?** No confirmation method is perfect, so providers should always use a combination of clinical assessment and detection devices. Continuous waveform capnography is recommended by the American Heart Association as the most reliable method for confirming and monitoring correct placement of an ETT.[28] Waveform capnographers provide a quantitative measure of $ETCO_2$ as well as a distinct repeating waveform that facilitates continuous monitoring of ETT position, even in most cases of cardiac arrest.[28,29] An $ETCO_2$ waveform may be absent in cases of prolonged cardiac arrest or monitor malfunction, but good chest compressions and a viable patient will usually produce a detectible waveform. Colorimetric and nonwaveform exhaled $CO_2$ detectors are not as useful in cardiac arrest but are nearly 100% accurate for confirming correct ETT placement in patients who are not in cardiac arrest. Soft drinks in the stomach containing $CO_2$

may mimic the exhaled $CO_2$ from the lungs for a few breaths, the so-called Cola complication; this confounding result ought not to persist beyond six breaths.

There are several types of EDDs that detect esophageal intubation by creating negative pressure in the ETT, causing the walls of the esophagus to collapse around the tip of the ETT. Although these devices detect about 99% of esophageal intubations, and are better in cases of prolonged cardiac arrest, they are generally less accurate than $ETCO_2$ devices.

It would be reasonable to believe that visualization of the ETT entering the larynx is a reliable method of verifying correct ETT position, but has been shown that additional confirmation methods are necessary, even when experienced providers place the ETT. Auscultation of the chest for breath sounds and of the epigastrium for absence of air entry into the stomach and observation of chest motion during ventilation are common but notoriously inaccurate methods of confirming correct ETT placement. Looking for condensation inside the ETT is a completely unreliable method for confirming correct placement.

None of these techniques alone guarantee correct placement, and as many of them as possible should be used in every case.

## REFERENCES


1. Buis ML, Maissan IM, Hoeks SE, et al. Defining the learning curve for endotracheal intubation using direct laryngoscopy: a systematic review. *Resuscitation*. 2016;99:63–71.
2. Sagarin MJ, Barton ED, Chng YM, et al; National Emergency Airway Registry Investigators. Airway management by US and Canadian emergency medicine residents: a multicenter analysis of more than 6,000 endotracheal intubation attempts. *Ann Emerg Med*. 2005;46(4):328–336.
3. Mort TC. Emergency tracheal intubation: complications associated with repeated laryngoscopic attempts. *Anesth Analg*. 2004;99(2):607–613, table of contents.
4. Sakles JC, Chiu S, Mosier J, et al. The importance of first pass success when performing orotracheal intubation in the emergency department. *Acad Emerg Med*. 2013;20(1):71–78.
5. Sakles JC, Mosier J, Chiu S, et al. A comparison of the C-MAC video laryngoscope to the Macintosh direct laryngoscope for intubation in the emergency department. *Ann Emerg Med*. 2012;60(6):739–748.
6. Michailidou M, O'Keeffe T, Mosier JM, et al. A comparison of video laryngoscopy to direct laryngoscopy for the emergency intubation of trauma patients. *World J Surg*. 2015;39(3):782–788.
7. Sakles JC, Patanwala AE, Mosier JM, et al. Comparison of video laryngoscopy to direct laryngoscopy for intubation of patients with difficult airway characteristics in the emergency department. *Intern Emerg Med*. 2014;9(1):93–98.
8. Kaplan MB, Ward DS, Berci G. A new video laryngoscope-an aid to intubation and teaching. *J Clin Anesth*. 2002;14(8):620–626.
9. O'Shea JE, Thio M, Kamlin CO, et al. Videolaryngoscopy to teach neonatal intubation: a randomized trial. *Pediatrics*. 2015;136(5):912–919.
10. Viernes D, Goldman AJ, Galgon RE, et al. Evaluation of the GlideScope direct: a new video laryngoscope for teaching direct laryngoscopy. *Anesthesiol Res Pract*. 2012;2012:820961.
11. Howard-Quijano KJ, Huang YM, Matevosian R, et al. Video-assisted instruction improves the success rate for tracheal intubation by novices. *Br J Anaesth*. 2008;101(4):568–572.
12. Driver BE, Prekker ME, Moore JC, et al. Direct versus video laryngoscopy using the C-MAC for tracheal intubation in the emergency department, a randomized controlled trial. *Acad Emerg Med*. 2016;23(4):433–439.
13. Cormack RS, Lehane J. Difficult tracheal intubation in obstetrics. *Anaesthesia*. 1984;39(11):1105–1111.
14. Adnet F, Baillard C, Borron SW, et al. Randomized study comparing the "sniffing position" with simple head extension for laryngoscopic view in elective surgery patients. *Anesthesiology*. 2001;95(4): 836–841.

15. Levitan RM, Mechem CC, Ochroch EA, et al. Head-elevated laryngoscopy position: improving laryngeal exposure during laryngoscopy by increasing head elevation. *Ann Emerg Med*. 2003;41(3):322–330.
16. Brodsky JB, Lemmens HJ, Brock-Utne JG, et al. Anesthetic considerations for bariatric surgery: proper positioning is important for laryngoscopy. *Anesth Analg*. 2003;96(6):1841–1842; author reply 2.
17. Brodsky JB, Lemmens HJ, Brock-Utne JG, et al. Morbid obesity and tracheal intubation. *Anesth Analg*. 2002;94(3):732–736.
18. Collins JS, Lemmens HJ, Brodsky JB, et al. Laryngoscopy and morbid obesity: a comparison of the "sniff" and "ramped" positions. *Obes Surg*. 2004;14(9):1171–1175.
19. Levitan RM, Kinkle WC, Levin WJ, et al. Laryngeal view during laryngoscopy: a randomized trial comparing cricoid pressure, backward-upward-rightward pressure, and bimanual laryngoscopy. *Ann Emerg Med*. 2006;47(6):548–555.
20. Tamura M, Ishikawa T, Kato R, et al. Mandibular advancement improves the laryngeal view during direct laryngoscopy performed by inexperienced physicians. *Anesthesiology*. 2004;100(3):598–601.
21. Combes X, Le Roux B, Suen P, et al. Unanticipated difficult airway in anesthetized patients: prospective validation of a management algorithm. *Anesthesiology*. 2004;100(5):1146–1150.
22. Green DW. Gum elastic bougie and simulated difficult intubation. *Anaesthesia*. 2003;58(4):391–392.
23. Henderson JJ. Development of the 'gum-elastic bougie'. *Anaesthesia*. 2003;58(1):103–104.
24. Noguchi T, Koga K, Shiga Y, et al. The gum elastic bougie eases tracheal intubation while applying cricoid pressure compared to a stylet. *Can J Anaesth*. 2003;50(7):712–717.
25. McNelis U, Syndercombe A, Harper I, et al. The effect of cricoid pressure on intubation facilitated by the gum elastic bougie. *Anaesthesia*. 2007;62(5):456–459.
26. Arino JJ, Velasco JM, Gasco C, et al. Straight blades improve visualization of the larynx while curved blades increase ease of intubation: a comparison of the Macintosh, Miller, McCoy, Belscope and Lee-Fiberview blades. *Can J Anaesth*. 2003;50(5):501–506.
27. American Society of Anesthesiologists Task Force on Management of the Difficult Airway. Practice guidelines for management of the difficult airway: an updated report by the American Society of Anesthesiologists Task Force on Management of Difficult Airway. *Anesthesiology*. 2003;98:1269–1277.
28. Neumar RW, Otto CW, Link MS, et al. Part 8: adult advanced cardiovascular life support: 2010 American Heart Association Guidelines for Cardiopulmonary Resuscitation and Emergency Cardiovascular Care. *Circulation*. 2010;122(18 suppl 3):S729–S767.
29. Silvestri S, Ralls GA, Krauss B, et al. The effectiveness of out-of-hospital use of continuous end-tidal carbon dioxide monitoring on the rate of unrecognized misplaced intubation within a regional emergency medical services system. *Ann Emerg Med*. 2005;45(5):497–503.

Chapter 14

# Video Laryngoscopy

John C. Sakles and Aaron E. Bair

## INTRODUCTION

Historically, direct laryngoscopy (DL) has been the primary method of performing tracheal intubation in the emergency department (ED). When utilizing DL, the goal is to compress and distract the tissues of the upper airway so that a direct line of sight can be achieved between the operator's eye and the laryngeal inlet. Due to anatomic limitations, this can technically be very difficult and is simply not possible in some patients. Therefore, laryngoscopes were developed which could allow intubation to be completed by looking around the obstructing tissues rather than relying on their displacement. The introduction of fiber-optics into medicine helped to spur the development of rigid fiber-optic laryngoscopes such as the Bullard laryngoscope. These devices were essentially rigid laryngoscopes that incorporated a fiber-optic bundle and an eyepiece that allowed the operator to effectively see around the tongue. These fiber-optic laryngoscopes were clever in their design but required significant operator expertise to use them effectively. The inherent limitations of fiber-optics, such as their small field of view, requirement of an ocular eyepiece, lens fogging, and easy contamination, restricted their widespread use. When video cameras became miniaturized to the point where they could be placed onto a laryngoscope blade, new opportunities for laryngoscopy developed. Dr. John A. Pacey developed the first commercially available video laryngoscope (VL), the GlideScope, which has been in clinical use since 2001. The GlideScope incorporated a micro-video camera on the distal portion of the blade that connected to an external monitor via a cable. The video camera provided an indirect view of the airway and allowed intubation to be performed by using the video monitor. Since that time, numerous VLs have been developed and are in clinical practice. These devices differ considerably in their design. Some use conventional Macintosh curved blades, whereas others use hyperangulated blades. Some require freehand delivery of the tube by the operator, whereas others have a built-in channel guide for tube placement. Some have an external monitor connected to the laryngoscope by a cable, whereas others have a monitor attached directly to the laryngoscope handle. Some use disposable single-use blades, whereas others use reusable blades that can undergo high-level disinfection. What they all have in common is that they provide an indirect view of the laryngeal inlet, displaying the relevant anatomy on a video monitor allowing intubation to be performed without having to move any of the obstructing tissue out of the way. Additionally, the viewing angle is greatly increased over what is usually experienced with DL (10° vs. 60° with VL). Due to the many differences in design, a general overview of the use of VLs will be presented, followed by specific information for each device.

## CLASSIFICATION OF VLs

The wide array of VLs can be fundamentally classified as standard geometry Macintosh blades and hyperangulated blades. Further, the hyperangulated blades can be further divided into those that have a tube guide and those that do not (see Table 14-1).

## ADVANTAGES OF VL

VLs have many advantages over DL:

1. Obviate the need for direct line of sight to airway
2. Magnify the view of the airway
3. Require less force to intubate
4. Allow assistants to see and help with the procedure
5. Allow supervising practitioners to supervise procedure (even remotely)
6. Allow for recording of photos and videos which can be used for documentation and teaching

TABLE 14-1 Classification of VLs

| Standard Geometry Macintosh Blade | Blade Sizes | Attached Screen | Reusable/ Disposable | Pediatric Version |
|---|---|---|---|---|
| C-MAC | Mac 2, 3, 4<br>Miller 0, 1 | Yes (requires special module) | R and D | Yes |
| GVL Titanium MAC | MAC T3, T4<br>MAC S3, S4 | No | R<br>D | |
| GVL Direct | Mac 3.5 | No | R | No |
| McGRATH MAC | Mac 2, 3, 4 | Yes | D | No |
| Venner AP Advance | Mac 3, 4 | Yes | D | No |
| **Hyperangulated Blade** | | | | |
| Channeled | | | | |
| King Vision | Adult | Yes | D | No |
| Pentax AWS | Adult | Yes | D | No |
| Venner AP Advance | Adult | Yes | D | No |
| Vividtrac | Adult | No | D | No |
| Unchanneled | | | | |
| GVL Titanium T3, T4<br>GVL Titanium S3, S4 | T3, T4<br>S3, S4 | No | R<br>D | |
| C-MAC D-blade | Adult | No | R | Yes |
| McGRATH MAC X-blade | Adult | Yes | D | No |
| CoPilot VL | Adult | No | D | No |

## BASIC TECHNIQUE FOR VL

VL in general requires a different technique than DL. There are three important aspects to understanding VL. The following points apply generally to the technique of VL.

### Visualization

With VLs, in contrast to DLs, the operator does not need to displace the tongue, but instead can look around it. Thus, there is no need to use the blade to sweep the tongue to the left as with DL. Instead the operator must use a midline approach. The VL should be inserted directly down the midline and advanced slowly while curling it around the base of the tongue. When introducing the blade it should be kept high and pressed against the tongue to avoid dipping the tip into the posterior oropharynx where it can get contaminated from pooled secretions. Once the epiglottis is identified, the tip of the blade should be advanced into the vallecula and a gentle lifting/rocking (primarily rocking) motion applied. The goal is to see the larynx in the top half of the screen. This leaves the bottom half of the screen available for visualizing the advancement of the endotracheal tube (ETT). A common mistake is to continue advancing the VL once an adequate view of the larynx is achieved. The problem that this creates is that it lifts the larynx higher and tilts it as well, making tube delivery much more difficult, and sometimes impossible.

### Tube Delivery

Once an appropriate view of the larynx is achieved, the next goal is to direct the tube to the vocal cords. Since the tongue is not being displaced, the operator must direct the tube around the curve to reach what is being seen on the screen. An angulated stylet is needed for this. It is recommended to conform the styletted tube to match the curvature of the blade. Verathon makes a proprietary stylet called the GlideRite that is a rigid, curved stylet similar to the acute angle of the GlideScope blade. It is recommended that this stylet be used for *any* hyperangulated VLs. When it is time to introduce the tube into the patient's mouth, the operator must take their attention away from the monitor and look at the patient. The tube is inserted into the patient's mouth under direct observation. If the operator is still looking at the screen and not observing tube introduction directly, there is risk of damaging the structures of the upper airway such as the soft palate, tonsillar pillars, or posterior pharyngeal wall. After the tube is introduced under direct vision, the operator can then turn their attention back to the screen to see the tube as it enters from the right-hand side on the video monitor. At this point, the operator should begin to orient the tip of the tube so it points at the glottic opening. This should be done early and can be accomplished by rotating the tube to a vertical position and thereby making the angle at the end of the ETT point upward at the glottic inlet. The operator can continue to advance the tube to the laryngeal inlet by using the screen as a guide. The operator should attempt to pass the tube through the vocal cords as far as initially possible. Typically, some resistance will be encountered as the tip of the tube hits the anterior tracheal wall.

### Tube Advancement

Once the tube passes the vocal cords and enters the trachea, the highly curved styletted tube will impinge on the anterior tracheal wall. At this point the stylet must be partially withdrawn by the operator or assistant so the tip of the tube will straighten out. The operator's thumb can be used to withdraw the stylet a few centimeters back. The GlideRite stylet has a specially designed tab on it to facilitate this maneuver. It is important to recognize that the GlideRite stylet cannot be pulled straight out like a conventional malleable stylet. If this is attempted it will likely pull the tube out with it. The GlideRite stylet has an extreme curve and is very rigid and thus must be withdrawn from the tube in an arc over the patient's chest to match its natural curvature.

## COMPLICATIONS OF VL

When used properly, VLs are very safe and effective devices. Improper use, however, can result in untoward complications. For example, if the operator does not look at the patient while inserting the tube it is possible to traumatize the upper airway and even perforate some of these structures. When using a VL it can sometimes take longer to intubate because of difficulty directing the tube to what is being seen on the screen. This can be remedied by having the VL blade at the appropriate depth in the patient and using an appropriately shaped stylet.

## GLIDESCOPE

The GlideScope was the first VL introduced into clinical practice and has undergone many modifications, with multiple units now available. The following is a description of the currently available units (**Figs. 14.1A** and **B**).

### GlideScope AVL

The original GlideScope video laryngoscope (GVL) consists of a micro-video camera encased within a sharply angulated blade, a rechargeable video liquid crystal display (LCD) monitor, and a video cable that transmits the image. The monitor can be mounted on a mobile stand or attached to any available pole with a C-clamp. The laryngoscope portion of the GVL consists of a combined handle and laryngoscope blade that are made from durable medical-grade plastic. The video camera is placed in a recess midway along the undersurface of the laryngoscope blade, partially protecting it from contamination from bodily secretions. In addition, the GVL incorporates an antifog mechanism that heats the lens around the video camera, thereby decreasing condensation during laryngoscopy. There are four blade sizes for the GVL (GVL-2 through GVL-5). The GVL-2 is designed for small children (2 to 10 kg), whereas the GVL-5 is meant to overcome anatomic challenges seen with morbidly obese patients. The GVL size 3 and 4 blades are appropriate for small adults and large adults, respectively. Additionally, neonatal sizes are available with the single-use, Cobalt version. Because the GVL does not incorporate an ETT guide or stylet connected to the device, ETTs of any size can be used.

The laryngoscope attaches to a portable LCD monitor through a video cable that also carries power to light-emitting diodes (LEDs) mounted alongside the video camera. The monitor has a video-out port that requires a proprietary cable to connect to the composite video input, allowing the image to be transmitted to another monitor or recording device. The monitor can be rotated to the optimal viewing angle, and the cradle rests on a mobile telescoping pole that allows easy adjustment of the height of the monitor. The unit is powered by standard alternating current or its backup rechargeable lithium battery. The battery can provide 90 minutes of continuous use and has a low-battery indicator light to warn the operator that the unit must be plugged in.

### GlideScope Ranger

The GlideScope Ranger is a rugged, portable, battery-operated GlideScope unit designed for field use. It is operational in a wide variety of temperatures, humidity, and altitudes and weighs roughly 2 lb (0.9 kg), making it very portable. It uses a 3.5-in (9 cm) LCD screen that allows good image clarity even when used outdoors. The Ranger can be used with a reusable blade or disposable Cobalt blades.

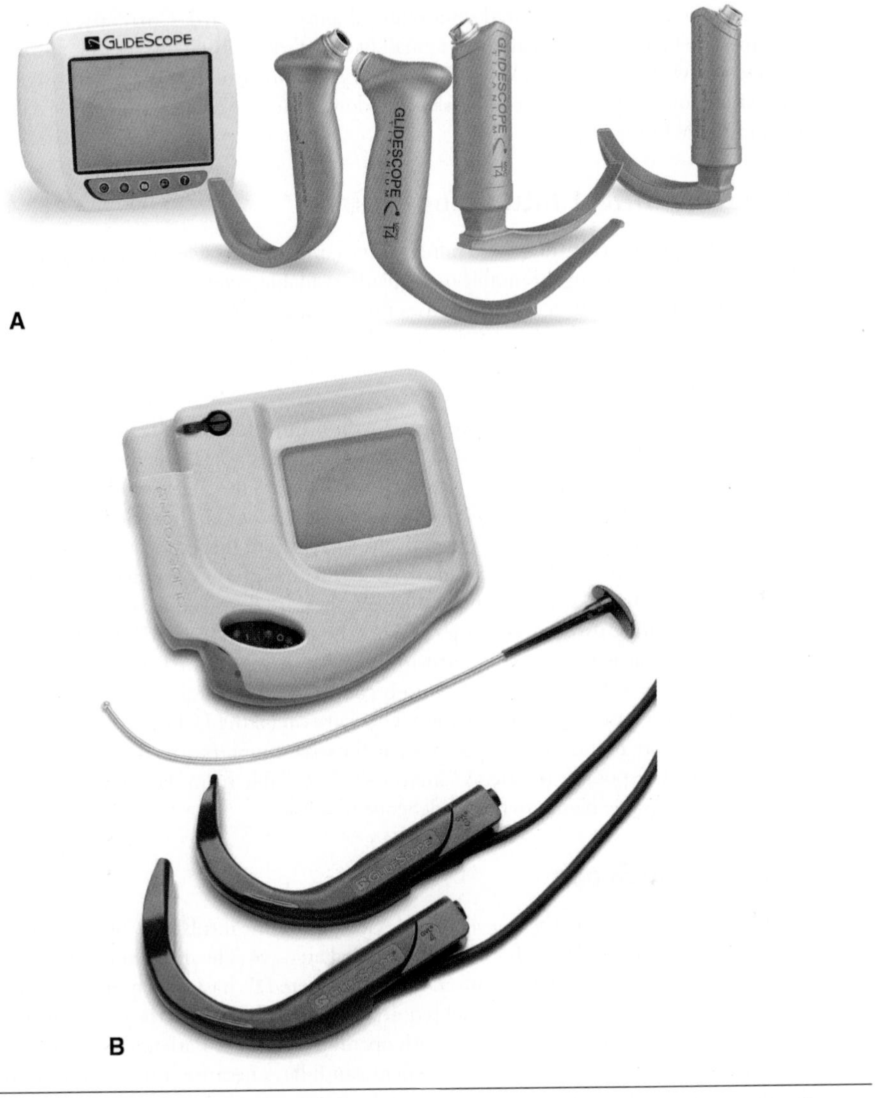


● **FIGURE 14-1. GlideScope. A:** The GlideScope Titanium series showing both the reusable hyperangulated T3 and T4 blades, and the reusable standard geometry Mac T3 and Mac T4 blades. **B:** The portable GlideScope Ranger.

The rechargeable lithium polymer battery provides 90 minutes of continuous use. The GlideScope Ranger is contained within a soft neoprene case for protection.

## GlideScope Cobalt

The GlideScope Cobalt is a disposable single-use version of the original GlideScope. The Cobalt consists of a flexible video baton that houses the micro-video camera that inserts into a disposable clear plastic protective blade, called the Stat. The Cobalt video baton may connect to either of two different video displays. The original Cobalt used the same color video LCD monitor as the GVL; however, this has largely been replaced by a newer version, the Cobalt Advanced Video Laryngoscope, which uses a high-definition video baton and digital video display. The monitor has similar dimensions to the original unit but has the benefit of a built-in tutorial as well as image and video clip acquisition that can be stored on a removable memory card. Currently, there are two baton sizes and five blade sizes available. The small baton works with Stat sizes 0, 1, and 2, and the large baton works with size 3 and 4 blades. The primary advantage of the Cobalt is its single-use design—eliminating logistic problems, costs, risks, and downtime associated with high-level disinfection of the traditional GlideScope.

## GlideScope Direct Intubation Trainer

The GlideScope Direct Intubation Trainer, as its name implies, was developed to help teach practitioners DL. There is a single reusable metal blade available, size Mac 3.5. The operator can perform DL with this device while a supervisor uses the screen to help guide them.

## GlideScope Titanium

The GlideScope Titanium is the newest product line introduced in the GlideScope series and consists of several different VLs. The GlideScope Titanium is a lightweight, low-profile GlideScope that is made of titanium. It comes in two varieties. There is the Titanium LoPro T3 and T4 which are based upon the hyperangulated GlideScope design and are in fact made of titanium. They are suitable for small and large adults, respectively. In addition, there are conventionally shaped Macintosh versions called the MAC T3 and MAC T4. Although they are shaped liked a conventional Mac blade to give them a more comfortable feel, they are designed to only be used as a VL. They are not intended to be used as DL blades because the camera on the undersurface partially obstructs the direct view that is necessary to perform DL with them. At the time of this writing, however, the manufacturer is developing a Macintosh combo VL/DL blade. All four titanium blades are also available in plastic single-use versions. These are called the LoPro S3 and S4 and MAC S3 and MAC S4. They are identical in design to their reusable counterparts, with the exception that they are composed of disposable plastic. A "smart cable" available from the manufacturer is required to connect the disposable blades to the GlideScope monitor.

## Using a GlideScope

The GlideScope is intended as an everyday device for routine intubation and can also be considered as an alternative airway device for difficult or failed airways. The distal angulation makes it ideally suited to visualize and intubate an anterior larynx where DL has proven unsuccessful. Because the handle has a narrow profile and does not require direct visualization of the larynx through the mouth, it is useful when cervical mobility or mouth opening is limited. Patients in whom it is desirable to minimize movement of the neck are excellent candidates because little force is needed to expose the glottis with the laryngoscope blade. The GlideScope generally performs well in the presence of secretions, blood, and vomitus, and thus is a good choice even in these circumstances.

The GlideScope is used in the following manner to perform tracheal intubation (**Fig. 14-2**). The handle is grasped with the left hand, in the same fashion as a conventional laryngoscope, and the tip of the laryngoscope blade is gently inserted into the mouth, in the midline, under direct vision. The critical point here is to keep the handle in the midline as you enter further into the mouth, noting key midline structures, such as the uvula, as you advance. There is no sweeping of the tongue to the left as is done with conventional laryngoscopy. It is difficult to identify landmarks if the blade is off the midline. As soon as the tip of the laryngoscope blade passes the teeth, the operator should direct his or her attention to the video monitor and use the landmarks on the video screen to navigate to the glottic aperture. As mentioned earlier, the uvula will be seen if the blade is correctly situated in the midline. The operator should then continue to gently advance the blade down the tongue and past the uvula, with a slight elevating motion until the epiglottis is seen. At that point, it is best to continue advancing the blade into the vallecula, with some gentle upward force, to indirectly lift the epiglottis out of the way. The blade should ultimately be seated in the vallecula, much in the same way that a Macintosh blade is used. The intubator should be cautious not to place the blade too close to the glottic aperture. Although this may result in a larger, more obvious view of the target, it

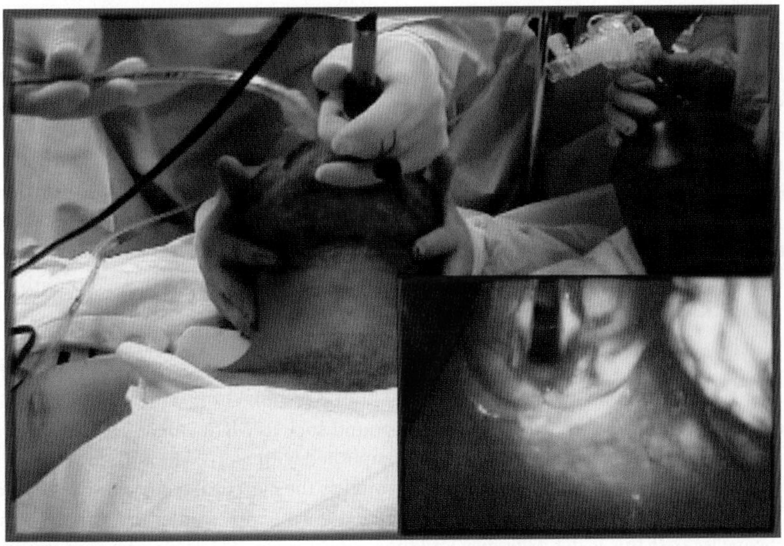

● **FIGURE 14-2. GlideScope in Clinical Use.** The standard reusable GlideScope being used to intubate a blunt trauma patient in the emergency department. The front of the cervical collar has been removed and an assistant is maintaining in-line cervical stabilization. An excellent view of the laryngeal inlet has been achieved, but the operator has inserted the blade too far, causing elevation and tilting of the larynx which will make tube delivery much more difficult.

ultimately makes ETT passage more challenging. The best view to complete intubation is one where the airway is seen somewhat "off in the distance" with the epiglottis visualized on the monitor. If the glottic view is insufficient, often a gentle tilt of the handle will expose it fully, in contrast to the lifting motion with a conventional laryngoscope. If the glottic aperture still cannot be exposed, the blade can be withdrawn slightly, placed under the epiglottis, and used like a Miller blade to physically displace the epiglottis up and out of the way. This motion can tilt the larynx more sharply, making advancement of the tube into the trachea technically more challenging. When an optimal glottic view is obtained, the operator again looks into the mouth, to insert the ETT with a stylet curved to match the curve of the GVL blade, alongside the blade. When the tube is placed where desired, the operator again views the video monitor to guide advancement of the tube into the glottis. Thus, intubation with the GlideScope can be thought of as occurring in four steps. For two of these steps, the operator views the video monitor; for the other two, the operator looks into the patient's mouth.

Identifying and exposing the glottis generally is easy using the GlideScope. However, advancing the ETT toward the image of the glottis displayed on the video screen can still be challenging. Negotiating the oropharynx and traversing the glottis with an acutely shaped ETT can be technically difficult for two reasons. First, the GlideScope blade is angulated at 60°, and thus, the angle of attack of the tube is quite steep. The second issue is that using the screen to navigate to the glottis requires a form of hand–eye coordination that is different from traditional DL. The critical factor in getting the tube to enter the trachea is configuring the ETT into a shape that conforms to that of the GlideScope blade so that the ETT is able to follow the same trajectory as the blade. Under direct vision, the operator places the tip of the ETT in the corner of the right side of the patient's mouth with the tube nearly parallel to the ground (operator's hand at the 2- to 3-o'clock position) and advances the tube into position alongside the GVL blade. When the tube is felt to be well positioned, that is, vertically oriented and parallel to the blade handle, the operator looks at the screen and advances the tube along its curved axis to guide it into the laryngeal inlet, with the curvature heading anteriorly toward the airway. The manufacturer has developed a preformed rigid reusable ETT stylet (GlideRite Rigid Stylet) that is intended to provide an optimal curve and angle of approach to the glottis. If this stylet is not available, a malleable stylet can be shaped into a similar 60° curve. When the glottis is entered, the stylet is withdrawn several centimeters to reduce the rigidity of the sharply angulated distal tip of the tube, facilitating advancement into the trachea. Withdrawal of the stylet may be done by an assistant or by the intubator, particularly if using the proprietary stylet as it has a flange designed to be actuated by the operator's thumb. If the tube continues to impinge on the anterior trachea, the GlideScope can be withdrawn about 2 cm, causing the larynx to drop down, lessening the angle of approach and thus facilitating further advancement of the tube. Additionally, the ETT can sometimes become engaged on the arytenoids or the anterior tracheal wall because of the steep anterior angle through the glottis. Using a soft tapered tip ETT, such as the proprietary Parker ETT, can help overcome this issue and facilitate intubation by easing entry of the tube through the glottic inlet.

The only absolute contraindication to use of the GlideScope is restricted mouth opening less than the thickness of the blade or inaccessible oral access such as can be seen with severe angioedema of the tongue.

The GlideScope GVL laryngoscope blade/handle unit must be cleaned and disinfected after each use. Gross contaminants and large debris can be scrubbed off with a surgical scrub brush or enzymatically removed with a proteolytic compound such as Medzyme. Laryngoscope blades must undergo high-level disinfection. This can be accomplished with Steris, Sterrad, ethylene oxide, or Cidex solutions, containing glutaraldehyde. On older models the electrical connector cap should be placed over the contact port on the laryngoscope handle to prevent corrosion of the contacts. On the newer GlideScope models this is not necessary and the connector can be left open during sterilization. The only method of sterilization that is absolutely contraindicated is autoclaving, which involves exposure of the device to very high temperatures that will damage the electronic components of the video camera.

## C-MAC

The C-MAC VL system (Karl Storz, Tuttlingen, Germany) uses a complementary metal-oxide semiconductor (CMOS) micro-video camera, which provides an enhanced field of view and resists fogging. The device also incorporates a video recording system, with controls on the handle, which supports both teaching and quality control. The C-MAC is powered by a rechargeable lithium battery, permitting 90 minutes of operation without a power source. The system comprises a variety of blades that accommodate the video camera, which connects through a single cable to a 7-in (17.8 cm) video screen, with straightforward controls (**Figs. 14-3A** and **B**). The monitor supports removable memory that allows capture and storage of both still images and video clips. One series of the C-MAC blades maintains standard Macintosh geometry and can be used for DL as well as VL. Since more traditional laryngoscopic mechanics are used, the trajectory from the mouth to the glottic opening is fairly straight and thus a rigid preformed stylet is not required. Tube insertion tends to be easier with the C-MAC than with the GlideScope because the stylet is shaped as for conventional laryngoscopy, thus permitting more direct insertion and avoiding the impingement on the anterior trachea that occurs with the GlideScope. In fact, when using the C-MAC, the operator can direct the tube along the curvature of the blade, using the flange as a guide, without obstructing the view of the airway. Currently, there are several blades available. The standard C-MAC blades are available in Macintosh size 2, 3, and 4 and Miller size 0 and 1. A difficult airway blade called the D-blade is also available (in both adult and pediatric sizes), with a hyperangulated curve and narrow profile similar to the GlideScope. This is intended to improve glottic visualization in difficult laryngoscopy situations where there are limitations with the standard geometry of Macintosh-based curvatures. The C-MAC system also has a range of disposable blades. This system utilizes a video baton in which clear plastic blades are placed.

The C-MAC monitor is portable and can be placed on any flat surface near the bedside, but is likely most useful when mounted on a pole and used in conjunction with a mobile stand. A compact version of the C-MAC (the pocket monitor) has a 2.4-in monitor directly attached to the handle, thus eliminating cables and external. As is the case for other VLs, the C-MAC blades cannot be autoclaved because this will damage the electronic circuitry of the micro-video camera. However, most other types of high-level disinfection such as Steris, Sterrad, and Cidex are acceptable.

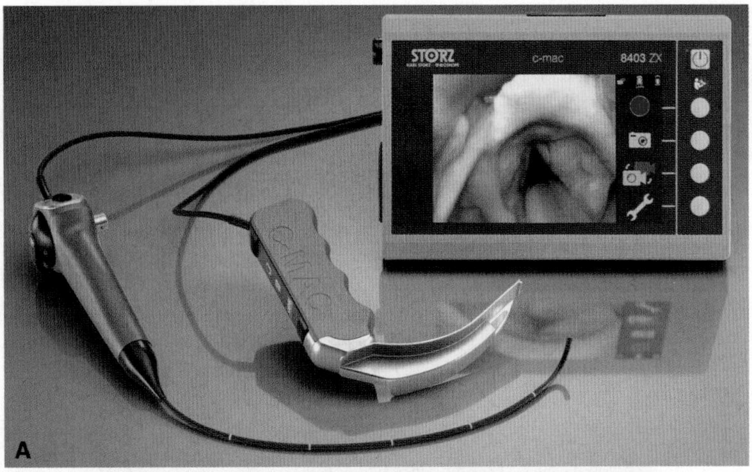


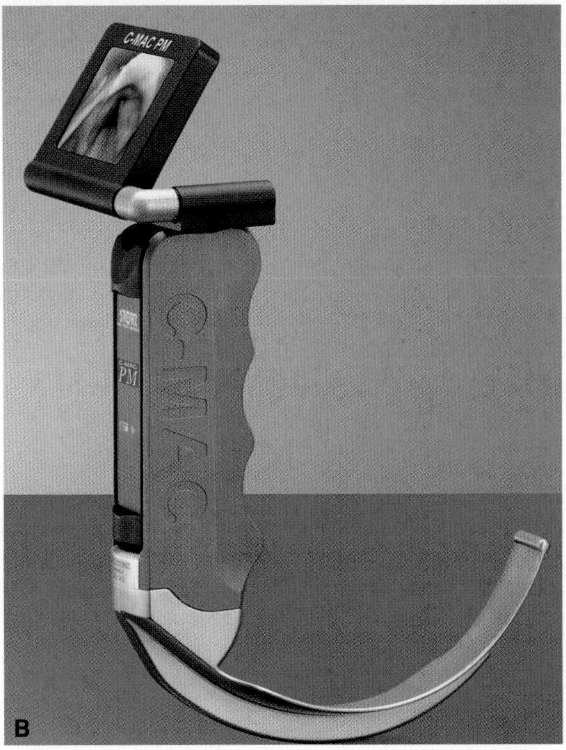


● **FIGURE 14-3. C-MAC. A:** The C-MAC system with both a rigid Mac blade and a flexible scope attached. **B:** The portable C-MAC pocket monitor (PM).

## Using a C-MAC

The C-MAC can be plugged into any wall outlet, or can be used cordless if the battery is charged. The video cartridge slides into the laryngoscope handle and the video cable plugs into the back of the monitor. There is a power switch on the monitor. The image autofocuses and image clarity is automatically maximized. Antifog is not required once the device has warmed for 90 seconds. The blade can be inserted like a traditional Macintosh blade when being used as a teaching device, but

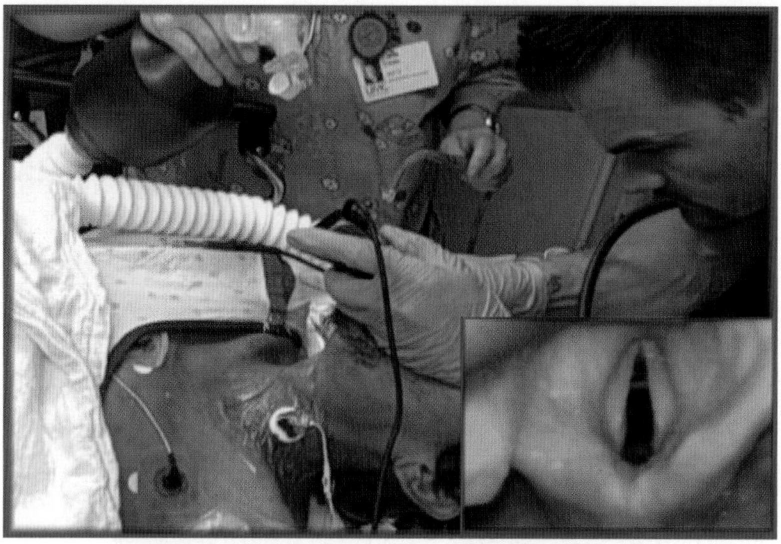

● **FIGURE 14-4. C-MAC in Clinical Use.** The C-MAC being used to intubate a patient with penetrating trauma in the emergency department.

for VL, it is inserted in the midline because the placement of the video camera makes the traditional tongue sweep unnecessary. The operator inserts the blade until the distal tip is past the uvula, and then advances in the midline while observing the screen until the epiglottis comes into view. The blade tip is placed within the vallecula (usual) or under the epiglottis (alternative) to provide visualization of the glottic inlet (**Fig. 14-4**). The angle of attack is less acute than with the GlideScope, and the tube is curved in a shape similar to that used for conventional DL.

### Summary

As is the case for the GlideScope, the Storz C-MAC is another dramatic improvement over DL. The system is simple to learn and use, has autofocus and antifogging capabilities, and provides a wide field of view for intubation. The system is useful as a primary VL for routine and difficult intubations, the latter being facilitated by the D-blade, and also as a training aid, with the trainee performing a conventional DL and the instructor viewing the image on the screen.

## MCGRATH MAC VL

A newer version of the McGRATH VL, called the McGRATH MAC, is based on the original McGRATH Series 5, but has several important differences (**Fig. 14-5**). Foremost, rather than using a highly angulated blade, the McGRATH MAC, as its name implies, uses a curvature akin to the Macintosh blade. The McGRATH MAC, therefore, can be used to perform DL. As for the Series 5, the McGRATH MAC uses a camera stick, onto which disposable plastic blades, which are provided in sizes 2, 3, and 4, are placed. There is no heat-based antifogging system on the McGRATH MAC, but the blades have a hydrophilic polymer optical surface that resists condensation. The screen on the McGRATH MAC is a 2.5-in (6.3 cm), vertically oriented monitor, and the system uses a proprietary 3.6-V lithium disposable battery. The battery has a runtime of 250 continuous minutes, and an indicator on the bottom of the video monitor image counts down the exact number of minutes left on the battery.

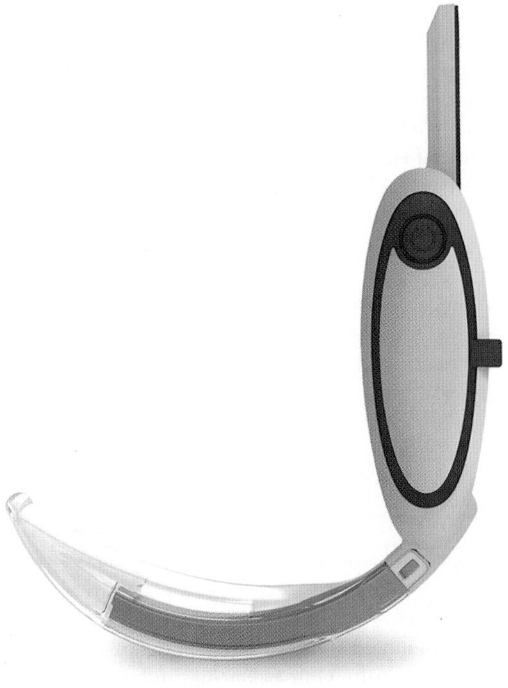

● **FIGURE 14-5. Side profile of the McGRATH MAC VL.**

## Using a McGRATH MAC

There is little setup needed for the McGRATH MAC, and once the disposable blade is placed on the camera stick and the device turned on, it is ready for use (**Fig. 14-6**). Similar to the other VLs, the McGRATH MAC is inserted into the patient's mouth in the midline. The tip of the blade is

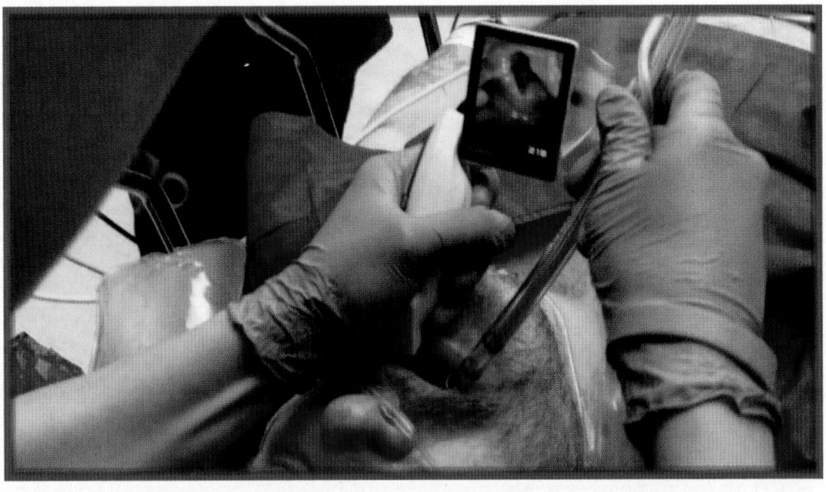

● **FIGURE 14-6. McGRATH MAC in Clinical Use.** The McGRATH MAC being used to intubate a patient with an overdose in the emergency department. There is no video-out port on the device so the photograph of the attached monitor was taken. An excellent view of the larynx is obtained with the epiglottis, vocal cords, and arytenoids visible.

then guided into the vallecula and tilted to lift the epiglottis anteriorly, similar to a conventional Macintosh blade. Once a clear view of the airway appears on the LCD screen, the operator looks back into the mouth to insert the acutely curved styletted tube. The tube is advanced into the trachea while visualizing the process on the video screen. After intubation, the disposable blade is removed and discarded while the handle is cleaned with an antiseptic wipe. When using the X-blade the technique must be modified to that used with other hyperangulated blades. Use of a hyperangulated stylet such as the GlideRite is recommended.

### Summary

The McGRATH is a compact, easy-to-use, intuitive device. The device is comfortable in the operator's hand and does not require prolonged setup time. However, the blade is narrower than the other devices, and for patients with large tongues, this can hinder the operator's view. Without the application of antifogging solution, the blade sometimes fogs during laryngoscopy.

## KING VISION

The King Vision video laryngoscope (KVL) from King Systems is another option in the VL field (**Fig. 14-7**). This is a unique integrated blade and display device with a 2.4-in (6.1 cm) diagonal reusable high-definition color organic LED screen that sits atop a plastic staff, onto which a variety of single-use blades can be mounted. The screen has antiglare properties and a high refresh rate for smooth image motion, provides autowhite balancing, and offers a 160° field of view. Additionally, the monitor maintains an upright image regardless of whether the blade is held upright or upside down. Blades with and without an integrated tube channel are available and are made of high-quality polycarbonate plastic. Both house a CMOS microcamera and LED light source and are disposable. A new disposable version is now available that contains a central flexible video wand that fits into a single-use clear plastic blade cover. At this time the sizes of the blades are all intended for use in adults. The device is battery operated, lightweight, water resistant, and ultraportable. With three fresh alkaline AAA batteries, it can operate for 90 minutes, and a warning light informs the operator that power is low. Additionally an integrated power management system with auto-shutoff helps preserve battery life. There is a video-out port on the device that can be connected to a proprietary

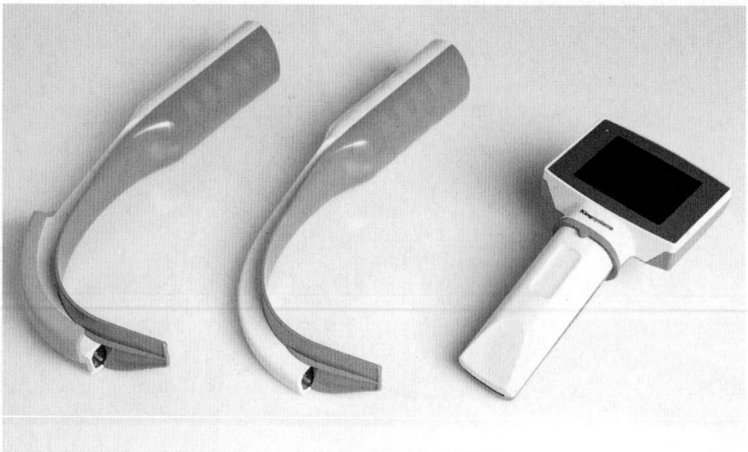

● **FIGURE 14-7. King Vision.** The King Vision video laryngoscope showing both the disposable channeled (left) and unchanneled blades and the reusable monitor.

video cable that terminates in a composite plug. Thus the display can be outputted to a larger video monitor or recorded on a video recording device.

## Using a King Vision

The intubator should select a blade, either with or without a tube channel, and plug the reusable screen into the top of the blade. The KVL is rather long, and in some patients it will be difficult to insert the device into the mouth because the video screen impinges on the chest wall as it is rotated forward during insertion. There are two options to overcome this problem. One is to insert only the blade into the mouth initially, and then plug the video screen into it after the insertion. The other option is to insert the KVL into the mouth while the whole unit is rotated 90° clockwise. Then after insertion, the device is rotated back 90° counterclockwise so that it is in the patient's midline. If a blade with tube channel is used, a lubricated ETT should be preloaded into the device before insertion. After power up, the KVL is inserted into the midline of the mouth, similar to others in this class of devices, and advanced gently with only slight lifting force used to visualize the laryngeal inlet (**Fig. 14-8**). Once the vocal cords are visualized, the tube is advanced forward, down the channel, and into the airway. It is critical to rotate the ETT counterclockwise in the channel as you advance it toward the glottic inlet. This will prevent the ETT from engaging and getting blocked by the right arytenoid. If a nonchanneled blade is used, then a standard ETT with a preformed curved, malleable stylet or the GlideRite stylet can be used and inserted in a similar fashion to a GlideScope intubation. Again, when inserting the tube into the mouth, the operator should be looking at the patient, not at the video screen. The tube should enter the right corner of the patient's mouth and is rotated counterclockwise until it is well proximated to the scope. The operator then looks at the video screen to identify the tip of the tube, and the tube is advanced through the glottis. Once the intubation is complete, the blade is discarded and the reusable screen can be cleaned with an aseptic wipe.

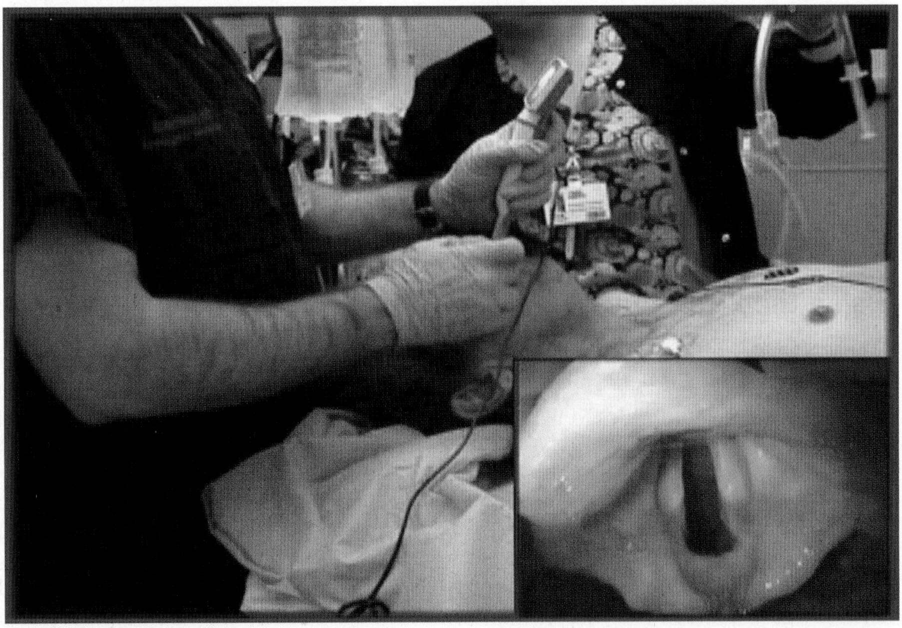

● **FIGURE 14-8. King Vision in Clinical Use.** The unchanneled King Vision being used to intubate a patient with altered mental status in the emergency department.

## Summary

The KVL is a lightweight, device that incorporates CMOS chip technology into a disposable blade design. The two blade configurations (channeled and unchanneled) give the device a great deal of flexibility as operators with different skill sets can choose the blade that works best for them. The cost of this device is considerably less than the other VLs on the market.

# PENTAX AIRWAY SCOPE

The Pentax Airway Scope (AWS) is a compact, portable VL that has a screen attached to it. Two versions are currently available: the original Pentax AWS-100 and a newer modified version called the Pentax AWS-200. The Pentax AWS consists of two components. The first is an unconventional handle with a more linear design that encompasses a monitor screen, power button, battery compartment, video-out port, locking connection ring for the disposable blade, and a flexible cable that houses the light source and charge-coupled device (CCD) micro-video camera that provides 90° of visualization. There is a disposable sleeve available that covers and protects the reusable handle from contamination. The second component is a polycarbonate Lexan disposable blade (P-Blade) that incorporates an ETT channel and 12F suction port. The blade does not feature a heat-based antifogging mechanism, but the optical portion of the blade is coated with a chemical to prevent fogging. When initially released, only a single adult size blade was available, but now there are four different blades that can be used with the Pentax AWS. There are two adult blades, a standard profile blade called the ITL-S and a low-profile blade called the ITL-L. There are also two pediatric blades available, ITL-P which can be used in children and the ITL-N which can be used in neonates. The ETT can be preloaded alongside the disposable blade with clips that hold the tube in place. The AWS has a green targeting reticle that can be displayed on the LCD screen to guide the user into the correct position for ETT placement. This targeting reticle is sometimes helpful as the side-mounted ETT does not advance into the true center of the field of view. The 2.4-in (6.1 cm) color LCD monitor is attached to the handle and can be tilted into various positions to allow easier viewing. The AWS has video output capabilities, allowing the image to be transmitted to an external video monitor or recording device. Two AA 1.5-V batteries provide approximately 60 minutes of continuous operation. A low-battery indicator flashes to alert the operator when 5 minutes of battery life remains. The AWS has a protective soft carrying case with preformed foam compartments to house the scope, video cables, and extra batteries.

The AWS is solidly built of strong plastic and stainless steel. It is somewhat bulkier than the three devices discussed earlier in this chapter. The unit is water resistant and portable, making it a reasonable option for prehospital use.

## Using the Pentax AWS

There is little setup necessary for the AWS. A disposable blade is locked onto the video cable, a lubricated ETT is loaded, the optional plastic sheath is secured, and the device is turned on and ready for use (**Fig. 14-9**). The operator may activate the targeting reticle on the LCD by pressing the on–off button. Antifog solution is recommended for use because the Lexan plastic resists fogging but does not eliminate it. The device is inserted into the mouth and advanced in the midline along the posterior pharyngeal wall, resulting in elevation of the epiglottis (**Fig. 14-10**). Unlike some of the other VLs, the blade of the AWS must be used to lift the epiglottis directly. This requires tilting the tip of the blade downward, which risks contamination of the optics because of pooled secretions in the oropharynx. If the tip of the blade is placed in the vallecula, the tube will engage the epiglottis as it emerges from the channel and the intubation will not be successful. The reticle is "aimed" at the vocal cords for appropriate position. The reduction in ETT maneuverability requires the AWS to be positioned correctly in front of the glottic inlet and decreases the operator flexibility to manipulate the ETT and the laryngoscope independently. Therefore, the operator does not use a stylet or provide manual control over the distal portion of the ETT. The ETT is advanced from the channel

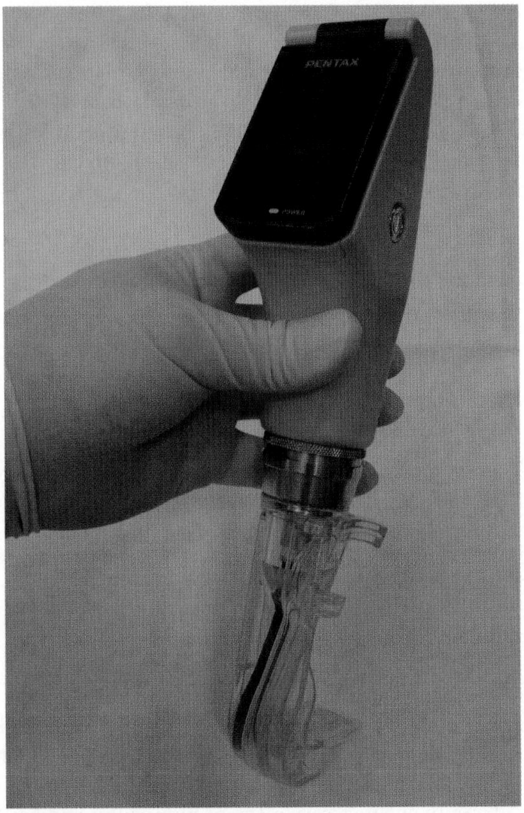


● **FIGURE 14-9.** Pentax AWS S-100.

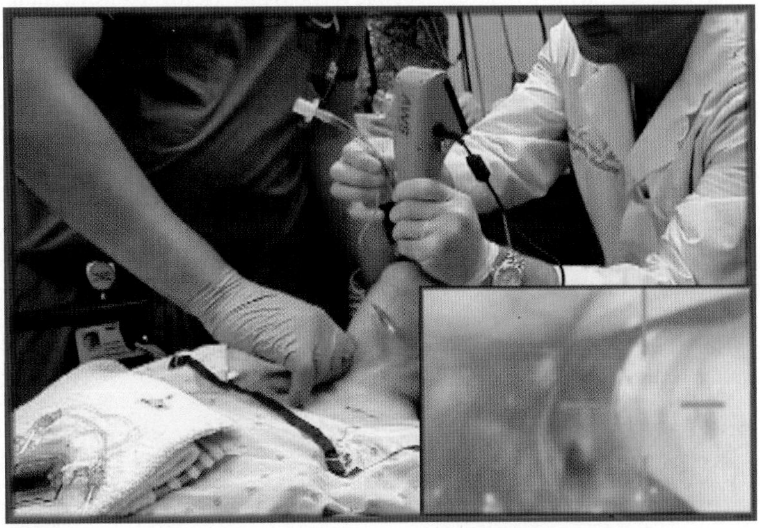

● **FIGURE 14-10. Pentax AWS in Clinical Use.** The Pentax AWS being used to intubate a patient with respiratory failure in the emergency department. Note that the tip of the blade is lifting up the epiglottis, which is necessary so that tube delivery down the guide is successful. The green reticle is slightly off center from the laryngeal inlet and the scope should be rotated to left slightly prior to attempting to advance the tube. A lubricated, unstyletted tube is being advanced down the guide and is about to pass between the vocal cords, which are not fully abducted.

through the vocal cords. If there is difficulty advancing the tube into the laryngeal inlet, a bougie can be advanced through the tube into the larynx and then used as a guide to facilitate tube passage. The AWS has the option of recording the intubation through the video output port and a proprietary RCA cable. This feature allows recording of the entire intubation for later viewing and teaching purposes. The AWS can be rinsed in water without submersion and wiped clean. The protective sheath and disposable blade make the AWS easy to clean and quickly ready for another intubation.

### Summary

The Pentax AWS is a lightweight, integrated device that incorporates CCD chip technology into a disposable blade design.

## OTHER VLs

The VL market is growing at an explosive rate, with new VLs being introduced all the time (Intubrite, Vividtrac, CoPilot VL, Venner AP Advance). There is currently insufficient research available to evaluate their effectiveness for emergency intubation, but their general characteristics are listed in **Table 14-1**.

## CONCLUSION

The technology fundamental to VLs is progressing at a rapid pace, and VL provides a superior glottic view with less force than does DL. VL is a first-line technique for both routine and difficult airways. The video-assisted laryngoscopes outperform conventional laryngoscopes, especially in those patients with reduced mouth opening, cervical spine immobility, and head and facial trauma. Most users report that only a handful of VLs are necessary before they adopt VL as their everyday device, and this has been confirmed by research studies that have demonstrated a more rapid learning curve for VL than DL. Several models have disposable versions that greatly reduce cleaning time and the potential spread of infectious agents. Additional areas where these devices are particularly helpful include confirmation of ETT placement for patients in whom tube location is in question, visualization of upper airway obstructions and foreign material, and aiding in difficult tube exchanges. Most important, all video-assisted laryngoscopes allow real-time feedback for assistance or airway management education. The instructor can provide advice for successful intubation while allowing the operator to maintain control of the scope.

DL for the purpose of endotracheal intubation was introduced into clinical medicine almost a century ago. Since then, little has changed in its application and performance. The development of VLs over the last decade is a significant advancement in the field of laryngoscopy and intubation. Based upon the current literature, VLs appear to be more effective tools than DL for emergency intubations. They are associated with enhanced laryngeal views, high first pass success, low esophageal intubation rates, and low complication rates. All airway managers should be familiar with and comfortable using video laryngoscopy.

## PEARLS FOR VL USE

- Always use a midline approach
- Stay high in the mouth to avoid contamination from the posterior pharynx
- Avoid advancing the blade too close to the larynx
- Use an appropriately curved, rigid stylet
- Back out the stylet slowly as the tube is being advanced down the trachea

## EVIDENCE

- **What is known about the role of VLs in the ED?** The literature comparing VL to DL in the ED has consistently shown that VL is superior to, or at least equal to DL for emergency intubation. A randomized trial by Driver et al.[1] found that the first pass success was 92% for the C-MAC and 86% for DL, although this difference did not achieve statistical significance. In an observational study by Sakles et al.,[2] the C-MAC was shown to have a higher first pass success and overall success than the Macintosh DL. In patients with difficult airway characteristics in the ED, Sakles et al.[3] found that use of the GlideScope or C-MAC resulted in a higher first pass success than DL. Sakles[4] also found that in patients with a failed first intubation attempt in the ED, the C-MAC was superior to the DL in achieving successful intubation on the second attempt. When used by emergency medicine residents, VL resulted in significantly fewer esophageal intubations than DL (1% vs. 5%).[5] Sakles et al. also found that the learning curve for VL was much better than that for DL, with emergency medicine residents increasing their first pass success with GlideScope by 16% (from 74% to 90%) over a 3-year training period but only by 4% (69% to 73%) with the DL.[6] VL use is increasing over time. Results from the National Emergency Airway Registry covering 10 years of ED airway management and more than 17,500 adult intubations showed that VL is now used in approximately half of all ED intubation first attempts.[7]
- **What is known about the role of VLs in the intensive care unit (ICU)?** The literature on ICU patients suggests that VLs are superior to DL for intubation of the critically ill. In a randomized study, Silverberg et al. compared the GlideScope to DL for intubation of critically ill patients by pulmonary fellows.[8] Rapid-sequence intubation was not used during this study, arguably affected DL performance more than VL, however the authors reported a first pass success with the GlideScope of 74% compared to 40% with the DL. There were no esophageal intubations in the GlideScope group but 7% in the DL group. Hypes et al. have performed the largest study on VL use in the ICU and their propensity score analysis demonstrated that VL was associated with a higher first pass success, lower incidence of oxygen desaturation, and a lower incidence of esophageal intubation.[9]
- **What is known about the role of VLs in the prehospital setting?** There are limited data on VL use in the prehospital setting, but the existing literature is very supportive. Wayne et al.[10] compared the GlideScope to DL in an urban EMS system and found that paramedics were able to intubate successfully with fewer attempts when using the GlideScope. Jarvis et al.[11] performed a study comparing the King Vision to DL in their EMS system. They found an increased first pass success when the King Vision was used compared to DL (74% vs. 44%), as well as an increased overall success with the King Vision (92% vs. 65%). Boehringer et al.[12] found that when the C-MAC pocket monitor was incorporated into their aeromedical flight program, first pass success improved from 75% to 95% and overall success improved from 95% to 99%.

## REFERENCES


1. Driver BE, Prekker ME, Moore JC, et al. Direct versus video laryngoscopy using the C-MAC for tracheal intubation in the emergency department, a randomized controlled trial. *Acad Emerg Med.* 2016;23(4):433–439.
2. Sakles JC, Mosier J, Chiu S, et al. A comparison of the C-MAC video laryngoscope to the Macintosh direct laryngoscope for intubation in the emergency department. *Ann Emerg Med.* 2012;60(6): 739–748.
3. Sakles JC, Patanwala AE, Mosier JM, et al. Comparison of video laryngoscopy to direct laryngoscopy for intubation of patients with difficult airway characteristics in the emergency department. *Intern Emerg Med.* 2014;9(1):93–98.

4. Sakles JC, Mosier JM, Patanwala AE, et al. The C-MAC(R) video laryngoscope is superior to the direct laryngoscope for the rescue of failed first-attempt intubations in the emergency department. *J Emerg Med.* 2015;48(3):280–286.
5. Sakles JC, Javedani PP, Chase E, et al. The use of a video laryngoscope by emergency medicine residents is associated with a reduction in esophageal intubations in the emergency department. *Acad Emerg Med.* 2015;22(6):700–707.
6. Sakles JC, Mosier J, Patanwala AE, et al. Learning curves for direct laryngoscopy and GlideScope(R) video laryngoscopy in an emergency medicine residency. *West J Emerg Med.* 2014;15(7):930–937.
7. Brown CA 3rd, Bair AE, Pallin DJ, et al. Techniques, success, and adverse events of emergency department adult intubations. *Ann Emerg Med.* 2015;65(4):363.e1–370.e1.
8. Silverberg MJ, Li N, Acquah SO, et al. Comparison of video laryngoscopy versus direct laryngoscopy during urgent endotracheal intubation: a randomized controlled trial. *Crit Care Med.* 2015;43(3):636–641.
9. Hypes CD, Stolz U, Sakles JC, et al. Video laryngoscopy improves odds of first attempt success at intubation in the ICU: a propensity-matched analysis. *Ann Am Thorac Soc.* 2016;13:382–390.
10. Wayne MA, McDonnell M. Comparison of traditional versus video laryngoscopy in out-of-hospital tracheal intubation. *Prehosp Emerg Care.* 2010;14(2):278–282.
11. Jarvis JL, McClure SF, Johns D. EMS intubation improves with king vision video laryngoscopy. *Prehosp Emerg Care.* 2015;19(4):482–489.
12. Boehringer B, Choate M, Hurwitz S, et al. Impact of video laryngoscopy on advanced airway management by critical care transport paramedics and nurses using the CMAC pocket monitor. *Biomed Res Int.* 2015;2015:821302.

Chapter 15

# Optical and Light-Guided Devices

Julie A. Slick

## INTRODUCTION

Traditional laryngoscopes require the operator to achieve a direct line of site of the glottis by aligning the oral, pharyngeal, and laryngeal axes (Chapter 13). Video laryngoscopes capitalize on a video camera, which is mounted on a rigid blade, to circumvent the need for a straight line of sight, while providing superior views of the glottis and surrounding spaces (Chapter 14). Optically enhanced devices are those laryngoscopes that allow the operator to visualize the glottis without creating a straight line of sight, but without using video or fiber-optic technology. The glottic view is obtained by the use of less expensive optics consisting of combinations of prisms, mirrors, and lenses. The relatively inexpensive cost of the technology is one of the major benefits of these devices when compared with the more expensive fiber-optic and video devices. Many of these devices also offer video capability through attachable video cameras. The addition of video capability provides a magnified view of the glottis, and enhances education by allowing other providers to visualize what the airway manager is observing. There are only two true optical devices of relevance to emergency airway management, the Airtraq and the Truview.

## DEVICES

### Airtraq

#### *Components*

The Airtraq is a single-use, disposable laryngoscope system that provides the operator with a magnified view of the glottic structures. The Airtraq is now available in two models: the single-use, all-in-one, ready-to-use Airtraq SP and the two-piece Airtraq Avant with reusable optics and single-use blade. The Airtraq SP comes in four sizes for conventional orotracheal intubations, with two additional special application devices. The conventional devices begin with size 0/Infant, using endotracheal tube (ETT) sizes 2.5 to 3.5, up through size 3/Regular, using ETT sizes 7.0 to 8.5 (**Fig. 15-1**). Both of the Avant blades and the conventional orotracheal SP devices have an ETT channel in which the ETT is preloaded before insertion. The channel guides the ETT directly toward the glottic

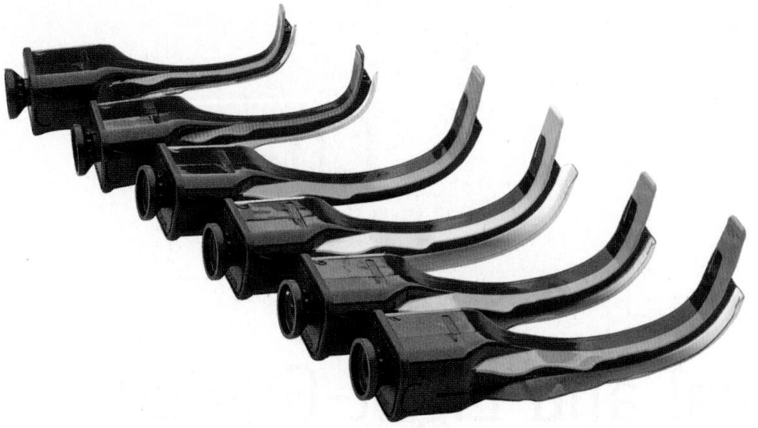

● **FIGURE 15-1. Airtraq SP Devices.** Sizes range from Infant/size 0, the gray-colored blade in the background, to Regular/size 4, the light blue device in the foreground. The orange device is the nasotracheal intubation device that lacks the tube channel, and the pale yellow device is the double-lumen device with the larger endobronchial tube channel.

opening (**Fig. 15-2**). Airtraq also offers Airtraq SP Nasotracheal that lacks the ETT channel and is intended for use during nasotracheal intubation. This device is inserted through the mouth to facilitate nasotracheal intubations with the assistance of glottic visualization. An additional specialty device, the Airtraq SP Double Lumen has a larger channel that will accommodate double-lumen endobronchial tubes. The Airtraq devices have a relatively narrow profile. The minimal mouth opening required is 16 mm for the Airtraq size 3 and 15 mm for the Airtraq size 2.

All of the Airtraq SP devices are made of plastic and are designed for single use. They cannot be cleaned or sterilized, and they will not function properly if this is attempted. This single-use attribute makes the Airtraq SP particularly suitable for field use by both emergency medical services (EMS) and military personnel. The devices are powered by three AAA batteries, which will provide approximately 90 minutes of operating time. The shelf life is approximately 2 years. The Airtraq SP is turned on by pressing a button on the top of the unit that illuminates a low-heat light-emitting diode. The device has a built-in antifog mechanism. A rubber eyepiece is connected to the optical

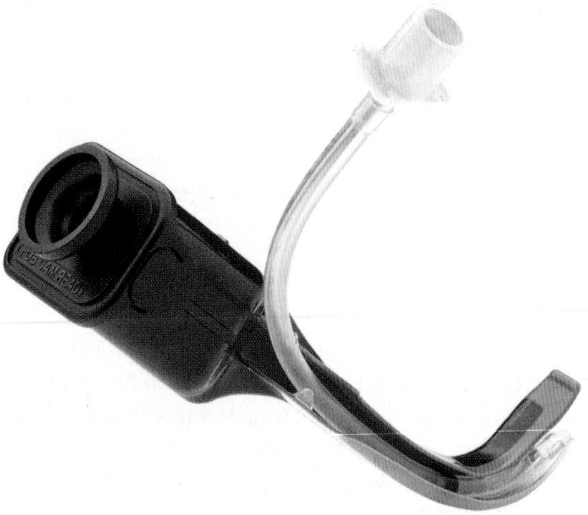

● **FIGURE 15-2. Airtraq SP Size 1/Pediatric.** This device with the ETT channel accepts tube sizes 4.0 to 5.5.

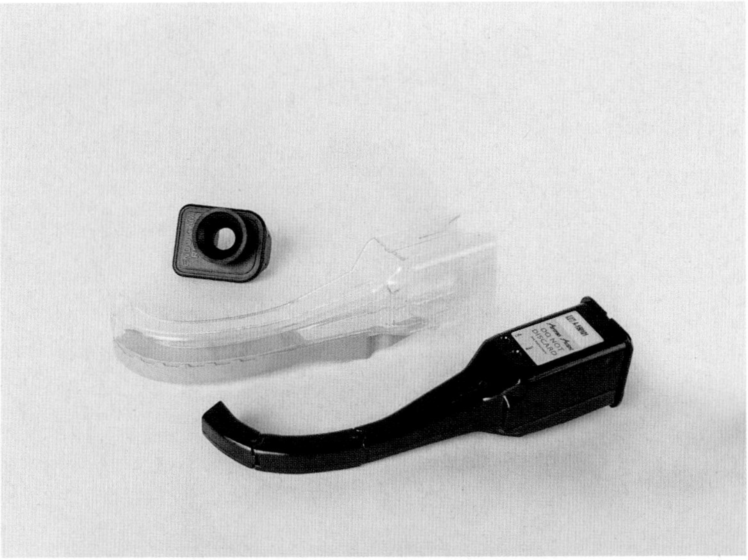

**FIGURE 15-3.** Airtraq Avant including the reusable optic device and the disposable blade and eyepiece.

channel. This rubber eyepiece can be removed and replaced with an optional video composite unit that will allow transmission of the optical image to a wired or wireless video monitor.

The Airtraq Avant offers an alternative option with essentially the same operation. The Avant employs a reusable, articulated optic component that is paired with a disposable blade (**Fig. 15-3**). The optical component has a rechargeable battery with a service life of approximately 100 minutes of continuous on time. This equates to roughly 40 to 50 intubations (**Fig. 15-4**). The Airtraq SP battery life is approximately 40 minutes, with the shelf life of the self-contained unit being 3 years. The Airtraq Avant reusable optics component is placed in a docking station for charging and storage, where the number of remaining uses is displayed. The display will also show an error code if the optics have become damaged. The Airtraq Avant has two disposable blade sizes that can be used in conjunction with the reusable optics. The blades are size 2 and size 3 and are identical in size to the number 2 and 3 blades of the fully disposable Airtraq SP units. The mouth opening required for both Avant blades is slightly larger at 17 mm.

### *Operation*

Both Airtraq devices require very little setup time. The Airtraq SP is simply removed from its protective packaging and turned on. The light will begin blinking while the antifog warms up the lens. The light will glow steady after about 30 seconds when the device is ready for use. The Airtraq Avant blade is similarly removed from its protective packaging and then placed over the reusable optic unit that has been removed from the docking station. When the optics are inserted into the blade the light will start blinking, and will glow steady when the device is fully operational. The Airtraq SP comes fully ready to use with the eyecup attached. The Avant blade is packaged with a disposable eyecup that is placed over the proximal end of the optics once inserted into the blade. A separate rechargeable Wi-Fi camera head can be purchased for use with the adult sizes of both the SP and the Avant. If the Wi-Fi camera is used, it supplants the eyecup on both devices. The ETT should be lightly lubricated and preloaded into the ETT channel. No stylet is used. The anterior surface of the Airtraq blade, which will come in contact with the tongue, can be lubricated to help facilitate passing the device around the tongue. The Airtraq should be placed into the mouth using a midline approach. Gentle outward traction may be applied to the tongue using the operator's free hand, if necessary, to ensure that the tongue is not pushed into the hypopharynx. As with all

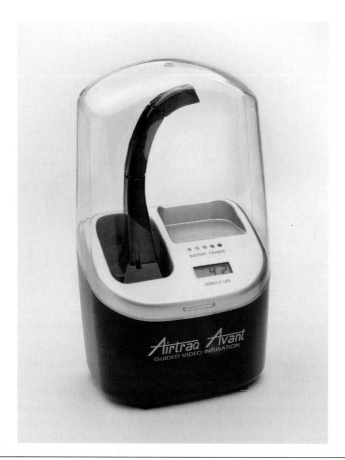


● **FIGURE 15-4. Airtraq Avant Optics Docking Station.** Battery charge and remaining service life are easily visualized.

optical and video devices, gentle and thorough suctioning of secretions is recommended before insertion of the device. The device should be kept high in the oropharynx, opposed to the surface of the tongue, to avoid contacting any pooled secretions posteriorly. As the Airtraq is advanced, the operator visualizes the epiglottis through the eyepiece and continues to move the device forward into the vallecula. When the vallecula is entered, the Airtraq is lifted in the vertical plane to elevate the epiglottis and align the vocal cords within the center of the optical field (**Fig. 15-5**). The ETT is slowly advanced through the vocal cords and then disengaged from the device and the Airtraq is removed. If the ETT is obstructed by the epiglottis or arytenoids, the entire device is manipulated to better align the ETT position with the glottic entrance. The Airtraq can be pulled back slightly and rotated along its longitudinal axis to help align the glottic structures. Alternatively, the epiglottis can be lifted directly by the Airtraq blade through a straight blade approach to appropriately align the glottic structures. However, this technique can somewhat distort the anatomy and is not the recommended approach.

If the Wi-Fi camera head is used in lieu of the eyecup, the operator will be provided a larger view of the anatomical structures, while maintaining a safe distance from the patient (**Fig. 15-5**). The Wi-Fi camera can also share real-time images with enabled Apple and Android devices. Airtraq additionally offers a phone adapter that can be used instead of the eyecup or Wi-Fi camera head for visualization of the airway. The phone adapter is compatible with most smartphones. The standard eyecups are also compatible with most endoscopy camera heads, offering another alternative for visualization.

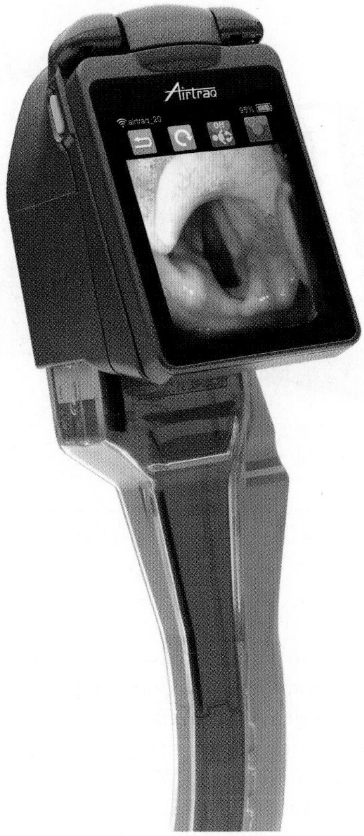


● **FIGURE 15-5.** Airtraq Avant with the optional Airtraq Wi-Fi camera head in place of the eyepiece.

### *Summary*

The Airtraq optical laryngoscope is a lightweight, inexpensive device that may have very practical applications in emergency airway management. Two models of this device are now offered, along with several viewing options. These devices require very little setup, making them extremely portable and offering added benefits for field and other "out of the department" applications. The optical device with the eyecup alone offers a clear image of the glottis. The addition of the video capability provides a magnified image with greater detail for improved visualization and obvious educational benefits. Although significantly different from standard direct laryngoscopes, the device is reasonably easy to learn and use in the emergency and difficult airway settings.

## Truphatek Truview Laryngoscopes

### *Components*

Truphatek manufactures two optical laryngoscopes, each with video capabilities. The Truview EVO2 is the older of the two devices; it has now essentially been replaced by the Truview PCD that was introduced in 2010. The Truview uses a conventional laryngoscope handle, which gives the device a familiar feel. The blades are the more unique parts of these devices. The blades are markedly angled near their midpoint and incorporate a telescope-like device with an angulated, prism-like, distal lens to provide the view of the difficult anterior airway (**Fig.15-6**). The blades are available in five sizes, allowing intubation from neonate to the morbidly obese adult. The low-profile blades require minimal mouth opening. They are made of stainless steel and can be easily cleaned and sterilized.

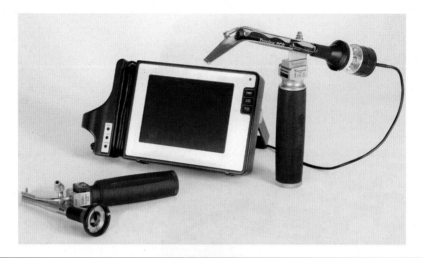

● **FIGURE 15-6.** The Truview PCD optical laryngoscope with video camera attached to the eyepiece of one of the blades.

The device can be awkward to use, as the eyepiece is designed to be viewed with the operator's eye at a distance of 2 ft (0.6 m) from the lens. Although this can provide a clear view of the glottic structures, the image appears small and distant when viewed in this manner. The system is much more capable when an optional video camera is affixed to the proximal lens of the telescope. A proprietary high-definition camera feeds to a 5-in (12.7 cm) digital liquid crystal display screen. Additionally, the eyepiece will also accept universal 32-mm endoscopic camera heads to be viewed on a nonproprietary external monitor. Either of the methods provides a significantly better image than is obtained without video enhancement, and allows for other providers to see what the operator sees.

The Truview blades also incorporate oxygen ports through which oxygen can be delivered at 5 L per minute. The oxygen flow is directed at the distal portion of the optical system to potentially clear secretions from the lens and to prevent fogging. This apneic diffusion oxygenation may provide for longer time to desaturation in the truly difficult airway (see Chapters 5 and 20). Patients who may experience rapid desaturation such as young children, pregnant women, obese patients, and those with acute or chronic respiratory illness might benefit from this feature. The device also comes with a preformed OptiShape stylet that mimics the blade shape to facilitate ETT placement, but a standard stylet may also be used.

### *Operation*

The setup time is for the device is minimal. The blade is connected to the handle, and oxygen tubing is connected to the oxygen port. Oxygen flow rate should be set at 5 L per minute. Antifog solution may be applied to the distal lens to minimize fogging. The operator should either use the preformed OptiShape stylet or configure the standard stylet to the shape of the Truview blade. The blade is placed in the midline of the patient's mouth and advanced until the handle is 2 to 3 cm from the patient's lips. Very little or no neck manipulation is required. The operator then looks through the eyepiece at a comfortable standing position to visualize the glottic structures. Small adjustments may be made to optimize the view. If the video attachment is used, the operator will look at the monitor to visualize the magnified glottic inlet. The technique for insertion of the ETT is similar to that for the GlideScope. The ETT is inserted at the right corner of the patient's mouth in a horizontal plane. It is then rotated clockwise 90° toward midline during advancement to place the tip of the ETT at the glottic inlet. The ETT is advanced through the vocal cords. The stylet and the laryngoscope are then removed, and tube placement is confirmed.

### *Summary*

The Truview PCD provides a unique, inexpensive option for difficult airway management. This third-generation optical laryngoscope offers definite improvements over its predecessors, particularly with the addition of enhanced video capabilities. Visualization can be difficult without the optional video camera. Magnified video images eliminate the difficulty of navigating toward the glottic structures with such a small field of view. The addition of the oxygen port may add benefit to this device for those patients prone to rapid desaturation.

## CONCLUSION

The Airtraq and the Truview PCD offer good glottic views without the need to obtain a direct line of sight. They do so more economically than their video or fiber-optic competitors by using simple optics with prisms and mirrors, but do so at the cost of some reduction in performance and image quality. The Airtraq device functions very well without the need for video enhancement, but the Truview PCD is difficult to use without the attached video system. Both devices have been subjected to several clinical trials (see evidence below), and have fared well in these limited studies. From a visualization perspective, the Airtraq provides generally better images than the Truview PCD, but each device has its strengths and weaknesses. Further study is required to clarify the roles for these devices in routine and difficult airway management.

## EVIDENCE

- **Is the Airtraq device better than a direct laryngoscope for patients predicted to be difficult intubations?** There have been several trials over the past few years that have evaluated the success of intubations in elective surgical patients using the Airtraq device versus the conventional Macintosh laryngoscope. A study by Koh et al.[1] placed surgical patients into Philadelphia cervical collars to simulate patients with cervical spine injury. The patients were randomized to the Airtraq group or the Macintosh group and compared regarding the ease of intubation and hemodynamic stability. The Airtraq proved to be superior with a 96% success rate on first intubation attempt versus 40% in the Macintosh group.

  A study by Ndoko et al. looked at intubation success rates in morbidly obese surgical patients in a similar comparison of the two devices. This study showed less time to intubation with the Airtraq than with the Macintosh laryngoscope at 24 and 56 seconds, respectively. Consequently, $Spo_2$ was better maintained in the Airtraq group than in the Macintosh laryngoscope group, with one and nine patients, respectively, demonstrating decline of $Spo_2$ to 92% or less.[2]
- **Is it easy to learn how to use the Airtraq?** In a study by DiMarco et al.,[3] first-year residents with no intubating experience attempted intubation on at least six patients with the Airtraq and an equal number of patients with the Macintosh. A more rapid acquisition of skills was observed in the Airtraq group as evidenced by time to intubation. The device was also judged to be easier to use by the residents.
- **How does the Airtraq perform in the prehospital setting?** Trimmel et al.[4] studied 212 patients requiring intubation in a prehospital setting. Anesthesiologists or emergency physicians responding with EMS intubated the patients. When the Airtraq was used as first-line airway device ($n$ = 106) versus direct laryngoscopy ($n$ = 106), success rate was 47% versus 99%, respectively ($p < 0.001$). The reasons for failed Airtraq intubation were related to the optical characteristic of the device (i.e., impaired sight resulting from blood and vomitus, $n$ = 11) or to presumed handling problems (i.e., cuff damage, tube misplacement, or inappropriate visualization of the glottis, $n$ = 24). This European study stands alone in its finding of a high failure rate using the Airtraq.

- **Does the Truview improve glottic view as compared to the Macintosh laryngoscope?** In a random crossover study by Li et al.,[5] 120 elective surgical patients in China underwent laryngoscopy with either a Macintosh or the Truview and assigned a Cormack–Lehane (C–L) grade by the intubator. They then underwent laryngoscopy with the other device and were intubated. Time to intubation was recorded for the second device used. The results showed that the Truview improved the glottic view of 87.5% of patients with a C–L view grade >1 by direct laryngoscopy. Another study by Miceli et al.[6] using mannequins to simulate patients with tongue swelling and neck stiffness also showed that a better C–L view was obtained with the Truview.
- **How does the time to intubation with the Truview compare to times seen with the Macintosh laryngoscope?** The study by Li et al.[5] showed that the time to intubation in the Truview group was longer by an average of 17 seconds, which likely is of no clinical significance. The mannequin study by Miceli et al.[6] also showed no significant difference in time to intubation or ease of tracheal tube placement.

## REFERENCES


1. Koh JC, Lee JS, Lee YW, et al. Comparison of the laryngeal view during intubation using Airtraq and Macintosh laryngoscopes in patients with cervical spine immobilization and mouth opening limitation. *Korean J Anesthesiol*. 2010;59(5):314–318.
2. Ndoko SK, Amathieu R, Tual L, et al. Tracheal intubation of morbidly obese patients: a randomized trial comparing performance of Macintosh and Airtraq laryngoscopes. *Br J Anaesth*. 2008;100(2):263–268.
3. DiMarco P, Scattoni L, Spinoglio A, et al. Learning curves of the Airtraq and the Macintosh laryngoscopes for tracheal intubation by novice laryngoscopists: a clinical study. *Anesth Analg*. 2011;112(1):122–125.
4. Trimmel H, Kreutziger J, Fertsak G, et al. Use of the Airtraq laryngoscope for emergency intubation in the prehospital setting: a randomized control trial. *Crit Care Med*. 2011;39(3):489–493.
5. Li JB, Xiong YC, Wang XL, et al. An evaluation of the Truview EVO2 laryngoscope. *Anaesthesia*. 2007;62:940–943.
6. Miceli L, Cecconi M, Tripi G, et al. Evaluation of new laryngoscope blade for tracheal intubation, Truview EVO2: a manikin study. *Eur J Anaesthesiol*. 2008;25(6):446–449.

Chapter 16

# Flexible Endoscopic Intubation

Alan C. Heffner and Peter M.C. DeBlieux

## INTRODUCTION

Tracheal intubation over a flexible endoscope is an invaluable technique in airway management, particularly in patients for whom standard laryngoscopy and orotracheal intubation are anticipated to be difficult or impossible. Endoscopic devices may be used for both diagnostic evaluation of the upper airway and tracheal intubation.

## INDICATIONS AND CONTRAINDICATIONS

Indications for flexible endoscopic intubation (FEI) in emergency airway management generally are identified during the LEMON evaluation for the difficult airway (see Chapter 2) and include the following:

- Patients who fail the 3-3-2 rule (restricted mouth opening, small mandible, or high larynx) or exhibiting a grade 4 Mallampati score.
- Inadequate oral access, recognized during first assessment of the 3-3-2 rule, is a strong predictor of difficult or impossible orotracheal intubation via conventional means. Examples include wired mandible, trismus, temporomandibular joint disease, tongue and oral floor space-occupying lesions (i.e., angioedema, hematoma, oral infection).
- Distorted upper airway anatomy often precludes visualization by direct or video laryngoscopy and prevents appropriate seating of blind extraglottic airway devices. Examples include pharyngeal abscess, neck or posterior oropharyngeal trauma or hematoma, and base of tongue or laryngeal tumor.
- The patient with laryngeal trauma or suspected tracheal disruption. In these cases, intubation with continuous visualization without neuromuscular blockade is recommended. The endoscope meets this indication.
- The patient for whom strict cervical spine immobility is required, particularly if the airway is predicted to be difficult. Rigid cervical collar and halo brace immobilization are the most common examples. However, severe cervicothoracic kyphosis also poses difficult positioning for most alternative airway interventions.
- The patient with morbid obesity, especially when coupled with additional markers of difficult orotracheal intubation.
- Failed intubation in the "can't intubate, can oxygenate" scenario, when time permits and immediate patient deterioration or evolving airway disease is not anticipated.

Contraindications to endoscopic intubation are mostly relative and may include the following:

- Excessive blood and secretions in the upper airway have the potential to obscure the indirect view of FEI. Some experienced bronchoscopists transilluminate their way into the trachea, then verify tracheal position via the endoscope, but this is highly operator dependent and requires advanced flexible endoscopic skill.
- Endoscopy in the context of high-grade laryngeal or tracheal obstruction, as with foreign bodies or malignancy, may precipitate total airway obstruction. In patients with high-grade supraglottic airway obstruction and impending complete airway closure, the delays and risks of precipitating laryngospasm or complete airway obstruction may argue against endoscopic intubation in favor of cricothyrotomy.
- Inadequate oxygenation by bag and mask (can't intubate, can't oxygenate scenario) does not permit endoscopic intubation because of time constraints of this critical situation.

# TECHNIQUE

## Overview

Once FEI is recognized as the intended airway technique, the best route must be selected. Outside of disease-related issues, the nasotracheal approach is considered technically easier because the nose maintains the endotracheal tube (ETT) and endoscope in the midline and the nasopharynx provides a panoramic and unobstructed view of the periglottic structures. The time required for topical anesthesia of the nose and use of smaller ETTs are significant drawbacks. The oral route typically accommodates a larger standard sized ETT but requires more technical dexterity. Oral intubating airways are a great asset to maintain midline position and control the tongue. Although either technique can be used with minimal topical anesthesia during an immediate crisis, the oral route is better tolerated when time does not allow for thorough topicalization.

### *Patient Preparation*

Although the emergency difficult or failed airway situation does not usually permit lengthy preparation, a methodical approach aims to provide psychological and pharmacologic patient preparation in a 10- to 20-minute window. Awake FEI generally includes the following patient preparation steps:

- Patient psychological preparation: Good communication with explanation of the procedure improves cooperation with less need for procedural sedation.
- Antisialogogue administration: Glycopyrrolate 0.005 mg per kg IM or IV, at least 10 to 20 minutes in advance of the procedure, reduces secretions to enhance visualization and improve efficacy of topically applied local anesthesia.
- Anesthetize the upper airway: Good anesthesia facilitates endoscopy and manipulation of the upper airway. FEI may be tolerated with limited anesthesia when patient condition mandates immediate intervention (see Chapter 23).
- Procedural sedation: Hypnosis should be used if needed with careful titration to sustain airway patency and spontaneous ventilation. Cooperative patients and those with critical airway compromise may not require or tolerate any sedation for FEI.

## Scope Selection

Instrument selection for emergency airway endoscopy is important. Affordable and durable scopes are available from a variety of manufacturers. Flexible endoscopes have several clinical uses including:

- Tracheal intubation, both nasal and oral
- Diagnostic nasopharyngoscopy and laryngoscopy
- Oropharyngeal foreign body identification

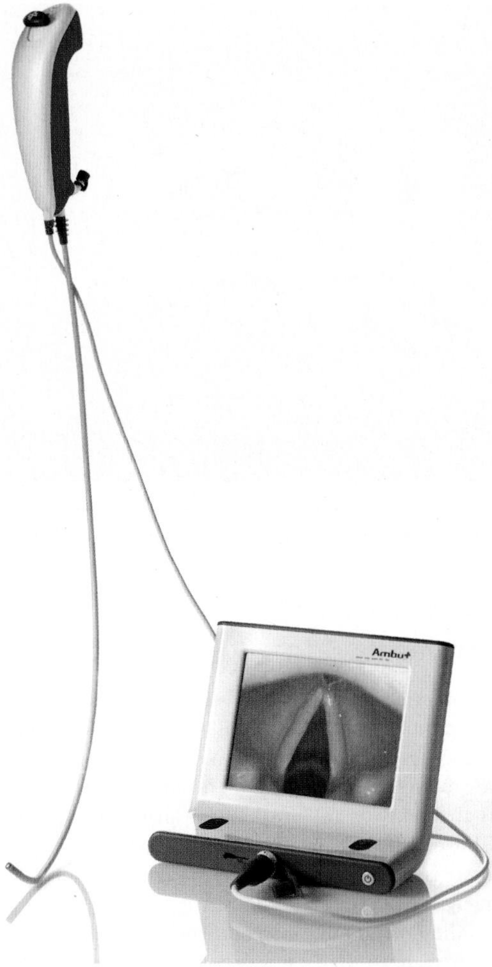

● **FIGURE 16-1.** The Ambu aScope is a single-use, flexible intubating scope.

The scope should be of sufficient caliber and stiffness to guide passage of an ETT through the curves of the airway without kinking and resist being pulled from the trachea. Standard full length (60 cm) adult bronchoscopes are generally recommended for emergency department and critical care use given their availability and breadth of use. These scopes also have the benefit of a working channel for local anesthetic injection, suctioning, and pulmonary lavage. Insufflation of oxygen through the working channel has been recommended to maintain oxygenation and disperse secretions but is now relatively contraindicated following cases of gastric insufflation and perforation. High-risk patients with marginal oxygen saturations may benefit, however, from supplemental oxygenation and may receive 5 L per minute flow through the device. The low flow rate minimizes the risk of injury while supplying oxygen and mitigating the risk of hypoxia.

Endoscopes with battery-powered, portable, self-contained light sources are compact and may be preferable for emergency applications. Single-use, disposable flexible intubating scopes are also available in the market (**Fig. 16-1**).

Some endoscope manufacturers produce intubation-specific devices with enhanced stiffness that allows small scope caliber (3- to 4-mm tip diameter) to be used for diagnostic work or endoscopic intubation. Neonatal and pediatric endoscopes (2- to 3-mm tip diameter) are also available. It is important to note that 40 cm scopes for pediatric use or nasopharyngoscopy are not long enough to permit adult endoscopic intubation.

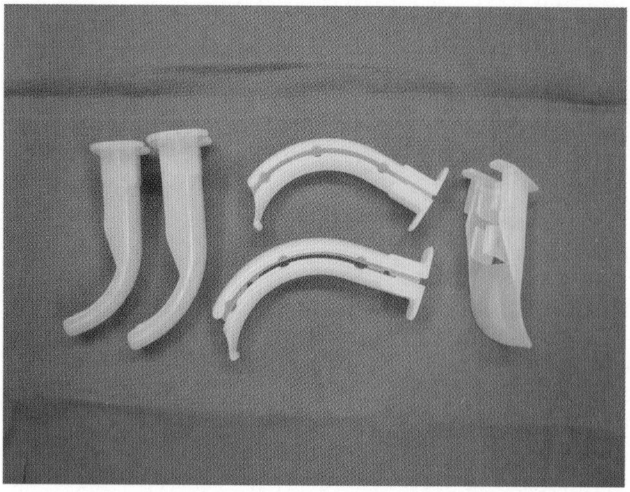

● **FIGURE 16-2.** Three examples of oral intubation airways: Williams airway (**left**), Berman breakaway airway (**center**), and Ovassapian guide (**right**).

## Care of the Instrument

Some general precautions are necessary to prevent damage to the delicate fiber-optic bundles in a scope and similar precautions are prudent even with the less damage-prone video endoscopes:

- Do not drop the scope
- Use a bite-block to protect the scope. Oral intubation airway guides incorporate this feature (e.g., Williams airway, Berman "breakaway" airway, Ovassapian airway) and are valuable aids to successful FEI (**Fig. 16-2**). The Rapid Oral Tracheal Intubation Guidance System (ROTIGS) airway is a novel device design that guides the ETT and manages the tongue to avoid gagging (**Fig. 16-3**).
- Avoid acute bending or kinking the endoscope, especially when advancing the ETT over the scope into the trachea.

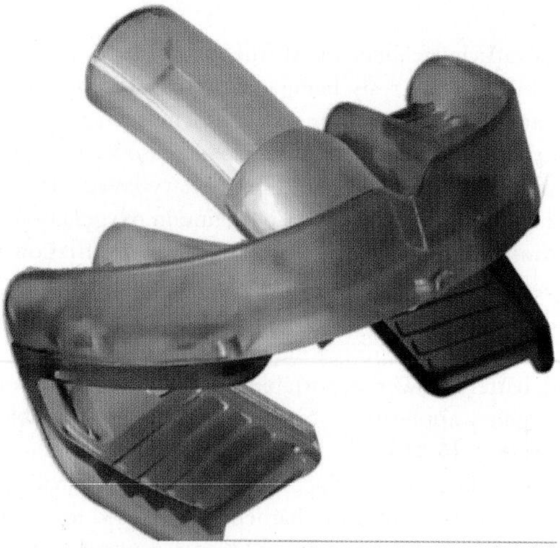

● **FIGURE 16-3. ROTIGS:** Rapid Oral Tracheal Intubation Guidance System.

- If rotation of the ETT during intubation is necessary, rotate the ETT and the scope as a unit.
- Lubricate the ETT by applying local anesthetic agent or other water-soluble lubricant to facilitate removal of the scope after the ETT is placed. Lubricating the scope cord may make it slippery and difficult to manipulate.
- Do not flex the endoscope tip against undue resistance in order to manipulate the direction of the ETT or to retract tissue.
- Clean the device, including the working channel, immediately after use. Delayed flushing can lead to semisolid deposits and the development of infectious biofilms. The best routine is to suction 1 L of saline through the device immediately after use. Manufacturers and endoscopy units provide instructions for acceptable cleaning routines.

## Technique of FEI

The endoscope has two main components: a body (hand piece) housing the controls and port access and a long flexible cord, containing video or fiber-optic components (**Fig. 16-4**). Scope tip control is simple: flexion forward and backward is achieved in a single vector with the thumb toggle on the body of the endoscope. The index finger activates the suction feature. Clockwise and counterclockwise long-axis endoscope rotation is achieved via wrist rotation. Flexing and extending the wrist moves the flexed endoscope tip left and right. The cord must be held straight to optimize this maneuver. Slack in the cord prevents wrist motion from being translated to the endoscope tip.

The dominant hand may be used to manage the endoscope body and controls or the distal cord at the interface with the patient and ETT, whichever is more comfortable. Holding the endoscope body in the hand ipsilateral to the dominant eye facilitates keeping the cord straight. Some also advocate holding the body of the scope in the left hand to provide clearance of the light source cable and suction tubing, which exit on the left of the scope body.

The endoscope view may be monitored via scope eyepiece or video screen. Many EDs do not have a video-capable system, so this description assumes the operator is viewing via the eyepiece. As a general rule, visual targets should be maintained in the center of the field of view, especially as the scope is advanced. The hand holding the cord gently advances or retracts the scope. Move toward the target slowly, using small manipulations of the toggle and wrist rotation to maintain the glottic inlet in the center of the visual field. The operator should move the hands and arms, and not the torso, to manipulate the endoscope. Hand–eye coordination needed for successful endoscopic intubation has been likened to the coordination of video game play.

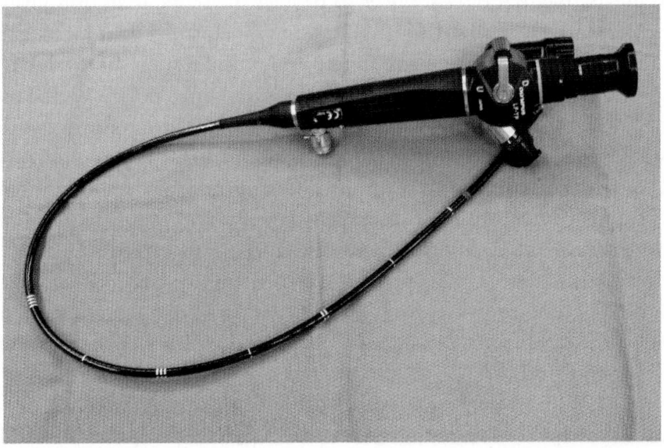

● **FIGURE 16-4. A Standard Adult Flexible Endoscopic Intubating Scope.** Note the white marks denoting 10, 15, 20, 25, 30, 35, and 40 cm on the cord of the scope.

Patient preparation for endoscopy depends on the time available. Generally, endoscopy supplies should be in a state of rapid readiness on the difficult and failed airway cart:

1. Gather all equipment (preferably preassembled on a tray):
   a. Topical airway anesthesia supplies and equipment, including three slip-tip or Luer-Lok syringes (type of syringe needed depends on the scope's make and model), 10 mL syringes loaded with 3 to 5 mL of 2% to 4% aqueous lidocaine to inject into the airway via the scope working port as needed. The remaining syringe should be filled with air flush to propel the anesthetic the length of the working port
   b. Endoscope, ETTs, oral airways, bite blocks
   c. Tonsil suction
   d. Lubricant and antifog solution
   e. Back-up airway management equipment as indicated in case of patient deterioration and need for rapid alternative intervention
2. Obtain an able and knowledgeable assistant, preferably one who is very familiar with this procedure.
3. Prepare the patient:
   a. Discuss the procedure steps prior to and during the procedure
   b. Antisialogogue, such as glycopyrrolate 0.005 mg/kg intramuscularly or intravenously, allowing sufficient time for this to work (minimum 10 minutes). This should be administered at first recognition of the procedure to allow time for effect
   c. Vasoconstrict the nose with a topical agent if the nasal route is desired
   d. Apply local, topical airway anesthesia (see Chapter 23)
   e. Optimize preoxygenation prior to procedure initiation
   f. Apply sedation if needed
4. Lubricate the inside and outside of the ETT. Lubricating the scope makes it slippery and difficult to manipulate.
5. Place the tip of the scope in a bottle of warmed saline or in a warmed blanket for 1 minute to prevent fogging. In addition, apply antifog solution if available.
6. Operator positioning is a matter of personal preference and patient tolerance. Most patients with respiratory distress or distorted upper airway anatomy need to be maintained in an upright sitting position. As such, stand up straight at the side of the bed facing the patient. Endoscopy can also be achieved from the head of the bed in the supine patient.
7. *Insert the endoscope through the preinserted ETT.*
8. Oral technique: Stay in the midline, stay in the midline, stay in the midline! *Mount the ETT within the oral intubating airway* ensuring that the tip of the ETT is flush with the tip of the airway. Insert the airway and ETT into the mouth as a single unit. The assistant must maintain the airway in the midline and avoid inserting the device too deeply. A conventional bite-block is a lesser alternative that only services to protect the scope if an oral intubating airway is not available. Alternatively, a 10 mL syringe can be transformed into a makeshift intubation guide by removing the plunger and cutting the tip end of the syringe, at the 1 mL mark, with trauma sheers. Rest a finger in the airway to maintain a reference point as you hold the cord with the index finger and thumb. Asking the patient to protrude the tongue or gentle tongue traction or jaw thrust by an assistant can help open the oropharynx to facilitate endoscopic view. If the patient is supine, placing the patient in the upright sitting position also makes the tongue less of an issue.
9. Nasal technique: Soften the ETT by placing it in warm water before inserting it. It may be helpful to dilate the chosen vasoconstricted and anesthetized nostril by gently and slowly inserting increasingly larger nasopharyngeal airways or a lubricated and gloved small finger into the nostril before inserting the ETT. This allows the operator to identify the largest and most patent nare. *Advance the lubricated ETT to the posterior nasopharynx and insert the endoscope through the preinserted ETT.*
10. The assistant should aspirate oral secretions with tonsil suction as needed. Avoid unessential suctioning of the airway as secretions may soil the endoscope tip and view. The working channel of the scope may provide insufficient suction to clear secretions during the procedure, especially if they are thick or tenacious. If the tip becomes soiled or fogged and obscures clear vision, touch the tip gently against the mucosa to clear it.

11. Get your bearings. *Recognize that the endoscopic view is inverted when the procedure is performed while facing the patient.* Upon passing the scope through the preinserted ETT, slowly advance the scope while looking for recognizable structures. The base of tongue and epiglottis are the most common first reference points.
12. Once the vocal cords are recognized, monitor opening and closing cadence with respiration. If time allows, inject 2 mL of 2% to 4% aqueous lidocaine through the working channel onto the larynx to obtund cough and closure reflexes. Position the scope in the center of the glottis and quickly advance the scope through the cords during inspiration. Ask the patient to inhale if they are cooperative.
13. If you are lost at any point, withdraw the scope until you identify a recognizable landmark.
14. Once through the vocal cords, advance the scope while confirming tracheal rings of the airway. Stop just above the carina to avoid invoking cough.
15. Advance the ETT over the scope into the trachea, being careful not to kink the scope. A conventional laryngoscope may be used to straighten the angle of approach, but rarely is required, except in the supine patient. Gentle rotation of the scope and ETT unit may be necessary if the ETT catches on the arytenoids. Newer ETT tip designs may facilitate passage of the ETT through the cords (e.g., Parker tube).

## COMPLICATIONS

Complications with emergency FEI are uncommon and typically are related to respiratory decompensation because of the course of disease, sedative administration, or airway manipulation. A back-up plan with appropriate alternative airway supplies should always be staged and ready prior to procedure initiation. Mucosal damage to the airway including epistaxis is usually mild, and damage to the vocal apparatus is possible but rare. The most frequent complication is damage to the scope from biting, twisting, kinking, or dropping. Inadvertent bronchial intubation can occur if the carina is misidentified or not appreciated.

## EVIDENCE

- **How common is FEI in emergency department patients?** FEI is an uncommon procedure during emergency airway management. From 2002 through the end of 2012, more than 17,500 adult intubations were recorded in the NEAR database. Approximately 1% of all encounters were managed with a flexible endoscope.[1]
- **What is the learning curve for emergency FEI?** There are no data, with emergency providers, that has established the expected learning curve for FEI. What we know is that intubating over an endoscope, nasally and orally, is a well-established technique for managing difficult airways. It is recognized as an important skill in emergency medicine training. Oddly, it is not an ACGME-required skill for emergency medicine residents. FEI is a technical challenge that requires initial training, and then skill maintenance to maintain speed and success. Manual dexterity in manipulating the endoscope is essential to performing endoscopic intubation in a timely fashion. This skill is best learned by attending endoscopic intubation workshops with expert instruction, and then practicing on intubation manikins or high-fidelity human patient simulators before attempting intubation in patients with difficult airways. Manufacturers of endoscopes often provide training videos, product support personnel, and manikins to support this endeavor.

  The requisite psychomotor skills cannot be developed without dedicated practice, and lack of training, practice, and experience constitute the most common cause of failed endoscopic intubation. A reasonable level of dexterity in bronchoscopic manipulation can be achieved within 3 to 4 hours of independent practice using an intubation model. The technique can also be learned in real-life situations by performance of diagnostic nasopharyngoscopy, for indications such as severe sore throat, upper odynophagia, foreign body sensation, hoarseness, and other upper airway conditions.

Gaining experience in routine cases is invaluable before one is required to perform endoscopic intubation in crisis. Patients requiring semi-emergent, but controlled emergency intubation for nonhypoxemic respiratory failure without anticipated difficult airway features are appropriate candidates for endoscopic intubation, with the confidence of back-up RSI.

## REFERENCES

1. Brown CA 3rd, Bair AE, Pallin DJ, et al. Techniques, Success, and Adverse Events of Emergency Department Adult Intubations. *Ann Emerg Med*. 2015;65(4):363–370.e1.

Chapter 17

# Fiberoptic and Video Intubating Stylets

Cheryl Lynn Horton and Julie A. Slick

## INTRODUCTION

Fiber-optic and video intubating stylets are novel intubating devices that permit visualization of the glottis by way of an image conveyed to an eyepiece or video screen from a distally positioned video or fiber-optic image source. Therefore, they do not require a direct line of sight from the operator's eye to the glottis, as must occur for successful direct laryngoscopy. Distinct from the video laryngoscopes (see Chapter 14) and optical devices (Chapter 15), the fiber-optic and video stylets are intended to have the endotracheal tube (ETT) mounted directly over them, as for any conventional stylet, and are used to guide the tube through the cords and into the trachea under continuous visualization. Unlike flexible fiber-optic devices, these devices are rigid or semirigid and include a fiber-optic bundle or video apparatus enclosed in a preformed, curved steel stylet. They are designed to navigate around the tongue and traverse the hypopharynx to visualize laryngeal structures, often with minimal mouth opening or neck mobility. Their use may offer advantages in patients with anatomic impediments to direct laryngoscopy, such as a high larynx, cervical spine immobility, or limited mouth opening. Also, rigid stylets do not have any control mechanisms like their flexible fiber-optic counterparts and thus are typically easier to maneuver, especially for nonexperts. Rigid stylets have nonmalleable curved metal sheaths, the shape of which cannot be altered, whereas semirigid devices, although not flexible, can be bent slightly to alter their angulation and thus fit the particular airway geometry of each patient.

Semirigid fiber-optic stylets include the Clarus Shikani optical stylet (SOS) and the Clarus Levitan scope (Clarus Medical, Minneapolis, MN). The predominant semirigid video stylet is the Clarus Video System (CVS). Rigid stylets include the Bonfils Retromolar Intubation Fiberscope (Karl Storz Endoscopy, Tuttlingen, Germany) and the Video Rigid Flexible Laryngoscope (RIFL) (AI Medical Devices, Inc., Williamston, MI). New intubating stylets, all similar in shape and principle, are appearing on the market regularly.

These devices are unusual emergency department (ED) tools and are not a routine part of emergency airway management; however, they have potential as adjunctive devices for the difficult airway especially when mouth opening is limited, as a method of awake intubation, or as rescue devices for the failed airway. They may also serve an expanding role in airway training because they all have video displays or are easily adapted for video by attachment of an eyepiece video camera adapter that transmits images to a video monitor.

The prototypical fiber-optic intubating stylet is the Clarus Shikani; therefore, more time is devoted to its description, proper use, advantages, and contraindications. The other devices are similar in their core design and application, and are therefore described in less detail, highlighting specific features and differences.

## SEMIRIGID STYLETS

### Clarus Shikani Optical Stylet

The Clarus Shikani is a semirigid stylet containing fiber-optic bundles for light and image transmission (**Fig. 17-1**). The stylet, rounded distally to an angle of about 70° to 80°, ends proximally in a high-resolution, fixed-focus eyepiece. The adult stylet can accommodate ETTs of 5.5 mm internal diameter (ID) or larger. A pediatric version is available and accommodates tubes of 3.0 to 5.0 mm ID. A bright halogen light is powered from the attached handle, which holds four AA batteries, but the stylet is also compatible with green specification fiber-optic laryngoscope handles or remote light sources through a fiber-optic cable. A camera can be attached to the eyepiece and the image displayed on a video monitor for teaching purposes. Additionally, a proprietary eyepiece adapter is available that can hold a variety of smartphones displaying images when the phone is in camera mode (**Fig. 17-2**). A push button power switch can be found on the top of the handle. An adjustable tube stop is mounted on the proximal portion of the stylet to hold the ETT in the desired position and prevent the tip of the stylet from protruding from the distal end of the ETT. The tube stop incorporates an oxygen port, permitting insufflation of oxygen during laryngoscopy. This helps prevent contamination of the tip of the stylet and can mitigate oxygen desaturation during prolonged intubation attempts. The malleable distal section of the stylet can be adjusted by hand, increasing or decreasing the angle of the bend to conform to the patient's anatomy. The manufacturer also sells a stylet bending guide that helps to bend the stylet in a smooth curve and helps avoid damage to the fiber-optic bundles by bending it too acutely.

To prepare the Clarus Shikani, an ETT is loaded on the stylet, with the distal end of the stylet positioned just proximal to the ETT tip, and stabilized in this position by adjusting the tube stop proximally. Lubrication of the stylet will facilitate tube withdrawal when the intubation is completed, but care should be taken not to contaminate the tip of the scope, which can obscure the image. Before insertion, the stylet tip should be warmed with either warm saline or a warm blanket. Antifog

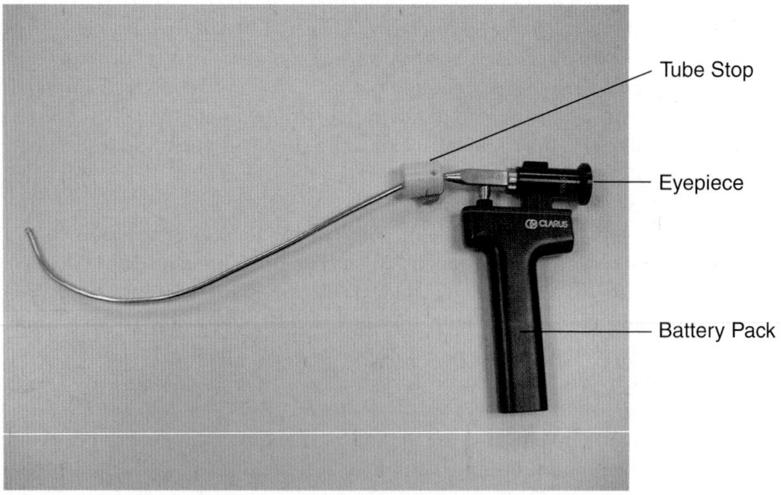


**FIGURE 17-1.** Shikani optical stylet.

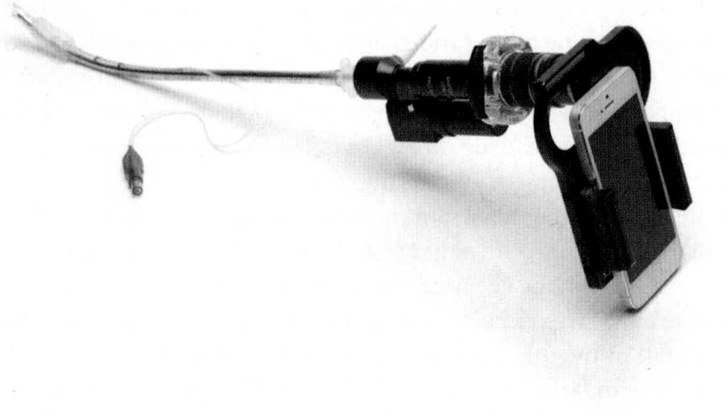

● **FIGURE 17-2.** Levitan optical stylet with optional eyepiece attachment for holding smartphones.

solution should be applied to minimize fogging during the intubation attempt. The device is held by the fingertips and thumb of the dominant hand, with the handle cradled in the web space between the thumb and index finger and the pads of all other fingers resting on the anterior part of the eyepiece and proximal stylet. Despite its appearance, the handle should not be gripped in the hand, but is properly held in the fashion demonstrated in **Figure 17-3**. The ETT–stylet combination is then inserted into the mouth in the midline and advanced into the hypopharynx under direct vision, not by using the eyepiece. The entire stylet is then advanced along its curve gently around the base of the tongue. A firm jaw lift/tongue pull during insertion will lift the soft tissues of the upper airway and create some anatomic space through which to navigate the scope. The operator should begin to visualize glottic structures through the eyepiece as the tip navigates the base of the tongue. The epiglottis should quickly come into view. Guide the stylet under the epiglottis to visualize the laryngeal inlet. The operator should then attempt to advance the tip of the stylet through the cords. Typically, the operator can advance the scope 1 to 2 cm into the laryngeal inlet. A common error is to advance the fiber-optic tip too far into the hypopharynx as it is inserted, giving a view of the posterior aspect of the hypopharynx or upper esophagus. To avoid this, ensure that the primary motion of the scope is initially rotation around the tongue and not advancement into the hypopharynx. If no anatomic

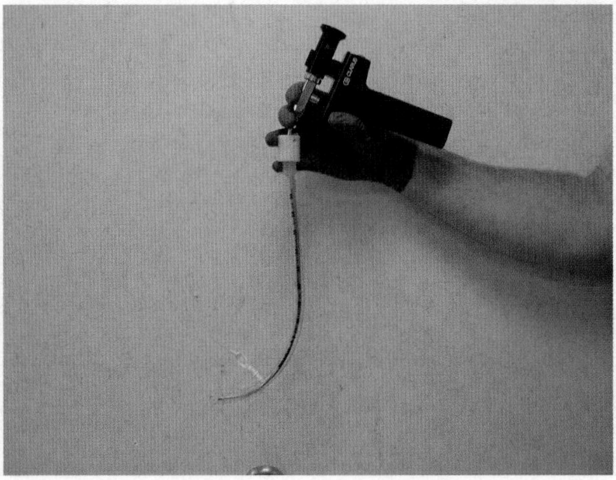

● **FIGURE 17-3.** Shikani optical stylet—in hand.

structures are recognized in the initial insertion, it is best to withdraw the stylet, ensure positioning in the midline, ensure proper elevation of the tongue and mandible, and attempt slow reinsertion, identifying the epiglottis or other laryngeal structures as the assembly is advanced. As with other intubating stylets, the instrument can be used in conjunction with direct laryngoscopy. For example, when an unanticipated grade 3 direct laryngoscopy (epiglottis only) occurs, the Clarus Shikani can be inserted under the epiglottis during direct laryngoscopy, and the glottic opening can then be located by looking through the eyepiece. When the stylet is used as an adjunct to direct laryngoscopy, an assistant may help loosen the tube from the tube stop and advance the ETT into the trachea under the guidance of the operator. With either technique, the ETT–stylet is advanced through the cords as the operator looks through the eyepiece, and then the ETT is held in place as the stylet is withdrawn by the operator, using a large circular motion, in an arc initially upward toward the ceiling in the axis of the proximal end of the tube, and then continuing toward the patient's chest and feet, following the curve of the stylet to facilitate removal (**Fig. 17-4**). Tube placement confirmation is with end-tidal carbon dioxide ($CO_2$), auscultation, and chest radiography, as for any other methods of intubation.

The Clarus Shikani is advertised as being useful for the management of difficult and routine airways, with the video and smartphone capability facilitating larger image displays, airway management supervision, and teaching. In the teaching setting, coupling the device with a video system can greatly enhance success by allowing the instructor to help guide and, if necessary, reorient the learner.

The primary limitation of the Clarus Shikani is its inability to maintain clear vision occasionally because of fogging or the presence of secretions or blood. Fogging can be greatly reduced by warming the lens and applying antifog solution, as described previously. Although secretions, vomitus, or blood can obscure the distal lens of the scope, two key design elements come into play:

1. The patient is typically supine, and with the jaw thrust and tongue pull, most of the manipulation of the scope is occurring anterior to the location of the pooled liquids.
2. If the lens becomes obscured and cannot be cleared, it is quickly and easily removed, wiped, and reinserted in a matter of seconds.

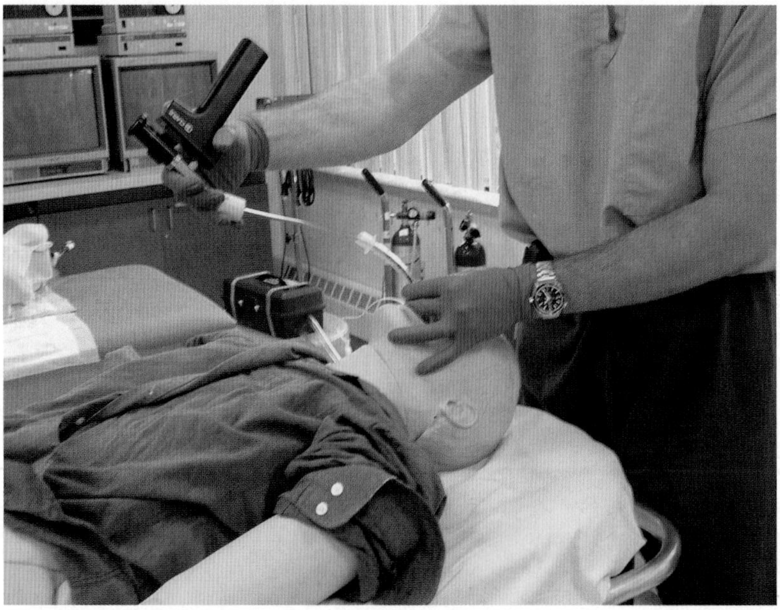

**FIGURE 17-4.** Removal of a Shikani optical stylet.

As with all video laryngoscopy and video stylet systems, it is recommended that the patient be suctioned prior to laryngoscopy using a jaw thrust and tongue pull. Performing this simple maneuver prior to inserting any video device into the mouth may greatly reduce the risk of obscuring the lens with secretions.

Occasionally, the glottis cannot be visualized using the scope, and in such cases, adjustment of the scope's curvature (usually increasing the angle, but sometimes decreasing it) provides an improved "angle of attack."

## Clarus Video System

The CVS (Clarus Medical, Minneapolis, MN) is a video reincarnation of the Clarus Shikani (**Fig. 17-5**). It is the same shape and design as the Clarus Shikani but has some new features that make it a superior device. Most importantly, a camera and a 4 in (10 cm) liquid crystal display (LCD) screen replace fiber-optic bundles and the eyepiece on the Clarus Shikani. The stylet is more malleable at the end than the SOS, making it adjustable for individual airway anatomy. The stylet can be removed from the handle and display unit, making it efficient to clean and disinfect. During intubation, the operator stands upright and looks at the screen instead of having to bend forward with the eye opposed to the eyepiece. The screen swivels, making it easy for the operator to adjust the viewing angle during the intubation. Another novel feature of the CVS is the presence of a red light-emitting diode (LED) on the tip of the fiber-optic stylet. This provides transillumination through the soft tissues of the anterior neck during intubation and thus can potentially be useful as a guide or "locator" if the lens gets contaminated and the operator cannot see the airway. The CVS in effect can be used like a lit stylet, with tracheal entry being signified by a strong glow of red light through the anterior neck. The CVS also has a video-out port allowing the operator to display the image of the airway on a larger monitor or connect one's smartphone to a video adaptor to capture, store, and share video images. Instead of using disposable batteries like the Clarus Shikani, the CVS uses an internal rechargeable battery system that provides hours of power under typical conditions.

## Clarus Levitan

The Clarus Levitan scope is a short, semirigid fiber-optic stylet intended to be used in concert with a standard laryngoscope. Its preformed shape is similar to other intubating stylets but with a gentler curve (approximately 45°); however, it can be gently bent to meet the unique geometry of most airways (**Fig. 17-6**). It has a handle with a small battery pack that powers an LED to provide illumination. A screw-down cap, rather than a push button, is used to activate the light source. The eyepiece is at the proximal end of the stylet, near the top of the battery pack. The mechanics of the Clarus Levitan are

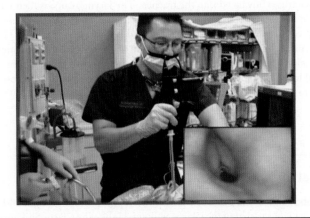

**FIGURE 17-5.** Clarus video system in use with screen image in lower right.

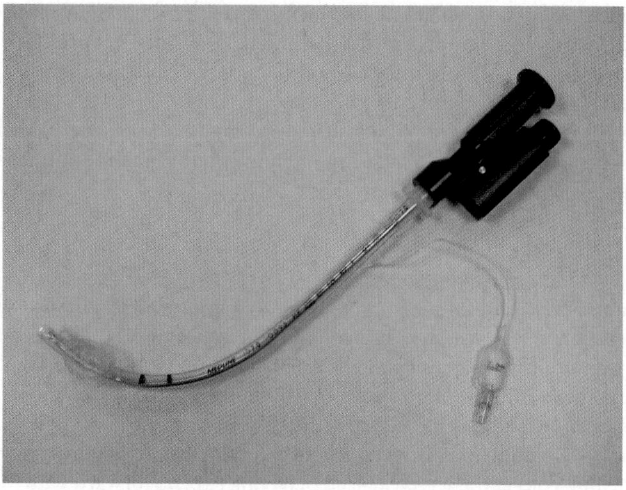

● **FIGURE 17-6.** Levitan/FPS scope.

similar to that of the Clarus Shikani, with one important difference: the Clarus Levitan is *intended* to be used with a standard laryngoscope. The ETT should be cut to 26 cm because the stylet is shorter than a standard ETT. The ETT is held in place by inserting it into a round, nonadjustable tube stop near the body of the scope. As with all intubating fiber-optic stylets, the distal end of the stylet is positioned within 0.5 cm of the ETT tip because positioning more proximally in the ETT obscures the view through the lens and results in severe "tunnel vision."

Unlike the Clarus Shikani, the oxygen port is on the distal part of the handle and there is no adjustable tube stop. A flow of 5 L per minute is intended to clear secretions and prevent hypoxia during laryngoscopy and tube placement. However, this practice has been reported to be rarely associated with gastric insufflation and perforation during flexible fiber-optic–assisted intubation and should be used with caution and low oxygen flow rates.

The Clarus Levitan scope is intended to be of particular benefit in patients with Cormack–Lehane grade 3 view on direct laryngoscopy. If a poor view is obtained by direct laryngoscopy, the operator positions the Clarus Levitan scope with mounted ETT so the tip of the scope is under the proximal tip of the epiglottis, acting, in essence, like a bougie with an eyepiece. The operator then looks through the eyepiece to visualize the laryngeal inlet (**Fig. 17-7**). When the vocal cords are seen, the entire apparatus is advanced into the trachea. The laryngoscope is then removed. The stylet is removed while the tube is well immobilized in a fashion similar to that described for the Clarus Shikani. Tube confirmation is done in the standard fashion with immediate end-tidal $CO_2$ detection and the typical clinical assessment. In the event that laryngoscopy identifies a grade 4 view, the lack of the epiglottis as a landmark greatly impairs the utility of the scope. In such cases, the scope might be used to search for the epiglottis, which, if found, might allow repositioning of the direct laryngoscope to achieve a grade 3 view.

## RIGID STYLETS

### Bonfils Retromolar Intubation Fiberscope

The Bonfils fiber-optic stylet uses high-grade fiber-optic bundles for light and image transmission in a manner analogous to that of the Clarus Shikani. Unlike the Clarus Shikani, which is inserted in the midline of the mouth, the Bonfils is intended to be used with a right paraglossal or retromolar

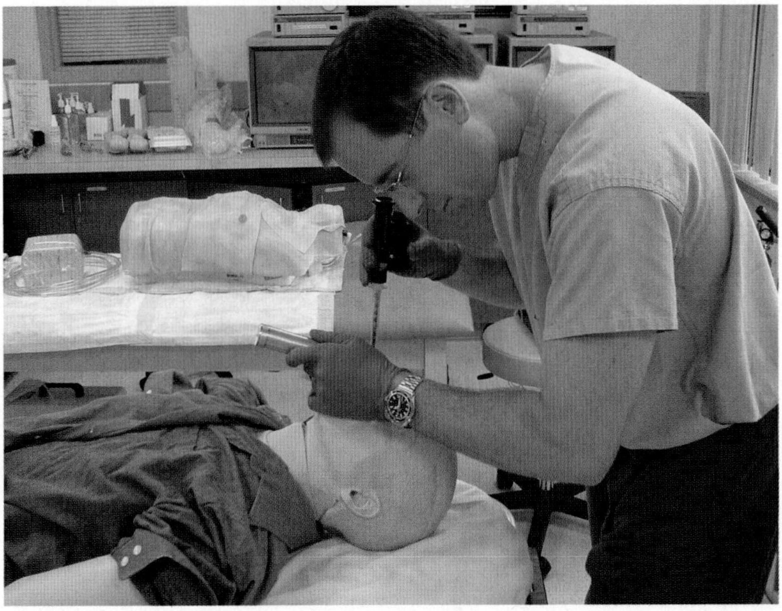

**FIGURE 17-7.** Levitan/FPS scope in use with standard direct laryngoscope.

approach, capitalizing on the proximity of the glottis to the third (most posterior) molar (**Fig. 17-8**). The Bonfils has been used extensively in Europe; however, in North America it is predominantly an operating room adjunct and is rarely, if ever, used by emergency physicians. Video laryngoscopes have largely replaced these tools for difficult airway management. There is insufficient evidence to draw conclusions about its performance in ED patients.

## Video RIFL

The Video RIFL is a hybrid intubating device with a rigid stylet that ends in a flexible tip that can be dynamically and continuously adjusted with a proximal lever up to a 135° angle (**Fig. 17-9**). It incorporates a complementary metal oxide semiconductor distal chip imaging system and a real-time

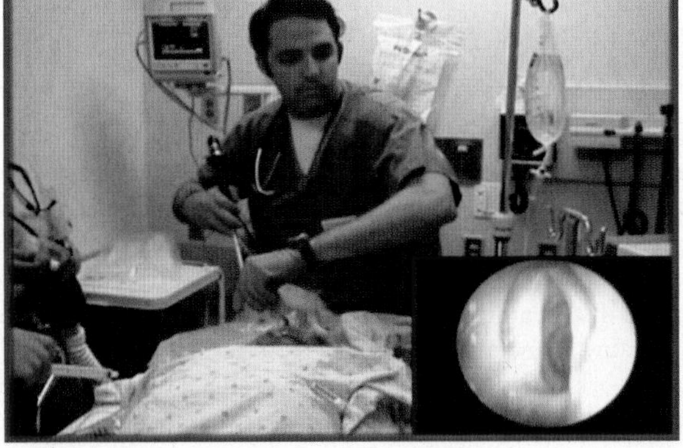

**FIGURE 17-8.** Bonfils retromolar intubation fiberscope with screen image at lower right.

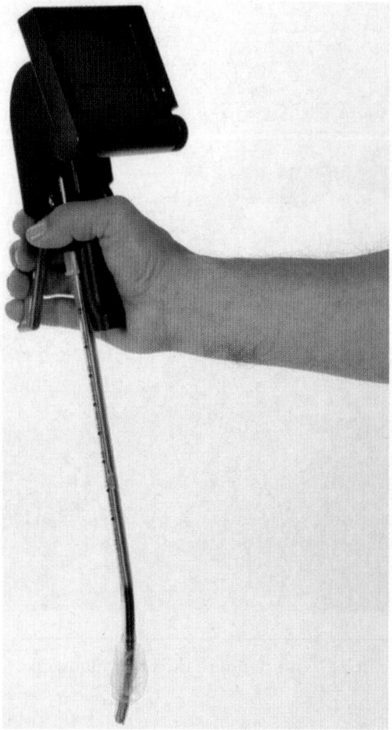

● **FIGURE 17-9.** Video rigid intubation fiber-optic laryngoscope. (Courtesy of AI Medical Devices Inc.).

articulation tip to combine features desired in flexible fiber-optic bronchoscopes as well as video laryngoscopes. The handle features a portable inline LCD, an integrated composite video output access for use with a monitor or recording device, and a self-contained power supply in addition to the lever that controls flexion of the distal tip. The manufacturer's literature states that it is intended for use in difficult airways and awake intubations, and can be used both with and without direct laryngoscopy, but clinical experience with the device is too limited to specify its role at the time of this writing. The Video RIFL uses a bright LED light source and can accommodate an ETT size of 6.5 and higher. There is no pediatric model. The RIFL can be sterilized with Steris or Cidex ortho-phthalaldehyde.

## SUMMARY

Intubating optical stylets are useful adjunctive devices for emergency airway management. The clear design advantages offered by these thin, curved, and sometimes malleable or controllable stylets have the potential to make both routine and difficult intubations more successful and safer. The primary advantage is the elimination of the need to create a straight line of sight from outside the patient's mouth to the glottic aperture, the major barrier to successful direct laryngoscopy. By positioning the "viewing port" at the distal end of a stylet, these optical intubating stylets offer a great advantage over direct laryngoscopy, allowing the operator to "steer" the distal end of the ETT through the cords. Considerable work needs to be done to fully evaluate these devices in the emergency arena; however, it seems reasonable that many of the benefits seen in anesthesia literature would apply to patients requiring emergency airway management.

## EVIDENCE

- **Do we have any proof that the Clarus Shikani is superior to direct laryngoscopy?** Most existing studies are relatively small reports in the anesthesia literature using healthy elective surgical patients, but studies in the emergency medicine literature are emerging. Shikani first described use of the Clarus Shikani in the management of difficult airways in adults and children undergoing elective otolaryngologic surgery.[1] Only a single case report describes use of the Clarus Shikani in emergency airway management, where it was successfully used for an awake intubation of an obese patient with chronic obstructive pulmonary disease.[2] Reports of use in pediatrics have been confined to difficult airway management in the OR.[3] A clear role in the care of trauma patients has not been elucidated, but one study shows that the Clarus Shikani causes less C-spine motion than Macintosh direct laryngoscopy.[4] In a study of simulated difficult tracheal intubation in manikins, the Clarus Shikani outperformed the gum elastic bougie, achieving higher success rates and shorter intubation times.[5]
- **Are there any studies supporting the use of the Clarus Levitan?** Similar to other optical devices, there is little literature besides case studies describing the use of the Clarus Levitan scope in emergency airway management. A study comparing the Clarus Levitan and the bougie as adjuncts to direct laryngoscopy in manikin-simulated difficult airways found them both equally effective in simulated Cormack–Lehane grade 3a views, but the Clarus Levitan was significantly more effective than the bougie in facilitating intubation of a Cormack–Lehane grade 3b view.[6] In a similar study on 34 elective anesthesia patients with simulated grade 3 laryngoscopy, the bougie and the Clarus Levitan performed similarly. The Clarus Levitan was limited by secretions obscuring the lens and the bougie by failing to hold its shape.[7] One study compared intubations with the Clarus Levitan and direct laryngoscopy in normal and simulated difficult airways where patients were placed in cervical collars. Both groups had similar laryngoscopic views and intubation times.[8] In another study of human subjects, a single operator modified the Clarus Levitan into an S-shape and successfully intubated 300/301 patients, with a mean intubation time of 23 seconds without using a direct laryngoscope.[9] These results likely cannot be generalized, though, and we recommend using the Clarus Levitan only with conventional direct laryngoscopy.
- **Should the Bonfils Retromolar Intubation Fiberscope be used for emergency airway management?** There have been multiple OR-based studies published involving the Bonfils fiberscope. A European case series reported on six prehospital intubations, the majority being difficult intubations, with all six patients successfully intubated on the first attempt.[10] In another study of 76 normal patients placed in a cervical collar before induction with intubation, the Bonfils was successful more frequently and with a shorter intubation time when compared with direct laryngoscopy.[11] One recent study compared the Bonfils fiberscope with the GlideScope Cobalt video laryngoscope for pediatric intubations and found the Bonfils to have better glottic views and shorter intubation times.[12] Several studies have shown the utility of the Bonfils in awake intubations on patients with difficult airways, demonstrating that it is well tolerated and highly successful (96.6%) in this setting even by inexperienced anesthesia operators.[13,14] In summary, there are several small, OR-based studies showing that the Bonfils has some utility in managing adult and pediatric difficult airways; however, at this time, we cannot recommend the Bonfils for ED use given the lack of ED-specific data, the complexity and expense of the equipment, and limited familiarity with and access to this device.
- **Is there any evidence supporting the use of the Video RIFL?** One recent study compared the Video RIFL to a flexible fiber-optic bronchoscope for difficult intubations and found intubations were faster using the RIFL and required fewer airway assist maneuvers.[15]
- **Is there a comprehensive analysis of the performance of fiber-optic stylets and nonstandard laryngoscopes versus direct laryngoscopy?** One study attempted a quantitative review and meta-analysis of the performance of nonstandard laryngoscopes and rigid fiber-optic intubation aids but was limited by data heterogeneity, which the authors deemed too difficult to

interpret. There are no definitive studies in nonsimulated environments that compare these alternative airway devices to make recommendations of success rates, ease of use, and time to intubation.[16] There have been several review articles written updating the advances and utility of these devices in airway management.[17,18] Overall, the role of fiber-optic intubating stylets in emergency airway management has yet to be clearly defined, but appears to have utility especially as an adjunct in managing the difficult airway.

## REFERENCES


1. Shikani AH. New "seeing" stylet-scope and method for the management of the difficult airway. *Otolaryngol Head Neck Surg*. 1999;120:113–116.
2. Kovacs G, Law AJ, Petrie D. Awake fiberoptic intubation using an optical stylet in an anticipated difficult airway. *Ann Emerg Med*. 2007;49(1):81–83.
3. Shukry M, Hanson RD, Koveleskie JR, et al. Management of the difficult pediatric airway with Shikani optical stylet. *Paediatr Anaesth*. 2005;15(4):342–345.
4. Turkstra TP, Pelz DM, Shaikh AA, et al. Cervical spine motion: a fluoroscopic comparison of Shikani optical stylet vs. Macintosh laryngoscope. *Can J Anaesth*. 2007;54(6):441–447.
5. Evans A, Morris S, Petterson J, et al. A comparison of the Seeing Optical Stylet and the gum elastic bougie in simulated difficult tracheal intubation: a manikin study. *Anaesthesia*. 2006;61(5):478–481.
6. Kovacs G, Law JA, McCrossin C, et al. A comparison of a fiberoptic stylet and a bougie as adjuncts to direct laryngoscopy in a manikin-simulated difficult airway. *Ann Emerg Med*. 2007;50(6):676–685.
7. Greenland KB, Liu G, Tan H, et al. Comparison of the Levitan FPS Scope and the single-use bougie for simulated difficult intubation in anaesthetised patients. *Anaesthesia*. 2007;62(5):509–515.
8. Kok T, George RB, McKeen D, et al. Effectiveness and safety of the Levitan FPS Scope™ for tracheal intubation under general anesthesia with a simulated difficult airway. *Can J Anaesth*. 2012;59(8):743–750.
9. Aziz M, Metz S. Clinical evaluation of the Levitan Optical Stylet. *Anaesthesia*. 2011;66(7):579–581.
10. Byhahn C, Meininger D, Walcher F, et al. Prehospital emergency endotracheal intubation using the Bonfils intubation fiberscope. *Eur J Emerg Med*. 2007;14(1):43–46.
11. Byhahn C, Nemetz S, Breitkreutz R, et al. Brief report: tracheal intubation using the Bonfils intubation fibrescope or direct laryngoscopy of patients with a simulated difficult airway. *Can J Anaesth*. 2008;55:232–237.
12. Kaufmann J, Laschat M, Hellmich M, et al. A randomized controlled comparison of the Bonfils fiberscope and the GlideScope Cobalt AVL video laryngoscope for visualization of the larynx and intubation of the trachea in infants and small children with normal airways. *Paediatr Anaesth*. 2013;23(10)913–919.
13. Corbanese U, Possamai C. Awake intubation with the Bonfils fibrescope in patients with difficult airway. *Eur J Anaesthesiol*. 2009;26(10):837–841.
14. Abramson SI, Holmes AA, Hagberg CA. Awake insertion of the Bonfils Retromolar Intubation Fiberscope in five patients with anticipated difficult airways. *Anesth Analg*. 2008;106(4):1215–1217.
15. Alvis BD, King AB, Hester D, et al. Randomized controlled pilot trial of the rigid and flexing laryngoscope versus the fiberoptic bronchoscope for intubation of potentially difficult airway. *Minerva Anesthesiol*. 2015;81(9):946–950.
16. Mihai R, Blair R, Kay H, et al. A quantitative review and meta-analysis of performance of non-standard laryngoscopes and rigid fibreoptic intubation aids. *Anaesthesia*. 2008;63(7):745–760.
17. Pott LM, Murray WB. Review of video laryngoscopy and rigid fiberoptic laryngoscopy. *Curr Opin Anaesthesiol*. 2008;21(6):750–758.
18. Hurford W. The video revolution: a new view of laryngoscopy. *Respir Care*. 2010;55:1036–1045.

Chapter 18

# Blind Intubation Techniques

Michael T. Steuerwald, Darren A. Braude, and Steven A. Godwin

## DESCRIPTION

Blind intubation techniques are those methods of airway management that result in passage of an endotracheal tube (ETT) through the larynx and into the trachea without any visualization of the glottic structures. Pertinent examples of such procedures include blind nasotracheal intubation (BNTI), digital tracheal intubation (DTI), and blind passage of an ETT through an extraglottic device (EGD).

BNTI relies on visual and auditory cues to distinguish tracheal versus esophageal tube passage, whereas DTI depends on the provider's ability to use tactile senses to distinguish airway anatomy as the tube is inserted. Blind passage of an ETT through an EGD is discussed in Chapter 10.

## BLIND NASAL INTUBATION

### Historical Perspective

Whereas BNTI was once a commonplace procedure for emergency intubation, it has now been relegated to a novelty in many settings. With the advent of medication-facilitated airway management (MFAM) and technologies such as video laryngoscopes, flexible intubating endoscopes, extraglottic airways, and noninvasive positive-pressure ventilation (NIPPV), the need for performing BNTI has virtually vanished. In addition, ICUs are generally unwilling to manage nasally intubated patients because the smaller tubes required for passage make ventilation and pulmonary toilet more difficult, and there is an increased risk of sinusitis. The "original" indication for BNTI in emergency airway management was for the patient in whom intubation was deemed necessary but who still had intact airway protective reflexes and MFAM was not available. Today, such patients would likely be managed with rapid sequence intubation (RSI) or NIPPV. There was also a long-held but now debunked belief that BNTI was preferable in the setting of confirmed or suspected cervical injury because of less perceived periprocedural cervical spine movement.

### Indications and Contraindications

BNTI may still be considered in those situations where intubation is clearly indicated and either (1) RSI is not permitted by scope of practice or (2) RSI is contraindicated because of predicted airway difficulty, and the equipment or expertise for awake oral or visualized nasal intubation is not available. Unfortunately, success rates for BNTI never came close to those for RSI even when it was commonly performed; it is undoubtedly even lower now. Therefore, providers who are attempting BNTI must be ready to perform a surgical airway if unsuccessful.

BNTI is achieved by using some cue to recognize that the patient's spontaneous airflow is traveling through the ETT after blind passage, and therefore, the procedure should not be attempted in the apneic patient or the chemically paralyzed patient. It is relatively contraindicated in combative patients; in those with anatomically disrupted or distorted airways (e.g., neck hematoma, upper airway tumor); in the context of severe facial trauma with suspected basal skull fracture; in upper airway infection, obstruction, or abscess (e.g., Ludwig's angina, epiglottitis); and in the presence of coagulopathy. It is also a poor choice for patients with hypoxemic respiratory failure who cannot be adequately oxygenated during a protracted nasal intubation attempt.

## Technique

1. *Preoxygenate* the patient with 100% oxygen.
2. *If the patient is awake, explain the procedure*. This is a crucial step that is often neglected. If the patient becomes combative during intubation, the attempt must cease because epistaxis, turbinate damage, or even pharyngeal perforation may ensue. A brief, reassuring explanation of the procedure, its necessity, and anticipated discomfort may avert this undesirable situation.
3. *Choose the nostril to be used*. Inspect the interior of the naris, with particular reference to the septum and turbinates. It may help to occlude each nostril in turn and listen to the flow of air through the orifices. If there appears to be no clear favorite, the right naris should be selected because it better facilitates passage of the tube, with the leading edge of the bevel laterally placed.
4. *Instill a topical vasoconstrictor* (i.e., phenylephrine or oxymetazoline) spray into each nostril. This may reduce the risk of epistaxis and make tube passage easier, though the evidence is limited. Atomization with a commercially available device may be the most desirable method of application. It may also be helpful to soak two or three cotton-tipped applicators in the vasoconstrictor solution and place them gently and fully into the naris until the tip touches the nasopharynx; this provides vasoconstriction at the area that is often most difficult to negotiate blindly with the ETT.
5. *Insert a nasal airway lubricated with 2% lidocaine jelly* into the selected naris. This helps to dilate the nasal passage and distribute the anesthesia. If there is ample time, some providers prefer to start with a smaller size and then sequentially replace these with larger diameter nasopharyngeal airways (NPAs) to "dilate up" to the size of the ETT to be used.
6. *Consider anesthesia of the posterior oropharynx* if time permits. The posterior cavity may be sprayed with 4% lidocaine or a similar spray; a commercially available "wand-style" atomization device may be the best choice for this application. An alternative is to nebulize 3 mL of 4% aqueous lidocaine solution in a standard small-volume nebulizer (see Chapter 23).
7. *Select the appropriate ETT*. A specialized ETT such as the Endotrol (Covidien; Mansfield, MA) tube may be extremely helpful. These tubes have a "pulley-like" apparatus built into them to allow anterior deflection of the tip of the tube at the will of the operator (**Fig. 18-1A, B**). In general, the tube should be the largest one that will fit through the nostril without inducing significant trauma, or 6.0 to 7.0 mm in most adults. Test the ETT cuff for leaks in the usual manner. You may consider warming the tube as for a standard endoscopic nasal intubation only if you are using an Endotrol-type ETT. If you are using a standard ETT, warming may make it too floppy to deflect far enough anteriorly.
8. *Prepare capnography* that will be used for tube guidance (**Fig. 18-2**).
9. *Lubricate the tube generously* using any appropriate ETT lubricant.
10. *Position the patient appropriately*. The awake patient will usually be seated while the unconscious patient will usually be supine. In either situation, a sniffing or ramped position should be assumed unless contraindicated. Positioning the head as for oral intubation is worthwhile, if possible. The so-called "ear to sternal notch" position, with the neck flexed on the body and the head extended on the neck, optimizes the alignment of the mouth and pharynx (in the adult patient) with the vocal cords and trachea (see Chapter 13). A small folded towel may be placed behind the

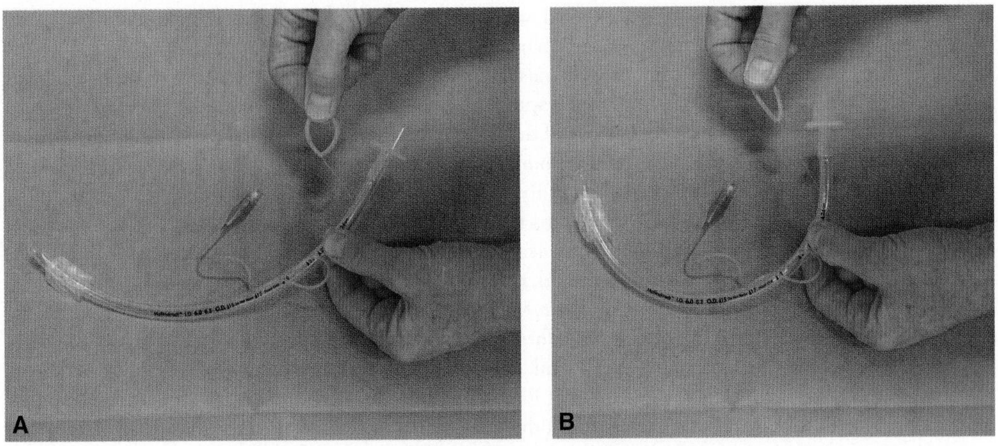

● **FIGURE 18-1. A:** The Endotrol tube, without flexion applied. **B:** The Endotrol tube, with flexion applied.

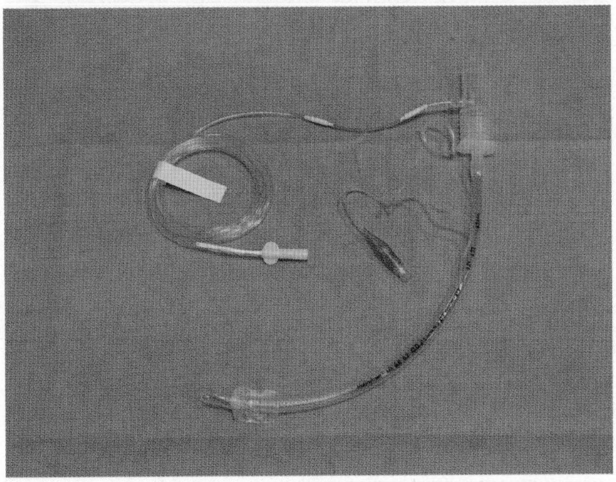

● **FIGURE 18-2.** An Endotrol tube, with waveform capnography equipment attached.

patient's occiput to help maintain this relationship. Care must be taken to avoid overextension of the atlanto-occipital joint, however, which can cause the tube to pass anteriorly to the epiglottis.

11. *Position yourself.* For a seated subject, the provider should position themselves where there is access and/or on whichever side they feel most comfortable to simultaneously manipulate the larynx, tube, and pulley mechanism. For the unconscious (but breathing) subject, it is often easiest to position yourself immediately above the patient's head.
12. *Consider sedation.* Some patients may benefit from cautious intravenous administration of a sedative or dissociative agent prior to BNTI (see Chapter 23).
13. *Remove the NPA and consider final dilation.* The operator can consider inserting a gloved and lubricated little finger into the chosen nostril as deeply as possible to check for patency and to dilate the nostril to accept the tube.
14. *Insert the ETT.* Gently insert the ETT into the nostril with the leading edge of the bevel lateral (i.e., "bevel out" or "bevel away" from the septum) to theoretically minimize the risk of epistaxis. For consistency, the remainder of this discussion assumes a bevel out, right naris intubation, which orients the natural curve of the ETT with the natural curve of the airway without rotation. The major nasal airway is located below the inferior turbinate and the placement of the ETT should

follow the floor of the nose backward, with the tip directed slightly caudad to follow the gently downsloping floor of the nose (see Chapter 4). This entire process should be performed slowly and with meticulous care. Once the nasal portion of the airway is navigated, inciting epistaxis is unlikely. When the tip of the tube approaches the posterior pharynx, resistance will often be felt, particularly if the leading edge of the ETT enters the depression in the nasopharynx where the Eustachian tube enters. At this point, it is possible to penetrate the nasopharyngeal mucosa with the ETT and dissect submucosally if care is not taken (see Chapter 4). Often, rotating the proximal end of the ETT 90° toward the left nostril once this resistance is felt will facilitate "turning the corner" by orienting the leading edge of the ETT away from the depression. Once the oropharynx is successfully entered, restore the tube to the original orientation and proceed.

15. *Advance the tube with capnography detector attached*. Carefully observe for a normal square waveform morphology (**Fig. 18-3**). Loss of waveform indicates esophageal positioning. If using an Endotrol tube, the ring may be manipulated while monitoring for the best possible waveform. A Beck Airway Airflow Monitor (BAAM; Great Plains Ballistics; Donaldsonville, LA) has often been used historically as an adjunct to provide audible feedback—louder whistling indicates the larynx has been approached or entered while cessation of whistling indicates esophageal passage (**Fig. 18-4**). Our preference is for capnographic guidance though this has not been subjected to rigorous evaluation.

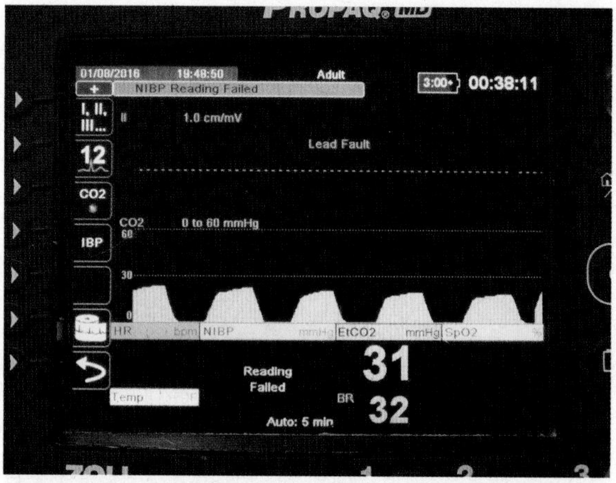


● **FIGURE 18-3.** A waveform capnogram with normal morphology.

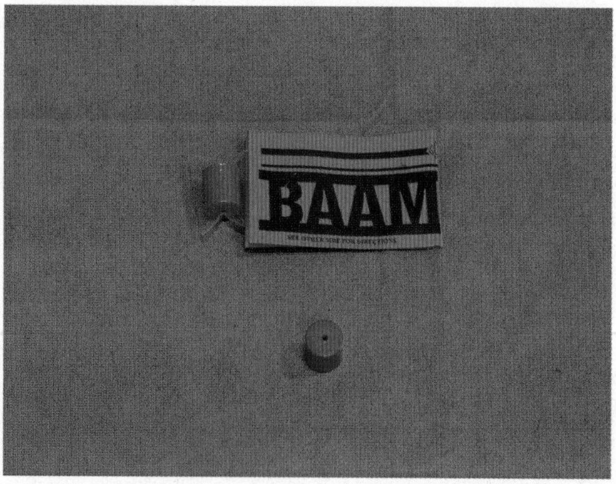


● **FIGURE 18-4.** A BAAM device.

16. *Advance tube into larynx*. Monitor respirations and capnography and advance the tube gently another 3 or 4 cm into the larynx during patient inspiration while applying laryngeal pressure with the hand not advancing the tube. The vocal cords abduct during inspiration and are most widely separated at this time.
17. *Determine if the trachea has been entered*.
    a. If the trachea is entered, a series of long, wheezy coughs will usually emanate from the patient immediately and the capnography waveform will still be present.
    b. If the esophagus is entered, withdraw the tube until an $ETCO_2$ waveform is regained before attempting again. Consider repositioning the patient's head if not contraindicated, first with additional extension. Pay close attention to the amount of pressure applied to the Endotrol ring. Note that, at most, only 60% to 70% of BNTI will succeed on the first attempt. If the intubation is proving extremely difficult, consider the various troubleshooting options below or abandon the attempt.
18. *Adjust tube depth*. Assess for an audible air leak, lost volume on the ventilator, and a square capnographic waveform—a tube in the hypopharynx will generate a waveform but will likely exhibit morphology that is "more peaked." Note that an appropriately positioned tube will be 3 cm deeper when measured at the nares than if it were measured at the lip after an oral intubation.
19. *Routine tube confirmation and postintubation management*.

### Troubleshooting

- If available, the first best means of troubleshooting involves passage of a flexible endoscope to convert a blind procedure into a visualized procedure (see Chapter 16). The rest of this section will presume this technology is not available.
- Convert to an Endotrol tube if available and not used initially.
- If the tube has met with a "dead end" it may be anterior to the cords or abutted against the anterior wall of the trachea—it may be possible to determine tube position by palpation—and slight withdrawal of the tube followed by slight flexion of the head may facilitate passage along with capnography guidance. If it is believed that the tube is off to the left or right, withdraw the tube, flex the head slightly if possible, and either twist the proximal end of the ETT or turn the head slightly in the direction to which the distal tip of the tube is believed to be off midline.
- Inflation of the cuff as the tube lies in the oropharynx may aid in alignment of the ETT with the glottic opening. The tube is then advanced until it meets resistance at the cords, and then the cuff is deflated before being pushed through the cords during inspiration. Inflation of the cuff is felt to lift the end of the tube away from the esophagus and into alignment with the vocal cords. This should not be necessary when using an Endotrol tube.
- Change to a new tube, perhaps one that is 0.5 to 1.0 mm internal diameter smaller. The tube often becomes warm and soft during the intubation attempt and is no longer capable of being appropriately manipulated.
- Grasp the tongue with a piece of gauze and pull it forward, or sit the patient up if possible, to improve the angle at the back of the tongue.
- Abandon the attempt. Prolonged attempts are associated with hypoxemia and glottic edema caused by local trauma. Either condition can worsen the situation substantially. Repeated attempts are not significantly more successful than the first. In 10% to 20% of cases, BNTI will simply not be possible.

## DIGITAL TRACHEAL INTUBATION

DTI is a blind tactile intubation technique in which the operator uses his or her fingers to direct an ETT into the larynx.

## Indications and Contraindications

DTI has mostly been described or recommended for airway situations in which laryngoscopy equipment fails or is unavailable, such as the tactical and military environment, difficult patient positioning, or because of extensive secretions obscuring visualization. Evidence for this procedure is primarily limited to cadaver and mannequin studies and case reports. Most such cases may also be managed with an EGD so it is rare that DTI would be the only or best option available. When performing DTI, the patient must be paralyzed or comatose, or at least sufficiently obtunded to prevent a biting injury to the operator.

## Technique

1. The right-handed operator stands on the patient's right side. Have an assistant use a gauze sponge to gently but firmly retract the tongue.
2. An ETT without a stylet should be tried first as this leaves the ETT tip most flexible and more easily deflected, digitally, into the larynx. If the operator's hand and fingers are short and unable to reach the glottic inlet, then a preshaped ETT with a standard malleable stylet can be used. Insert a stylet in the ETT and bend the ETT/stylet at a 90° angle just proximal to the cuff, and place the ETT/stylet into the mouth. Alternatively, use of an endotracheal introducer (e.g., bougie) has been described.
3. Slide the index and long fingers of the right hand palm down along the tongue positioning the ETT/stylet on the palmar surface of the hand.
4. Identify the tip of the epiglottis with the tip of the long finger and direct it anteriorly.
5. Use the index finger to gently direct the ETT/stylet or bougie into the glottic opening. If a bougie is used, tracheal positioning should be confirmed in the usual manner and then the ETT passed over it into the trachea.
6. Confirm ETT placement in the usual manner.

## Success Rates and Complications

Perhaps the most substantial limitation in performing this technique successfully is the length of the operator's fingers relative to the patient's oropharyngeal dimensions. Biting injuries or unintentional dental injuries to the hand with the risk of infectious disease transmission may occur. The technique has only infrequently been reported and most authors agree that some degree of experience is needed to perform this technique in an efficient and effective manner. There are insufficient data to report a reliable expected success rate.

# EVIDENCE

- **How often is BNTI performed in the emergency department (ED)?** Because RSI has become the method of choice for intubation of emergency patients, fewer physicians routinely perform BNTI. In a large multicenter registry of more than 17,500 adult ED intubations, Brown et al.[1] reported 162 nasal intubations, 99 utilizing a flexible endoscope; 63 (0.35%) were performed without a device (BNTI). Overall first attempt success for nasal intubation was 65%.
- **How successful is BNTI when performed by prehospital providers?** In a recent meta-analysis by Hubble and colleagues, approximately 57,000 cases of prehospital airway management were examined. Overall, the BNTI success rate for nonphysician clinicians was 75.9%.[2]
- **Can BNTI be performed in patients with facial trauma?** Historically, facial trauma was believed to be an absolute contraindication for BNTI because of the perceived associated risk of intracranial placement in the presence of cribriform plate disruption. At least one study has been published evaluating the risk of BNTI in the presence of facial trauma. This retrospective review of 311 patients with intubation in the presence of facial fractures found

that 82 patients underwent BNTI.[3] The authors found no episodes of intracranial placement, significant epistaxis requiring nasal packing, esophageal intubation, or osteomyelitis. Overall, the data are limited and, in general, this practice is strongly discouraged. In dire circumstances when no alternative is available, it may be attempted regardless of facial trauma but clinicians should be aware of the possible complications.

- **What maneuvers can aid successful blind nasal intubation?** A number of improvements to the technique for passage of the nasotracheal tube through the oropharynx and into the glottis have been suggested over the years. The most studied and successful aid to BNTI appears to be the addition of cuff inflation during passage of the tube through the oropharynx until the outlet abuts the glottic opening. A prospective randomized trial evaluating successful BNTI with the cuff inflated vs. deflated technique demonstrated the inflated cuff technique to be superior. The results showed that 19/20 (95%) patients were intubated with the cuff inflated. In contrast, only 9/20 (45%) patients were intubated with the cuff deflated.[4] A separate study compared success rates for BNTI and flexible bronchoscope in patients with an immobilized cervical spine with the American Society of Anesthesiologists Class I (ASA I) and ASA II status airways while undergoing elective surgery. The authors reported that there was no significant difference in success rates between the groups. The study concluded that ETT cuff inflation could be used as an alternative to flexible bronchoscopy in patients with an immobilized cervical spine,[5] but this conclusion is not warranted by this small study, and both techniques are highly operator dependent. Other studies have demonstrated increased success with BNTI using a neutral head position[6] and ETTs with directional tip control.[7]
- **Should waveform capnography be used to improve BNTI success?** To the authors' knowledge, there has not been a clinical trial comparing BNTI with, and without, use of this technology. Thus, recommendations for their use in BNTI represent expert opinion only.

## REFERENCES


1. Brown C III, Bair A, Pallin D, et al. Techniques, success, and adverse events of emergency department adult intubations. *Ann Emerg Med*. 2015;65:363–370.
2. Hubble MW, Brown L, Wilfong DA, et al. A meta-analysis of prehospital airway control techniques part I: orotracheal and nasotracheal intubation success rates. *Prehosp Emerg Care*. 2010;14(3):377–401.
3. Rosen CL, Wolfe RE, Chew SE, et al. Blind nasotracheal intubation in the presence of facial trauma. *J Emerg Med*. 1997;15:141–145.
4. Van Elstraete AC, Pennant JH, Gajraj NM, et al. Tracheal tube cuff inflation as an aid to blind nasotracheal intubation. *Br J Anaesth*. 1993;70:691–693.
5. Van Elstraete AC, Mamie JC, Mehdaoui H. Nasotracheal intubation in patients with immobilized cervical spine: a comparison of tracheal tube cuff inflation and fiberoptic bronchoscopy. *Anesth Analg*. 1998;87(2):400–402.
6. Chung Y, Sun M, Wu H. Blind nasotracheal intubation is facilitated by neutral head position and endotracheal tube cuff inflation in spontaneously breathing patients. *Can J Anaesth*. 2003;50(5):511–513.
7. O'Connor RE, Megargel RE, Schnyder ME, et al. Paramedic success rate for blind nasotracheal intubation is improved with the use of an endotracheal tube with directional tip control. *Ann Emerg Med*. 2000;36:328–332.

Chapter 19

# Surgical Airway Management

Aaron E. Bair and David A. Caro

## INTRODUCTION

Surgical airway management is defined as the creation of an opening to the trachea by invasive, surgical means, to provide ventilation and oxygenation. However, there may be some confusion engendered by use of the term *surgical airway management*. In some contexts the discussions are limited to open surgical techniques. For the purposes of discussion in this chapter, surgical airway management includes cricothyrotomy (both open and wire-guided techniques), percutaneous transtracheal ventilation (PTV), and placement of a surgical airway using a cricothyrotome (a device intended to place a surgical airway percutaneously, usually in one or two steps, without performance of a formal cricothyrotomy). Each category of surgical airway technique is described in detail in the sections that follow.

### Description

Cricothyrotomy is the establishment of a surgical opening through the cricothyroid membrane with placement of a cuffed tracheostomy tube or endotracheal tube (ETT) into the trachea.

A cricothyrotome is a kit or device that is intended to establish a surgical airway without resorting to formal cricothyrotomy. These kits use two basic approaches. One approach relies on the Seldinger technique, in which the airway is accessed through a small needle through which a flexible guide wire is passed. The airway device, with a dilator, is then passed over this guide wire and into the airway in a manner analogous with that of central line placement by the Seldinger technique. The other technique relies on the direct percutaneous placement of an airway device without the use of a Seldinger technique. There have been no clinical studies to date demonstrating the superiority of one approach over another or of any of these devices over formal surgical cricothyrotomy. However, certain attributes of the devices make them intuitively more, or less, hazardous for insertion (see the "Evidence" section).

### Indications and Contraindications

The primary indication for cricothyrotomy is when a failed airway has occurred (see Chapters 2 and 3) and the patient cannot be adequately oxygenated despite optimal attempts with BMV or an extraglottic device. A second indication is a method of primary airway management in patients for whom intubation is contraindicated or believed to be impossible with another available device (e.g., fiber optic scope, lighted stylet, intubating laryngeal mask airway) that otherwise would have been likely to successfully secure the airway. Thus, cricothyrotomy should be thought of as a rescue technique in most circumstances, and only infrequently will it be used as the primary method of airway management. An example of a circumstance in which cricothyrotomy is the primary method of airway management is the patient with severe facial trauma in whom access through the mouth or nose would be too time consuming or impossible. This patient requires immediate airway management because of the risk of aspiration of blood and secretions, and cricothyrotomy is indicated.

The primary hurdle to performing cricothyrotomy is simply recognizing when it is necessary to proceed with surgical airway management, thereby abandoning further attempts at laryngoscopy or the use of an alternative device. Rapid sequence intubation (RSI) is so successful that cricothyrotomy is often viewed as a method of last resort to be undertaken only after multiple noninvasive attempts or techniques have failed. However, the relentless, unsuccessful pursuit of a noninvasive airway delays the initiation of a surgical airway, greatly increasing the likelihood of hypoxic injury to the patient. This fact is particularly true in the "*can't* intubate, *can't* oxygenate" (CICO) circumstance, when surgical airway management is indicated and must not be delayed for attempts using other devices.

In deciding to initiate surgical airway management, there are a few fundamental considerations:

1. Will accessing the cricothyroid membrane be *effective*? In other words, will an incision at the level of the cricothyroid membrane bypass the obstruction and solve the problem? If the obstructing lesion is significantly distal to the cricothyroid membrane, performing a cricothyrotomy is a critical waste of time (see Chapter 36).
2. Will the patient's anatomy or pathologic process make cricothyrotomy *difficult* to perform? Placement of the initial skin incision is based on palpating the pertinent anatomy. If adiposity, burns, trauma, or infection make this procedure difficult, then the strategy should be adjusted accordingly. A mnemonic for difficult cricothyrotomy (SMART) is shown in **Box 19-1** and is discussed in Chapter 2.
3. Which *type* of invasive technique is best in the particular circumstances (i.e., open surgical or percutaneous)? This consideration takes into account provider preference based on previous experience, equipment availability, and patient characteristics. Needle cricothyrotomy (PTV) is preferred in children <10 years of age (see Chapter 26). In obese patients, subcutaneous tissue may obscure landmarks, making needle localization difficult (see Chapter 40). For these patients, often an open surgical cricothyrotomy is a better choice.

Contraindications to surgical airway management are few and, with one exception, are relative. That one exception is young age. Children have a small, pliable, mobile larynx and cricoid cartilage, making cricothyrotomy extremely difficult. For children 10 years of age or younger, needle cricothyrotomy is the surgical airway technique of choice (see Chapter 26). Relative contraindications include preexisting laryngeal or tracheal pathology such as tumor, infections, or abscess in the area in which the procedure will be performed; hematoma or other anatomical destruction of the landmarks that would render the procedure difficult or impossible; coagulopathy; and lack of operator expertise.

**BOX 19-1**

**SMART mnemonic for difficult cricothyrotomy.**

**S**urgery
**M**ass
**A**ccess/**A**natomy
**R**adiation
**T**rauma

Cricothyrotomy has been performed successfully after systemic thrombolytic therapy. Cricothyrotomy has a high success rate when performed in the emergency department (ED) setting. The presence of an anatomical barrier, in particular, should prompt consideration of alternative techniques that might result in a successful airway. However, in cases in which no alternative method of airway management is likely to be successful or timely enough, cricothyrotomy should be performed. The same principles apply for both the cricothyrotome and PTV.

The cricothyrotomes have not been demonstrated to improve success rates or time to completion, or to decrease complication rates when compared with surgical cricothyrotomy. As with formal cricothyrotomy, experience, skill, knowledge of anatomy, and adherence to proper technique are essential for success when a cricothyrotome is used.

## TECHNIQUE

### Anatomy and Landmarks

The cricothyroid membrane is the anatomical site of access in the emergent surgical airway, regardless of the technique used. It has several advantages over the trachea in the emergent setting. The cricothyroid membrane is more anterior than the lower trachea, and there is less soft tissue between the membrane and the skin. There is less vascularity and therefore less chance of significant bleeding.

The cricothyroid membrane is identified by first locating the laryngeal prominence (notch) of the thyroid cartilage. Approximately one fingerbreadth below the laryngeal prominence, the membrane may be palpated in the midline of the anterior neck, as a soft depression between the inferior aspect of the thyroid cartilage above and the hard cricoid ring below. The relevant anatomy may be easier to appreciate in males because of the more prominent thyroid notch. The thyrohyoid space, which lies high in the neck between the laryngeal prominence and the hyoid bone, should also be identified. This will prevent the misidentification of the thyrohyoid membrane as the cricothyroid membrane, which would lead to misplacement of the incision. We would emphasize that recent literature suggests that identification of the cricothyroid membrane may be more difficult than previously assumed (see "Evidence" section). As landmark identification is critical in any of these approaches, it merits learning and practicing proper landmark identification. The cricothyroid membrane is disproportionately smaller in children because of a greater overlap of the thyroid cartilage over the cricoid cartilage, which is one reason cricothyrotomy is not recommended in children 10 years or younger.

Unfortunately, the same anatomical or physiologic abnormalities (i.e., trauma, morbid obesity, and congenital anomalies) that necessitated surgical airway may also hinder easy palpation of landmarks. One way of estimating the location of the cricothyroid membrane is by placing four fingers on the neck, oriented longitudinally, with the small finger in the sternal notch. The membrane is approximately located under the index finger and can serve as a point at which the initial longitudinal incision is made. Except as described later in the technique for the rapid four-step technique (RFST) of cricothyrotomy, a vertical skin incision is preferred, especially if anatomical landmarks are not readily apparent. Palpation through this vertical incision can then confirm the location of the cricothyroid membrane. Alternatively, identification may be facilitated by using a locator needle, attached to a syringe containing saline or lidocaine. Aspiration of air bubbles suggests entry into the airway, but it will not distinguish between the cricothyroid membrane and a lower tracheal placement.

### The No-Drop Technique

The cricothyrotomy instrument set should be simple, consisting of only the equipment necessary to complete the procedure. A sample listing of recommended contents of a cricothyrotomy tray is shown in **Box 19-2**. Commercial kits that also contain the instruments required for a cricothyrotomy (**Fig. 19-1**) are available.

**BOX 19-2**

## Recommended contents of cricothyrotomy tray.

- Trousseau dilator
- Tracheal hook
- Scalpel with no. 11 blade
- Cuffed, nonfenestrated, no. 4 tracheostomy tube
- Optional equipment: several 4 × 4 gauze sponges, two small hemostats, and surgical drapes

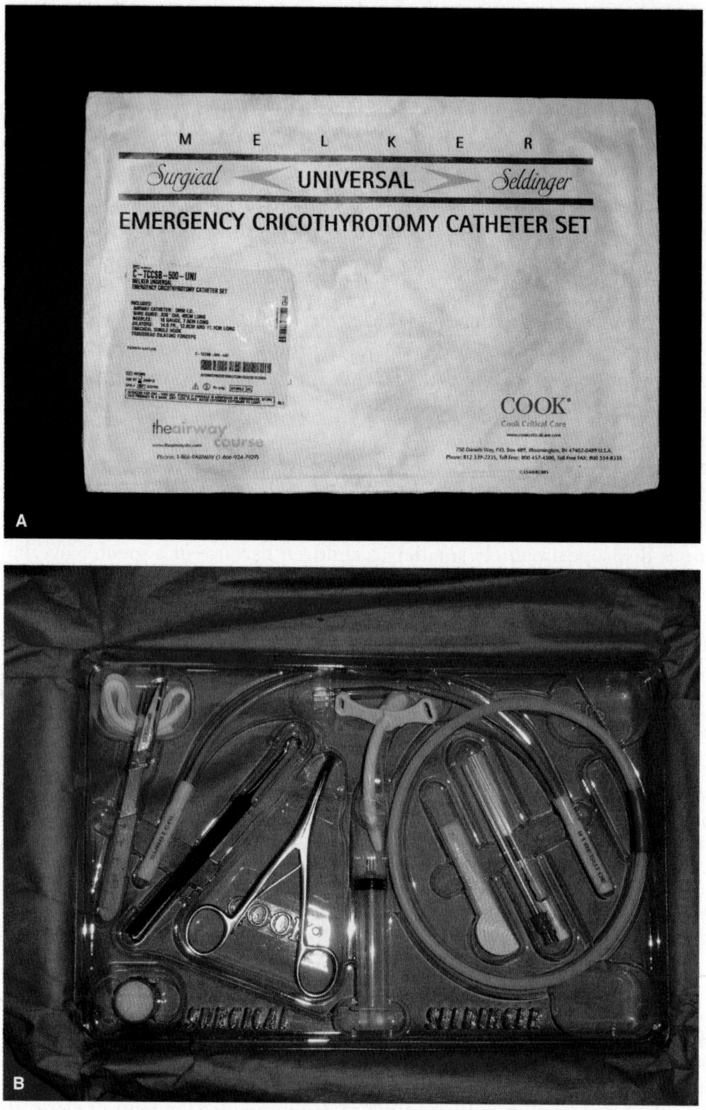


● **FIGURE 19-1. A:** Universal Emergency Cricothyrotomy Catheter Set (Cook Critical Care, Bloomington, IN). **B:** Opened set containing cuffed tracheostomy tube, as well as equipment for both open surgical and Seldinger techniques.

1. *Identify the landmarks.* The practitioner moves to their dominant hand side of the patient (i.e., a right-handed practitioner moves to the right of the patient). The cricothyroid membrane is then identified by the nondominant hand using the landmarks described previously (**Fig. 19-2**). Be aware that the cricothyroid membrane might not be clearly identifiable by palpation. If in doubt, it is better to err by starting lower (more inferiorly) in the neck.
2. *Prepare the neck.* If time permits, apply appropriate antiseptic solution. Local anesthesia is desirable if the patient is conscious. Infiltration of the skin and subcutaneous tissue of the anterior neck with 1% lidocaine solution will provide adequate anesthesia. If time permits and the patient is conscious and responsive, anesthetize the airway by injecting lidocaine by transcricothyroid membrane puncture (see Chapter 23). The patient will cough briefly, but the airway will be reasonably anesthetized and further cough reflexes suppressed.
3. *Immobilize the larynx.* Throughout the procedure, the larynx must be immobilized (**Fig. 19-3**). This is best done by placing the thumb and long finger of the nondominant hand on opposite sides of the superior laryngeal horns, the posterior superior aspect of the laryngeal cartilage. With the thumb and long finger thus placed, the index finger is ideally positioned anteriorly to relocate and reidentify the cricothyroid membrane at any time during the procedure.
4. *Incise the skin.* Using the dominant hand, a 2-cm vertical midline skin incision is performed (**Fig. 19-4**). Care should be taken to avoid cutting the deeper structures of the neck. The cricothyroid membrane is separated from the outside world only by skin, subcutaneous tissue, and anterior cervical fascia. An overly vigorous incision risks damage to the larynx, cricoid cartilage, and the trachea. The practitioner should expect venous bleeding at this point in the procedure, which will obscure the view of the cricothyroid membrane. Once the skin is opened, safely withdraw the scalpel blade away from the immediate area so as not to injure yourself or other personnel.
5. *Reidentify the membrane.* With the thumb and long finger maintaining immobilization of the larynx, the index finger can now palpate the anterior larynx, the cricothyroid membrane, and

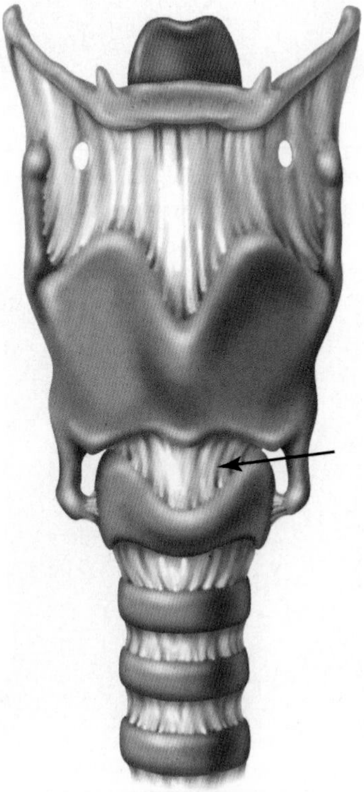

● **FIGURE 19-2. Anatomy of the Larynx.** The cricothyroid membrane (*arrow*) is bordered above by the thyroid cartilage and below by the cricoid cartilage.

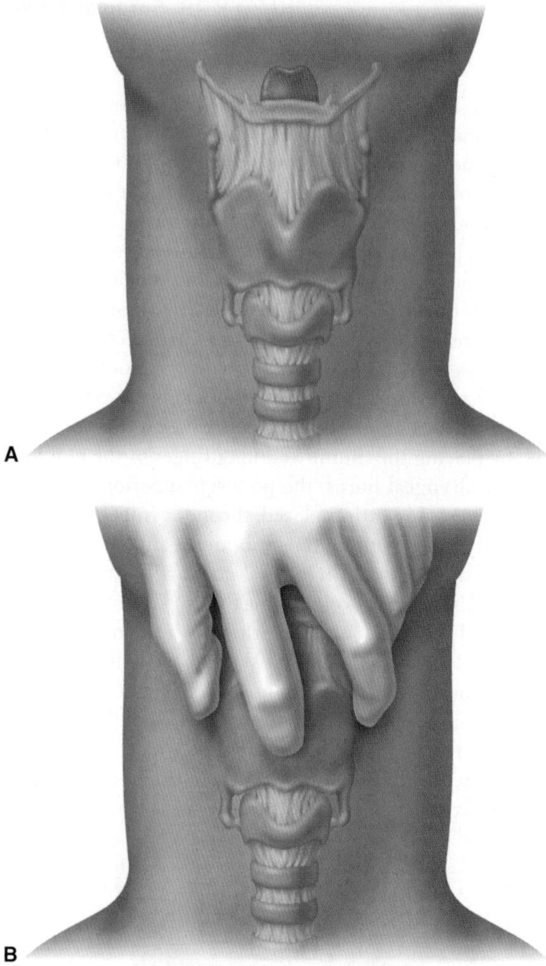


● **FIGURE 19-3.** **A:** Surface anatomy of the airway. **B:** The thumb and long finger immobilize the superior cornu of the larynx; the index finger is used to palpate the cricothyroid membrane.

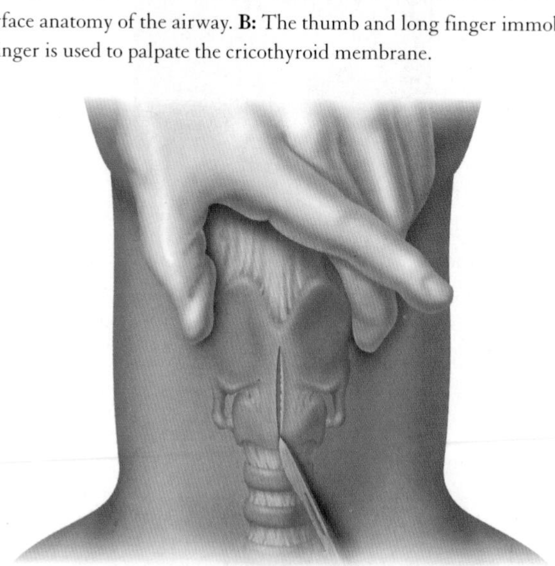

● **FIGURE 19-4.** With the index finger moved to the side but continued firm immobilization of the larynx, a vertical midline skin incision is made, down to the depth of the laryngeal structures.

the cricoid cartilage without any interposed skin or subcutaneous tissue (**Fig. 19-5**). With the landmarks thus confirmed, the index finger can be left in the wound by placing it on the inferior aspect of the anterior larynx, thus providing a clear indicator of the superior extent of the cricothyroid membrane.

6. *Incise the membrane.* The cricothyroid membrane should be incised in a horizontal direction, with an incision at least 1 cm long (**Fig. 19-6A**). It is recommended to try to incise the lower half of the membrane rather than the upper half because of the relatively cephalad location of the superior cricothyroid artery and vein; however, this may be unrealistic in the emergent setting (**Fig. 19-6B**).
7. *Insert the tracheal hook.* With the scalpel blade still inside the cricothyroid membrane incision, the tracheal hook is rotated so that it is oriented in the transverse plane, passed through the incision, and then rotated again so the hook is oriented in a cephalad direction. The hook is then applied to the inferior aspect of the thyroid cartilage, and gentle upward and cephalad traction is applied to bring the airway immediately out to the skin incision (**Fig. 19-7**). If an assistant is available, this hook may be passed to the assistant to maintain immobilization of the larynx. At this point in the procedure, the scalpel blade can be put down and away from the immediate area so as not to injure yourself or other personnel.
8. *Insert the Trousseau dilator.* The Trousseau dilator may be inserted in one of two ways. One method is to insert the dilator well in through the incision, directing the blades of the dilator longitudinally down the airway. The second method, which is preferred, is to insert the dilator minimally into the anterior wound with the blades oriented superiorly and inferiorly, allowing the dilator to open and enlarge the vertical extent of the cricothyroid membrane incision, which

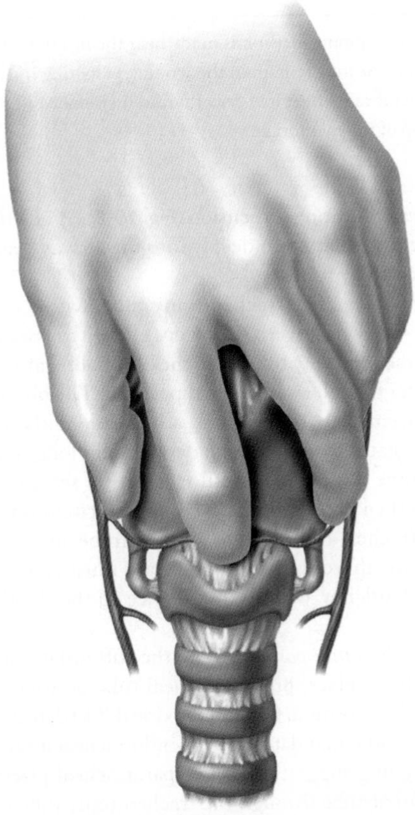

● **FIGURE 19-5.** With the skin incised, the index finger can now directly palpate the cricothyroid membrane.

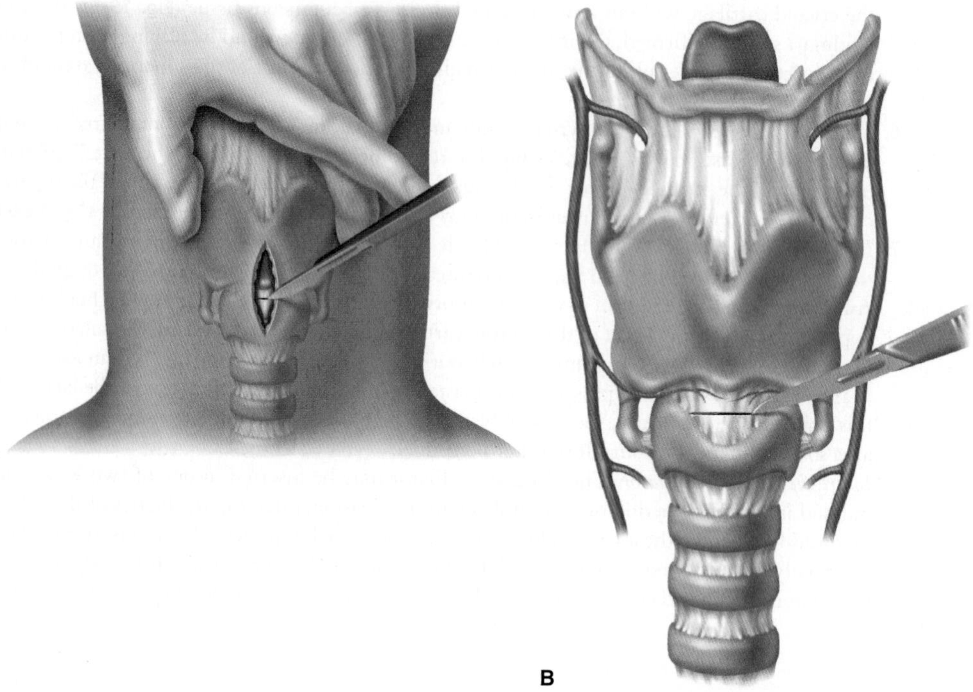

A B

● **FIGURE 19-6. A:** A horizontal membrane incision is made near the inferior edge of the cricothyroid membrane. The index finger may be moved aside or may remain in the wound, palpating the inferior edge of the thyroid cartilage, to guide the scalpel to the membrane. **B:** A low cricothyroid incision avoids the superior cricothyroid vessels, which run transversely near the top of the membrane.

is often the anatomically limiting dimension (**Fig. 19-8**). When this technique is used, care must be taken not to insert the dilator too deeply into the airway because it will impede subsequent passage of the tracheostomy tube.

9. *Insert the tracheostomy tube.* The tracheostomy tube, with its inner cannula in situ, is gently inserted through the incision between the blades of the Trousseau dilator. An alternate approach is to first insert the tracheostomy tube with the blunt obturator in situ and then replace it with the inner cannula after the tube is in its final position. The blunt obturator can provide smooth insertion during placement. As the tube is advanced gently following its natural curve, the Trousseau dilator is rotated to allow the blades to orient longitudinally in the airway (**Fig. 19-9**). The tracheostomy tube is advanced until it is firmly seated against the anterior neck. The Trousseau dilator is then carefully removed. If a tracheostomy tube is not readily available, a small gauge endotracheal tube (size 6.0 - 6.5) can be advanced over a bougie inserted into the opening in the cricothyroid membrane. Care must be taken to advance each only a few centimeters, as the tendency will be to advance to the depth one would usually advance through the mouth.
10. *Inflate the cuff, and confirm tube position.* With the cuff inflated and while the practitioner holds the tracheostomy tube in place, proper tracheal tube position can be confirmed by the same methods as for oral ETT position. Carbon dioxide ($CO_2$) detection will reliably indicate correct placement of the tube and is mandatory, as for endotracheal intubation. Immediate subcutaneous emphysema with bagging suggests probable paratracheal placement. If doubt remains, rapid insertion of a nasogastric tube through the tracheostomy tube will result in easy passage if the tube is in the trachea and obstruction if the tube has been placed through a false passage into the tissues of the neck. Auscultation of both lungs and the epigastric area is also recommended, although esophageal placement of the tracheostomy tube is exceedingly unlikely. Once these

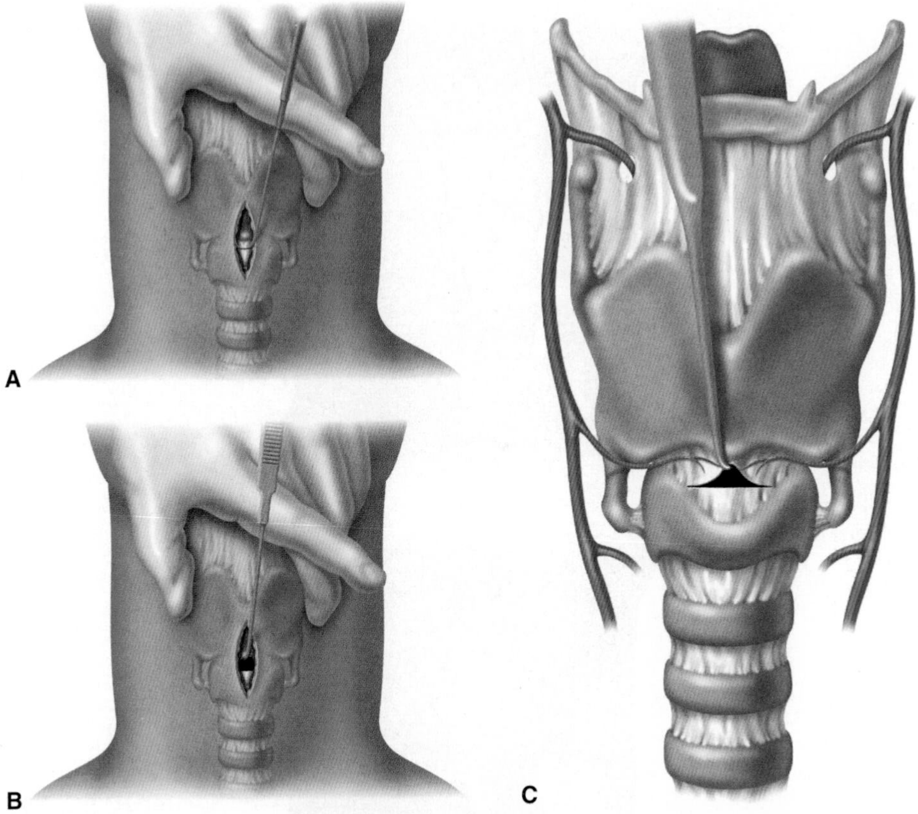


● **FIGURE 19-7. A:** The tracheal hook is oriented transversely during insertion. **B and C:** After insertion, cephalad traction is applied to the inferior margin of the thyroid cartilage.

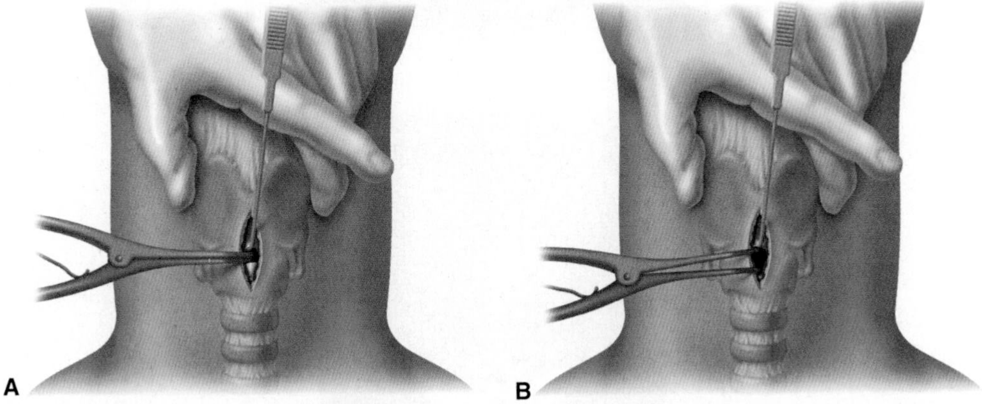


● **FIGURE 19-8. A:** The Trousseau dilator is inserted a short distance into the incision. **B:** In this orientation, the dilator enlarges the opening vertically, the crucial dimension.

measures confirm placement, secure the tube to the neck either by tracheal tube tape or by suturing it into position. Chest radiography should then be performed to assist in the assessment of tube placement and to evaluate for the presence of barotrauma. Pneumothorax is also possible, but far less likely than the placement of the tube paratracheally.

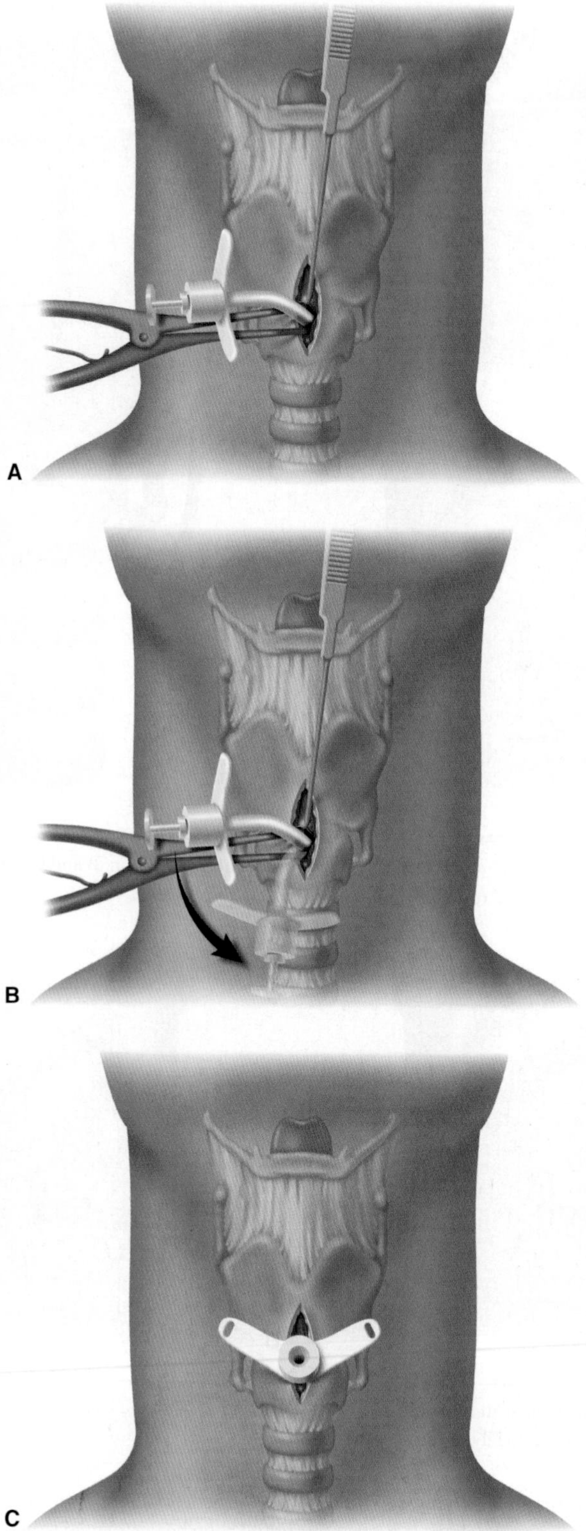


● **FIGURE 19-9.** **A:** Insertion of the tracheostomy tube. **B:** Rotation of the Trousseau dilator to orient the blades longitudinally in the airway facilitates passage of the tracheostomy tube. **C:** Tracheostomy tube fully inserted, instruments removed.

## The Rapid Four-Step Technique

This cricothyrotomy method has been adopted at some centers as it abbreviates the procedure and may reduce time to oxygenation. As with all techniques, the patient should be maximally oxygenated and, if given sufficient time, the anterior neck may be prepared and locally anesthetized as for the no-drop method. One distinguishing feature of this technique is that it can be performed from a *position at the head of the bed*. Thus, it does not require the intubator to change position in a scenario where the bed space is likely to be crowded and chaotic. The RFST for cricothyrotomy proceeds sequentially as follows:

1. *Palpate and identify landmarks.* The cricothyroid membrane should be identified as described previously (**Fig. 19-10**). If the key landmarks are unable to be identified by palpation through the soft tissue, then a vertical skin incision is required to permit accurate identification.
2. *Make skin incision.* Once the pertinent palpable anatomy is identified, the cricothyroid membrane is incised. If the anatomy is fully appreciated through the intact skin, and there is certainty about landmarks and location, then incise the skin and cricothyroid membrane simultaneously with a single horizontal incision of approximately 1.5 cm in length (**Fig. 19-11A**). For this type of incision, a no. 20 scalpel yields an incision that requires little widening. The intention of the initial incision is to puncture the skin and cricothyroid membrane simultaneously. If the anatomy is not readily and unambiguously identified through the skin, then an initial 2 cm vertical incision should be created to allow more precise palpation of the anatomy and identification of the cricothyroid membrane. In either situation, the cricothyroid membrane is incised with the no. 20 blade that is maintained in the airway, while a tracheal hook (preferably a blunt hook) is placed parallel to the scalpel on the caudad side of the blade (**Fig. 19-11B**). The hook is then rotated to orient it in a caudad direction to put gentle traction on the cricoid ring. The scalpel is then removed from the airway. At no time during this procedure is the incision left without instrument control of the airway. This detail is particularly important in a scenario where the patient still has the ability to respond or swallow. The newly created opening could be irretrievably lost if the airway is uncontrolled and moves relative to the skin incision. This is a technique that relies exclusively on palpation of key structures. Bleeding will inevitably obscure visualization of the anatomy. No time should be wasted using suction or gauze or manipulating the overhead lighting.
3. *Apply traction.* The tracheal hook that has been rotated caudally and is controlling the cricoid ring is now used to lift the airway toward the skin incision. This action provides modest stoma dilation. The direction of traction should be "up and away" and should feel reminiscent of laryngoscopy. Importantly, at this time the whole larynx should be lifted and controlled by the hook. If the hook placement is incorrect, it will often be apparent as the hook will simply be

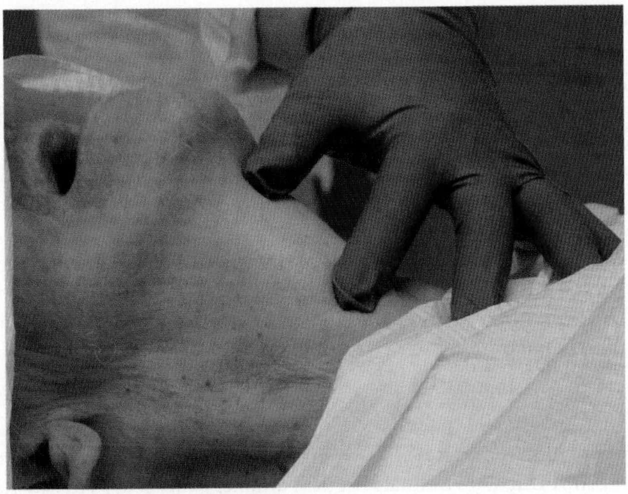

● **FIGURE 19-10. Palpation.** The operator's thumb is on the hyoid bone, while the cricothyroid membrane is identified using the index finger.

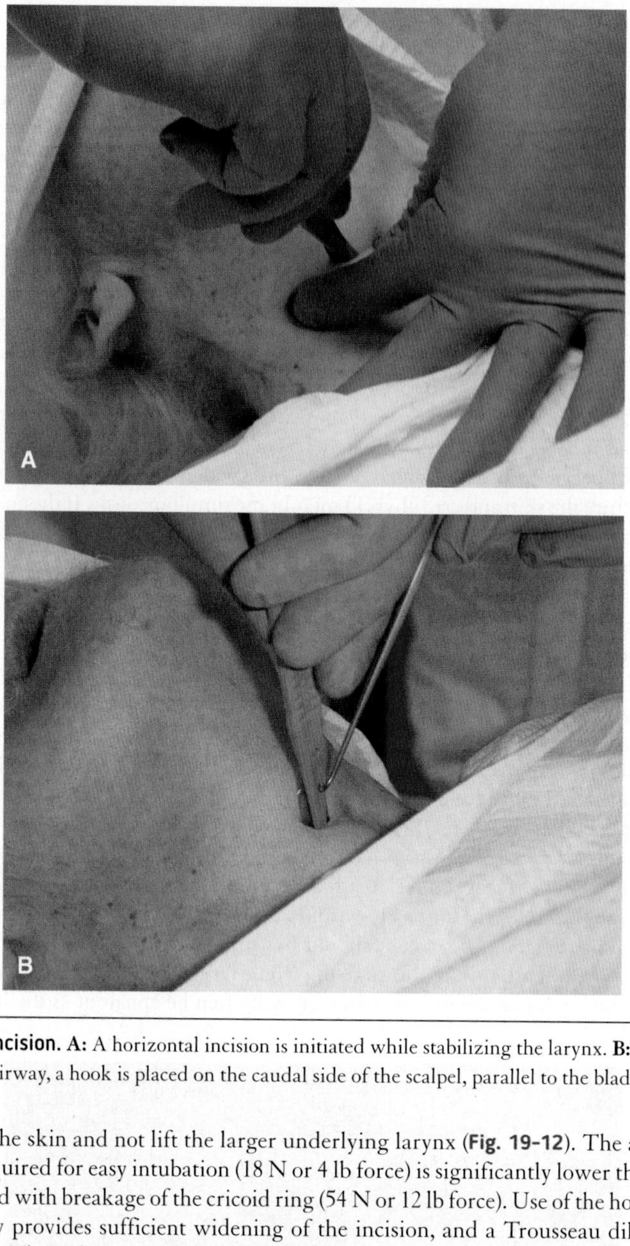

● **FIGURE 19-11. Incision. A:** A horizontal incision is initiated while stabilizing the larynx. **B:** Before removing the scalpel from the airway, a hook is placed on the caudal side of the scalpel, parallel to the blade.

tenting the skin and not lift the larger underlying larynx (**Fig. 19-12**). The amount of traction force required for easy intubation (18 N or 4 lb force) is significantly lower than the force that is associated with breakage of the cricoid ring (54 N or 12 lb force). Use of the hook in this direction generally provides sufficient widening of the incision, and a Trousseau dilator is usually not required. The technique of pulling the airway upward in this way also minimizes the possibility of intubating the pretracheal potential space.

4. *Intubate.* With adequate control of the airway using the hook placed on the cricoid ring, ETT is readily placed into the airway and secured (**Fig. 19-13**). Confirmation techniques proceed as described in the no-drop technique. A bougie can also be inserted at this point to aid passage of a small caliber standard ETT.

## Complications

Because of the high success rate of RSI, cricothyrotomy is infrequently performed in EDs, so reports of complications are difficult to evaluate. In the National Emergency Airway Registry (NEAR III) study, only 0.3% of more than 17,500 adult ED intubations required a rescue cricothyrotomy.

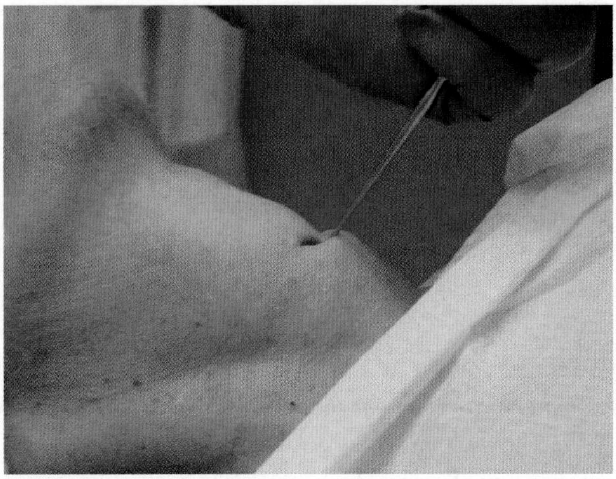

● **FIGURE 19-12. Traction.** The hook is applied to the cricoid ring and lifted.

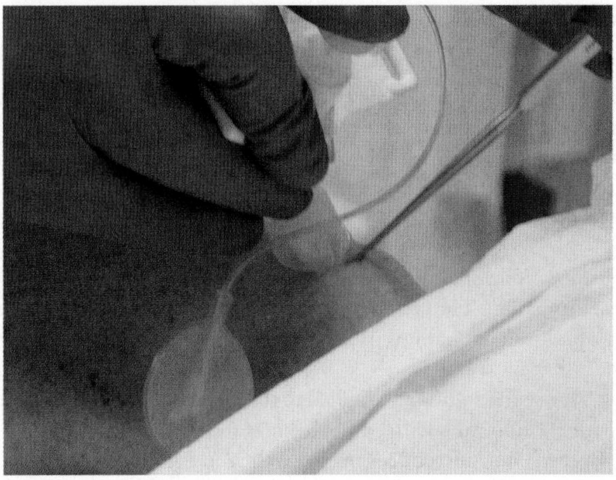

● **FIGURE 19-13. Intubation.** The tracheostomy tube is passed into the incision as the hook stabilizes the cricoid ring.

The most important complication for the patient in the context of surgical airway management is when delayed decision-making after initial intubation failure leads to prolonged, ineffective intubation attempts that result in hypoxic injury. Failure to rapidly place the tracheostomy tube into the trachea or misplacement of the tube into the soft tissues of the neck is more a failure of technique than a complication and must be recognized immediately, as is the case with any misplaced ETT. Complications such as pneumothorax, significant hemorrhage requiring operative intervention, laryngeal or tracheal injury, and infection and long-term complications, such as subglottic stenosis or permanent voice change, are relatively infrequent. In general, the incidence of all complications, immediate and delayed, and major or minor, is approximately 20%, although published reports range from 0% to 54%. Emergency cricothyrotomy has higher complication rate than elective cricothyrotomy. However, most of these complications are minor, particularly when compared with the consequences of a failed airway.

There is insufficient evidence to determine whether the overall complication rate is lower when the traditional no-drop technique of cricothyrotomy is used versus the RFST. **Box 19-3** lists complications of surgical airway management.

**BOX 19-3**

**Complications of surgical airway management.**

Hemorrhage
Pneumomediastinum
Laryngeal/tracheal injury
Cricoid ring laceration
Barotrauma (especially when jet ventilation is used)
Infection
Voice change
Subglottic stenosis

## Alternatives to Open Surgical Techniques

### *Seldinger Technique*

When an alternative to open cricothyrotomy is desired, we recommend using a Seldinger technique. The Melker Universal Emergency Cricothyrotomy Catheter Set uses a modified Seldinger technique to assist in the placement of a tracheal airway (**Fig. 19-14**). This method is similar to the one commonly used in the placement of central venous catheters and offers some familiarity to the operator uncomfortable with or inexperienced in the surgical cricothyrotomy techniques described previously. Devices that incorporate an inflatable cuff are recommended (**Fig. 19-14B**).

1. *Identify landmarks.* The operator is positioned at the head of the bed, similar to positioning for endotracheal intubation. The cricothyroid membrane is then identified by the method described earlier. The nondominant hand is used to control the larynx and maintain identification of the landmarks.
2. *Prepare neck.* Antiseptic solution is applied to the anterior neck, and if time permits, infiltration of the site with 1% lidocaine with epinephrine is recommended.
3. *Insert locator needle.* The introducer needle is then inserted into the cricothyroid membrane in a slightly caudal direction (**Fig. 19-14C**). The needle is attached to a syringe and advanced with the dominant hand, while negative pressure is maintained on the syringe. The sudden aspiration of air indicates placement of the needle into the tracheal lumen.
4. *Insert guide wire.* The syringe is then removed from the needle. A soft-tipped guide wire is inserted through the needle into the trachea in a caudal direction (**Fig. 19-14D**). The needle is then removed, leaving the wire in place. Control of the wire must be maintained at all times.
5. *Incise skin.* A small skin incision is then made adjacent to the wire. This facilitates passage of the airway device through the skin (**Fig. 19-14E**). Alternatively, the skin incision may be made vertically over the membrane before insertion of the needle and guide wire.
6. *Insert the airway and dilator.* The airway catheter (3 to 6 mm internal diameter [ID]) with an internal dilator in place is inserted over the wire into the trachea (**Fig. 19-14F**). If resistance is met, the skin incision should be deepened and a gentle twisting motion applied to the airway device as it is firmly seated in the trachea (**Fig. 19-14G**). The wire and dilator are then removed together while taking care to hold the tracheal tube in position (**Fig. 19-14H**).
7. *Confirm tube location.* If the device has a cuff, inflate it at this time. Tube location is confirmed in the usual manner, including mandatory end-tidal $CO_2$ detection. The airway must then be secured properly. The devices are radiopaque on radiographs.

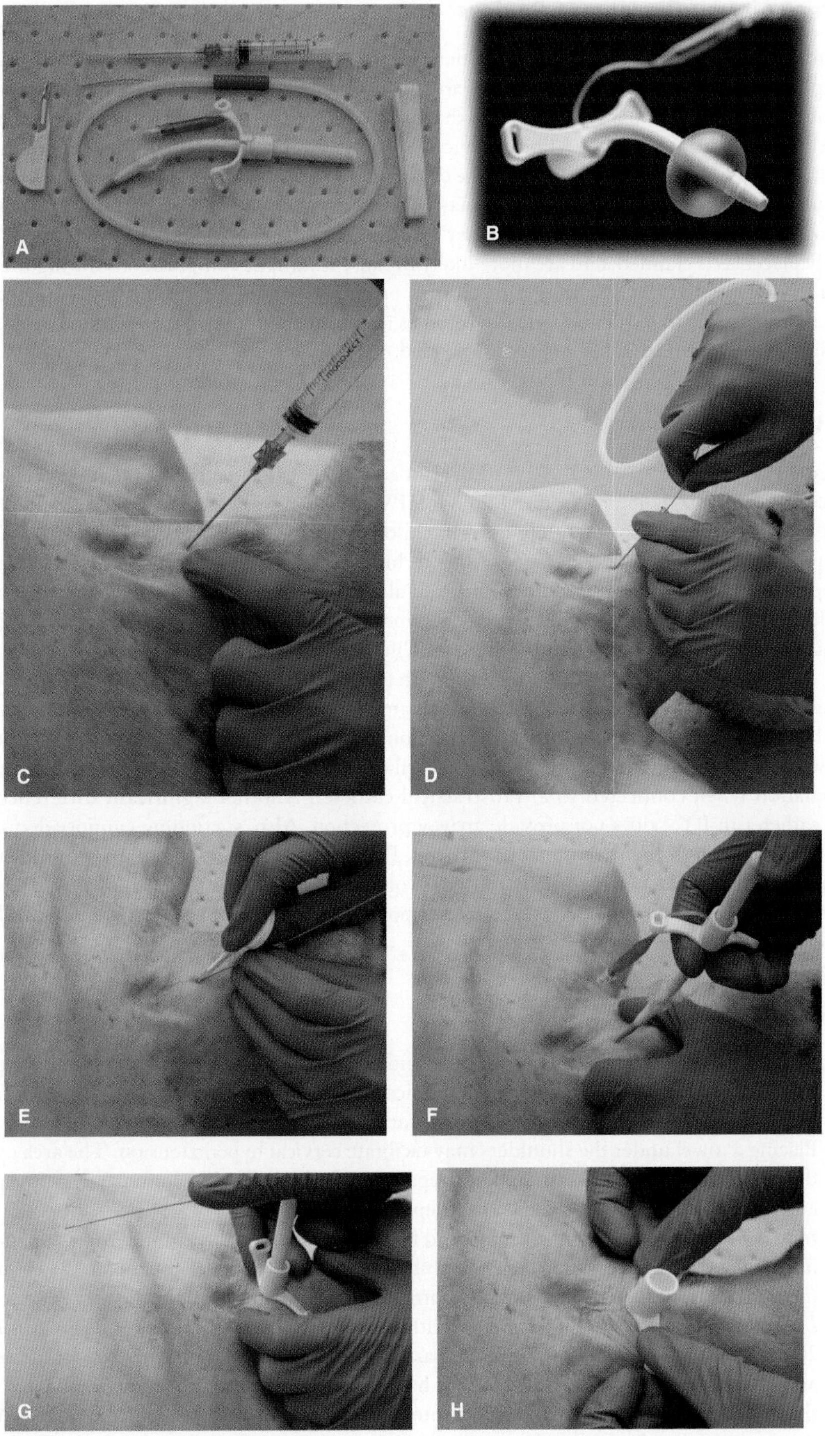

● **FIGURE 19-14. A:** Kit contents. **B:** Cuffed tube. **C:** Needle insertion. **D:** Wire placement through needle. **E:** Small incision. **F:** Airway with dilator inserted with wire guidance. **G:** Airway inserted to the hub using a gentle twisting motion. **H:** Wire and dilator removed as one (Melker Universal Cricothyrotomy Kit, Cook Critical Care, Bloomington, IN).

### *Direct Airway Placement Devices*

Numerous commercial cricothyrotome devices are available. These purport to place an airway simply and rapidly, but none of these has an adequate safety and performance record to warrant a recommendation for emergency use, and the incidence of injury to the airway is higher than when a Seldinger technique is used. These devices, such as Nu-Trake and Petrarch, generally involve multiple steps in the insertion, using a large device that functions as both introducer and airway. The details of the operation of these devices may be obtained from the manufacturer and are provided as inserts with the kits. These devices offer no clear advantage in technique, are rarely (if ever) as easily placed as is claimed, and are more likely to cause traumatic complications during their insertion than those that use a Seldinger technique, primarily because of the cutting characteristics of the airway device. In particular, cricothyrotomes recommended for children should be approached with extreme caution and are not recommended.

### *PTV Technique*

Needle cricothyrotomy with PTV is a surgical airway that may be used to temporize the CICO situation, particularly in children. Although PTV is virtually never used in adult patients in the emergency setting, and very rarely even in children, it is a simple, relatively effective means of supporting oxygenation. Advantages of this technique over cricothyrotomy may include speed, a simpler technique, and less bleeding. PTV can also provide an alternative for operators unable to perform a cricothyrotomy. Age is not a contraindication to PTV, which is the invasive airway of choice for children younger than 10 years (see Chapter 26).

Several other aspects of this technique that differ from cricothyrotomy are important to consider. To provide ventilation, supraglottic patency must be maintained to allow for exhalation. In the case of complete upper airway obstruction, air stacking from PTV will cause barotrauma. New novel devices such as the Ventrain ventilation device, allows for gas elimination during exhalation when connected to a transtracheal catheter. Another significant difference is that the catheter in PTV does not provide airway protection. Also, suctioning cannot adequately be performed through the percutaneous catheter. PTV has been associated with a significant incidence of barotrauma, particularly with the use of high-flow oxygen, and is rarely used as a rescue device. PTV is therefore best considered a temporizing means of rescue oxygenation until a more definitive airway can be obtained.

## Procedure

**a.** *Identify the landmarks*. The anatomy and landmarks used in needle cricothyrotomy are identical to those described previously for a surgical cricothyrotomy. The best approach is from the head of the bed. If there are no contraindications, the head of the patient should be extended. Placing a towel under the shoulders may facilitate cervical hyperextension. The area overlying the cricothyroid membrane should be prepared with an antiseptic solution and, if time permits, anesthetized with 1% lidocaine and epinephrine.

**b.** *Immobilize the larynx*. Use the thumb and the middle fingers of the nondominant hand to stabilize the larynx and cricoid cartilage while using the index finger to palpate the cricothyroid membrane. It is essential to maintain control of the larynx throughout the procedure.

**c.** *Insert transtracheal needle*. A large-bore intravenous (IV) catheter (12G to 16G) is attached to a 20-mL syringe, which may be empty or partially filled with water or saline to identify aspirated air bubbles. A 15° angle can be created by bending the needle/catheter combination 2.5 cm from the distal end of the IV catheter, or a commercially available catheter can be used (**Fig. 19-15A**). A commercial catheter may be preferred because it is reinforced with wire coils to prevent kinking (**Fig. 19-16**). The dominant hand holds the syringe with the needle directed caudally in the long axis of the trachea at a 30° angle to the skin (**Fig. 19-15B**). While maintaining negative pressure on the syringe, the needle is inserted through the cricothyroid membrane into the trachea. As soon as the needle enters the trachea, the syringe will easily fill with air. If a liquid

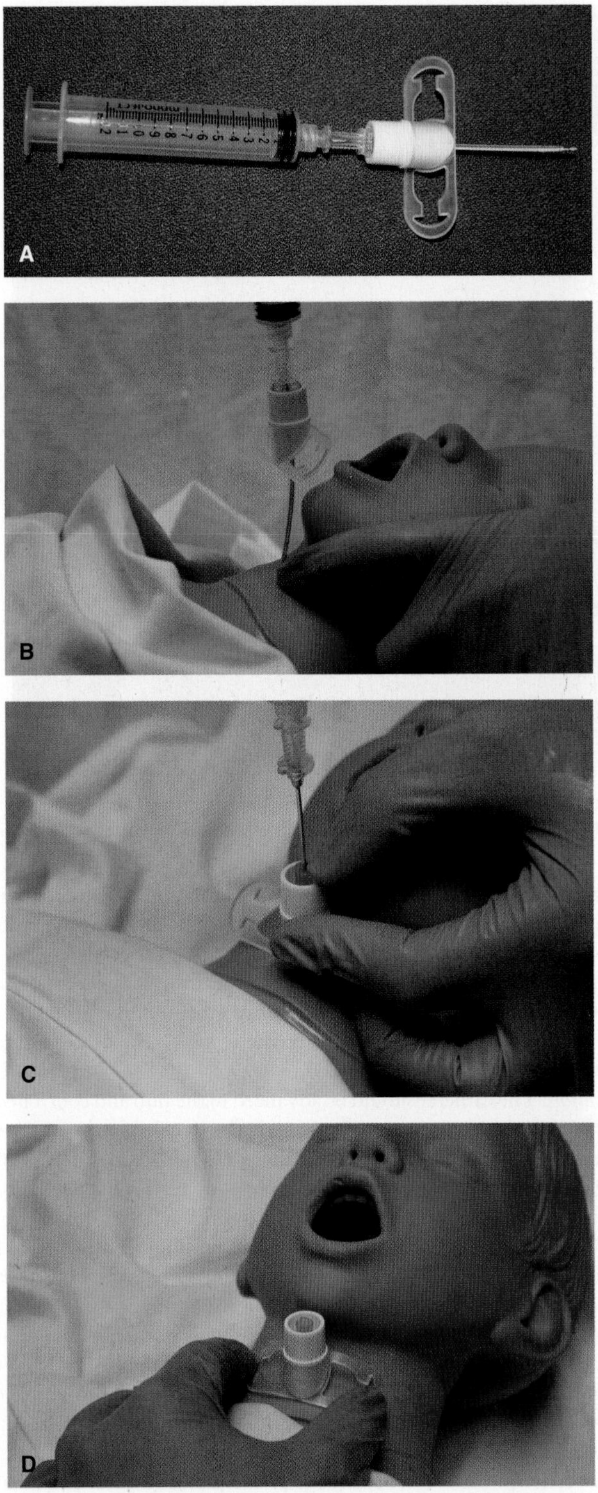


● **FIGURE 19-15.** **A:** Catheter for jet ventilation. **B:** Needle insertion. **C:** Removal of needle. **D:** Tracheostomy catheter placed.

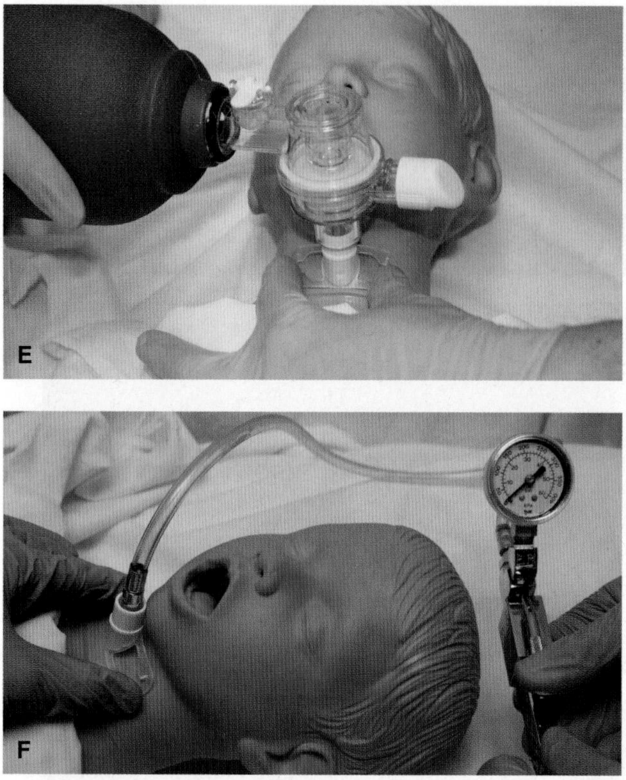


● **FIGURE 19-15. *(continued)*** **E:** Oxygenation with bag. **F:** Oxygenation with jet ventilator (Acutronic, Germany).

is used, bubbles will appear. Any resistance implies that the catheter remains in the tissue. In the awake patient, lidocaine may be used in the syringe and then injected into the tracheal lumen to suppress the cough reflex.

**d.** *Advance catheter*. Once entry into the trachea is confirmed, the catheter can be advanced. The needle may be partially or completely withdrawn before advancement; however, the needle should not be advanced with the catheter. A small incision can assist with catheter advancement if there is resistance at the skin.

**e.** *Confirm location*. The catheter should be advanced to the hub and controlled by hand at all times. Air should be reaspirated to confirm once again the location of the catheter within the trachea.

**f.** *Connect to bag or jet ventilation*. The catheter may be connected to a bag ventilator using either a preexisting adapter or the adapter from a 3-0 pediatric ETT, which will fit a Luer lock if there is only a Luer lock present (**Fig. 19-15E**). Placing an ETT adapter directly to the Luer lock might kink the catheter, so the use of a short IV extension tubing set attached to the catheter hub will allow the adapter to be easily placed while maintaining its patency. For jet ventilation, the catheter is connected to the female end of the tubing of the jet ventilation system by a Luer lock. The hub should not be secured in place by anything other than a human hand until a definitive airway is established (**Fig. 19-15F**). Firm, constant pressure must be applied by hand to ensure that proper positioning is maintained and to create a seal at the skin to minimize air leak.

**g.** *Perform jet ventilation*. In the adult, the jet ventilation system should be connected to an oxygen source of 50 psi with a continuously adjustable regulator to allow the pressure to be titrated so the lowest effective pressure (often about 30 psi) required to safely deliver a tidal volume is used. In general, inspiration is <1 second followed by 3 seconds of expiration. Because the gas flow through a 14G needle at 50 psi is 1,600 mL per second, <1 second of inspiratory time is required for an adequate tidal volume in a normally compliant lung. Recent research demonstrates that effective oxygenation may occur with considerably less than 30 psi pressure, and the lowest pressure that results in effective oxygenation should be used. Exhalation depends on the elastic recoil of the lung, which is a relatively low-driving pressure. Therefore, the recommended inspiratory-to-expiratory ratio (I:E) is 1:3. It is important to maintain upper airway patency to allow for exhalation and avoid air trapping and barotrauma. All patients should have an oral and nasal airway placed. For small adults and children, oxygen pressure should be downregulated to less than 20 to 30 psi, if possible. For children younger than 5 years, a bag should be used for ventilation, connected to the catheter using the ETT adapter from a 3.0-mm-ID ETT. The pop-off valve should be deactivated in order to generate high enough pressure for forward flow (see Chapter 26).

## Equipment

A regulator to control the driving pressure is optional but recommended. This device is particularly useful where barotrauma is a concern and in pediatrics, where the inspiratory pressures should be reduced to less than 20 to 30 psi, if possible. Although a system can be assembled inexpensively from readily available materials, a commercially made, preassembled system is recommended. The reliability and control inherent in the commercial devices are well worth the marginal increase in cost.

A PTV system can also be connected to a low-flow portable oxygen tank when circumstances require mobility. When the flow is set at 15 L per minute and no flow is allowed, the pressure temporarily increases to 120 psi. Once flow is released, high flow occurs momentarily and then rapidly decreases to the steady state of 5 to 10 psi. Adequate tidal volumes may be achieved through a 14G catheter in the first 0.5 seconds. A shorter I:E ratio of 1:1 is recommended.

Another setup using manual ventilation with a self-inflating reservoir bag has been described, using standard equipment found in any ED. Bag ventilation may be connected directly to the percutaneous transtracheal catheter in two ways. The male end of a 15-mm ETT adapter from a 3-mm-ID ETT will fit directly into the catheter. Alternatively, the male end of a plungerless 3-mL syringe will fit into the catheter, and the male end of an 8-mm-ID ETT adapter will then be inserted into the female end of the empty syringe. Ventilation is temporary at best, and partial arterial $CO_2$ pressure will increase at a rate 2 to 4 mm Hg per minute. Even the simple assembly of this system is more time consuming to be done during the event, so it must be preassembled. This arrangement may have particular utility in the pediatric patient younger than 5 years when excessive pressures may be delivered through a PTV device, even when a regulator to control inspiratory pressures is available. In general, children younger than 5 years should receive PTV through a ventilation bag; children of age 5 to 12 years receive ventilation by bag or using PTV at less than 30 mm Hg; and those older than 12 years to adult receive ventilation at a pressure range from 30 to 50 mm Hg. A catheter of less than 3 mm ID will be insufficient to adequately oxygenate the adult patient using a bag, and 50 psi pressurized oxygen is required.

a. *Transtracheal catheters*. A large-bore IV catheter is acceptable. The proper placement is made easier by placing a small angle 2.5 cm from the tip. Commercially available devices include precurved (Acutronic, Germany) and nonkinkable wire-coiled (Cook Critical Care, Bloomington, IN) catheters (**Figs. 19-15A** and **19-16**). The wire-coiled catheter will not kink when bent; therefore, it provides a more secure airway.
b. *PTV systems*. The PTV system consists of a high-pressure oxygen source (usually central wall oxygen pressure of 50 psi), high-pressure oxygen tubing, a regulator to control the driving pressure, an on–off valve to control inspiratory time, high-pressure tubing, and a Luer lock to connect to the catheter (**Fig. 19-17**).

## Complications Specific to PTV

There is insufficient experience with PTV to properly identify, quantify, or classify complications. Insufflation of gases at high pressure has significant likelihood of inflicting injury to the airway

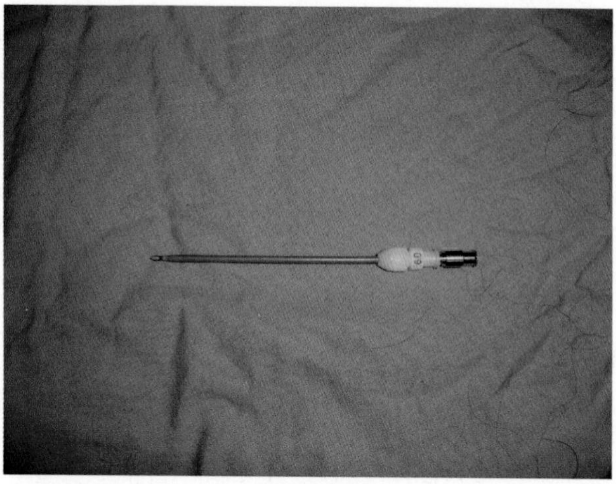

● **FIGURE 19-16.** Nonkinkable wire-coiled transtracheal jet ventilation catheter (Cook Critical Care, Bloomington, IN).

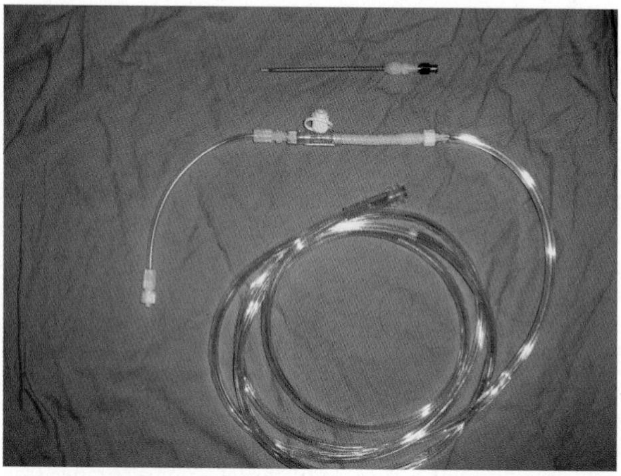

● **FIGURE 19-17.** Disposable jet ventilator system with high-pressure oxygen tubing, on–off valve, and PVC tubing with Luer lock. Note that this device does not include a pressure regulator (Cook Critical Care, Bloomington, IN).

mucosa or deeper tissues and must be undertaken with extreme caution. Known complications of PTV include the following:

a. Subcutaneous emphysema
b. Barotrauma including mucosal emphysema
c. Reflex cough with each ventilation (may be aborted with lidocaine)
d. Catheter kinking
e. Obstruction from blood or mucus
f. Esophageal puncture
g. Mucosal damage if nonhumidified gas is used

## TIPS AND PEARLS

- Surgical airway management is rarely the method of first choice for patients requiring emergency airway management. However, there is a population of patients for whom surgical airway management can make the difference between life and death. Therefore, providers for patients requiring emergency airway management must be proficient with surgical airway management.
- Although appealing on the surface, there may be little advantage to using a Seldinger-based method rather than a formal, surgical cricothyrotomy set. Time of performance of the procedure, complication rates, degree of difficulty, and success rates are all comparable. Seldinger technique devices that use a cuffed tube are preferable. Personal preference should also guide selection. The faculty of "The Difficult Airway Course: Emergency" have advised (although receive no money) on the design of a kit that offers the instruments and equipment to perform either the Seldinger percutaneous cricothyrotomy or an open cricothyrotomy, using a cuffed tube for both methods (Melker Universal Emergency Cricothyrotomy Catheter Set, Cook Critical Care, Bloomington, IN; **Fig. 19-1**).
- There is no evidence that any cricothyrotome can be placed with acceptable success and safety in a child younger than 10 to 12 years, regardless of the design of the device or the claims of the manufacturer.
- PTV is virtually never indicated in the adult patient for rescue of a failed emergency airway. The establishment of a more functional surgical airway using a percutaneous technique or by formal cricothyroidotomy is vastly preferable. However, in children younger than 10 years, the opposite is true. In this age group, PTV is the primary invasive airway management method of choice. Despite the rarity of use of PTV in the ED, centers providing emergency care to children should have a PTV set readily available and providers should be familiar with how to connect and use it. The wire-coiled catheter designed for the PTV cannula resists kinking and so is preferable to a standard IV catheter.
- Of the methods described in this chapter, only a formal surgical cricothyrotomy and variations of the recently modified Melker set result in the placement of a cuffed tube within the trachea. The other techniques described here must be considered temporary at best. Placement of a tracheostomy tube or ETT through a formal surgical cricothyrotomy incision results in a definitive airway for the patient.
- The No.4 cuffed tracheostomy tube, despite having a variable ID that depends on manufacturer and type, can be used for virtually all cases of adult cricothyrotomy in the ED. The tube is of adequate size to provide ventilation in virtually all circumstances, and its outside dimensions are such that it will almost always be easily inserted.

## EVIDENCE

- **When is a surgical airway indicated and how often is it performed?** The failed airway algorithm (see Chapter 3) suggests that cricothyrotomy should be considered in a "*can't* intubate, *can* oxygenate" situation, when it is clear that alternative approaches have failed or are judged likely to fail. However, it helps to recognize that a given provider attempting laryngoscopy may have a certain "emotional inertia" when it comes to changing strategies. First, one must acknowledge that a laryngoscopist may not want to recognize that his or her laryngoscopy has failed. In addition, the hesitancy to perform an infrequently used technique may conspire to tempt the provider to have just "one more look." Such perseveration on a single method of intubation can have disastrous results. Although some rescue devices may serve as a bridge in some circumstances, anatomy and urgency often preclude their use, and insistence on attempting to try alternative devices in a desaturating CICO patient can be disastrous. In all likelihood, the main complication associated with cricothyrotomy or other invasive airways is not placing one soon enough. Cricothyrotomy is an infrequent procedure in ED populations. In a recent report from the NEAR III, overall, a surgical airway was used in 0.5% of 17,583 adult ED intubations. It was used as rescue technique in only 0.3%. In a recent pediatric report from the same registry, not a single surgical airway was recorded in more than a 1,000 pediatric intubations.[1,2]

- **Which technique (open or percutaneous) is best?** There is limited literature that effectively compares different techniques of invasive surgical airway management. The relatively rare performance of an emergency surgical airway, compounded with the urgency of the circumstance, may explain the absence of any controlled clinical trials comparing techniques in the emergency setting. As such, the current level of evidence for or against a particular technique exists as expert consensus based on collective experience, limited descriptive series, or studies in cadaveric and animal models. Cadaveric studies have compared the percutaneous, wire-guided technique to the traditional open, or no-drop, technique in cadavers with variable results.[3–5] The recent National Audit Project suggests that open techniques are more successful than percutaneous.[6] There is insufficient evidence to promote either RFST or no-drop technique for open cricothyrotomy as the *best* technique. Each approach has its share of expert champions and challengers. The choice of the RFST against the no-drop method will be made by the operator on the basis of training, experience, and judgment, and either approach is acceptable, each having some advantages and disadvantages and neither being clearly superior. Although the no-drop technique has been used successfully for decades, the RFST is proposed to be an improvement over the no-drop technique based on the following:
  - The RFST requires only one person to perform the procedure, whereas, ideally, the no-drop technique requires *two* people (i.e., one operator and one assistant).
  - The RFST can be readily performed from the head of the bed.
  - The RFST can be performed with fewer pieces of equipment (scalpel and tracheal hook only).

The major downside to the RFST is that it relies on a single horizontal incision and proper identification of the cricothyroid membrane, which may be more difficult than previously assumed.[7–10]

- **What is the best technique for locating the cricothyroid membrane?** In one study involving ED patients, physician volunteers were randomized to one of three techniques: a general palpation technique, the four-finger sternal notch approach, or an evaluation based on neck skin creases. The cricothyroid membrane was located independently by ultrasound. All techniques performed poorly, with success rates ranging from 46% to 62%.[7] Anesthesiologists have similar challenges. In one study of resident and staff anesthesia providers in Canada, success rates by general palpation ranged from 24% to 72%. Women and obese patients produced the lowest rates of accurate identification.[8] Ultrasound has been shown to be easy and accurate in locating and identifying the cricothyroid membrane and should be used, when time permits, to identify the cricothyroid membrane in patients with poor external landmarks.[11,12]
- **Is there a role for surgical airways in the prehospital setting?** Although its use is rare, cricothyrotomy has been widely taught and employed in the prehospital environment. The data are limited and preclude any firm recommendation on this practice. A recent position paper on the use of alternate airways in the out-of-hospital setting, from the National Association of EMS Physicians, also concluded that there is insufficient evidence to either support or refute the need for all agencies to have a surgical airway technique available.[13] If cricothyrotomy is to be used in an emergency medical services system, training, skill retention, individual case review, and system-wide quality management are essential. A field cricothyrotomy might be viewed as analogous to a police officer discharging a firearm. Each event is significant and worthy of thoughtful review.

## REFERENCES

1. Brown CA 3rd, Bair AE, Pallin DJ, et al. Techniques, success, and adverse events of emergency department adult intubations. *Ann Emerg Med*. 2015:65(4);363 e1–370 e1.

2. Pallin DJ, Dwyer RC, Walls RM, et al. Techniques and trends, success rates, and adverse events in emergency department pediatric intubations: a report from the National Emergency Airway Registry. *Ann Emerg Med*. 2016;67(5):610–615.
3. Benkhadra M, Lenfant F, Nemetz W, et al. A comparison of two emergency cricothyroidotomy kits in human cadavers. *Anesth Analg*. 2008;106:182.
4. Schaumann N, Lorenz V, Schellongowski P, et al. Evaluation of Seldinger technique emergency cricothyroidotomy versus standard surgical cricothyroidotomy in 200 cadavers. *Anesthesiology*. 2005;102:7.
5. Schober P, Hegemann MC, Schwarte LA, et al. Emergency cricothyrotomy-a comparative study of different techniques in human cadavers. *Resuscitation*. 2009;80:204.
6. Cook TM, Woodall N, Ferk C; on behalf of the Fourth National Audit Project. Major complications of airway management in the UK: results of the fourth national audit project of the Royal College of Anaesthetists and the Difficult Airway Society. Part I: anesthesia. *Br J Anaesth*. 2011;106:617–631.
7. Bair AE, Chima R. The inaccuracy of using landmark techniques for cricothyroid membrane identification: a comparison of three techniques. *Acad Emerg Med*. 2015;22:908–914.
8. Aslani A, Ng SC, Hurley M, et al. Accuracy of identification of the cricothyroid membrane in female subjects using palpation: an observational study. *Anesth Analg*. 2012;114:987–992.
9. Lamb A, Zhang J, Hung O, et al. Accuracy of identifying the cricothyroid membrane by anesthesia trainees and staff in a Canadian institution. *Can J Anaesth*. 2015;62:495–503.
10. Dinsmore J, Heard AMB, Green RJ, et al. The use of ultrasound to guide time-critical cannula tracheotomy when anterior neck airway anatomy is unidentifiable. *Eur J Anaesthesiol*. 2011;28(7):506–510.
11. Kristensen MS, Teoh WH, Rudolph SS. et al. A randomised cross-over comparison of the transverse and longitudinal techniques for ultrasound-guided identification of the cricothyroid membrane in morbidly obese subjects. *Anesthesia*. 2016;71(6):675–683.
12. Kristensen MS, Teoh WH, Rudolph SS. Ultrasonographic identification of the cricothyroid membrane: best evidence, techniques, and clinical impact. *Br J Anesth*. 2016;117:i39–i48.
13. O'Connor RE. Alternate airways in the out-of-hospital setting: position statement of the National Association of EMS Physicians. *Prehosp Emerg Care*. 2007;11(1):54–55.

# Section V

# Pharmacology and Techniques of Airway Management

Chapter 20

# Rapid Sequence Intubation

Calvin A. Brown III and Ron M. Walls

## INTRODUCTION

### Definition

Rapid sequence intubation (RSI) is the administration, after preoxygenation and patient optimization, of a potent induction agent followed immediately by a rapidly acting neuromuscular blocking agent (NMBA) to induce unconsciousness and motor paralysis for tracheal intubation. The technique is predicated on the fact that the patient has not fasted before intubation and, therefore, is at risk for aspiration of gastric contents. The preoxygenation phase begins before drug administration and permits a period of apnea to occur safely between the administration of the drugs and intubation of the trachea without the need for positive-pressure ventilation. Likewise, preintubation optimization is a step focused on maximizing patient hemodynamics and overall physiology before RSI drugs are given and is designed predominantly to protect against circulatory collapse during or immediately after the intubation. In other words, the purpose of RSI is to render the patient unconscious and paralyzed and then to intubate the trachea, with the patient as oxygenated and physiologically optimized as possible, without the use of bag-mask ventilation, which may cause gastric distention and increase the risk of aspiration. The Sellick maneuver (posterior pressure on the cricoid cartilage to occlude the esophagus and prevent passive regurgitation) has been shown to impair glottic visualization in some cases, and the evidence supporting its use is dubious, at best. As in the fourth edition, we no longer recommend routine use of this maneuver during emergency intubation.

### Indications and Contraindications

RSI is the cornerstone of emergency airway management and is the technique of choice when emergency intubation is indicated, and the patient does not have difficult airway features felt to contraindicate the use of an NMBA (see Chapters 2 and 3). When a contraindication to succinylcholine is present, rocuronium should be used as the NMBA (see Chapter 22). Some practitioners eschew the use of succinylcholine and routinely use rocuronium for all intubations; this is a matter of preference, for there are both pros and cons to this approach.

# TECHNIQUE

RSI can be thought of as a series of discrete steps, referred to as the seven Ps. Although conceptualizing RSI as a series of individual actions is helpful when teaching or planning the technique, most emergency intubations require that several steps, especially leading up to tube placement, occur simultaneously. In this latest edition, *preintubation optimization* has replaced *pretreatment* as the third "P" in RSI because a critical reappraisal of the available evidence behind pretreatment agents has failed to identify high-quality studies or clear patient benefit, except when these agents are used to optimize the patient's physiologic state to better tolerate the medications, intubation, and positive-pressure ventilation. Otherwise, adding unnecessary drugs contributes to procedural inefficiencies and introduces the potential for adverse drugs reactions and dosing errors. The seven Ps of RSI are shown in **Box 20-1**.

## Preparation

Before initiating the sequence, the patient is thoroughly assessed for difficulty of intubation (see Chapter 2). Fallback plans in the event of failed intubation are established, and the necessary equipment is located. The patient is in an area of the emergency department that is organized and equipped for resuscitation. Cardiac monitoring, BP monitoring, and pulse oximetry should be used in all cases. Continuous waveform capnography provides additional valuable monitoring information, particularly after intubation, and should be used whenever possible. The patient should have at least one, and preferably two, secure, well-functioning intravenous (IV) lines. Pharmacologic agents are drawn up in properly labeled syringes. Vital equipment is tested. A video laryngoscope, if available, should be brought to the bedside and tested for image clarity whether or not it is to be used on first attempt. If a direct laryngoscope is to be used, the blade of choice is affixed to the laryngoscope handle and clicked into the "on" position to ensure that the light functions and is bright. The endotracheal tube (ETT) of the desired size is prepared, and the cuff is tested for leaks. If difficult intubation is anticipated, a tube 0.5 mm or less in internal diameter (ID) should also be prepared. Selection and preparation of the tube, as well as the use of the intubating stylet and bougie, are discussed in Chapter 13. Throughout this preparatory phase, the patient is receiving preoxygenation and optimization measures, if appropriate, as described in the next two sections.

## Preoxygenation

Preoxygenation is essential to the "no bagging" principle of RSI. Preoxygenation is the establishment of an oxygen reservoir within the lungs, blood, and body tissue to permit several minutes of apnea to occur without arterial oxygen desaturation. The principal reservoir is the functional residual capacity in the lungs, which is approximately 30 mL per kg. Administration of 100% oxygen for 3 minutes replaces this predominantly nitrogenous mixture of room air with oxygen, allowing several minutes

**BOX 20-1**

**The seven Ps of RSI.**

1. Preparation
2. Preoxygenation
3. Preintubation Optimization
4. Paralysis with induction
5. Positioning
6. Placement with proof
7. Postintubation management

of apnea time before hemoglobin saturation decreases to <90% (**Fig. 20-1**). Similar preoxygenation can be achieved much more rapidly by having the patient take eight vital capacity breaths (the greatest volume breaths the patient can take) while receiving 100% oxygen.

Obese patients are best preoxygenated when placed upright and oxyhemoglobin desaturation is significantly delayed if oxygen is continuously administered at 5 to 15 L per minute by nasal cannula throughout the intubation sequence. The highest flow rate the patient will tolerate, with a goal of 15 L per minute, should be used. The evidence for "apneic oxygenation" will be presented at the end of this chapter. Even in non-obese patients, desaturation can be mitigated through continuous administration of oxygen at 5 to 15 L per minute during apnea. There is little downside to providing nasal cannula oxygen during the apneic phase of intubation for all emergency department intubations, however we consider it essential for patients predicted to rapidly desaturate.

The time to desaturation for an individual patient varies. Children, morbidly obese patients, chronically ill patients (especially those with cardiopulmonary diseases), and late-term pregnant women desaturate significantly more rapidly than an average healthy adult.

Note the bars indicating recovery from succinylcholine paralysis on the bottom right of Figure 20-1. This demonstrates the fallacy of the oft-cited belief that a patient will recover sufficiently from succinylcholine-induced paralysis to breathe on his or her own before sustaining injury from hypoxemia, even if intubation and mechanical ventilation are both impossible. Although many healthy patients with normal body habitus will recover adequate neuromuscular function to breathe on their own before catastrophic desaturation, many others, including almost all children and a majority of patients intubated for emergency conditions, will not, and even those who do are dependent on optimal preoxygenation before paralysis.

A healthy, fully preoxygenated 70-kg adult will maintain oxygen saturation at >90% for 8 minutes, whereas an obese adult will desaturate to 90% in <3 minutes. A 10-kg child will desaturate to 90% in <4 minutes. The time for desaturation from 90% to 0% is even more important and is much shorter. The healthy 70-kg adult desaturates from 90% to 0% in <120 seconds, and the small child

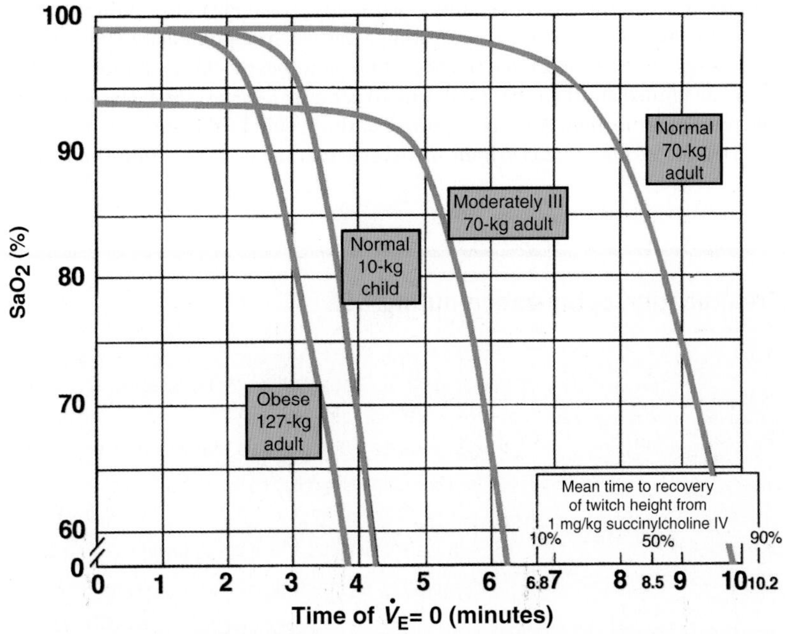


● **FIGURE 20-1. Time to Desaturation for Various Patient Circumstances.** (From Benumof J, Dagg R, Benumof R. Critical hemoglobin desaturation will occur before return to an unparalyzed state following 1 mg/kg IV succinylcholine. *Anesthesiology*. 1997;87:979.)

does so in 45 seconds. A late-term pregnant woman is a high oxygen user, has a reduced functional residual capacity, and has an increased body mass, so she desaturates quickly in a manner analogous to that of the obese patient. Particular caution is required in this circumstance because both the obese patient and the pregnant woman may also be difficult to intubate and to bag-mask ventilate.

Most emergency departments do not use systems that are capable of delivering 100% oxygen. Typically, emergency department patients are preoxygenated using the "100% non-rebreather mask," which delivers approximately 65% to 70% oxygen depending on fit, oxygen flow rate, and respiratory rate (see Chapter 5). In physiologically well patients in whom difficult intubation is not anticipated, this percentage is often sufficient and adequate preoxygenation is achieved. However, higher inspired fractions of oxygen are often desirable and can be delivered by active breathing through the demand valve of bag-mask systems equipped with a one-way exhalation valve. Recent evidence suggests preoxygenation performed with an Ambu bag is superior to face mask oxygen. Specially designed high-concentration oxygen delivery devices such as high-flow nasal cannula (HFNC), capable of providing both positive end-expiratory pressure and up to 70 L per minute of oxygen flow through specially designed nasal prongs, have been used for preparatory oxygenation, although the role of HFNC for emergency department (ED) patients is not defined. Available evidence from intensive care unit patients is mixed on its ability to prevent desaturation during urgent inpatient intubations. Oxygen delivery is discussed in detail in Chapter 5. The use of pulse oximetry throughout intubation enables the physician to monitor the level of oxygen saturation eliminating guesswork.

## Preintubation Optimization

Patients may be challenging to intubate for anatomic reasons such as airway obstruction or reduced neck mobility. Additionally, overall airway management can be made more complex by dramatic perturbations in vital signs and patient physiology. Although septic shock, severe myocardial depression, or an inability to preoxygenate in and of themselves do not make the act of laryngoscopy and tracheal tube placement more difficult, they can contribute to operator stress and patient morbidity by drastically compressing the time available to safely intubate or by placing the patient at risk for hypoxic injury or peri-intubation circulatory collapse after receiving induction agents. Preintubation optimization involves identifying and mitigating areas of cardiopulmonary vulnerability that may complicate resuscitative efforts, even if tracheal intubation goes quickly and smoothly. If the need for intubation is not immediate, then abnormal hemodynamic parameters should be normalized as much as possible prior to intubation. A simple example of this would be the insertion of a chest tube for a patient with tension pneumothorax to improve oxygenation and perfusion before initiating intubation.

BOX 20-2

### Preintubation optimization during RSI.

| | |
|---|---|
| Fentanyl | When sympathetic responses should be blunted (e.g., increased ICP, aortic dissection, intracranial hemorrhage, cardiac ischemia) |
| Fluids or Blood | Hypotension from bleeding, dehydration, sepsis, etc. |
| Pressors (Epinephrine or Neo-Synephrine) | Hypotension refractory to fluid challenge |
| BiPAP/CPAP | Hypoxia refractory to face mask oxygen |
| Tube Thoracostomy | Identified or suspected tension pneumothorax |

These steps should be addressed for all intubations when time and resources allow.
ICP = Intracranial pressure
Bi-PAP = Bi-level positive airway pressure
CPAP = Continuous positive airway pressure

Common aspects of abnormal patient physiology that should be identified and addressed during this step are shown in **Box 20-2**. The most commonly encountered physiologic problem is hypotension. Bleeding, dehydration, sepsis, and primary cardiac pathology are common emergency conditions that can complicate patient management, despite successful placement of the ETT. All induction agents can potentiate peripheral vascular dilation and myocardial depression and patients who present with depressed cardiac function, low intravascular volume, or poor vascular tone can suffer profound refractory shock or circulatory collapse after RSI drugs are administered, particularly when positive-pressure ventilation further compromises venous return. Isotonic fluids, blood products, and pressor agents may be used, time permitting, to support blood pressure and increase pharmacologic options for RSI. Oxygenation efforts are reassessed during this step and escalated if necessary. Hypertensive crises can also be prevented or treated with sympatholytic agents (fentanyl) prior to laryngeal manipulation and tube placement, both known to result in a sympathetic surge during intubation.

## Paralysis with Induction

In this phase, a rapidly acting induction agent is given in a dose adequate to produce prompt loss of consciousness (see Chapter 21). Administration of the induction agent is immediately followed by the NMBA, usually succinylcholine (see Chapter 22). If succinylcholine is contraindicated, rocuronium should be used. Both the induction agent and the NMBA are given by IV push. RSI does not involve the slow administration of the induction agent or a titration-to-end point approach. The sedative agent and dose are selected with the intention of rapid IV administration of the drugs. Although rapid administration of the induction agent can increase the likelihood and severity of side effects, especially hypotension, the entire technique is predicated on rapid loss of consciousness, rapid neuromuscular blockade, and a brief period of apnea without interposed assisted ventilation before intubation. Therefore, the induction agent is given as a rapid push followed immediately by a rapid push of the NMBA. Within several seconds of the administration of the induction agent and NMBA, the patient will begin to lose consciousness, and respiration will decline, and then cease.

## Positioning

After 20 to 30 seconds, the patient is induced, apneic and becoming flaccid. If succinylcholine has been used as the NMBA, fasciculations will be observed during this time. The oxygen mask and nasal cannula used for preoxygenation remain in place to prevent the patient from acquiring even a partial breath of room air. At this point, the patient is positioned optimally for intubation, with consideration for cervical spine immobilization in trauma. The bed should be at sufficient height to comfortably perform laryngoscopy, although this is much more an issue for direct than for video laryngoscopy. The patient should be transitioned fully to the head of the bed and, if appropriate, the head should be elevated and extended. Some patients will be sufficiently compromised that they require assisted ventilation continuously throughout the sequence to maintain oxygen saturations over 90%. Such patients, especially those with profound hypoxemia, are ventilated with bag and mask at all times except when laryngoscopy is occurring. Patients predicted to rapidly desaturate (morbid obesity, suboptimal starting oxygen saturations) will maintain high oxygen saturations longer if they receive oxygen at 5 to 15 L per minute through nasal cannula throughout laryngoscopy. The highest nasal cannula flow rate the patient can tolerate while awake should be used. The flow rate can then be increased to as much as 15 L per minute after the patient is unconscious. When bag-mask ventilation is performed on an unresponsive patient, the application of Sellick maneuver may minimize the volume of gases passed down the esophagus to the stomach, possibly decreasing the likelihood of regurgitation.

## Placement with Proof

At 45 seconds after the administration of the succinylcholine, or 60 seconds if rocuronium is used, test the patient's jaw for flaccidity and intubate. Strict attention to robust preoxygenation endows most patients with *minutes* of safe apnea time, allowing the intubation to be performed gently and carefully. Multiple attempts, if needed, are often possible without any need to provide additional oxygenation by bag and mask. Tube placement is confirmed as described in Chapter 12. End-tidal carbon dioxide ($ETCO_2$) detection is mandatory. A capnometer, such as a colorimetric $ETCO_2$ detector, is sufficient for this purpose. We recommend the use of continuous quantitative capnography, if available, as this provides additional and ongoing information.

## Postintubation Management

After placement is confirmed, the ETT is secured in place. Mechanical ventilation should be initiated as described in Chapter 7. A chest radiograph should be obtained to assess pulmonary status and ensure that mainstem intubation has not occurred. Hypotension is common in the postintubation period and is often caused by diminished venous blood return as a result of the increased intrathoracic pressure that attends mechanical ventilation, exacerbated by the hemodynamic effects of the induction agent. Although this form of hypotension is often self-limited and responds to IV fluids, persistent or profound hypotension may indicate a more ominous cause, such as tension pneumothorax or impending circulatory collapse. If significant hypotension is present, the management steps in **Table 20-1** should be considered.

Long-term sedation is generally indicated. The intubating clinician should pay close attention to postintubation sedation as recent ED-based research suggests that sedation is either not administered or given in low doses in as many as 18% of patients intubated after using neuromuscular blockade. Long-term paralysis, however, is generally avoided, except when necessary. Use of a sedation scale, such as the Richmond Agitation Sedation Scale, to optimize patient comfort helps guide decision-making regarding the necessity of neuromuscular blockade (**Box 20-3**). Sedation and analgesia are administered to reach the desired level, and neuromuscular blockade is used only if the patient then requires it for management. Use of a sedation scale prevents the use of neuromuscular blockade for patient control when the cause of the patient's agitation is inadequate sedation. A sample sedation protocol is shown in **Figure 20-2**. Maintenance of intubation and mechanical ventilation requires both sedation and analgesia, and these can be titrated to patient response. Propofol has become the agent of choice for ongoing sedation in mechanically ventilated patients, especially for those with neurologic conditions. Propofol is preferable because it can be discontinued or decreased with rapid recovery of consciousness. Propofol infusion can be started at 25 to 50 μg/kg/minute and titrated. An initial bolus of 0.5 to 1 mg per kg may be given if rapid sedation is desired. Analgesia is required, as above, because propofol is not an analgesic. Secondary sedation strategies might include midazolam 0.1 to 0.2 mg per kg, combined

**TABLE 20-1 Hypotension in the Postintubation Period**

| Cause | Detection | Action |
|---|---|---|
| Pneumothorax | Increased peak inspiratory pressure [PIP], difficulty bagging, decreased breath sounds, and decreasing oxygen saturation | Immediate thoracostomy |
| Decreased venous return | Especially in patients with high PIPs secondary to high intrathoracic pressure or those with marginal hemodynamic status before intubation | Fluid bolus and treatment of airway resistance (bronchodilators); increase the inspiratory flow rate to allow increased expiratory time; try $\downarrow V_T$, respiratory rate, or both if $Spo_2$ is adequate, and decrease the dose of sedation agent(s) |
| Induction agents | Other causes excluded | Fluid bolus and decrease the dose of sedation agent(s) |
| Cardiogenic | Usually in compromised patient; ECG; exclude other causes | Fluid bolus (caution), pressors, and decrease the dose of sedation agent(s) |

BOX 20-3

## Richmond agitation sedation scale.

| Score | Term | Description | |
|---|---|---|---|
| +4 | Combative | Overtly combative, violent, and immediate danger to staff | |
| +3 | Very agitated | Pulls or removes tube(s) or catheter(s) and is aggressive | |
| +2 | Agitated | Frequent nonpurposeful movement and fights ventilator | |
| +1 | Restless | Anxious but movements not aggressive and vigorous | |
| 0 | Alert and calm | | |
| −1 | Drowsy | Not fully alert, but has sustained awakening (eye opening/eye contact) to *voice* (>10 s) | Verbal stimulation |
| −2 | Light sedation | Briefly awakens with eye contact to *voice* (<10 s) | Verbal stimulation |
| −3 | Moderate sedation | Movement or eye opening to *voice* (but no eye contact) | Verbal stimulation |
| −4 | Deep sedation | No response to voice, but movement or eye opening to *physical* stimulation | Physical stimulation |
| −5 | Unarousable | No response to *voice* or *physical* stimulation | Physical stimulation |

## Procedure for Richmond Agitation Sedation Scale Assessment

1. Observe patient.
   a. Patient is alert, restless, or agitated. **(score 0 to +4)**
2. If not alert, state patient's name and *say* to open eyes and look at speaker.
   b. Patient awakens with sustained eye opening and eye contact. **(score −1)**
   c. Patient awakens with eye opening and eye contact, but not sustained. **(score −2)**
   d. Patient has any movement in response to voice but no eye contact. **(score −3)**
3. When no response to verbal stimulation, physically stimulate patient by shaking shoulder and/or rubbing sternum.
   e. Patient has any movement to physical stimulation. **(score −4)**
   f. Patient has no response to any stimulation. **(score −5)**

Adapted from Sessler CN, Gosnell M, Grap MJ, et al. The Richmond Agitation-Sedation Scale: validity and reliability in adult intensive care patients. *Am J Respir Crit Care Med.* 2002;166:1338–1344; and Ely EW, Truman B, Shintani A, et al. Monitoring sedation status over time in ICU patients: the reliability and validity of the Richmond Agitation Sedation Scale (RASS). *JAMA.* 2003;289:2983–2991.

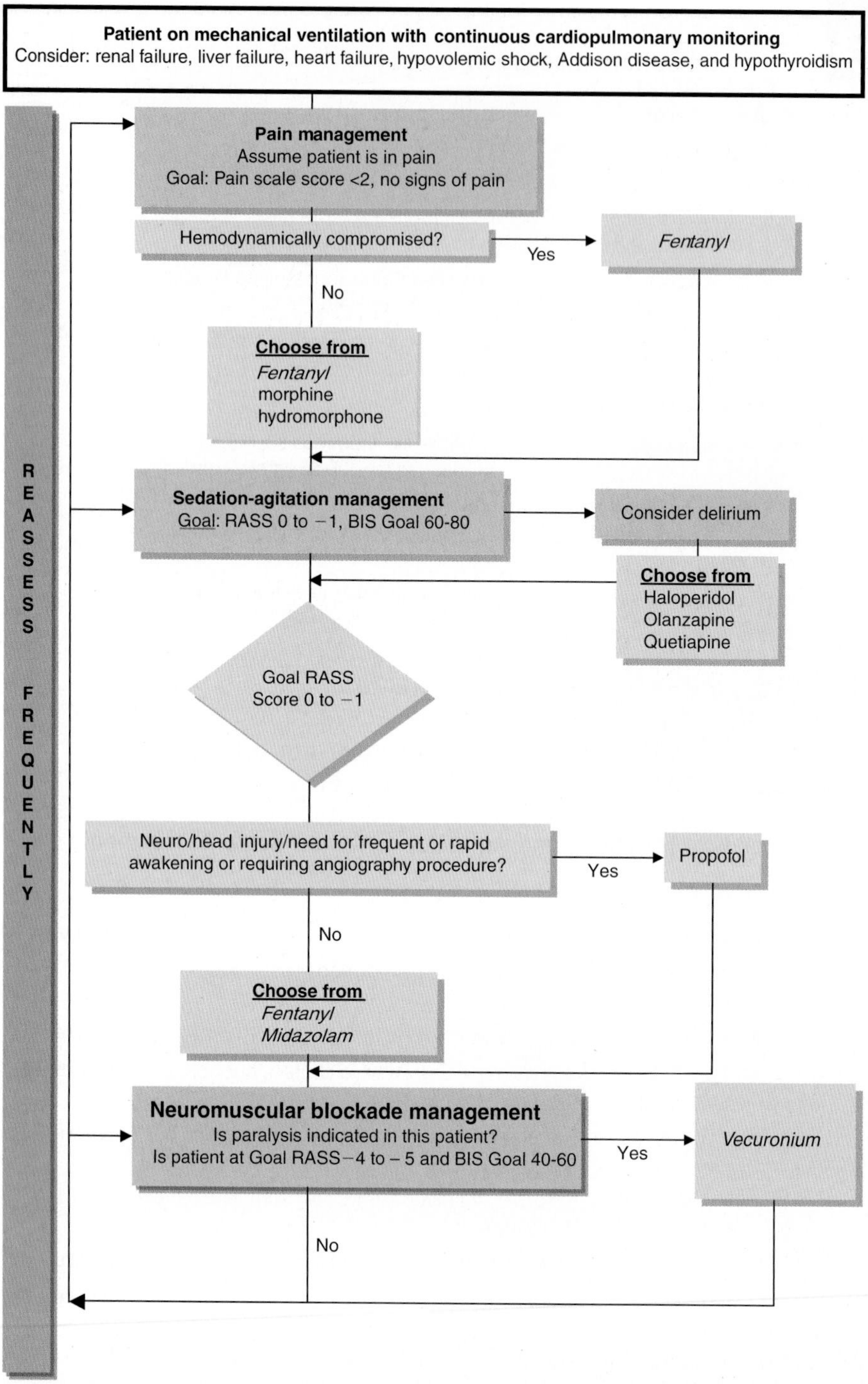


● **FIGURE 20-2. Postintubation Management Protocol Using the RASS Score.** See also Box 20-3 for description of the Sedation Scale (RASS). BIS, Bispectral Index. (The protocol, adapted with permission, was developed for use at Brigham and Women's Hospital, Boston, MA.)

with an analgesic such as fentanyl 2 μg per kg, morphine 0.2 mg per kg, or hydromorphone (Dilaudid) 0.03 mg per kg. Fentanyl may be preferable because of its superior hemodynamic stability. When an NMBA is required, a full paralytic dose should be used (e.g., vecuronium 0.1 mg per kg). Sedation and analgesia are difficult to titrate when the patient is paralyzed, and "topping up" doses should be administered regularly, before physiologic stress (hypertension and tachycardia) is evident.

## Timing the Steps of RSI

Successful RSI requires a detailed knowledge of the sequence of steps to be taken and also of the minimum time required for each step to achieve its purpose. The duration of time from preparation to administration of RSI medications is variable and depends on the clinical scenario. Although some patients may require an airway immediately, such as in a case of rapidly progressing anaphylaxis, some patients will have no immediate threat to oxygenation and ventilation but present with profound hypotension, and the clinician may spend additional time on fluid resuscitation and hemodynamic optimization before proceeding with RSI drugs. Preoxygenation requires at least 3 minutes for maximal effect. If necessary, eight vital capacity breaths can accomplish equivalent preoxygenation in <30 seconds. If a hypertensive crisis exists, fentanyl for sympatholysis should be given 3 minutes before the administration of the sedative and NMBA. The pharmacokinetics of the sedatives and neuromuscular blockers would suggest that a 45-second interval between administration of these agents and initiation of endotracheal intubation is optimal, extending to 60 seconds if rocuronium is used. Onset may be delayed if the patient's condition results in poor cardiac output as drug delivery will be affected. Thus, the entire sequence of RSI can be described as a series of timed steps. For the purposes of discussion, *time zero* is the time at which the sedative agent and NMBA are pushed. If the need for intubation is not immediate and standard preparatory steps can be taken, then the operator needs a minimum of 5 to 15 minutes to accomplish a safe and efficient team response with a defined rescue plan, sufficient preoxygenation, and physiologic optimization. As already mentioned, the timeline leading up to administration of RSI drugs can vary greatly based on the urgency for tube placement and patient stability. A hypotensive blunt trauma patient with an open femur fracture and an unstable pelvis, but no immediate threat to the airway, may need 20 to 30 minutes in order to establish IV access and begin saline and blood product resuscitation before intubation can take place safely. Therefore, although there are minimum time requirements for certain preintubation steps, preparation for RSI may take longer if a patient requires physiologic optimization prior to intubation, or may be shortened if the intubation is highly emergent. The recommended sequence is shown in Table 20-2.

TABLE 20-2 Rapid Sequence Intubation

| Time | Action (Seven Ps) |
|---|---|
| Zero minus 10+ min | **P**reparation: *Assemble all necessary equipment, drugs, etc.* |
| Zero minus 10+ min (at least 3 min) | **P**reoxygenation |
| Zero minus 10+ min | **P**reintubation optimization |
| Zero | **P**aralysis with induction: *Administer induction agent by IV push, followed immediately by paralytic agent by IV push* |
| Zero plus 30 s | **P**ositioning: *Position patient for optimal laryngoscopy; continue oxygen supplementation at 5 L per min by nasal cannula after apnea ensues* |
| Zero plus 45 s | **P**lacement with proof: *Assess mandible for flaccidity; perform intubation; confirm placement* |
| Zero plus 1 min | **P**ostintubation management: *Long-term sedation with paralysis only if indicated* |

**TABLE 20-3 RSI for Healthy 80-kg Patient**

| Time | Action (Seven Ps) |
|---|---|
| Zero minus 10+ min | **P**reparation |
| Zero minus 10+ min | **P**reoxygenation |
| Zero minus 10+ min | **P**re*intubation optimization: None indicated* |
| Zero | **P**aralysis with induction: *Etomidate 24 mg IV push; succinylcholine 120 mg IV push* |
| Zero plus 20–30 s | **P**ositioning: *Position patient for optimal laryngoscopy; continue oxygen supplementation at 5–15 L per min* |
| Zero plus 45 s | **P**lacement with proof: *Confirm with $ETCO_2$, physical examination* |
| Zero plus 1 min | **P**ostintubation management: *Long-term sedation/paralysis as indicated* |

An example of RSI performed for a generally healthy 40-year-old, 80-kg patient is shown in Table 20-3. Other examples of RSI for particular patient conditions are in the corresponding sections throughout this manual.

## Success Rates and Adverse Events

RSI has a very high success rate in the emergency department, approximately 99% in most modern series. The National Emergency Airway Registry (NEAR), an international multicenter study of >17,500 adult emergency department intubations, reported a first-attempt success of 85% when RSI was used. RSI success rates are higher than those for other emergency airway management methods. The ultimate success rate was 99.4% for all encounters. RSI was the principal approach, used in 85% of all first attempts. The NEAR investigators classify events related to intubation as follows:

- Immediate complications such as witnessed aspiration, broken teeth, airway trauma, and undetected esophageal intubation
- Technical problems such as mainstem intubation, cuff leak, and recognized esophageal intubation
- Physiologic alterations such as pneumothorax, pneumomediastinum, cardiac arrest, and dysrhythmia

This system allows witnessed complications to be identified and all adverse events to be captured, but avoids the incorrect attribution of various technical problems (e.g., recognized esophageal intubation or tube cuff failure) or physiologic alterations (e.g., cardiac arrest in a patient who was *in extremis* before intubation was undertaken and which may or may not be attributable to the intubation) as complications. Overall, the peri-intubation event rate is low, recorded in approximately 12%, with the most common being recognized esophageal intubation (3.3%) followed by hypotension (1.6%). Hypotension and alterations in heart rate can result from the pharmacologic agents used or from stimulation of the larynx with resultant reflexes. Other studies have reported consistent results. The most catastrophic complication of RSI is unrecognized esophageal intubation, which is rare in the emergency department, but occurs with alarming frequency in some prehospital studies. This situation underscores the importance of confirming tube placement. It is incumbent on the person who performs RSI to be able to establish an airway and maintain mechanical ventilation. This process may require a surgical airway as the final rescue from a failed oral intubation attempt (see Chapter 3). Aspiration of gastric contents can occur but is uncommon. Overall, the true complication rate of RSI in the emergency department is low and the success rate is exceedingly high, especially when one considers the serious nature of the illnesses for which patients are intubated, as well as the limited time and information available to the clinician performing the intubation.

### Delayed Sequence Intubation

When a patient is persistently hypoxemic or at risk for precipitous oxyhemoglobin desaturation, and is unable to cooperate with providers in achieving oxygenation, it may be appropriate to temporarily pause during the intubation sequence to focus on maximizing preoxygenation. This approach has been called delayed sequence intubation or DSI, and is predicated on failure of the ability to preoxygenate using usual methods. The fundamental difference between DSI and what we describe as preintubation optimization is that, for the latter, all measures are taken before an induction agent is given. With the DSI technique, an induction agent is given first, in hopes of facilitating oxygenation of a combative or agitated patient. The technique involves administration of a dissociative dose of ketamine (1 mg per kg IV) followed by several minutes of oxygenation using a non-rebreather face mask or pressure support mask ventilation (such as bilevel positive airway pressure [BL-PAP] or continuous positive airway pressure). When oxygenation is felt to be optimal, the operator pushes the NMBA and intubates as for RSI. One case series of approximately 60 ED and ICU patients showed a significant improvement in pre- and post-DSI saturations using this strategy. Additionally, no desaturation events were reported, even in high-risk patients. Although this process seems to have promise, it has not been validated in general ED environments, and has not been compared with conventional RSI for outcomes, including complications. Although it is reasonable to use this approach in selected cases, we prefer undertaking oxygenation as part of patient optimization whenever possible, then performing the RSI swiftly, as outlined above.

## EVIDENCE

- **What is the optimal method for preoxygenation?** Standard preoxygenation has traditionally been achieved by 3 minutes of normal tidal volume breathing of 100% oxygen. Pandit et al.[1] showed that eight vital capacity breaths achieves similar preoxygenation to that of 3 minutes of normal tidal volume breathing, and that both of these methods are superior to four vital capacity breaths. The time to desaturation of oxyhemoglobin to 95% is 5.2 minutes after eight vital capacity breaths versus 3.7 minutes after 3 minutes of tidal volume breathing and 2.8 minutes after four vital capacity breaths.[2,3] Preoxygenation of normally sized healthy patients can produce an average of 6 to 8 minutes of apnea time before desaturation to 90% occurs, but the times are much less (as little as 3 minutes) in patients with cardiovascular disease, obese patients, and small children.[4]

  Recent evidence suggests that preoxygenation with either flush-flow rate oxygen or an Ambu bag should be done whenever possible as oxygenation is superior to that accomplished by face mask with 15 L per minute oxygen flow.[5] Sufficient recovery from succinylcholine paralysis cannot be relied on before desaturation occurs, even in properly preoxygenated healthy patients.[4] Term pregnant women also desaturate more rapidly than nonpregnant women do and desaturate to 95% in $<3$ minutes, compared with 4 minutes for nonpregnant controls. Preoxygenating in the upright position prolongs desaturation time in nonpregnant women to 5.5 minutes, but does not favorably affect term pregnant patients.[2,6] HFNC systems are specially designed nasal oxygen delivery systems able to deliver up to 60 to 70 L per minute oxygen flow. In ICU patients, the results have been mixed with regard to HFNC's ability to effectively preoxygenate prior to urgent intubation or stave off desaturation compared with face mask oxygen.[7,8] A randomized controlled trial of HFNC vs. high-flow face mask oxygen in hypoxic ICU patients being preoxygenated for intubation showed no difference in desaturation rates ($Sao_2 < 80\%$).[7] However, Miguel-Montanes et al.[8] looked at 100 patients with starting saturations less than 80% who were preoxygenated with either non-rebreather face mask oxygen or HFNC and found that preintubation saturations were higher in the HFNC group (when measured at 5- and 30-minute intervals) and the face mask group had seven times the number of desaturation events during intubation.

- **How should obese patients be preoxygenated?** Obese patients desaturate more rapidly than nonobese patients.[4] Two techniques have emerged that maximize the time to desaturation for obese patients. First, preoxygenation of the morbidly obese (body mass index > 40 kg per m$^2$) in the 25° head-up position achieves higher arterial oxygenation saturations and significantly prolongs desaturation time to 92%, to about 3.5 minutes versus 2.5 minutes over those patients preoxygenated in the supine position.[9] Second, providing continuous oxygen by nasal cannula during the apneic phase is known to prolong maintenance of high oxyhemoglobin saturation in normal body habitus patients. In one study, despite preoxygenation using only four vital capacity breaths, 15 patients receiving 5 L per minute of oxygen through a nasopharyngeal catheter did not desaturate at all, maintaining oxyhemoglobin saturations of 100% for 6 minutes, versus their "no oxygen" comparison group, which desaturated to 95% in an average of approximately 4 minutes.[10] In obese patients, the effect may be even more important because of the rapid desaturation these patients otherwise exhibit. When obese patients receive continuous oxygen at 5 L per minute during the apneic phase of intubation, desaturation is delayed to about 5¼ versus 3.75 minutes for a nonoxygenated comparison group, and 8/15 oxygenated patients versus 1/15 nonoxygenated patients maintained oxyhemoglobin saturation of 95% or higher for 6 minutes.[11] Surprisingly, although the use of noninvasive positive-pressure ventilation for preoxygenation of obese patients shortened the time required for preoxygenation, it did not prolong the time to desaturation to 95%.[12] For all obese patients, we recommend the use of continuous apneic oxygenation with nasal cannula at 5 to 15 L per minute flow rate. For nonobese patients, continuous oxygenation also makes sense, particularly if the airway is anticipated to be difficult. Early investigations evaluated the effect of continuous nasal oxygenation at 5 L per minute flow; however, some have suggested turning the nasal cannula flow rate up to 15 L per minute.[13] Healthy volunteers are able to tolerate this rate of oxygen through standard nasal cannula; however, sick, agitated patients may not. On balance, it is reasonable to turn the flow-up rate up to the highest tolerable level for each patient and then up to 15 L per minute once induced. Noninvasive positive-pressure ventilation can be helpful in oxygenating patients with morbid obesity or physiologic shunts and may be employed if ambient pressure oxygenation is not adequate.[14,15]
- **What is the evidence for Delayed Sequence Intubation?** The term *delayed sequence intubation* is meant to describe the act of sedating patients with ketamine at a dose of 1 mg per kg IV for the purposes of facilitating preoxygenation either by face mask or BL-PAP. One case series of both ICU and ED patients showed an average improvement of 9% in oxygen saturation from a pre-DSI saturation of 90% to post-DSI saturation of 99%. There were no desaturation events, even in high-risk patients.[16] This study suggests this approach is successful in ICU and high-intensity EDs with specially trained personnel who are comfortable using ketamine and have the staff to closely monitor patients after ketamine is administered. There are not enough data to recommend this for all ED settings.
- **What are the hemodynamic consequences of RSI?** The combination of acute illness, hemorrhage, dehydration, sepsis, and the vasodilatory effects of induction agents makes peri-intubation hypotension a common event. One retrospective review of 336 emergency department intubations found that significant peri-intubation hypotension occurred 23% of the time.[17] Patients with peri-intubation hypotension were more likely elderly, suffering from chronic obstructive pulmonary disease, or were in shock upon arrival and, not surprisingly, went on to have significantly higher in-hospital mortality. In a separate review, the same investigators found the rate of peri-intubation cardiac arrest occurred in 4.2% of all encounters, with two-thirds occurring within 10 minutes of receiving RSI medications.[18] A before and after ICU study showed that a strategy using effective preloading, cardio-stable drug selection, and early use of vasopressors resulted in significantly lower rates of cardiac arrest, refractory shock, and critical hypoxemia.[19] These studies form the current basis for our recommendation to maximize patient physiology prior to RSI.
- **Sellick maneuver:** A meta-analyses of the studies of Sellick maneuver showed that there is no solid evidence supporting its routine use during RSI.[20] Similarly, a 2010 study of 402 trauma patients suggests that, at the least, the maneuver has as much potential for harm as for good.[21]

Sellick maneuver may be applied improperly or not at all during a significant proportion of emergency department RSIs.[22] Even when applied by experienced practitioners, Sellick maneuver can increase peak inspiratory pressure and decrease tidal volume or even cause complete obstruction during bag-mask ventilation.[23] The practice, though, is so embedded in emergency medicine and anesthesia cultures that practitioners have been slow to abandon it.

- **Is RSI superior to intubation with sedation alone?** This is also discussed in the evidence section for Chapter 22. The most powerful evidence supporting the use of an NMBA in addition to an induction agent comes from dosing studies of NMBAs, of which there are many. The results uniformly are the same. Intubation is more successful because of better intubating conditions when an NMBA is used, when compared to the use of an induction agent alone. These results are even more compelling when one realizes that the depth of anesthesia in these studies is invariably deeper than that obtained with use of a single dose of an induction agent for emergency intubation. In a study of 180 general anesthesia patients, 0% of patients who received no succinylcholine had excellent intubating conditions versus 80% of patients receiving 1.5 mg per kg of succinylcholine.[24] Seventy percent of the "no NMBA" group had intubating conditions characterized as "poor." In a different study by the same investigators, "acceptable" intubating conditions were achieved in 32% of patients with general anesthesia but no NMBA versus over 90% of patients receiving any effective dose of succinylcholine.[25] Bozeman et al.[26] compared the use of etomidate alone to etomidate plus succinylcholine in a prehospital flight paramedic program and found that RSI outperformed etomidate-alone intubations by all measures of ease of intubation. Bair et al.[27] analyzed 207 (2.7%) failed intubations among 7,712 intubations in the NEAR registry and found that the greatest proportion of rescue procedures (49%) involved the use of RSI to achieve intubation after failure of oral or nasotracheal intubation by non-RSI methods. Results from the second phase of the NEAR project reporting on 8,937 emergency department adult intubations showed that RSI was associated with a first-attempt success rate of 82%, whereas sedation-alone intubations were successful only 76% of the time.[28] In the following NEAR III report of 17,583 adult intubations, RSI was the most successful method (85%) and significantly higher than intubations facilitated by sedatives alone (76%).[29]
- **What about RSI for children?** In 1,053 pediatric intubations from phase III of the NEAR project, the vast majority of intubations (81%) were performed using RSI, with a first-attempt success rate of 85%, higher than sedation-facilitated intubations or those intubated without medications.[30] A study of 105 children younger than 10 years (average age, 3 years) who underwent RSI with etomidate as the induction agent showed stable hemodynamics and high success and safety profiles.[31]

## REFERENCES


1. Pandit JJ, Duncan T, Robbins PA. Total oxygen uptake with two maximal breathing techniques and the tidal volume breathing technique: a physiologic study of preoxygenation. *Anesthesiology*. 2003;99:841–846.
2. Baraka AS, Taha SK, Aouad MT, et al. Preoxygenation: comparison of maximal breathing and tidal volume breathing techniques. *Anesthesiology*. 1999;91:612–616.
3. Ramez Salem M, Joseph NJ, Crystal GJ, et al. Preoxygenation: comparison of maximal breathing and tidal volume techniques. *Anesthesiology*. 2000;92:1845–1847.
4. Benumof JL, Dagg R, Benumof R. Critical hemoglobin desaturation will occur before return to an unparalyzed state following 1 mg/kg intravenous succinylcholine. *Anesthesiology*. 1997;87(4):979–982.
5. Groombridge C, Chin CW, Hanrahan B, et al. Assessment of common preoxygenation strategies outside of the operating room environment. *Acad Emerg Med*. 2016 [Epub ahead of print].
6. Hayes AH, Breslin DS, Mirakhur RK, et al. Frequency of haemoglobin desaturation with the use of succinylcholine during rapid sequence induction of anaesthesia. *Acta Anaesthesiol Scand*. 2001;45:746–749.

7. Vourc'h M, Asfar P, Volteau C, et al. High-flow nasal cannula oxygen during endotracheal intubation in hypoxemic patients: a randomized controlled clinical trial. *Intensive Care Med.* 2015;41(9):1538–1548.
8. Miguel-Montanes R, Hajage D, Messika J, et al. Use of high-flow nasal cannula oxygen therapy to prevent desaturation during tracheal intubation of intensive care patients with mild-to-moderate hypoxemia. *Crit Care Med.* 2015; 43(3):574–583.
9. Dixon BJ, Dixon JB, Carden JR, et al. Preoxygenation is more effective in the 25 degrees head-up position than in the supine position in severely obese patients: a randomized controlled study. *Anesthesiology*. 2005;102(6):1110–1115.
10. Taha SK, Siddik-Sayyid SM, El-Khatib MF, et al. Nasopharyngeal oxygen insufflation following pre-oxygenation using the four deep breath technique. *Anaesthesia*. 2006;61(5):427–430.
11. Ramachandran SK, Cosnowski A, Shanks A, et al. Apneic oxygenation during prolonged laryngoscopy in obese patients: a randomized, controlled trial of nasal oxygen administration. *J Clin Anesth*. 2010;22(3):164–168.
12. Delay JM, Sebbane M, Jung B, et al. The effectiveness of noninvasive positive pressure ventilation to enhance preoxygenation in morbidly obese patients: a randomized controlled study. *Anesth Analg*. 2008;107(5):1707–1713.
13. Weingart SD, Levitan RM. Preoxygenation and prevention of desaturation during emergency airway management. *Ann Emerg Med*. 2012;59(3):165–175.
14. Baillard C, Fosse JP, Sebbane M, et al. Noninvasive ventilation improves preoxygenation before intubation of hypoxic patients. *Am J Respir Crit Care Med.* 2006;174:171–177.
15. De Jong A, Futier E, Millot A, et al. How to preoxygenate in operative room: healthy subjects and situations "at risk". *Ann Fr Anesth Reanim.* 2014;33:457–461.
16. Weingart SD, Trueger NS, Wong N, et al. Delayed sequence intubation: a prospective observational trial. *Ann Emerg Med*. 2015;65(4):349–355.
17. Heffner AC, Swords DS, Nussbaum ML, et al. Predictors of the complication of postintubation hypotension during emergency airway management. *J Crit Care*. 2012;27(6):587–593.
18. Heffner AC, Swords DS, Neale NM, et al. Incidence and factors associated with cardiac arrest complicating emergency airway management. *Resuscitation*. 2013;84(11):1500–1504.
19. Jaber S, Jung B, Come P, et al. An intervention to decrease complications related to endotracheal intubation in the intensive care unit: a prospective, multicenter study. *Intensive Care Med*. 2010;36(2):248–255.
20. Ellis DY, Harris T, Zideman D. Cricoid pressure in emergency department rapid sequence tracheal intubations: a risk-benefit analysis. *Ann Emerg Med*. 2007;50:653–665.
21. Harris T, Ellis DY, Foster L, et al. Cricoid pressure and laryngeal manipulation in 402 pre-hospital emergency anaesthetics: essential safety measure or a hindrance to rapid safe intubation? *Resuscitation*. 2010;81:810–816.
22. Olsen JC, Gurr DE, Hughes M. Video analysis of emergency medicine residents performing rapid-sequence intubations. *J Emerg Med*. 2000;18(4):469–472.
23. Allman KG. The effect of cricoid pressure application on airway patency. *J Clin Anesth*. 1995;7(3):197–199.
24. Naguib M, Samarkandi AH, El-Din ME, et al. The dose of succinylcholine required for excellent endotracheal intubating conditions. *Anesth Analg*. 2006;102(1):151–155.
25. Naguib M, Samarkandi A, Riad W, et al. Optimal dose of succinylcholine revisited. *Anesthesiology*. 2003;99(5):1045–1049.
26. Bozeman WP, Kleiner DM, Huggett V. A comparison of rapid-sequence intubation and etomidate-only intubation in the prehospital air medical setting. *Prehosp Emerg Care*. 2006;10(1):8–13.
27. Bair AE, Filbin MR, Kulkarni RG, et al. The failed intubation attempt in the emergency department: analysis of prevalence, rescue techniques, and personnel. *J Emerg Med*. 2002;23(2):131–140.

28. Walls RM, Brown CA 3rd, Bair AE, et al. Emergency airway management: a multi-center report of 8937 emergency department intubations. *J Emerg Med*. 2011;41(4):347–354.

29. Brown CA 3rd, Bair AE, Pallin DJ, et al. Techniques, success, and adverse events of emergency department adult intubations. *Ann Emerg Med*. 2015;65(4):363 e1–370 e1.

30. Pallin DJ, Walls RM, Brown CA 3rd. Techniques and success rates of pediatric emergency department intubations. *Ann Emerg Med*. 2016;67(5):610–615.

31. Guldner G, Schultz J, Sexton P, et al. Etomidate for rapid-sequence intubation in young children: hemodynamic effects and adverse events. *Acad Emerg Med*. 2003;10:134–139.

# Chapter 21

# Sedative Induction Agents

David A. Caro and Katren R. Tyler

## INTRODUCTION

Agents used to sedate, or "induce," patients for intubation during rapid sequence intubation (RSI) are properly called sedative induction agents because induction of general anesthesia is at the extreme of the spectrum of their sedative actions. In this chapter, we refer to this family of drugs as "induction agents." The ideal induction agent would smoothly and quickly render the patient unconscious, unresponsive, and amnestic in one arm/heart/brain circulation time. It would also provide analgesia, maintain stable cerebral perfusion pressure (CPP) and cardiovascular hemodynamics, be immediately reversible, and have few, if any, adverse physiologic effects. Unfortunately, such an induction agent does not exist. Most induction agents meet the first criterion because they are highly lipophilic and so have a rapid onset within 15 to 30 seconds of intravenous (IV) administration. Their clinical effects are also terminated quickly as the drug rapidly redistributes to less well-perfused tissues. However, all induction agents have the potential to cause myocardial depression and subsequent hypotension. These effects depend on the particular drug; the patient's underlying physiologic condition; and the dose, concentration, and speed of injection of the drug. The faster the drug is administered IV, the larger the concentration of drug that saturates organs with the greatest blood flow (i.e., brain and heart) and the more pronounced its effect. Because RSI requires rapid administration of a precalculated dose of an induction agent, the choice of drug and the dose must be individualized to capitalize on desired effects, while minimizing those that might adversely affect the patient. Some patients are so unstable that the primary goal is to produce amnesia rather than anesthesia because to produce the latter might lead to severe hypotension and organ hypoperfusion.

The most commonly used emergency induction agent is etomidate (Amidate), which is popular because of its rapid onset of action, relative hemodynamic stability, and widespread availability. Recent registry data suggest ketamine (Ketalar) and propofol (Diprivan) are the next two most commonly used induction agents, but both trail far behind etomidate. Midazolam is still used as an induction agent but should be considered a distant fourth option and only used if other agents are unavailable. It is less reliable in inducing anesthesia, has a slower onset of action, and is more likely to produce hypotension than either etomidate or ketamine. The ultra–short-acting barbiturates such as methohexital (Brevital) and the ultra–short-acting narcotics such as sufentanil are rare in the ED and will not be discussed in further detail in this chapter. Additionally, thiopental is no longer available in North America and is rarely used in other countries. The relatively selective $\alpha_2$-adrenergic agonist dexmedetomidine is not used as an RSI induction agent because it is not administered as a rapid bolus by IV push.

General anesthetic agents act through two principal mechanisms: (1) an increase in inhibition through activity at gamma-aminobutyric acid "A" (GABA) receptors (e.g., benzodiazepines, barbiturates, propofol, etomidate, isoflurane, enflurane, and halothane), and (2) a decreased excitation through *N*-methyl-D-aspartate (NMDA) receptors (e.g., ketamine, nitrous oxide, and xenon).

The IV induction agents discussed in this chapter share important pharmacokinetic characteristics. Induction agents are highly lipophilic and because the brain is a highly perfused, lipid-dense organ, a standard induction dose of each agent (with the exception of midazolam) in a euvolemic, normotensive patient will produce unconsciousness within 30 seconds. The blood–brain barrier is freely permeable to medications used to induce anesthesia. The observed clinical duration of each drug is measured in minutes because of the drugs' distribution half-life ($t_{1/2}\alpha$), characterized by distribution of the drug from the central circulation to well-perfused tissues, such as brain. The redistribution of the drug from brain to fat and muscle terminates its central nervous system (CNS) effects. The elimination half-life ($t_{1/2}\beta$, usually measured in hours) is characterized by each drug's reentry from fat and lean muscle into plasma down a concentration gradient leading to hepatic metabolism and renal excretion. Generally, it requires four to five elimination half-lives to completely clear the drug from the body.

The dosing of induction agents in nonobese adults should be based on ideal body weight (IBW) in kilograms; however, in clinical practice, the total body weight (TBW or actual body weight) is a close enough approximation to IBW for the purposes of dosing these agents. The situation is more complicated for morbidly obese patients, however. The high lipophilicity of the induction agents combined with the increased volume of distribution ($V_d$) of these drugs in obesity argues for actual body weight dosing. Opposing this, however, is the significant cardiovascular depression that would occur if such a large quantity of drug is injected as a single bolus. Balancing these two considerations, and given the paucity of actual pharmacokinetic studies in obese patients, the best approach is to use lean body weight (LBW) for dosing of most induction agents, decreasing to IBW if the patient is hemodynamically compromised, or for drugs with significant hemodynamic depression, such as propofol. LBW is obtained by adding 0.3 of the patient's excess weight (TBW minus IBW) to the IBW, and using the sum as the dosing weight. More details on drug dosing for obese patients is discussed in Chapter 40.

Aging affects the pharmacokinetics of induction agents. In elderly patients, lean body mass and total body water decrease while total body fat increases, resulting in an increased volume of distribution, an increase in $t_{1/2}\beta$, and an increased duration of drug effect. In addition, the elderly are more sensitive to the hemodynamic and respiratory depressant effects of these agents, and the induction doses should be reduced to approximately one-half to two-thirds of the dose used in their healthy, younger counterparts.

# ETOMIDATE

| Etomidate (Amidate) | | | | |
|---|---|---|---|---|
| **Usual emergency induction dose (mg/kg)** | **Onset (s)** | **$t_{1/2}\alpha$ (min)** | **Duration (min)** | **$t_{1/2}\beta$ (h)** |
| 0.3 | 15–45 | 2–4 | 3–12 | 2–5 |

## Clinical Pharmacology

Etomidate is an imidazole derivative that is primarily a hypnotic and has no analgesic activity. With the exception of ketamine, etomidate is the most hemodynamically stable of the currently available induction agents. It exerts its effect by enhancing GABA activity at the GABA–receptor complex. GABA receptors moderate the activity of inhibitory chloride channels, thus making neurons less excitable. Etomidate attenuates the underlying elevated intracranial pressure (ICP) by decreasing cerebral blood flow (CBF) and cerebral metabolic rate for oxygen ($CMRO_2$). Its hemodynamic stability preserves CPP. Etomidate is cerebroprotective (although not as much as other agents like the barbiturates); its hemodynamic stability and favorable CNS effects make it an excellent choice for patients with elevated ICP.

Etomidate does not release histamine and is safe for use in patients with reactive airway disease. However, it lacks the direct bronchodilatory properties of ketamine or propofol, which may be preferable agents in these patients.

### Indications and Contraindications

Etomidate has become the induction agent of choice for most emergent RSIs because of its rapid onset, its hemodynamic stability, its positive effect on $CMRO_2$ and CPP, and its rapid recovery. As with any induction agent, dosage should be adjusted in hemodynamically compromised patients. Etomidate is a U.S. Food and Drug Administration (FDA) pregnancy category C drug.

Etomidate is not FDA approved for use in children, but many series report safe and effective use in pediatric patients.

### Dosage and Clinical Use

In euvolemic and hemodynamically stable patients, the normal induction dose of etomidate is 0.3 mg per kg IV push. In compromised patients, the dose should be reduced commensurate with the patient's clinical status; reduction to 0.2 mg per kg is usually sufficient. In morbidly obese patients, the induction dose should be based on LBW, by using IBW, and adding a correction of 30% of the excess weight (see earlier).

### Adverse Effects

Pain on injection is common because of the diluent (propylene glycol) and can be somewhat mitigated by having a fast-flowing IV solution running in a large vein. Myoclonic movement during induction is common and has been confused with seizure activity. It is of no clinical consequence and generally terminates promptly as the neuromuscular blocking (NMB) agent takes effect.

The most significant and controversial side effect of etomidate is its reversible inhibition of adrenal cortisol production by blockade of 11-$\beta$-hydroxylase, which decreases both serum cortisol and aldosterone levels. This side effect occurs both with continuous infusions of etomidate in the ICU setting and with a single-dose injection used for emergency RSI. The risks and benefits of the use of etomidate in patients with sepsis are discussed in detail in the "Evidence" section at the end of the chapter.

## KETAMINE

| **Ketamine (Ketalar)** | | | | |
|---|---|---|---|---|
| **Usual emergency induction dose (mg/kg)** | **Onset (s)** | **$t_{1/2}\alpha$ (min)** | **Duration (min)** | **$t_{1/2}\beta$ (h)** |
| 1.5 | 45–60 | 11–17 | 10–20 | 2–3 |

### Clinical Pharmacology

Ketamine is a phencyclidine derivative that provides significant analgesia, anesthesia, and amnesia, with minimal effect on respiratory drive. The amnestic effect is not as pronounced as that seen with the benzodiazepines. Ketamine is believed to interact with the NMDA receptors at the GABA–receptor complex, promoting neuroinhibition and subsequent anesthesia. Action on opioid receptors accounts for its analgesic effect. Ketamine stimulates the release of catecholamines, activating the sympathetic nervous system, and augmenting heart rate and blood pressure (BP) in those patients who are not catecholamine depleted secondary to the demands of their underlying disease. Furthermore, increases in mean arterial pressure (MAP) may offset any rise in ICP, resulting in a relatively stable CPP. In addition to its catecholamine-releasing effect, ketamine directly relaxes bronchial smooth muscle, producing bronchodilation. Ketamine is primarily metabolized in the liver, producing one active metabolite, norketamine, which is metabolized and excreted in the urine.

### Indications and Contraindications

Ketamine is the induction agent of choice for patients with reactive airway disease who require tracheal intubation, and is also an excellent induction agent for patients who are hypovolemic, hypotensive, or hemodynamically unstable, including those with sepsis. In normotensive or hypertensive patients with ischemic heart disease, catecholamine release may adversely increase myocardial oxygen demand, but it is unlikely that this effect is detrimental in patients with significant hypotension, in whom additional catecholamine release may support the BP. Ketamine's preservation of upper airway reflexes makes it appealing for awake laryngoscopy and intubation in the difficult airway patient where the dose is titrated to effect. Concern has been raised regarding ketamine's effect on ICP, especially in the head-injured patient. Although it has been linked to mild increases in ICP, ketamine also increases MAP and therefore CPP. Ketamine has been increasingly used in head-injured patients, and no study to date has identified an increase in mortality when used in the head-injured patient. The pregnancy category of ketamine has not been established by the FDA, and so it is currently not recommended for use in pregnant women.

### Dosage and Clinical Use

The induction dose of ketamine for RSI is 1.5 mg per kg IV. In patients who are catecholamine depleted, doses more than 1.5 mg per kg IV may cause myocardial depression and exacerbate hypotension. Because of its generalized stimulating effects, ketamine enhances laryngeal reflexes and can increase pharyngeal and bronchial secretions. These effects may uncommonly precipitate laryngospasm, and may interfere with upper airway examination during awake intubation, but are generally not an issue during RSI. Atropine 0.01 mg per kg IV or glycopyrrolate (Robinul) 0.005 mg per kg IV may be administered 15 minutes before ketamine to promote a drying effect for awake intubation, when feasible. Ketamine is available in three separate concentrations: 10, 50, and 100 mg per mL. Care should be taken to verify which concentration is utilized during RSI to avoid inadvertent over- or underdosing.

### Adverse Effects

Hallucinations may occur on emergence from ketamine and are more common in adults than in children. Such emergence reactions occur infrequently in the emergency department as most patients are subsequently sedated with either a benzodiazepine or propofol, after the airway has been secured.

## PROPOFOL

| Propofol (Diprivan) | | | | |
|---|---|---|---|---|
| **Usual emergency induction dose (mg/kg)** | **Onset (s)** | **$t_{1/2}\alpha$ (min)** | **Duration (min)** | **$t_{1/2}\beta$ (h)** |
| 1.5 | 15–45 | 1–3 | 5–10 | 1–3 |

## Clinical Pharmacology

Propofol is an alkylphenol derivative (i.e., an alcohol) with hypnotic properties. It is highly lipid soluble. Propofol enhances GABA activity at the GABA–receptor complex. It decreases $CMRO_2$ and ICP. Propofol does not cause histamine release, but it does cause a reduction in BP through vasodilation and direct myocardial depression. The ensuing hypotension and resultant decrease in CPP may be detrimental in a compromised patient. The manufacturer recommends that rapid bolus dosing (either single or repeated) be avoided in patients who are elderly, debilitated, or American Society of Anesthesiologists Class III or IV in order to minimize undesirable cardiovascular depression, including hypotension. It must be used cautiously for emergency RSI in hemodynamically unstable patients.

## Indications and Contraindications

Propofol is an excellent induction agent in a stable patient. Its adverse potential for hypotension and reduction in CPP limits its role as a primary induction agent in emergent RSI, but it has been used successfully as an induction agent for reactive airway disease. There are no absolute contraindications to its use. Propofol is delivered as an emulsion in soybean oil and lecithin; patients who are allergic to eggs generally react to the ovalbumin and not to lecithin, so propofol is not contraindicated in patients with egg allergy. Propofol is a pregnancy category B drug, and has become the induction agent of choice in pregnant patients.

## Dosage and Clinical Use

The induction dose of propofol is 1.5 mg per kg IV in a euvolemic, normotensive patient. Because of its predictable tendency to reduce mean arterial BP, doses are reduced by one-third to one-half when propofol is given as an induction agent for emergency RSI in compromised or elderly patients.

## Adverse Effects

Propofol causes pain on injection, which can be attenuated by injecting the medication through a rapidly running IV in a large vein (e.g., antecubital). Premedication of the vein with lidocaine (2 to 3 mL of 1% lidocaine) will also minimize the pain of injection. Propofol and lidocaine are compatible in the same syringe and can be mixed in a 10:1 ratio (10 mL of propofol to 1 mL of 1% lidocaine). Propofol can cause mild clonus, and venous thrombophlebitis at the injection site may occasionally occur.

# BENZODIAZEPINES

**Short-Acting Benzodiazepines**

| | Usual emergency induction dose (mg/kg) | Onset (s) | $t_{1/2}\alpha$(min) | Duration (min) | $t_{1/2}\beta$(h) |
|---|---|---|---|---|---|
| Midazolam (Versed) | 0.2–0.3 | 60–90 | 7–15 | 15–30 | 2–6 |

## Clinical Pharmacology

Benzodiazepines bind to a drug-specific receptor of the GABA complex and act to increase the frequency with which inhibitory chloride channels open. This results in CNS depression manifested by amnesia, anxiolysis, muscle relaxation, sedation, anticonvulsant effects, and hypnosis. Although the benzodiazepines generally have similar pharmacologic profiles, they differ in selectivity, which makes their clinical usefulness variable. The benzodiazepines have potent, dose-related amnestic properties, perhaps their greatest asset for emergency indications. The three benzodiazepines of interest for emergency applications are midazolam (Versed), diazepam (Valium), and lorazepam (Ativan). Of the three, midazolam is the most lipid soluble and is the only benzodiazepine suitable for use as an induction agent for emergent RSI. However, midazolam's time to clinical effectiveness is much longer than is the case for any of the other commonly used induction agents. When IV midazolam is given as an anesthetic induction agent, induction of anesthesia occurs in approximately 1.5 minutes when narcotic premedication has been used, and in 2 to 2.5 minutes without narcotic premedication. Its pharmacokinetic attributes make it a poor induction agent, and it cannot be recommended for this purpose. Midazolam has one significant active metabolite, 1-hydroxy-midazolam, which may contribute to the net pharmacologic activity of midazolam. Clearance of midazolam is reduced in association with old age, congestive heart failure, and liver disease. The elimination half-life of midazolam ($t_{1/2}\beta$) may be prolonged in renal impairment. The benzodiazepines do not release histamine, and allergic reactions are very rare.

## Indications and Contraindications

The primary indications for benzodiazepines are to promote amnesia and sedation. In this regard, the benzodiazepines are unparalleled. Midazolam's primary use in the emergency department and elsewhere in the hospital is for procedural sedation. Lorazepam is used primarily for treatment of seizures and alcohol withdrawal, and both agents are used for sedation and anxiolysis in a variety of settings, including postintubation.

Because of their dose-related reduction in systemic vascular resistance and direct myocardial depression, dosage must be adjusted in volume-depleted or hemodynamically compromised patients. Studies have shown that the correct induction dose of midazolam, 0.3 mg per kg, is rarely used. Even at this dose, midazolam is a poor induction agent for emergent RSI because of delay in onset of action and adverse hemodynamic effects and should only be chosen if other agents are not available. All benzodiazepines are FDA pregnancy category D.

## Dosage and Clinical Use

Although midazolam is occasionally used as an induction agent in the operating room, we do not recommend its use for emergent RSI. Even in the correct induction dose for hemodynamically stable patients of 0.3 mg per kg IV push, the onset is slow, and so the drug is not suited for emergency applications. Midazolam should be reserved for sedative applications, and its use in emergency RSI is not advised because superior agents are readily available.

## Adverse Effects

With the exception of midazolam, the benzodiazepines are insoluble in water and are usually in solution in propylene glycol. Unless injected into a large vein, pain and venous irritation on injection can be significant.

# EVIDENCE

- **Is etomidate safe to use in septic patients?** Etomidate remains popular because of its simple dosing, reliable onset of action, and cardiovascular stability.[1–3] There is significant concern, however, about etomidate's inhibition of cortisol production and the potential to harm patients in septic shock that are potentially reliant on endogenous cortisol.

  A single dose of etomidate causes self-limited inhibition of adrenal hormone synthesis by reversibly blocking 11-$\beta$-hydroxylase in the adrenal cortex. The inhibition lasts 12 to

24 hours, and may extend as long as 72 hours in some patients.[1,4] What remains unclear is whether there are any significant clinical sequelae from the transient inhibition of adrenal hormonal synthesis in the critically ill patient, a condition dubbed critical illness relative corticosteroid insufficiency (CIRCI).[5–7] CIRCI, however, is more complicated than a simple reduction in circulating cortisol levels, and likely stems from a dysfunction at the level of the hypothalamic pituitary axis.[2,8]

There remains much debate as to the potential risks of etomidate. The literature is significantly divided for patients with sepsis or sepsis-like syndromes. Much of the data have emerged from observational studies,[2,9–13] post hoc analyses,[14,15] retrospective review articles,[16–23] and meta-analyses of these reports.[24,25] None of the articles used to raise suspicion about etomidate were designed or powered to look at its effects, and the literature we currently have results in diametrically opposing opinions supporting or refuting etomidate. Very few patients have been enrolled in randomized controlled trials. No large, randomized, prospective study that has been adequately powered to detect a small difference in mortality or in hospital, ICU, or ventilator length of stay has yet been performed.[4,18,19,21,26,27]

It is clear that some degree of adrenal insufficiency occurs in many patients with critical illness, but etomidate's role in sepsis mortality is a subject of much debate. For the emergency physician who relies upon etomidate for reasons stated above, there are three main choices in the patient with presumptive sepsis:

- *Avoid etomidate use entirely in patients who are presumed to be septic.* Ketamine has emerged as a comparable agent in sepsis, and may offer some advantage as it provides some sympathetic "kick" that might actually improve BP in some patients. Only ketamine provides hemodynamic stability comparable with etomidate.[9,11,28,29] Some advocates of etomidate avoidance emerged early in the debate,[14,15] but as further data have emerged, the possible risk of etomidate use in septic patients appears to have been overstated and clinical equipoise remains.[1,2,4,11,19,26] The risk of using etomidate must be balanced against the risk of an alternative agent.
- *Routinely administer glucocorticoids to patients with septic shock who have received etomidate.* Studies of supplemental corticosteroids in patients with sepsis have had equivocal results.[30–33] Although it has been posited that glucocorticoids should be given immediately after the administration of etomidate when the adrenal suppression is likely to be greatest,[14] there is no evidence that this approach improves patient outcome,[9,31,32] including the current Cochrane recommendation demonstrating a statistically insignificant trend toward improvement in patients with CIRCI that receive steroids.[34]
- *Communicating clearly to critical care staff that the patient was given a dose of etomidate for induction.* It is almost impossible to argue against this common sense approach.

- **Which induction agents are the most hemodynamically stable when used for RSI?** Although virtually all induction agents *could be used* for RSI, not all are appropriate. We want to avoid both patient awareness and hemodynamic compromise. The ideal induction agent in RSI will have rapid and reliable onset and few adverse effects.

Etomidate results in the least variation in BP and heart rate when compared with the other agents used for rapid induction of anesthesia.[3,20,23] The drug is delivered to the CNS in a timely and dependable manner. It is for these reasons that etomidate remains a standard choice for RSI.[35]

Ketamine offers several advantages as an induction agent in hemodynamically compromised patients. Ketamine is a sympathomimetic agent, increasing heart rate, arterial pressure, and cardiac output in animal models. There is significant clinical experience, and mounting research evidence, for using ketamine for RSI.[28,29,35–37] In 2009, Jabre et al.[11] published the largest clinical trial to date involving ketamine 2 mg per kg for RSI in adults, and comparing it to etomidate 0.3 mg per kg, both with succinylcholine as the NMB agent. There were no significant hemodynamic differences between the two groups. The study concluded that ketamine is a safe alternative to etomidate for endotracheal intubation in critically ill patients, and should be considered in those with sepsis. This study has been followed by others supporting the same conclusion.[26,28,29,36–38]

Benzodiazepines are generally not suitable as induction agents in RSI. Midazolam is 95% protein bound. Both midazolam and lorazepam require closure of an imidazole ring to have enough lipid solubility to cross the blood–brain barrier, which takes as long as 10 minutes. The benzodiazepines are well known to produce dose-dependent hypotension and are suspect for use in the RSI scenario in a patient with hemodynamic compromise.[35]

Propofol is a very popular induction agent for elective procedures, when the induction dose is titrated against the patient response. It is a poor choice of induction agent for RSI in hemodynamically compromised patients, who run the risk of further hemodynamic deterioration coupled with awareness during intubation.[35]

Likewise, dexmedetomidine is popular as a sedative infusion in the critical care setting, but has a limited role for RSI because it is typically titrated to effect and administered as a slow drip and not by rapid IV push.[39] This concern makes it more difficult to use and counterproductive if the goal is rapid sedation to facilitate RSI. In the hemodynamically unstable patient, ketamine or etomidate offers the most reliable method of rapidly achieving unconsciousness while limiting further hemodynamic compromise.

- **What is the risk of ketamine in the brain-injured patient?** Ketamine has been noted to increase ICP through increased CBF and excitatory effects on neurons. Following brain injury, there is a loss of cerebral autoregulation, and CBF is largely dependent on CPP, which in turn is largely dependent on MAP. Consequently, agents such as etomidate and ketamine that maintain MAP will maintain CBF. This is particularly true in patients with polytrauma where traumatic brain injury and shock may coexist.[35,40] The dangers of hypotension on the injured brain are well known, and avoiding hypotension in traumatic brain injury is a priority.[40] In ventilated patients with controlled ventilation, ketamine does not appear to increase ICP in some studies,[41] whereas at least one study does show mild increases in ICP with tracheal suctioning during ketamine use.[42] In addition to the neuroprotective effects of maintaining CBF through CPP, ketamine has also been found to have other neuroprotective properties.[40,41] Ketamine inhibits the NMDA receptor activation, reduces neuronal apoptosis, and reduces the systemic inflammatory response to tissue injury.[41] In the last few years, increasing clinical evidence of the safety of ketamine in brain-injured patients has emerged, and it is becoming increasingly clear that ketamine is likely not dangerous in brain-injured patients.[40,43] If the brain-injured patient is also hypotensive, then ketamine is an excellent choice.[38]
- **Is ketofol an appropriate agent for RSI?** Ketofol, a 1:1 mixture of ketamine and propofol, has gained popularity as a combination agent for procedural sedation. Both medications can be mixed in a single syringe, with the same total volume of anesthetic administered that typically would be dosed for a single one of the agents. The practitioner therefore gives a half-dose of each of the medications, with the sum of both causing a similar level of sedation as either alone at full dose. Theoretically, this will allow the benefits of both (amnesia and sedation), while the cardiovascular side effects counteract each other—in particular the maintenance of a normal BP and maintenance of protective airway reflexes. Ketofol has not yet been studied in-depth in the population of patients who require RSI, so evidence-based recommendations cannot be authoritative.[44,45]
- **When should sedation be started following RSI?** Sedation and analgesia must be addressed almost immediately following the use of RSI. Sedation is particularly important if a long-acting neuromuscular blocker such as rocuronium has been used for RSI, or the patient is at risk for being awake and paralyzed.[46–49] Sedative infusions can be prepared simultaneously with the RSI medications. Propofol is widely used as a sedative agent for intubated patients, but does not offer any analgesic properties.

## REFERENCES

1. Hohl CM, Kelly-Smith CH, Yeung TC, et al. The effect of a bolus dose of etomidate on cortisol levels, mortality, and health services utilization: a systematic review. *Ann Emerg Med*. 2010;56(2):105.e5–113.e5.

2. Dmello D, Taylor S, O'Brien J, et al. Outcomes of etomidate in severe sepsis and septic shock. *Chest*. 2010;138(6):1327–1332.
3. Song J, Lu Z, Jiao Y, et al. Etomidate anesthesia during ERCP caused more stable haemodynamic responses compared with propofol: a randomized clinical trial. *Int J Med Sci*. 2015;12(7):559–565.
4. Gu W, Wang F, Tang L, et al. Single-dose etomidate does not increase mortality in patients with sepsis: a systematic review and meta-analysis of randomized controlled trials and observational studies. *Chest*. 2015;147(2):335–346.
5. Bhatia R, Muraskas J, Janusek LW, et al. Measurement of the glucocorticoid receptor: relevance to the diagnosis of critical illness-related corticosteroid insufficiency in children. *J Crit Care*. 2014;29(4):691.e1–695.e5.
6. de Jong MFC, Molenaar N, Beishuizen A, et al. Diminished adrenal sensitivity to endogenous and exogenous adrenocorticotropic hormone in critical illness: a prospective cohort study. *Crit Care*. 2015;19:1.
7. Lim SY, Kwon YS, Park MR, et al. Prognostic significance of different subgroup classifications of critical illness-related corticosteroid insufficiency in patients with septic shock. *Shock*. 2011;36(4):345–349.
8. Gibbison B, Angelini GD, Lightman SL. Dynamic output and control of the hypothalamic-pituitary-adrenal axis in critical illness and major surgery. *Br J Anaesth*. 2013;111(3):347–360.
9. Ray DC, McKeown DW. Effect of induction agent on vasopressor and steroid use, and outcome in patients with septic shock. *Crit Care*. 2007;11(3):R56.
10. Baird CRW, Hay AW, McKeown DW, et al. Rapid sequence induction in the emergency department: induction drug and outcome of patients admitted to the intensive care unit. *Emerg Med J*. 2009;26(8):576–579.
11. Jabre P, Combes X, Lapostolle F, et al. Etomidate versus ketamine for rapid sequence intubation in acutely ill patients: a multicentre randomised controlled trial. *Lancet*. 2009;374(9686):293–300.
12. Archambault P, Dionne CE, Lortie G, et al. Adrenal inhibition following a single dose of etomidate in intubated traumatic brain injury victims. *CJEM*. 2012;14(5):270–282.
13. Cherfan AJ, Tamim HM, AlJumah A, et al. Etomidate and mortality in cirrhotic patients with septic shock. *BMC Clin Pharmacol*. 2011;11:22.
14. Annane D. ICU physicians should abandon the use of etomidate! *Intensive Care Med*. 2005;31(3):325–326.
15. Cuthbertson BH, Sprung CL, Annane D, et al. The effects of etomidate on adrenal responsiveness and mortality in patients with septic shock. *Intensive Care Med*. 2009;35(11):1868–1876.
16. Edwin SB, Walker PL. Controversies surrounding the use of etomidate for rapid sequence intubation in patients with suspected sepsis. *Ann Pharmacother*. 2010;44(7–8):1307–1313.
17. Kulstad EB, Kalimullah EA, Tekwani KL, et al. Etomidate as an induction agent in septic patients: red flags or false alarms? *West J Emerg Med*. 2010;11(2):161–172.
18. Hinkewich C, Green R. The impact of etomidate on mortality in trauma patients. *Can J Anaesth*. 2014;61(7):650–655.
19. Alday NJ, Jones GM, Kimmons LA, et al. Effects of etomidate on vasopressor use in patients with sepsis or severe sepsis: a propensity-matched analysis. *J Crit Care*. 2014;29(4):517–522.
20. Komatsu R, You J, Mascha EJ, et al. Anesthetic induction with etomidate, rather than propofol, is associated with increased 30-day mortality and cardiovascular morbidity after noncardiac surgery. *Anesth Analg*. 2013;117(6):1329–1337.
21. McPhee LC, Badawi O, Fraser GL, et al. Single-dose etomidate is not associated with increased mortality in ICU patients with sepsis: analysis of a large electronic ICU database. *Crit Care Med*. 2013;41(3):774–783.
22. Ehrman R, Wira C, Lomax A, et al. Etomidate use in severe sepsis and septic shock patients does not contribute to mortality. *Intern Emerg Med*. 2011;6(3):253–257.
23. Banh KV, James S, Hendey GW, et al. Single-dose etomidate for intubation in the trauma patient. *J Emerg Med*. 2012;43(5):e277–e282.

24. Gu H, Zhang M, Cai M, et al. Combined use of etomidate and dexmedetomidine produces an additive effect in inhibiting the secretion of human adrenocortical hormones. *Med Sci Monit*. 2015;21:3528–3535.
25. Chan CM, Mitchell AL, Shorr AF. Etomidate is associated with mortality and adrenal insufficiency in sepsis: a meta-analysis*. *Crit Care Med*. 2012;40(11):2945–2953.
26. Freund Y, Jabre P, Mourad J, et al. Relative adrenal insufficiency in critically ill patient after rapid sequence intubation: KETASED ancillary study. *J Crit Care*. 2014;29(3):386–389.
27. Morel J, Salard M, Castelain C, et al. Haemodynamic consequences of etomidate administration in elective cardiac surgery: a randomized double-blinded study. *Br J Anaesth*. 2011;107(4):503–509.
28. Patanwala AE, McKinney CB, Erstad BL, et al. Retrospective analysis of etomidate versus ketamine for first-pass intubation success in an academic emergency department. *Acad Emerg Med*. 2014;21(1):87–91.
29. Kim JY, Lee JS, Park HY, et al. The effect of alfentanil versus ketamine on the intubation condition and hemodynamics with low-dose rocuronium in children. *J Anesth*. 2013;27(1):7–11.
30. Sprung CL, Annane D, Keh D, et al; CORTICUS Study Group. Hydrocortisone therapy for patients with septic shock. *N Engl J Med*. 2008;358(2):111–124.
31. Jung B, Clavieras N, Nougaret S, et al. Effects of etomidate on complications related to intubation and on mortality in septic shock patients treated with hydrocortisone: a propensity score analysis. *Crit Care*. 2012;16(6):R224.
32. Payen J, Dupuis C, Trouve-Buisson T, et al. Corticosteroid after etomidate in critically ill patients: a randomized controlled trial. *Crit Care Med*. 2012;40(1):29–35.
33. Annane D, Sébille V, Charpentier C, et al. Effect of treatment with low doses of hydrocortisone and fludrocortisone on mortality in patients with septic shock. *JAMA*. 2002;288(7):862–871.
34. Annane D, Bellissant E, Bollaert PE, et al. Corticosteroids for treating sepsis. *Cochrane Database Syst Rev*. 2015;12:CD002243.
35. Morris C, Perris A, Klein J, et al. Anaesthesia in haemodynamically compromised emergency patients: does ketamine represent the best choice of induction agent? *Anaesthesia*. 2009;64(5):532–539.
36. Price B, Arthur AO, Brunko M, et al. Hemodynamic consequences of ketamine vs etomidate for endotracheal intubation in the air medical setting. *Am J Emerg Med*. 2013;31(7):1124–1132.
37. Sibley A, Mackenzie M, Bawden J, et al. A prospective review of the use of ketamine to facilitate endotracheal intubation in the helicopter emergency medical services (HEMS) setting. *Emerg Med J*. 2011;28(6):521–525.
38. Hughes S. Towards evidence based emergency medicine: best BETs from the manchester royal infirmary. BET 3: is ketamine a viable induction agent for the trauma patient with potential brain injury. *Emerg Med J*. 2011;28(12):1076–1077.
39. Calver L, Isbister GK. Dexmedetomidine in the emergency department: assessing safety and effectiveness in difficult-to-sedate acute behavioural disturbance. *Emerg Med J*. 2012;29(11):915–918.
40. Chang LC, Raty SR, Ortiz J, et al. The emerging use of ketamine for anesthesia and sedation in traumatic brain injuries. *CNS Neurosci Ther*. 2013;19(6):390–395.
41. Hudetz JA, Pagel PS. Neuroprotection by ketamine: a review of the experimental and clinical evidence. *J Cardiothorac Vasc Anesth*. 2010;24(1):131–142.
42. Caricato A, Tersali A, Pitoni S, et al. Racemic ketamine in adult head injury patients: use in endotracheal suctioning. *Critical Care*. 2013;17(6):R267.
43. Ballow SL, Kaups KL, Anderson S, et al. A standardized rapid sequence intubation protocol facilitates airway management in critically injured patients. *J Trauma Acute Care Surg*. 2012;73(6):1401–1405.
44. Erdogan MA, Begec Z, Aydogan MS, et al. Comparison of effects of propofol and ketamine-propofol mixture (ketofol) on laryngeal mask airway insertion conditions and hemodynamics in elderly patients: a randomized, prospective, double-blind trial. *J Anesth*. 2013;27(1):12–17.

45. Smischney NJ, Hoskote SS, Gallo de Moraes A, et al. Ketamine/propofol admixture (ketofol) at induction in the critically ill against etomidate (KEEP PACE trial): study protocol for a randomized controlled trial. *Trials*. 2015;16:177.

46. Watt JM, Amini A, Traylor BR, et al. Effect of paralytic type on time to post-intubation sedative use in the emergency department. *Emerg Med J*. 2013;30(11):893–895.

47. Johnson EG, Meier A, Shirakbari A, et al. Impact of rocuronium and succinylcholine on sedation initiation after rapid sequence intubation. *J Emerg Med*. 2015;49(1):43–49.

48. Korinek JD, Thomas RM, Goddard LA, et al. Comparison of rocuronium and succinylcholine on postintubation sedative and analgesic dosing in the emergency department. *Eur J Emerg Med*. 2014;21(3):206–211.

49. Kendrick DB, Monroe KW, Bernard DW, et al. Sedation after intubation using etomidate and a long-acting neuromuscular blocker. *Pediatr Emerg Care*. 2009;25(6):393–396.

# Chapter 22

# Neuromuscular Blocking Agents

David A. Caro and Erik G. Laurin

## INTRODUCTION

Neuromuscular blockade is the cornerstone of rapid sequence intubation (RSI), optimizing conditions for tracheal intubation while minimizing the risks of aspiration or other adverse physiologic events. Neuromuscular blocking agents (NMBAs) do not provide analgesia, sedation, or amnesia. As a result, they are paired with a sedative induction agent for RSI. Similarly, appropriate sedation is essential when maintaining neuromuscular blockade postintubation.

Cholinergic nicotinic receptors on the postjunctional membrane of the motor endplate play the primary role in stimulating muscular contraction. Under normal circumstances, the presynaptic neuron synthesizes acetylcholine (ACH) and stores it in small packages (vesicles). Nerve stimulation results in these vesicles migrating to the prejunctional nerve surface, rupturing and discharging ACH into the cleft of the motor endplate. The ACH attaches to the nicotinic receptors, promoting depolarization that culminates in a muscle cell action potential and muscular contraction. As the ACH diffuses away from the receptor, the majority of the neurotransmitter is hydrolyzed by acetylcholinesterase (ACHE). The remainder undergoes reuptake by the prejunctional neuron.

NMBAs are either agonists ("depolarizers" of the motor endplate) or antagonists (competitive agents, also known as "nondepolarizers"). Agonists work by persistent depolarization of the endplate, exhausting the ability of the receptor to respond. Antagonists, on the other hand, attach to the receptors and competitively block access of ACH to the receptor while attached. Because they are in competition with ACH for the motor endplate, antagonists can be displaced from the endplate by increasing concentrations of ACH, the end result of reversal agents (cholinesterase inhibitors such as neostigmine, edrophonium, and pyridostigmine) that inhibit ACHE and allow ACH to accumulate and reverse the block. The ideal muscle relaxant to facilitate RSI would have a rapid onset of action, rendering the patient paralyzed within seconds; a short duration of action, returning the patient's normal protective reflexes within 3 to 4 minutes; no significant adverse side effects; and metabolism and excretion independent of liver and kidney function.

## SUCCINYLCHOLINE

**Depolarizing (Noncompetitive) NMBA: Succinylcholine**

| Intubating Dose (mg/kg) | Onset (s) | $t_{1/2}\alpha$ (min) | Duration (min) | $t_{1/2}\beta$ (h) | Pregnancy Category |
|---|---|---|---|---|---|
| 1.5 | 45 | <1 | 6–10 | 2–5 | C |

Succinylcholine (SCh) comes closest to meeting the desirable goals listed earlier. Rocuronium's popularity is increasing possibly as a result of the adverse effects of SCh and, in pediatric patients, the specter of hyperkalemia from administering SCh to a child with an undiagnosed degenerative neuromuscular disorder. Recent registry data suggest SCh is still the most common NMBA for emergency RSI, although rocuronium use is becoming much more common. Recent Food and Drug Administration approval of sugammadex, a rocuronium reversal agent, may position rocuronium as the primary NMBA in the near future.

## Clinical Pharmacology

SCh is comprised of two molecules of ACH linked by an ester bridge and, as such, is chemically similar to ACH. It stimulates all nicotinic and muscarinic cholinergic receptors of the sympathetic and parasympathetic nervous system to varying degrees, not just those at the neuromuscular junction. For example, stimulation of cardiac muscarinic receptors can cause bradycardia, especially when repeated doses are given to small children. Although SCh can be a negative inotrope, this effect is so minimal as to have no clinical relevance. SCh causes the release of trace amounts of histamine, but this effect is also not clinically significant. Initially, SCh depolarization manifests as fasciculations, but this is followed rapidly by complete motor paralysis. The onset, activity, and duration of action of SCh are independent of the activity of ACHE and instead depend on rapid hydrolysis by pseudocholinesterase (PCHE), an enzyme of the liver and plasma that is not present at the neuromuscular junction. Therefore, diffusion away from the neuromuscular junction motor endplate and back into the vascular compartment is ultimately responsible for SCh metabolism. This extremely important pharmacologic concept explains why only a fraction of the initial intravenous (IV) dose of SCh ever reaches the motor endplate to promote paralysis. As a result, larger, rather than smaller, doses of SCh are used for emergency RSI. Incomplete paralysis may jeopardize the patient by compromising respiration while failing to provide adequate relaxation to facilitate tracheal intubation.

Succinylmonocholine, the initial metabolite of SCh, sensitizes the cardiac muscarinic receptors in the sinus node to repeat does of SCh, which may cause bradycardia that is responsive to atropine. At room temperature, SCh retains 90% of its activity for up to 3 months. Refrigeration mitigates this degradation. Therefore, if SCh is stored at room temperature, it should be dated and stock should be rotated regularly.

## Indications and Contraindications

SCh is the most commonly used NMBA for emergency RSI because of its rapid onset and relatively brief duration of action. A personal or family history of malignant hyperthermia (MH) is an absolute contraindication to the use of SCh. Inherited disorders that lead to abnormal or insufficient cholinesterases prolong the duration of the block and contraindicate SCh use in elective anesthesia, but are not ordinarily an issue in emergency airway management. Certain conditions, described in the "Adverse Effects" section, place patients at risk for SCh-related hyperkalemia and represent absolute contraindications to SCh. These patients should be intubated using rocuronium. Relative contraindications to the use of SCh are dependent on the skill and proficiency of the intubator and the individual patient's clinical circumstance. The role of difficult airway assessment in the decision regarding whether a patient should undergo RSI is discussed in Chapter 2.

## Dosage and Clinical Use

In the normal size adult patient, the recommended dose of SCh for emergency RSI is 1.5 mg per kg IV. During crash intubations when both residual muscular tone and impaired circulation may be present, we recommend increasing the dose to 2.0 mg per kg IV to compensate for reduced IV drug delivery. In a rare, life-threatening circumstance when SCh must be given intramuscularly (IM) because of inability to secure venous access, a dose of 4 mg per kg IM may be used. Absorption and delivery of drug will be dependent on the patient's circulatory status. IM administration may result in a prolonged period of vulnerability for the patient, during which respirations will be compromised, but relaxation is not sufficient to permit intubation. Active bag-mask ventilation will usually be required before laryngoscopy in this circumstance.

SCh is dosed on a total body weight basis. In the emergency department, it may be impossible to know the exact weight of a patient, and weight estimates, especially of supine patients, have been shown to be notoriously inaccurate. In those uncertain circumstances, it is better to err on the side of a higher dose of SCh to ensure adequate patient paralysis. The serum half-life of SCh is less than 1 minute, so doubling the dose increases the duration of block by only 60 seconds. SCh is safe up to a cumulative dose of 6 mg per kg. At doses >6 mg per kg, the typical phase 1 depolarization block of SCh becomes a phase 2 block, which changes the pharmacokinetic displacement of SCh from the motor endplate. Although the electrophysiologic features of a phase 2 block resemble that of a nondepolarizing or competitive block (train-of-four fade and post-tetanic potentiation), the block remains nonreversible. This prolongs the duration of paralysis but is otherwise clinically irrelevant. The risk of an inadequately paralyzed patient who is difficult to intubate because of an inadequate dose of SCh greatly outweighs the minimal potential for adverse effects from excessive dosing.

In children younger than 10 years, length-based dosing is recommended, but if weight is used as the determinant, the recommended dose of SCh for emergency RSI is 2 mg per kg IV, and in the newborn (younger than 12 months), the appropriate dose is 3 mg per kg IV. Some practitioners routinely administer atropine to children younger than 12 months who are receiving SCh, but there is no high-quality evidence to support this practice. There is similarly no evidence that it is harmful. When adults or children of any age receive a second dose of SCh, bradycardia may occur, and atropine should be readily available.

## Adverse Effects

The recognized side effects of SCh include fasciculations, hyperkalemia, bradycardia, prolonged neuromuscular blockade, MH, and trismus/masseter muscle spasm. Each is discussed separately.

### *Fasciculations*

Fasciculations are believed to be produced by stimulation of the nicotinic ACH receptors. Fasciculations occur simultaneously with increases in intracranial pressure (ICP), intraocular pressure, and intragastric pressure, but these are not the result of concerted muscle activity. Of these, only the increase in ICP is potentially clinically important.

The exact mechanisms by which these effects occur are not well elucidated. In the past, it was recommended that nondepolarizing agents be given in advance of SCh to mitigate ICP elevation, but there is insufficient evidence to support this practice.

The relationship between muscle fasciculation and subsequent postoperative muscle pain is controversial. Studies have been variable with respect to prevention of fasciculations and subsequent muscle pain. Although there exists a theoretical concern regarding the extrusion of vitreous in patients with open globe injuries who are given SCh, there are no published reports of this potential complication. Anesthesiologists continue to use SCh as a muscle relaxant in cases of open globe injury, with or without an accompanying defasciculating agent. Similarly, the increase in intragastric pressure that has been measured has never been shown to be of any clinical significance, perhaps because it is offset by a corresponding increase in the lower esophageal sphincter pressure.

### *Hyperkalemia*

Under normal circumstances, serum potassium increases minimally (0 to 0.5 mEq per L) when SCh is administered. In certain pathologic conditions, however, a rapid and dramatic increase in serum potassium can occur in response to SCh. These pathologic hyperkalemic responses occur by two distinct mechanisms: receptor upregulation and rhabdomyolysis. In either situation, potassium increase may approach 5 to 10 mEq per L within a few minutes and result in hyperkalemic dysrhythmias or cardiac arrest.

Two forms of postjunctional receptors exist: mature (junctional) and immature (extrajunctional). Each receptor is composed of five proteins arranged in a circular fashion around a common channel. Both types of receptors contain two $\alpha$-subunits. ACH must attach to both $\alpha$-subunits to open the channel and effect depolarization and muscle contraction. When receptor upregulation occurs, the mature receptors at and around the motor endplate are gradually converted over a 3- to 5-day period to immature receptors that propagate throughout the entire muscle membrane. Immature receptors are characterized by low conductance and prolonged channel opening times (four times longer than mature receptors), resulting in increasing release of potassium. Most of the entities associated with hyperkalemia during emergency use of SCh are the result of receptor upregulation. Interestingly, these same extrajunctional nicotinic receptors are relatively refractory to nondepolarizing agents, so larger doses of vecuronium, pancuronium, or rocuronium may be required to produce paralysis. This is not an issue in emergency RSI, where full intubating doses several times greater than the ED95 for paralysis are used.

Hyperkalemia may also occur with rhabdomyolysis, most often that associated with myopathies, especially inherited forms of muscular dystrophy. When severe hyperkalemia occurs related to rhabdomyolysis, the mortality approaches 30%, almost three times higher than that in cases of receptor upregulation. This mortality increase may be related to coexisting cardiomyopathy. SCh is a toxin to unstable membranes in any patient with a myopathy and should be avoided.

Patients with the following conditions are at risk of SCh-induced hyperkalemia:

**A.** Receptor Upregulation

- **a. Burns**—In burn victims, the extrajunctional receptor sensitization becomes clinically significant 3 to 5 days postburn. It lasts an indefinite period of time, at least until there is complete healing of the burned area. If the burn becomes infected or healing is delayed, the patient remains at risk for hyperkalemia. It is prudent to avoid SCh in burned patients beyond this window if any question exists regarding the status of their burn. The percent of body surface area burned does not correlate well with the magnitude of hyperkalemia. Significant hyperkalemia has been reported in patients with as little as 8% total body surface area burn (less than the surface of one arm), but this is rare. The majority of emergent intubations for burn patients are performed well within the safe 3- to 5-day window period. Should a later intubation become necessary, however, rocuronium or vecuronium provides excellent alternatives.
- **b. Denervation**—The patient who suffers a denervation event, such as spinal cord injury or stroke, is at risk for hyperkalemia from approximately the third day postevent, until 6 months postevent. Patients with progressive neuromuscular disorders, such as multiple sclerosis or amyotrophic lateral sclerosis, are perpetually at risk for hyperkalemia. Likewise, patients with transient neuromuscular disorders, such as Guillain-Barré syndrome or wound botulism, can develop hyperkalemia after day 3, depending on the severity of their disease. As long as the neuromuscular disease is dynamic, there will be augmentation of the extrajunctional receptors, which increases the risk for hyperkalemia. These specific clinical situations should be considered absolute contraindications to SCh during the designated time periods.
- **c. Crush injuries**—The data regarding crush injuries are scant. The hyperkalemic response begins about 3 days postinjury, similar to denervation, and persists for several months after healing seems complete. The mechanism appears to be receptor upregulation.
- **d. Severe infections**—This entity seems to relate to established, serious infections, usually in the ICU environment, and relative patient immobility that accompanies these conditions. The mechanism is receptor upregulation, but the initiating event is not established. Total body muscular disuse atrophy and chemical denervation of the ACH receptors, particularly related to long-term infusions of NMBAs, appear to drive the pathologic receptor changes. Again, the at-risk time period begins as early as 3 days after initiation of the infection and continues indefinitely as long as the disease process is dynamic. Any serious, prolonged, debilitating infection should prompt concern.

**B.** Myopathy

SCh is absolutely contraindicated in patients with inherited myopathies, such as muscular dystrophy. Myopathic hyperkalemia can be devastating because of the combined effects of receptor upregulation and rhabdomyolysis. This is a particularly difficult problem in pediatrics, when a child with occult muscular dystrophy receives SCh. SCh has a black box warning advising against its use in elective pediatric anesthesia, but it continues to be the muscle relaxant of choice for emergency intubation. Any patient suspected of a myopathy should be intubated with nondepolarizing muscle relaxants rather than SCh.

C. Preexisting Hyperkalemia

Hyperkalemia, per se, is not an absolute contraindication to SCh. There is little evidence that the normal SCh-induced potassium rise of 0 to 0.5 mEq per L is harmful in patients with preexisting hyperkalemia, but who are not otherwise at risk of severe SCh-induced hyperkalemia by one of the mechanisms described in the preceding section. In fact, there is only one published report that documents this phenomenon. Despite this lack of significant evidence, there is widespread concern that patients with hyperkalemia secondary to acute kidney injury or acidotic conditions like diabetic ketoacidosis are likely to exhibit cardiac dysrhythmias from SCh administration. The largest study that examined the use of SCh in patients with chronic renal failure (including documented hyperkalemia before intubation) failed to identify any adverse effects related to SCh. Therefore, a reasonable approach is to assume that SCh is safe to use in patients with preexisting hyperkalemia or renal failure unless the ECG (either monitor tracing or 12-lead ECG) shows evidence of myocardial instability from hyperkalemia (increased PR interval or prolongation of the QRS complex).

### Bradycardia

In both adults and children, repeated doses of SCh may produce bradycardia, and administration of atropine may become necessary.

### Prolonged Neuromuscular Blockade

Prolonged neuromuscular blockade may result from an acquired PCHE deficiency, a congenital absence of PCHE, or the presence of an atypical form of PCHE, any of the three of which will delay the degradation of SCh and prolong paralysis. Acquired PCHE deficiency may be a result of liver disease, chronic cocaine abuse, pregnancy, burns, oral contraceptives, metoclopramide, bambuterol, or esmolol. A 20% reduction in normal levels will increase apnea time about 3 to 9 minutes. The most severe variant (0.04% of population) will result in prolonged paralysis for 4 to 8 hours.

### Malignant Hyperthermia

A personal or family history of MH is an absolute contraindication to the use of SCh. MH is a myopathy characterized by a genetic skeletal muscle membrane abnormality of the Ry (ryanodine) receptor. It can be triggered by halogenated anesthetics, SCh, vigorous exercise, or emotional stress. Following the initiating event, its onset can be acute and progressive or delayed for hours. Generalized awareness of MH, earlier diagnosis, and the availability of dantrolene (Dantrium) have decreased the mortality from as high as 70% to less than 5%. Acute loss of intracellular calcium control results in a cascade of rapidly progressive events manifested primarily by increased metabolism, muscular rigidity, autonomic instability, hypoxia, hypotension, severe lactic acidosis, hyperkalemia, myoglobinemia, and disseminated intravascular coagulation. Temperature elevation is a late manifestation. The presence of more than one of these clinical signs is suggestive of MH.

Masseter spasm, once claimed to be the hallmark of MH, is not pathognomonic. SCh can promote isolated masseter spasm as an exaggerated response at the neuromuscular junction, especially in children.

The treatment for MH consists of discontinuing the known or suspected precipitant and the immediate administration of dantrolene sodium (Dantrium). Dantrolene is essential to successful resuscitation and must be given as soon as the diagnosis is seriously entertained. Dantrolene is a hydantoin derivative that acts directly on skeletal muscle to prevent calcium release from the sarcoplasmic reticulum without affecting calcium reuptake. The initial dose is 2.5 mg per kg IV, repeated every 5 minutes until muscle relaxation occurs or the maximum dose of 10 mg per kg is administered. Dantrolene is free of any serious side effects. In addition, measures to control body temperature, acid–base balance, and renal function must be used. All cases of MH require frequent monitoring of pH, arterial blood gases, and serum potassium. Immediate and aggressive management of hyperkalemia with the administration of calcium gluconate, glucose, insulin, and sodium bicarbonate may be necessary. Interestingly, full paralysis with nondepolarizing NMBAs will prevent SCh-triggered MH. MH has never been reported related to the use of SCh in the emergency department. The MH emergency hotline number is 1–800-MH-HYPER 1-800-644-9737 (United States and Canada) 24 hours a day, 7 days a week. Ask for "index zero." The e-mail address for the Malignant Hyperthermia Association of the United States (MHAUS) is mhaus@norwich.net, and the Website is www.mhaus.org.

### *Trismus/Masseter Muscle Spasm*

On occasion, SCh may cause transient trismus/masseter muscle spasm, especially in children. This manifests as jaw muscle rigidity associated with limb muscle flaccidity. Pretreatment with defasciculating doses of nondepolarizing NMBAs will not prevent masseter spasm. If masseter spasm interferes with intubation, an intubating dose of a competitive nondepolarizing agent (e.g., rocuronium 1 mg per kg) should be administered and will relax the involved muscles. The patient may require bag-mask ventilation until relaxation is complete and intubation is possible. Masseter spasm should prompt serious consideration of the diagnosis of MH (see previous discussion).

## COMPETITIVE NEUROMUSCULAR BLOCKING AGENTS

**Nondepolarizing (Competitive) NMBAs**

| | Intubating Dose (mg/kg) | Time to Intubation Level Paralysis (s) | Duration (min) | Pregnancy Category |
|---|---|---|---|---|
| Rocuronium | 1.0–1.2 | 60 | 40–60 | B |
| Vecuronium | 0.01 to prime, then 0.15 | 75–90 | 60–75 | C |

### Clinical Pharmacology

The nondepolarizing, or competitive, NMBAs compete with and block the action of ACH at the motor endplate's postjunctional, cholinergic nicotinic receptors. The blockade is accomplished by competitively binding to one or both of the $\alpha$-subunits in the receptor, preventing ACH access to both $\alpha$-subunits, which is required for muscle depolarization. This competitive blockade is characterized by the absence of fasciculations. It can be reversed by ACHE inhibitors that normally prevent the metabolism of ACH. ACHE inhibitors cause ACH reaccumulation at the motor endplate, which competes with the competitive NMBA and promotes muscular contraction.

For the most part, nondepolarizing NMBAs are eliminated by Hofmann degradation (atracurium and cisatracurium) or excreted unchanged in bile (vecuronium and rocuronium), although there is limited liver metabolism and renal excretion of both vecuronium and rocuronium. They are divided into two groups: the benzylisoquinoline compounds (e.g., D-tubocurarine, atracurium, and mivacurium) and the aminosteroid compounds (e.g., rocuronium and vecuronium). Of the two groups, the aminosteroid compounds are the only agents commonly used for emergency RSI and postintubation paralysis.

In general, the aminosteroid compounds do not release histamine and do not cause ganglionic blockade. They vary inversely regarding their potency and time to onset (more potent agents require longer time to onset), and they exhibit differences in their vagolytic effects (i.e., moderate in pancuronium, slight in rocuronium, and absent in vecuronium).

These compounds are further subdivided based on their duration of action, which is determined by their metabolism and excretion. None has the brief duration of action of SCh.

Pancuronium is longer lasting than vecuronium or rocuronium and is therefore a distant third choice for RSI. Although pancuronium is excreted primarily by the kidney, 10% to 20% is metabolized in the liver. Vecuronium is more lipophilic, hence more easily absorbed. It is eliminated primarily in bile and is very stable from a cardiovascular standpoint. Rocuronium is lipophilic and excreted in bile. We recommend rocuronium for emergency RSI, because its onset time and duration of action are the shortest of all nondepolarizing NMBAs.

The nondepolarizing NMBAs can be reversed by administering ACHE inhibitors such as neostigmine (Prostigmin) 0.06 to 0.08 mg per kg IV after significant (40%) spontaneous recovery has occurred. Atropine 0.01 mg per kg IV or glycopyrrolate (Robinul) 0.01 to 0.005 mg per kg IV can be given routinely to block excessive muscarinic stimulation (SLUDGE syndrome—Salivation, Lacrimation, Urination, Diarrhea, Gastrointestinal Upset, Emesis). Reversal of blockade is virtually never indicated following emergency airway management.

A new selective rocuronium reversal agent, sugammadex, is now approved for use in the United States. Its hollow, cone-shaped polysaccharide molecular structure encapsulates rocuronium, thereby reversing the neuromuscular block without the muscarinic side effects of the ACHE inhibitors. Spontaneous breathing is restored in approximately 1 minute, compared to more than 5 minutes with the ACHE inhibitors. In addition, sugammadex is rapidly effective, regardless of the extent of the neuromuscular block, and it is not necessary for any spontaneous recovery to occur before reversal is initiated. See "Evidence" section for details.

## Indications and Contraindications

The nondepolarizing NMBAs serve a multipurpose role in emergency airway management. Rocuronium is the preferred nondepolarizing NMBA for emergency RSI. If rocuronium is not available, then vecuronium is an alternative, although the longer onset time may be problematic. Any of the nondepolarizing agents are appropriate for maintenance of paralysis after intubation, when this is desired. The only contraindication to a nondepolarizing NMBA is known prior anaphylaxis to that agent. Patients with myasthenia gravis are sensitive to NMBAs and may experience greater, or more prolonged, paralysis at any given dose.

## Dosage and Clinical Use

Rocuronium, 1.0 to 1.2 mg per kg IV, is the most commonly used nondepolarizing NMBA for RSI. It produces intubation-level paralysis consistently within 60 seconds, especially when an adequate dose of induction (sedative) agent is used, because the induction agent also causes substantial relaxation. If rocuronium is not available, vecuronium can be given using a priming regimen. A priming dose of 0.01 mg per kg is given, followed 3 minutes later by an intubating dose of 0.15 mg per kg. Pancuronium is not recommended for emergency RSI because of its long onset time.

For postintubation management when continued neuromuscular blockade is desired, vecuronium 0.1 mg per kg IV or pancuronium 0.1 mg per kg IV is appropriate, in concert with adequate sedation (see Chapters 20 and 30). **Table 22-1** lists the onset and duration of action for routine paralyzing doses of all commonly used NMBAs. The onset times and durations are for the specific doses listed, which are lower than the doses used for intubation.

## Adverse Effects

Of the three aminosteroid compounds, pancuronium is the least expensive, but may be less desirable because it tends to produce tachycardia. The nondepolarizing NMBAs are generally less desirable for intubation than SCh because of delayed time to paralysis, prolonged duration of action, or both. Their onset can be shortened by administering the larger intubating dose (as opposed to the ED95 dose [**Table 22-1**] used for surgical paralysis), but this further prolongs the duration of action. Availability of the rapidly effective reversal agent sugammadex may greatly expand the role of nondepolarizing NMBAs in emergency RSI.

TABLE 22-1

**Onset and Duration of Action of Neuromuscular Blocking Drugs**

| Drug | Dose (mg/kg) | Time to Maximal Blockade (min) | Time to Recovery (min) 25% | 75% |
|---|---|---|---|---|
| **Quaternary amine** | | | | |
| SCh | 1.0 | 1.1 | 8 | 11 (90%) |
| **Aminosteroid compounds** | | | | |
| Pancuronium | 0.1 | 2.9 | 86 | — |
| Vecuronium | 0.1 | 2.4 | 44 | 56 |
| Rocuronium | 0.6 | 1.0 | 43 | 66 |

From Hunter JM. Drug therapy: new neuromuscular blocking drugs. *N Engl J Med.* 1995;332:1691–1699, with permission.

## EVIDENCE

- **What is the advantage to RSI with an NMBA versus intubation with deep sedation alone?** RSI with an NMBA is the current standard of care for emergency intubation. Multiple prospective studies and ED registry data confirm the high success rate of RSI with NMBAs when performed by experienced operators in both adult and pediatric emergency patients.[1–3]
- **Are any of the nondepolarizing NMBAs as good as SCh for emergency RSI?** Multiple studies have compared SCh with rocuronium and vecuronium for intubation. All have concluded that the two drugs are similar but not identical. Recent reviews comparing SCh and rocuronium for emergency department RSI by emergency physicians demonstrate no significant difference between intubation success with either agent.[4–9] The dose of rocuronium is critical to the success of RSI. The correct dose of rocuronium for RSI is 1.0 to 1.2 mg per kg, not 0.6 mg per kg as is commonly recommended. A 2015 Cochrane review concluded that 1.2 mg per kg gives equivalent intubating conditions as SCh, but the duration of action is longer than 1.0 mg per kg, and far longer than that of SCh.[7] The duration for the 1.0 mg per kg dose is 46 minutes.
- **What is the correct dose of SCh for RSI?** Intubating conditions are directly related to the dose of SCh used, with excellent intubating conditions in more than 80% of patients receiving 1.5 mg per kg or more of SCh.[10] Increasing the dose of SCh from 1.5 to 2 mg per kg increases the duration of action only from 5.2 to 7.5 minutes, reinforcing the notion that the half-life of SCh in vivo is about 1 minute. There is sufficient evidence that decreasing doses of SCh produce inferior intubating conditions. Therefore, we firmly recommend 1.5 mg per kg (or more) of SCh for emergent RSI.
- **What is the correct dose of rocuronium for RSI?** 1.0 to 1.2 mg per kg is the optimal dose of rocuronium for RSI.[4] This dose provides adequate intubating conditions and similar success rate as SCh.
- **SCh use in patients with open eye injuries.** SCh has been linked to an increase in intraocular pressure. However, there has never been a case report of vitreous extrusion following the use of SCh in a patient with an open globe injury. Therefore, we recommend that the NMBA for RSI in patients with open globe injury be selected as for any other patient.
- **SCh use in denervation injuries (stroke, Guillain–Barré syndrome, polio, spinal cord trauma, myasthenia gravis, etc.).** Denervation injuries cause a change in the number and function of junctional and extrajunctional ACH receptors as early as 3 to 5 days postinjury.[11,12] This can result in massive serum potassium increases that can cause cardiac arrest. SCh can be safely used up to 3 days postdenervation and then should be avoided until muscle atrophy is complete and the event is no longer dynamic.

- **SCh use in myopathic patients (muscular dystrophy, rhabdomyolysis, crush injuries, prolonged immobility, etc.)**. Information on this phenomena is scant. Myopathies cause hyperkalemia by a similar mechanism as denervation, that is, changes in ACH receptor function and density.[13] Congenital myopathies are considered an absolute contraindication to SCh; its use in patients with myopathies can result in rhabdomyolysis and resuscitation-resistant hyperkalemic arrest.[14,15] Hyperkalemia secondary to occult, undiagnosed myopathy must be considered in children who experience cardiac arrest after SCh.[16] When a patient with known rhabdomyolysis is encountered, SCh should be avoided.
- **SCh use in patients with preexisting hyperkalemia.** Few studies to date have examined the risk of SCh administration in hyperkalemic patients.[17] In a meta-analysis, Thapa and Brull identified four controlled studies of patients with and without renal failure, and there were no cases in which serum potassium increased by more than 0.5 mEq per L.[18] The largest series, involving more than 40,000 patients undergoing general anesthesia, identified 38 adults and children with hyperkalemia (5.6 to 7.6 mEq per L) at the time they received SCh. None of these patients had an adverse event, and the authors calculated that the maximum likelihood of an adverse event related to SCh in hyperkalemic patients is 7.9%.[17] The long-held dogma to avoid SCh in any patient with renal failure is not valid, and SCh's independence of renal excretion makes it an excellent agent to consider when renal function is impaired.[19,20] We recommend that when hyperkalemia is present, or believed to be present (e.g., patient with end-stage renal disease), and the ECG shows stigmata of cardiac instability from hyperkalemia (increased QRS duration), an alternative agent, such as rocuronium, should be used for RSI. Otherwise, renal failure, or nominal hyperkalemia (i.e., without ECG changes), is not a contraindication to SCh.
- **Sugammadex evidence**. The molecular shape of sugammadex allows it to encapsulate rocuronium and reverse neuromuscular blockade.[20] Early studies demonstrate safe and effective reversal of rocuronium neuromuscular blockade in <2 minutes.[8,21–24]

## REFERENCES

1. Brown CA 3rd, Bair AE, Pallin DJ, et al. Techniques, success, and adverse events of emergency department adult intubations. *Ann Emerg Med*. 2015;65(4):363.e1–370.e1.
2. Pallin DJ, Dwyer RC, Walls RM, et al. Techniques and trends, success rates, and adverse events in emergency department pediatric intubations: a report from the National Emergency Airway Registry. *Ann Emerg Med*. 2016;67:610.e1–615.e1.
3. Wilcox SR, Bittner EA, Elmer J, et al. Neuromuscular blocking agent administration for emergent tracheal intubation is associated with decreased prevalence of procedure-related complications. *Crit Care Med*. 2012;40(6):1808–1813.
4. Perry JJ, Lee JS, Sillberg VA, et al. Rocuronium versus succinylcholine for rapid sequence induction intubation. *Cochrane Database Syst Rev*. 2008;(2):CD002788. doi:10.1002/14651858.CD002788.pub2
5. Patanwala AE, Stahle SA, Sakles JC, et al. Comparison of succinylcholine and rocuronium for first-attempt intubation success in the emergency department. *Acad Emerg Med*. 2011;18(1):10–14.
6. Herbstritt A, Amarakone K. Towards evidence-based emergency medicine: best BETs from the manchester royal infirmary. BET 3: Is rocuronium as effective as succinylcholine at facilitating laryngoscopy during rapid sequence intubation? *Emerg Med J*. 2012;29(3):256–258.
7. Tran DTT, Newton EK, Mount VAH, et al. Rocuronium versus succinylcholine for rapid sequence induction intubation. *Cochrane Database Syst Rev*. 2015;(10):CD002788. doi:10.1002/14651858.CD002788.pub3
8. Sørensen MK, Bretlau C, Gätke MR, et al. Rapid sequence induction and intubation with rocuronium-sugammadex compared with succinylcholine: a randomized trial. *Br J Anaesth*. 2012;108(4):682–689.
9. Marsch SC, Steiner L, Bucher E, et al. Succinylcholine versus rocuronium for rapid sequence intubation in intensive care: a prospective, randomized controlled trial. *Crit Care*. 2011;15(4):R199. doi:10.1186/cc10367

10. Naguib M, Samarkandi AH, El-Din ME, et al. The dose of succinylcholine required for excellent endotracheal intubating conditions. *Anesth Analg*. 2006;102(1):151–155.
11. Martyn JA, White DA, Gronert GA, et al. Up-and-down regulation of skeletal muscle acetylcholine receptors. Effects on neuromuscular blockers. *Anesthesiology*. 1992;76(5):822–843.
12. Gronert GA, Theye RA. Pathophysiology of hyperkalemia induced by succinylcholine. *Anesthesiology*. 1975;43(1):89–99.
13. Smith CL, Bush GH. Anaesthesia and progressive muscular dystrophy. *Br J Anaesth*. 1985;57(11):1113–1118.
14. Gronert GA. Cardiac arrest after succinylcholine: mortality greater with rhabdomyolysis than receptor upregulation. *Anesthesiology*. 2001;94(3):523–529.
15. Larach MG, Rosenberg H, Gronert GA, et al. Hyperkalemic cardiac arrest during anesthesia in infants and children with occult myopathies. *Clin Pediatr*. 1997;36(1):9–16.
16. Schow AJ, Lubarsky DA, Olson RP, et al. Can succinylcholine be used safely in hyperkalemic patients? *Anesth Analg*. 2002;95(1):119–122, table of contents.
17. Thapa S, Brull SJ. Succinylcholine-induced hyperkalemia in patients with renal failure: an old question revisited. *Anesth Analg*. 2000;91(1):237–241.
18. Powell DR, Miller R. The effect of repeated doses of succinylcholine on serum potassium in patients with renal failure. *Anesth Analg*. 1975;54(6):746–748.
19. Koide M, Waud BE. Serum potassium concentrations after succinylcholine in patients with renal failure. *Anesthesiology*. 1972;36(2):142–145.
20. Sacan O, White PF, Tufanogullari B, et al. Sugammadex reversal of rocuronium-induced neuromuscular blockade: a comparison with neostigmine-glycopyrrolate and edrophonium-atropine. *Anesth Analg*. 2007;104(3):569–574. doi:10.1213/01.ane.0000248224.42707.48
21. Suy K, Morias K, Cammu G, et al. Effective reversal of moderate rocuronium- or vecuronium-induced neuromuscular block with sugammadex, a selective relaxant binding agent. *Anesthesiology*. 2007;106(2):283–288.
22. Groudine SB, Soto R, Lien C, et al. A randomized, dose-finding, phase II study of the selective relaxant binding drug, sugammadex, capable of safely reversing profound rocuronium-induced neuromuscular block. *Anesth Analg*. 2007;104(3):555–562. doi:10.1213/01.ane.0000260135.46070.c3
23. Sparr HJ, Vermeyen KM, Beaufort AM, et al. Early reversal of profound rocuronium-induced neuromuscular blockade by sugammadex in a randomized multicenter study: efficacy, safety, and pharmacokinetics. *Anesthesiology*. 2007;106(5):935–943. doi:10.1097/01.anes.0000265152.78943.74
24. Schaller SJ, Fink H. Sugammadex as a reversal agent for neuromuscular block: an evidence-based review. *Core Evid*. 2013;8:57–67.

Chapter 23

# Anesthesia and Sedation for Awake Intubation

Alan C. Heffner and Peter M.C. DeBlieux

## INTRODUCTION

Humans protect their airway at virtually any cost. It is generally impossible to even glimpse the glottis with a laryngoscope in a fully awake and aware patient. The "awake" methods of endoscopy referred to in the difficult airway algorithm are rarely performed without pharmacologic assistance. Even in patients who are unaware because of their illness, sensibilities must be attenuated by a combination of local anesthesia and systemic sedation in order to facilitate diagnostic and therapeutic airway laryngoscopy.

Focusing on emergency airway management, the "awake" intubation is frequently indicated in situations where abnormal airway anatomy or difficult laryngoscopy is suspected. As a general rule, local anesthesia is first optimized in order to limit potential untoward effects of systemic sedation. In uncooperative or decompensating patients, sedation may dominate over local anesthesia.

## DESCRIPTION

Awake laryngoscopy has two main roles, and both are applicable in patients with anticipated difficult intubation: (1) to determine whether intubation is feasible, thus facilitating a decision regarding the use of neuromuscular blockade to complete the procedure, and (2) to facilitate intubation, particularly in circumstances when the patient's airway is deteriorating as in angioedema, upper airway burns, or trauma, during which it is desirable to keep the patient breathing while intubation is accomplished.

An awake look intended to determine the feasibility of nasal or oral intubation can be accomplished in two ways. A flexible video or fiber-optic endoscope is inserted through the nostril to evaluate periglottic anatomy in patients with neck disease or acute injury to determine if nasal intubation or orotracheal intubation is feasible. This can be performed quickly with topical nasal anesthesia and minimal, if any, sedation.

The second approach engages a standard or video laryngoscope to perform laryngoscopy, with the intention of confirming glottic visualization. Awake rigid laryngoscopy is more stimulating and requires a greater degree of local anesthesia and sedation than does its flexible endoscopy counterpart. Concentrated local anesthesia of the mouth, oropharynx, and hypopharynx facilitates the procedure and minimizes the dose of systemic sedation required. If the glottis is adequately visualized, the airway manager may either proceed with awake intubation, or may withdraw the laryngoscope and perform rapid sequence intubation (RSI). The approach is dictated by the clinical circumstance.

- If the difficult airway is dynamic and evolving, then it is advisable to intubate the patient during the awake laryngoscopy, as the airway may deteriorate quickly or as a result of laryngoscopic manipulation. If there is reasonable concern that the airway might change, intubation should be attempted on the first good opportunity.
- If the difficult airway is subacute to chronic and is more a confounder to intubation than the primary reason for airway crisis (e.g., fixed cervical or maxillofacial disease), then the goal is to confirm feasibility of intubation. Glottis visualization is followed by laryngoscope withdrawal and proper RSI, with the knowledge that the airway is within reach and very unlikely to deteriorate between steps. Cases of slowly evolving, acute disease (e.g., infection and inhalation burn) are reasonable opportunities to take this same approach. Appropriate supplies and drugs are prepared before the first laryngoscopy to minimize delay to definitive RSI.

## INDICATIONS AND CONTRAINDICATIONS

Awake intubation is indicated when the airway manager is not confident that gas exchange will be assured by airway rescue techniques if the patient is rendered apneic (see Chapters 2 and 3). Although the difficult airway assessment defines an airway as potentially difficult if it meets any or all of a number of markers (LEMON), the degree of perceived difficulty and the decision whether to use an RSI technique or an awake approach depend both on the patient and experience and judgment of the clinician. Local anesthesia of the upper airway, with or without sedation, facilitates upper airway endoscopy even when intubation is not anticipated. Common indications include airway examination for foreign body, supraglottitis, hoarseness, stridor, and blunt or penetrating neck injury.

The only contraindication to the use of this strategy is a patient who mandates an immediate airway. Rapidly deteriorating airway situations require immediate management through other means, as there is insufficient time for patient preparation before intervention (see Chapter 3 discussion of the "forced to act" scenario). Adequate time and patient cooperation (usually with the use of anesthesia and sedation) are the most important limitations to awake endoscopy. In addition, copious airway secretions or blood thwarts efforts to effectively anesthetize the airway and may obscure the indirect view via endoscopy.

## LOCAL ANESTHESIA FACTORS

Local anesthesia of the airway may be achieved topically, by injection, or by combining both techniques. The selection of a local anesthetic agent depends on the properties of the agent and how it is supplied (concentration and preparation—aqueous, gel, or ointment). Potent local anesthesia may enable the airway to be visualized with little or no sedation. As a general rule, local anesthesia should be optimized before sedation is given to the high-risk patient selected for this technique.

Airway secretions are a barrier to topical anesthetics and are capable of diluting applied agents or washing them away from the intended target region. Antisialagogues are effective adjuncts to reduce secretion production and improve topical anesthesia and endoscopy conditions. The antimuscarinic agent glycopyrrolate (Robinul) is the preferred agent. The greatest drawback is time to effective drying, which is 10 to 20 minutes following intravenous (IV) administration (glycopyrrolate 0.005 mg per kg; usual adult dose 0.4 mg IV). Given sufficient time, even if only 10 minutes, it is advisable to administer glycopyrrolate to facilitate local anesthesia of the upper airway.

Lidocaine remains a favored drug for airway anesthesia because of its rapid onset (2 to 5 minutes to peak effect), safety, and widespread availability. Concentrations of 2% (20 mg per mL) to

4% (40 mg per mL) aqueous solutions are optimal for topical administration via nebulization. The addition of epinephrine provides no advantage.

Anesthetics applied to mucous membranes undergo rapid systemic absorption. The maximum safe dose of topical anesthetic applied to mucous membranes depends on the method and timing of administration. Although traditional dosage guidelines may be excessively conservative when drugs are administered by aerosol or atomizer, we recommend a maximum lidocaine dose of 4 mg per kg. This threshold is unlikely to be surpassed in large adults, but in small adults and children, the dose should be calculated before administration. As always, clinical judgment is required, and meticulous attention to detail is necessary when lidocaine is applied to the airway to achieve effective anesthesia without producing toxicity.

Aerosolization of aqueous lidocaine is easy and effective. Gas flow–directed nebulizers, as are used for inhalational therapy in asthma, are an effective first step to initiate broad (nasal, oral, and hypopharyngeal) local anesthesia during an emergency airway situation. Three milliliters of lidocaine can be administered over 10 minutes while additional agents and equipment are prepared. Augmentation with additional focused topical application is the norm.

Atomizers produce larger droplets than nebulizers. For topical anesthesia of the upper airway, atomizers are more rapid and effective than nebulizers. The DeVilbiss atomizer (**Fig. 23-1**) and mucosal atomization device (LMA North America, San Diego, CA) (**Fig. 23-2**) are two examples of commonly used atomizers.

Lidocaine is also available in gel and paste formulas, in a variety of concentrations, to permit direct local administration. Some combination of these formula applications is often warranted.

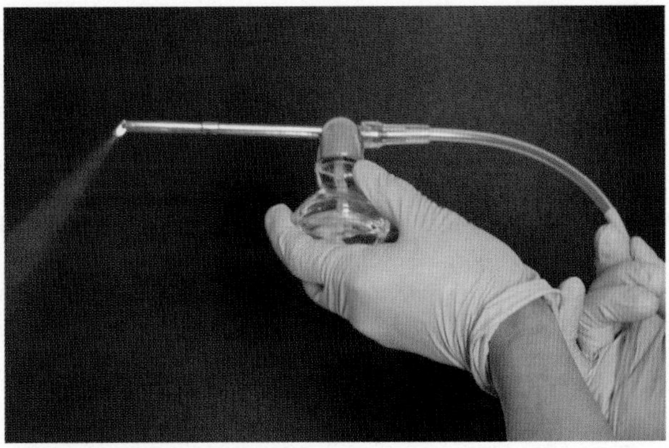

● **FIGURE 23-1. DeVilbiss Atomizer.**

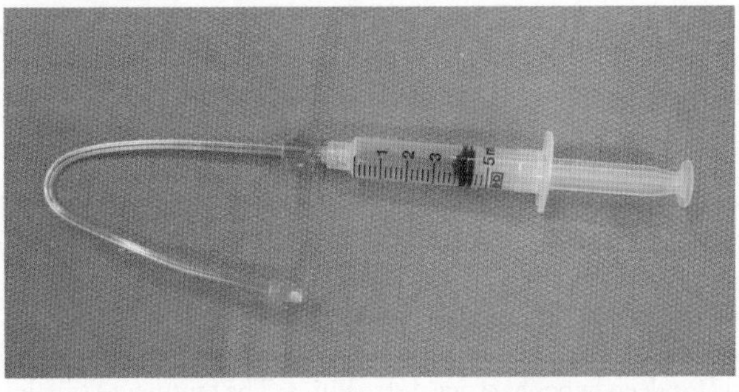

● **FIGURE 23-2. Mucosal Atomization Device.** The syringe forces the local anesthetic solution through the atomizing tip, resulting in a very fine mist that can be synchronized with the patient's inspiration.

## Nasal Anesthesia

The nasal mucosa is highly vascular and tends to bleed during manipulation. Topical vasoconstriction improves nasal passage caliber and may prevent epistaxis. Although evidence for this practice is not strong, there is little downside and generally no contraindication to its use. Phenylephrine (Neo-Synephrine) 0.5% or oxymetazoline (Afrin) 0.05% solution is sprayed and sniffed into each nostril 2 to 3 minutes before application of local anesthesia. Cocaine 4% (40 mg per mL) can also be used, although concerns about systemic toxicity have limited its availability of late. Virtually all local anesthetic agents are effective when used topically in the nose. If available, cocaine 4% and tetracaine 0.45% are particularly effective because of their tissue penetration and ability to eliminate deep pressure discomfort commonly associated with nasal manipulation. Lidocaine is also effective (discussed previously), although it is associated with burning dysesthesia and produces less deep anesthesia.

Commonly used techniques for focused nasal anesthesia include the following:

- Nebulize a mixture of 3 mL of 2% or 4% lidocaine with 1 mL of 1% phenylephrine.
- Atomize 1 mL of agent directly into the nostril while asking the patient to sniff.
- Inject viscous anesthetic gel (2 to 4 mL) into the nares with a small syringe while asking the patient to sniff. The gel can also be distributed throughout the nasal passage using a cotton dip applicator or through insertion of a nasopharyngeal airway. If intubation is planned, an endotracheal tube can be inserted with lidocaine gel applied to the outer surface of the distal tip.

## Oral Anesthesia

Topical anesthesia of the oral cavity focuses on the tongue to attenuate the gag response, and to reduce the discomfort associated with manipulation (e.g., grasping the tongue with gauze and pulling it forward to draw the epiglottis forward during endoscopic exam).

- The mouth is best anesthetized topically by having the patient gargle and swish with a 2% or 4% aqueous lidocaine solution. Gargling also augments anesthesia of the oro- and hypopharynx.
- "Butter" the tongue base with lidocaine paste or ointment applied with a tongue depressor. Apply 2 to 4 mL of 5% lidocaine evenly to the posterior base of the protruded tongue. Maintain the mouth open and tongue protruded for several minutes to allow the formula to melt down the base of the tongue toward the glottis. Manual control of tongue with gauze while asking the patient to pant "like a dog" facilitates this maneuver.
- An atomizer can also be used to spray the structures of the oral cavity.

## Oropharyngeal and Hypopharyngeal Anesthesia

The major sensory supply to the oropharynx and hypopharynx is the glossopharyngeal nerve (see Chapter 4). Although cooperative patients can gargle anesthetic to initiate the process, the best way to achieve dense local anesthesia to permit laryngoscopy or awake intubation is through a nerve block at the base of the palatopharyngeal arch (posterior tonsillar pillar; see Fig. 4-4). The following two techniques are commonly used:

- *Injection technique:* A 23G angled tonsillar needle with 1 cm of exposed needle tip is inserted 0.5 cm behind the midpoint of the posterior tonsillar pillar and directed laterally and slightly posteriorly (**Fig. 23-3**). Two mL of 2% lidocaine is deposited following a negative aspiration. Although this block is effective, it is not widely used because of the proximity of the carotid artery and risk of carotid injection in up to 5% of cases.
- *Topical technique:* The "butter" the tongue technique mentioned earlier provides effective anesthesia for deep hypopharyngeal structures. The ointment liquefies as it warms and runs down the base of the palatopharyngeal arch, penetrates the mucosa, and reaches the glossopharyngeal nerve. Distribution to the valleculae and pyriform recesses provides local anesthesia and blocks the internal branch of the superior laryngeal nerve, providing laryngeal anesthesia.

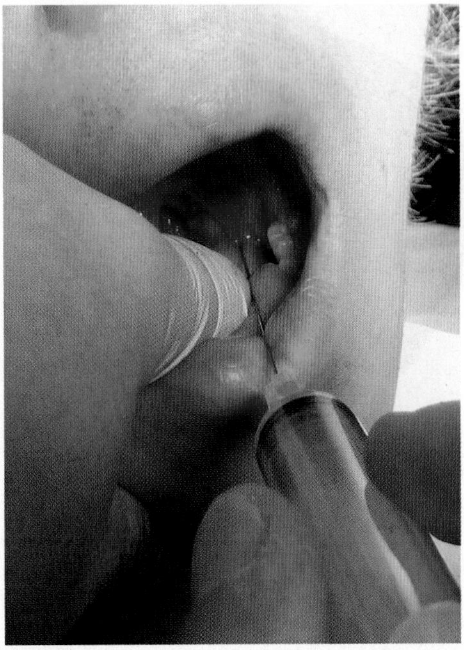

● **FIGURE 23-3. Glossopharyngeal Nerve Block.** Insertion point for a 23G angled tonsillar needle.

## Laryngeal Anesthesia

The drying imperative does not apply to the larynx. Topical local anesthesia of this structure can be provided using a manual spray device, an atomizer, or nebulizer to spray 2 to 4 mL of 4% aqueous lidocaine. Alternatively, one can block the superior laryngeal branch of the vagus nerve (see Fig. 4-6).

- The internal branch of the superior laryngeal nerve can be blocked as it runs just deep to the mucosa in the pyriform recess, using Jackson forceps to hold a cotton pledget soaked in 4% lidocaine against the mucosa for 1 minute (**Fig. 23-4**).
- This block can also be performed using an external approach to the nerve as it perforates the thyrohyoid membrane just below the greater cornu of the hyoid bone. A 21G to 25G needle is passed medially through the skin to contact the hyoid bone as posteriorly as possible. The needle is then walked caudad off the hyoid. Resistance may be appreciated as the thyrohyoid membrane is perforated. Following aspiration to rule out entry into the pharyngeal lumen or a vessel, 3 mL 2% lidocaine can be injected. If the hyoid cannot be palpated or if palpation produces undue patient discomfort, then the thyroid cartilage is used as a landmark. The needle is walked cephalad from a point on the thyroid cartilage, about one-third of the distance from the midline to the greater cornu. Complications include intra-arterial injection, hematoma, and airway distortion. One should have confidence in laryngeal anatomy and experience with this procedure before this approach is used.

## Tracheal Anesthesia

The trachea is best anesthetized topically. Drying is unnecessary. Local anesthetic agent can be sprayed into the trachea through handheld spray devices, atomizer, or nebulizer. Additional anesthetic can be applied through the working channel during flexible endoscopy.

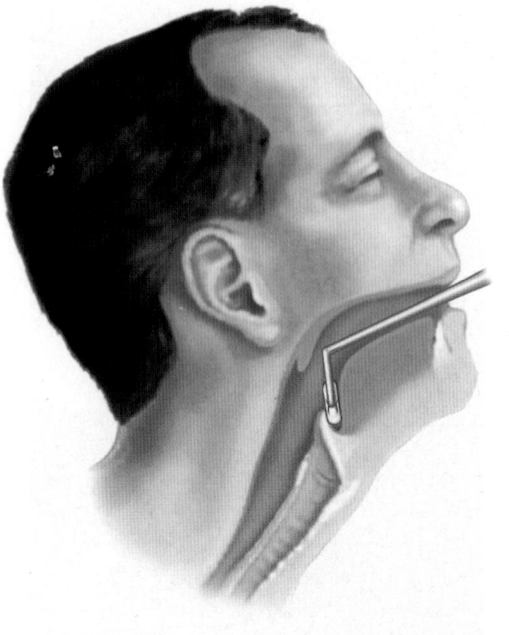

● **FIGURE 23-4. Use of Jackson Crossover Forceps to Perform a Transmucosal Superior Laryngeal Nerve Block.** A cotton pledget, soaked in 4% lidocaine, is held against the mucosa for about 1 minute.

- Tracheal and laryngeal anesthesia can be produced by puncturing the cricothyroid membrane and injecting local anesthetic agent directly into the trachea. A 5-mL syringe containing 3 mL of 4% lidocaine aqueous is attached to a 20G IV catheter-over-needle device. It may be helpful to cut the plastic cannula to 1.5 cm in length to minimize tracheal stimulation and cough. A small area of skin is anesthetized over the cricothyroid membrane using a 25G to 27G needle. The needle-cannula is then inserted into the trachea, while aspirating for air. Once the air column is entered, the plastic cannula is advance over the needle into the trachea. The needle is withdrawn and discarded. Lidocaine is injected at end exhalation with the subsequent inspiration and cough facilitating downward and upward spread of anesthetic.

## SEDATION TECHNIQUES

Awake endoscopy during an emergency airway situation frequently relies on some degree of IV titration of systemic sedation to supplement topical anesthesia. Mild-to-moderate sedation is typically required similar to that used for painful procedures, such as for reduction of a dislocated shoulder or drainage of a deep cutaneous abscess.

A variety of sedative-hypnotic medications may be used, including midazolam, propofol, etomidate, and ketamine. Agent selection depends on the clinical situation, medication availability, and airway manager experience with each medication. In general, it is best to achieve sedation for airway examination by the same methods used for other procedures so the airway manager is using familiar agents and doses. Deep anesthesia defeats the fundamental purpose of an awake approach to maintain spontaneous ventilation and active airway protection.

All agents classified as sedative-hypnotics (e.g., benzodiazepines, barbiturates, propofol, and etomidate) cause respiratory depression in a dose-dependent fashion. This is also true of opioids such as fentanyl and morphine, particularly when used in conjunction with sedative-hypnotic agents. Fragile patients with compensated respiratory failure may be rendered critically bradypneic or apneic with relatively small doses of these agents. Sedative and opioid analgesia also produce some degree of muscle relaxation. Patients with partial upper airway obstruction may progress to complete obstruction if these agents invoke a loss of critical upper airway muscle tone. The operator should always be prepared to proceed directly to a surgical airway (i.e., double setup situation) when sedation and local anesthesia are undertaken on a patient with partial or impending airway obstruction (see Chapter 36).

Ketamine is a unique dissociative agent that maintains muscle tone and spontaneous respirations when used at low to moderate doses. Doses exceeding 1 mg per kg IV may invoke respiratory and cardiovascular depression. Ketamine may also sensitize the larynx to laryngospasm in the face of laryngeal inflammation. The preservation of airway maintenance and spontaneous ventilation is important for this procedure, and ketamine is a preferred agent. Ketamine should be titrated in 25 mg aliquots IV until the patient can tolerate an awake look. The patient may be dissociated, continuing to breathe spontaneously while maintaining airway patency. Some authors advocate a combination of ketamine and propofol drawn up in the same syringe to make a concentration of 5 mg per mL of each (5 mL of 10 mg per mL ketamine plus 5 mL of 10 mg per mL propofol in a 10-mL syringe) titrated 1 to 2 mL at a time. Although this method administers two agents in a fixed combination, it appears to be effective and safe, and the two drugs are compatible in the same syringe. Alternatives include balanced use of a benzodiazepine (e.g., midazolam) and an opioid (e.g., fentanyl), or other agents used for painful, stimulating procedures. All agents require continuous vigilance with respect to airway patency and adequacy of ventilation.

Uncooperative or intoxicated patients may require chemical restraint before and during airway assessment. If hypoxia or severe respiratory distress is the cause of the combative behavior, an awake technique is neither advised nor likely to succeed. Haloperidol, a butyrophenone, is rapid acting such that IV doses of 2 to 5 mg in the adult can be carefully titrated to effect at 3- to 5-minute intervals.

Two additional newer agents show promise for awake endoscopy during emergency situations. Remifentanil is an ultra–short-acting opioid with rapid onset and offset, both measured in tens of seconds rather than minutes. There is a wide range of recommended dosing and a conservative starting dose should be considered. An IV bolus of 0.75 mcg per kg may precede the continuous infusion that is generally started at 0.05 to 0.1 mcg/kg/minute with subsequent titration to effect. Dosing should be calculated on lean body mass in morbidly obese patients and reduced by as much as 50% in the elderly. Anecdotally, remifentanil infusion appears to attenuate both the gag reflex and laryngeal reflexes, and can facilitate airway anesthesia. It may be particularly useful in patients with hyperactive gag reflexes, and in the presence of excess secretions.

Dexmedetomidine is an IV $\alpha_2$-agonist indicated for induction of general anesthesia and sedation during critical illness. It possesses desirable properties for awake endoscopy including rapid onset of hypnosis, analgesia, and amnesia without respiratory depression. Typical dosing is 1 mcg per kg IV load over 10 minutes followed by infusion at 0.1 mcg/kg/hour and titrated to effect. Supplemental doses of an alternative agent may be required. Bradycardia and hypotension are uncommon but important side effects.

## SUMMARY

- Effective topical anesthesia of the upper airways is most effective when the drug is applied to dry mucous membranes.
- For mucosal drying, we recommend glycopyrrolate (0.005 mg per kg IV) with a usual adult dose of 0.4 mg IV.
- When time allows, local anesthesia is first optimized in order to limit potential untoward effects of systemic sedation. Uncooperative or rapidly decompensating patients are exceptions where sedation may dominate over local anesthesia.
- The dissociated anesthesia and preserved respiratory drive produced with low to moderate dose IV ketamine (up to 1 mg per kg) make it a prime agent for awake endoscopy procedures.
- Systemic sedation should be titrated with extreme caution in patients with impending airway obstruction.

## EVIDENCE

- **Is there any evidence for the use of ketamine and propofol together?** "Ketofol," the combination of ketamine and propofol, for procedural sedation has emerged over the last decade. Fixed dose (1:1 mixture of ketamine 10 mg per mL and propofol 10 mg per mL) single-syringe mixtures are frequently used.[1,2] Although theoretically advantageous to limit dose-related adverse events of each agent, there are little data to support improved efficacy or safety over single-agent sedation. There are no specific data for use of this combination in airway management.
- **Can local anesthesia of the upper airway cause airway obstruction?** In the presence of preexisting airway compromise, topical anesthesia and instrumentation are associated with airway compromise resulting from dynamic airflow obstruction with or without associated laryngospasm.[3,4] Preparation for immediate surgical airway control is a necessity whenever one applies topical anesthesia or performs instrumentation of an inflamed, infected, or obstructed airway. In certain cases, awake cricothyrotomy or tracheostomy under local anesthesia is a reasonable option.
- **What is the evidence for dexmedetomidine use during awake airway procedures?** Rapid-onset hypnosis and amnesia without accompanying respiratory depression are primary sedation goals during awake airway maneuvers. As anticipated, the favorable pharmacologic profile of dexmedetomidine led to its application in patients with tenuous or difficult airways. Growing case reports and trial evidence support the safety and efficacy of dexmedetomidine as the primary and/or sole hypnotic agent to facilitate awake fiber-optic intubation.[5–7]

## REFERENCES


1. Willman EV, Andolfatto G. A prospective evaluation of "ketofol" (ketamine/propofol combination) for procedural sedation and analgesia in the emergency department. *Ann Emerg Med*. 2007;49(1):23–30.
2. Andolfatto G, Willman E. A prospective case series of single syringe ketamine-propofol (Ketofol) for emergency department procedural sedation and analgesia in adults. *Acad Emerg Med*. 2011;18(3):237–245.
3. Ho AM, Chung DC, To EW, et al. Total airway obstruction during local anesthesia in a non-sedated patient with a compromised airway. *Can J Anaesth*. 2004;51(8):838–841.
4. Ho AM, Chung DC, Karmakar MK, et al. Dynamic airflow limitation after topical anaesthesia of the upper airway. *Anaesth Intensive Care*. 2006;34(2):211–215.
5. Bergese SD, Candiotti KA, Bokesch PM, et al. A phase IIIb, randomized, double-blind, placebo controlled, multi-center study evaluating the safety and efficacy of dexmedetomidine for sedation during awake fiberoptic intubation. *Am J Ther*. 2010;17(6):586–595.
6. Bergese SD, Patrick Bender S, McSweeney TD, et al. A comparative study of dexmedetomidine with midazolam and midazolam alone for sedation during elective awake fiberoptic intubation. *J Clin Anesth*. 2010;22(1):35–40.
7. Johnston KD, Rai MR. Conscious sedation for awake fiberoptic intubation: a review of the literature. *Can J Anesth*. 2013;60:584–599.

# Section VI

# Pediatric Airway Management

Chapter 24

# Differentiating Aspects of the Pediatric Airway

Robert C. Luten and Nathan W. Mick

## THE CLINICAL CHALLENGE

Airway management in the pediatric population presents many potential challenges, including age-related drug dosing and equipment sizing, anatomical variation that continuously evolves as development proceeds from infancy to adolescence, and the performance anxiety that invariably accompanies the resuscitation of a critically ill child. Clinical competence in managing the airway of a critically ill or injured child requires an appreciation of age- and size-related factors, and a degree of familiarity and comfort with the fundamental approach to pediatric airway emergencies.

The principles of airway management in children and adults are the same. Medications used to facilitate intubation, the need for alternative airway management techniques, and the basic approach to performing the procedure are similar whether the patient is 8 or 80 years of age. There are, however, a few important differences that must be considered. These differences are most exaggerated in the first 2 years of life, after which the pediatric airway gradually develops more adult-like features.

In adults, recognition and management of the difficult airway is the principal skill to be mastered. During training and in actual practice, there is ample opportunity to master and maintain these skills. In pediatrics, this is not the case. The paucity of sick children encountered in training and actual practice makes attaining the same level of comfort difficult to achieve. Although the incidence of difficult pediatric airways encountered by emergency physicians is negligible, the challenge for the emergency physician is developing comfort in managing small children who have predictable differences in anatomy and physiology compared with older children and adults. This chapter will review those difference with the aim of simplifying them and making the key skills more easily learned and maintained.

## APPROACH TO THE PEDIATRIC PATIENT

### General Issues

A review of pediatric resuscitation processes defined elements of the mental (cognitive) burden of providers, when dealing with the unique aspects of critically ill children compared with adults.

Age- and size-related variables unique to children introduce the need for more complex, nonreflexive, or knowledge-based mental activities, such as calculating drug doses and selecting equipment. The concentration required to undertake these activities while under stress may subtract from other important mental activity such as assessment, evaluation, prioritization, and synthesis of information, referred to in the resuscitative process as critical thinking activities. The cumulative effect of these factors leads to inevitable time delays and a corresponding increase in the potential for decision-making errors in the pediatric resuscitative process. This is in sharp contrast to adult resuscitation, where drug doses, equipment sizing, and physiologic parameters are usually familiar to the provider, leading to more automatic decisions that free the adult provider's attention for critical thinking. In children, drug doses are based on weight and may vary by an order of magnitude depending on age (i.e., 3-kg neonate vs. a 30-kg 8-year-old vs. a 100-kg adolescent). The use of resuscitation aids in pediatric resuscitation significantly reduces the cognitive load (and error) related to drug dosing calculations and equipment selection by relegating these activities to a lower order of mental function (referred to as "automatic" or "rule based"). The results are reduced error, attenuation of psychological stress, and an increase in critical thinking time. Table 24-1 is a length-based, color-coded equipment reference chart (based on the "resuscitation guide" of Broselow–Luten) for pediatric airway management that eliminates error-prone strategies based on age and weight. Both equipment and drug dosing information are included in the Broselow–Luten system and can be accessed by a single length measurement or patient weight. This system is also available as part of a robust online resource (www.ebroselow.com).

## Specific Issues

### *Anatomical and Functional Issues*

The approach to the child with airway obstruction (the most common form of a difficult pediatric airway) incorporates several unique features of the pediatric anatomy.

1. Children obstruct more readily than adults do, and the pediatric airway is especially susceptible to airway obstruction resulting from swelling. (See Table 26-4 [Chapter 26] that outlines the effect of 1-mm edema on airway resistance in the infant [4-mm airway diameter] vs. the adult [8-mm airway diameter].) Nebulized racemic epinephrine causes local vasoconstriction and can reduce mucosal swelling and edema to some extent. For diseases such as croup, where the anatomical site of swelling occurs at the level of the cricoid ring, functionally the narrowest part of the pediatric airway, racemic epinephrine can have dramatic results. Disorders located in areas with greater airway caliber, such as the supraglottic swelling of epiglottitis or the retropharyngeal swelling of an abscess, rarely produce findings as dramatic. In these latter examples, especially in the epiglottitis, efforts to force a nebulized medication on a child may agitate the child, leading to increased airflow velocity and dynamic upper airway obstruction.
2. Noxious interventions can lead to dynamic airway obstruction and precipitate respiratory arrest, leading to the admonition to "leave them alone." The work of breathing in the crying child increases 32-fold, elevating the threat of dynamic airway obstruction and hence the principle of maintaining children in a quiet, comfortable environment during evaluation and management for upper airway obstruction (**Fig. 24-1A-C**).
3. Bag-mask ventilation (BMV) may be of particular value in the child with upper airway obstruction. Note in **Figure 24-1C** that efforts by the patient to alleviate the obstruction may actually exacerbate it, as increased inspiratory effort creates increased negative extrathoracic pressure, leading to collapse of the malleable extrathoracic trachea. The application of positive pressure through BMV causes the opposite effect by stenting the airway open and relieving the dynamic component of obstruction (**Fig. 24-1C, D**). This mechanism explains the recommendation to try BMV first as a temporizing measure, even if the patient arrests from obstruction. There have been numerous case reports of children with epiglottitis successfully being resuscitated utilizing BMV.
4. Apart from differences related to size, there are certain anatomical peculiarities of the pediatric airway. These differences are most pronounced in children <2 years of age, whereas children >8 years of age are similar to adults anatomically and the 2- to 8-year-old period is one of transition.

**TABLE 24-1** Equipment Selection

| | Pink[a] | Red | Purple | Yellow | White | Blue | Orange | Green |
|---|---|---|---|---|---|---|---|---|
| **Length (cm)-based pediatric equipment chart** | | | | | | | | |
| Weight (kg) | 6–7 | 8–9 | 10–11 | 12–14 | 15–18 | 19–23 | 23–31 | 31–41 |
| Length (cm) | 60.75–67.75 | 67.75–75.25 | 75.25–85 | 85–98.25 | 98.25–110.75 | 110.75–122.5 | 122.5–137.5 | 137.5–155 |
| ETT size (mm) | 3.5 cuff<br>3.0 uncuff | 3.5 cuff<br>3.0 uncuff | 4.0 cuff<br>3.0 uncuff | 4.5 cuff<br>4.0 uncuff | 5.0 cuff<br>4.5 uncuff | 5.5 cuff<br>5.0 uncuff | 6.0 cuff | 6.5 cuff |
| Lip-to-tip length (mm) | 10–10.5 | 10.5–11 | 11–12 | 12.5–13.5 | 14–15 | 15.5–16.5 | 17–18 | 18.5–19.5 |
| Laryngoscope size+blade | 1 straight | 1 straight | 1 straight | 2 straight | 2 straight | 2 straight or curved | 2 straight or curved | 3 straight or curved |
| Suction catheter | 8F | 8F | 8F | 8F–10F | 10F | 10F | 10F | 12F |
| Stylet | 6F | 6F | 10F | 10F | 10F | 10F | 14F | 14F |
| Oral airway (mm) | 50 | 50 | 60 | 60 | 60 | 70 | 80 | 80 |
| Nasopharyngeal airway | 14F | 14F | 18F | 20F | 22F | 24F | 26F | 30F |
| Bag/valve device | Infant | Infant | Child | Child | Child | Child | Child/adult | Adult |
| Oxygen mask | Newborn | Newborn | Pediatric | Pediatric | Pediatric | Pediatric | Adult | Adult |
| Vascular access | 22–24/23–25 | 22–24/23–25 | 20–22/23–25 | 18–22/21–23 | 18–22/21–23 | 18–20/21–23 | 18–20/21–22 | 16–20/18–21 |
| Catheter/ butterfly | Intraosseous | Intraosseous | Intraosseous | Intraosseous | Intraosseous | Intraosseous | | |
| NG tube | 5–8F | 5–8F | 8–10F | 10F | 10–12F | 12–14F | 14–18F | 18F |

(*continued*)

TABLE 24-1

## Equipment Selection (continued)

| | Pink[a] | Red | Purple | Yellow | White | Blue | Orange | Green |
|---|---|---|---|---|---|---|---|---|
| Urinary catheter | 5–8F | 5–8F | 8–10F | 10F | 10–12F | 10–12F | 12F | 12F |
| Chest tube | 10–12F | 10–12F | 16–20F | 20–24F | 20–24F | 24–32F | 24–32F | 32–40F |
| BP cuff | Newborn/infant | Newborn/infant | Infant/child | Child | Child | Child | Child/adult | Adult |
| LMA[b] | 1.5 | 1.5 | 2 | 2 | 2 | 2–2.5 | 2.5 | 3 |

Directions for use: (1) measure patient length with centimeter tape or with a Broselow tape; (2) using measured length in centimeters or Broselow tape measurement, access appropriate equipment column; (3) column for ETTs, oral and nasopharyngeal airways, and LMAs; always select one size smaller and one size larger than the recommended size.

[a]For infants smaller than the pink zone, but not preterm, use the same equipment as the pink zone.

[b]Based on manufacturer's weight-based guidelines:

| Mask size | Patient size (kg) |
|---|---|
| 1 | ≤5 |
| 1.5 | 5–10 |
| 2 | 10–20 |
| 2.5 | 20–30 |
| 3 | >30 |

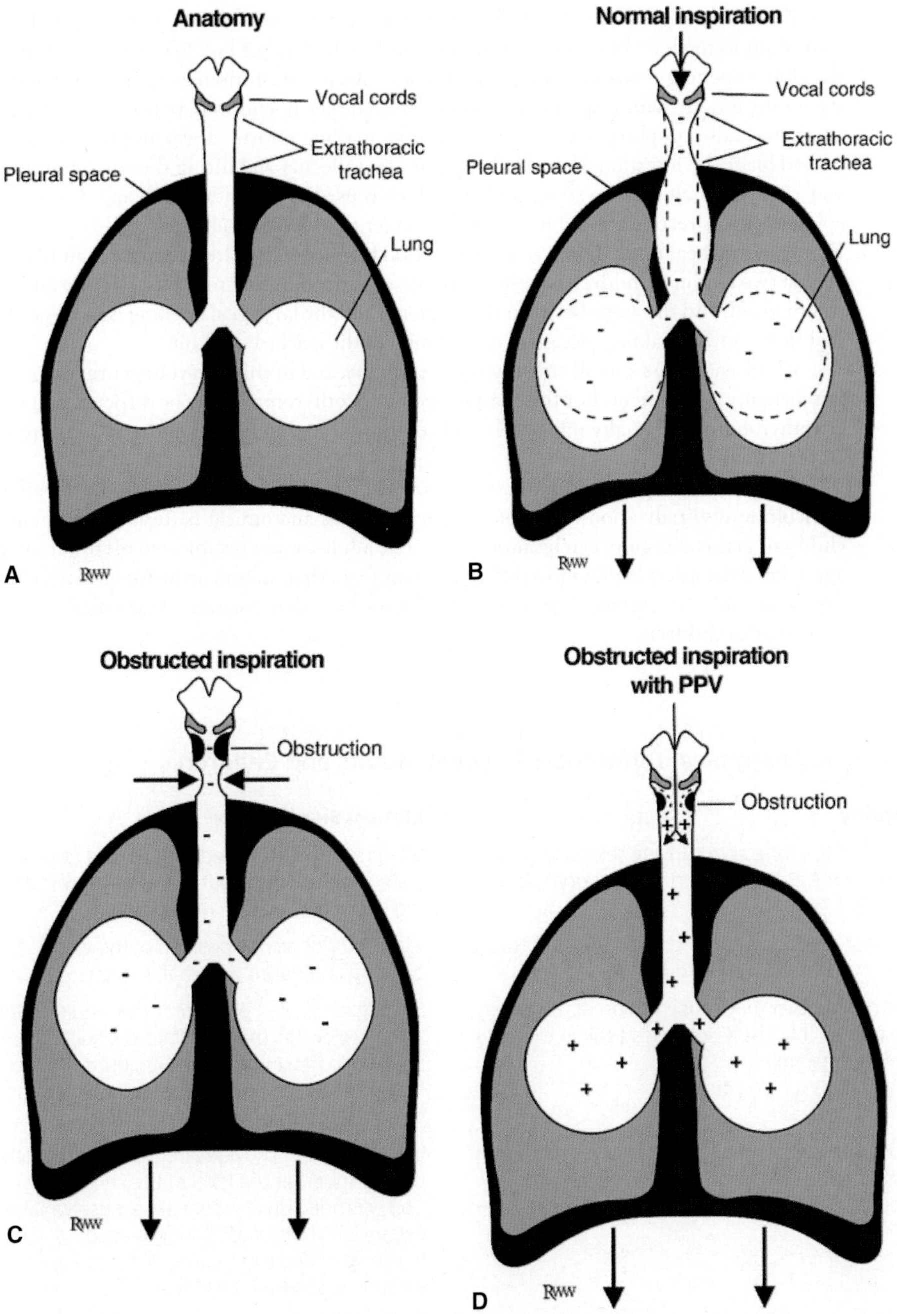


● **FIGURE 24-1. Intra- and Extrathoracic Trachea and the Dynamic Changes That Occur in the Presence of Upper Airway Obstruction.** **A:** Normal anatomy. **B:** The changes that occur with normal inspiration; that is, dynamic collapsing of the upper airway associated with the negative pressure of inspiration on the extrathoracic trachea. **C:** Exaggeration of the collapse secondary to superimposed obstruction at the subglottic area. **D:** Positive-pressure ventilation (PPV) stents the collapse/obstruction versus the patient's own inspiratory efforts, which increase the obstruction. (Adapted from Cote CJ, Ryan JF, Todres ID, et al., eds. *A Practice of Anesthesia for Infants and Children*. 2nd ed. Philadelphia, PA: WB Saunders; 1993, with permission.)

The glottic opening is situated at the level of the first cervical vertebra (C-1) in infancy. This level transitions to the level of C-3 to C-4 by age 7 and to the level of C-5 to C-6 in the adult. Thus, the glottic opening tends to be higher and more anterior in children as opposed to adults. The size of the tongue with respect to the oral cavity is larger in children, particularly infants. The epiglottis is also proportionately larger in a child, making efforts to visualize the airway with a curved blade, by insertion of the blade tip into the vallecula and lifting the epiglottis out of the way more difficult. Thus a straight blade, which is used to get underneath and directly lift the epiglottis up, is recommended in children younger than 3 years (**Table 24-2**).

5. Blind nasotracheal intubation is relatively contraindicated in children younger than 10 years for at least two reasons: Children have large tonsils and adenoids that may bleed significantly when traumatized, and the angle between the epiglottis and the laryngeal opening is more acute than that in the adult, making successful cannulation of the trachea difficult.

   Children possess a small cricothyroid membrane, and in children younger than 3 to 4 years, it is virtually nonexistent. For this reason, needle cricothyrotomy may be difficult, and surgical cricothyrotomy is virtually impossible and contraindicated in infants and small children up to 10 years of age.

   Although younger children possess a relatively high, anterior airway with the attendant difficulties in visualization of the glottic aperture, this anatomical pattern is consistent in all children, so this difficulty can be anticipated. The adult airway is subject to more variation and age-related disorders leading to a difficult airway (e.g., rheumatoid arthritis, obesity). Children are predictably "different," not "difficult." **Figure 24-2** demonstrates anatomical differences particular to children.

TABLE 24-2

## Anatomical Differences between Adults and Children

| Anatomy | Clinical Significance |
|---|---|
| Large intraoral tongue occupying relatively large portion of the oral cavity and proportionally larger epiglottis | Straight blade preferred over curved to push distensible anatomy out of the way to visualize the larynx and elevate the epiglottis |
| High tracheal opening: C-1 in infancy vs. C-3 to C-4 at age 7, C-5 to C-6 in the adult | High anterior airway position of the glottic opening compared with that in adults |
| Large occiput that may cause flexion of the airway, large tongue that easily collapses against the posterior pharynx | Sniffing position is preferred. The larger occiput actually elevates the head into the sniffing position in most infants and children. A towel may be required under shoulders to elevate torso relative to head in small infants |
| Cricoid ring is functionally the narrowest portion of the trachea as compared with the vocal cords in the adult | Uncuffed tubes provide adequate seal because they fit snugly at the level of the cricoid ring<br>Correct tube size is essential because variable expansion cuffed tubes are not used<br>If using a cuffed tube, careful monitoring of cuff inflation pressure is essential |
| Consistent anatomical variations with age with fewer abnormal variations related to body habitus, arthritis, chronic disease | Younger than 2 y, high anterior; 2–8 y, transition; and older than 8 y, small adult |
| Large tonsils and adenoids may bleed; more acute angle between epiglottis and laryngeal opening results in nasotracheal intubation attempt failures | Blind nasotracheal intubation not indicated in children; nasotracheal intubation failure |
| Small cricothyroid membrane landmark, surgical cricothyrotomy impossible in infants and small children | Needle cricothyrotomy recommended and the landmark is the anterior surface of the trachea, not the cricoid membrane |

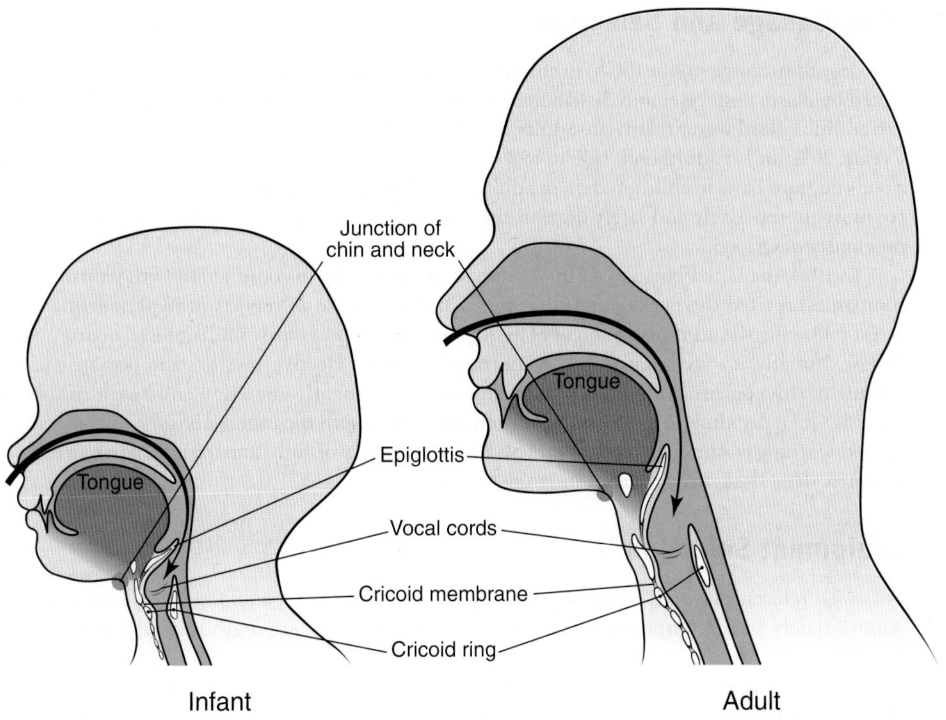


● **FIGURE 24-2.** The anatomical differences particular to children are (1) higher, more anterior position of the glottic opening (note the relationship of the vocal cords to the chin/neck junction); (2) relatively larger tongue in the infant, which lies between the mouth and glottic opening; (3) relatively larger and more floppy epiglottis in the child; (4) the cricoid ring is the narrowest portion of the pediatric airway versus the vocal cords in the adult; (5) position and size of the cricothyroid membrane in the infant; (6) sharper, more difficult angle for blind nasotracheal intubation; and (7) larger relative size of the occiput in the infant.

### *Physiologic Issues*

There are two important physiologic differences between children and adults that impact airway management (**Box 24-1**). Children have a basal oxygen consumption that is approximately twice that of adults. Coupled with a proportionally smaller functional residual capacity (FRC) to body weight ratio, these factors result in more rapid desaturation in children compared with adults, given an equivalent duration of preoxygenation. Rapid desaturation is most pronounced in children less than 24 months old. The clinician must anticipate and communicate this possibility to the staff and be prepared to provide supplemental oxygen by BMV if the patient's oxygen saturation drops below 90%.

BOX **24-1**

**Physiologic differences.**

| Physiologic Difference | Significance |
|---|---|
| Basal $O_2$ consumption is twice adult values (>6 mL/kg/min). Proportionally smaller FRC as compared with adults | Shortened period of protection from hypoxia for equivalent preoxygenation time as compared with adults. Infants and small children often require BMV while maintaining cricoid pressure to avoid hypoxia |

## Drug Dosage and Selection

The dose of succinylcholine (SCh) in children is different from that in adults. SCh is rapidly metabolized by plasma esterases and distributed to extracellular water. Children have a larger volume of extracellular fluid water relative to adults: at birth, 45%; at age 2 months, approximately 30%; at age 6 years, 20%; and at adulthood, 16% to 18%. The recommended dose of SCh, therefore, is higher on a per kilogram basis in children than in adults (2 vs. 1.5 mg per kg). All drug dosage determinations are most appropriately and safely done using resuscitation aids such as the Broselow–Luten system previously described.

In 1993, the U.S. Food and Drug Administration (FDA), in conjunction with pharmaceutical companies, revised the package labeling for SCh in the wake of reports of hyperkalemic cardiac arrest following the administration of SCh to patients with previously undiagnosed neuromuscular disease. Initially, it stated that SCh was contraindicated for elective anesthesia in pediatric patients because of this concern, although the wording was subsequently altered to embrace a risk–benefit analysis when deciding to use SCh in children. However, both the initial advisory warning and the revised warning continue to recommend SCh for emergency or full-stomach intubation in children. Pediatric drug doses are provided in Table 24-3.

## Equipment Selection

Table 24-1 references length-based recommendations for emergency equipment in pediatric patients. Appropriately sized equipment can be chosen with a centimeter length measurement or with a Broselow tape.

*A word of caution with respect to the storage of airway management equipment for children*: Despite best efforts (e.g., equipment lists or periodic checks), it is not uncommon for newborn equipment to be mixed in with or placed in proximity to the smallest pediatric equipment. This practice may lead to newborn equipment being used in older children for whom it may not function properly or may, in fact, be dangerous. Examples include the no. 0 laryngoscope blade,

TABLE 24-3 Drugs—Pediatric Considerations

| Drug | Dosage | Pediatric-Specific Comments |
|---|---|---|
| **Premedications** | | |
| Atropine | 0.02 mg/kg | An option <1 y of age |
| **Induction agents** | | |
| Midazolam | 0.3 mg/kg IV | Use 0.1 mg/kg if hypotensive |
| Thiopental | 3–5 mg/kg IV | Lower dose to 1 mg/kg or delete if perfusion poor |
| Etomidate | 0.3 mg/kg IV | |
| Ketamine | 2 mg/kg IV, 4 mg/kg IM | |
| Propofol | 2–3 mg/kg IV | |
| **Paralytics** | | |
| SCh | 2 mg/kg IV | Have atropine drawn up and ready |
| Vecuronium | 0.2 mg/kg IV | May increase to 0.3 mg/kg of vecuronium for RSI (0.1 mg/kg for maintenance of paralysis) |
| Rocuronium | 1.0 mg/kg IV | For RSI |

which is too short to allow visualization of the airway; the 250-mL newborn BMV, which provides inadequate ventilation volumes; and various other equipments, such as oral airways that can cause airway obstruction if too small, or a curved laryngoscope blade that may not reach and pick up the relatively large epiglottis, or effectively remove the large tongue from the laryngoscopic view of the airway (see **Table 24-4**).

1. **Endotracheal tubes**

   The correct endotracheal tube (ETT) size for the patient can be determined by a length measurement and by referring to the equipment selection chart. The formula (16 + age in years)/4 is also a reasonably accurate method of determining the correct tube size. However, the formula cannot be used in children younger than 1 year and is only useful if an accurate age is known, which cannot always be determined in an emergency. Either cuffed or uncuffed ETTs are acceptable in the younger pediatric age groups, and cuffed tubes are used for size 5.5 mm and up (**Fig. 24-3**). The admonition to avoid cuffed tubes in young infants is historical and in the past, there was an unacceptably high rate of subglottic stenosis resulting from failure to carefully monitor cuff pressures. Newer ETTs make it easier to monitor cuff pressures and can be safely used in infants and small children, provided clinicians recognize the following fact: A cuffed tube adds 0.5 mm to the internal diameter (ID), so a smaller than predicted (by 0.5 mm) tube may be required. The cuffed tube should be placed with the cuff deflated initially and inflated with the minimum volume of air needed to affect an adequate seal.

   When intubating a young child, there is a tendency to insert the ETT too far, usually into the right mainstem bronchus. Various formulas can be used to determine the correct insertion distance (e.g., tube size times 3; age/2 + 10). For example, a 3.5-mm ID tube should be inserted 3.5 × 3 = 10.5 cm at the lip. Alternatively, a length-based chart can be used. We recommend placing a piece of tape on the tube at the appropriate lip-to-tip centimeter line, which serves as a constant reminder of the correct position of the tip of the ET tube in the intubated patient.

TABLE 24-4 Dangerous Equipment

| Equipment | Problem |
|---|---|
| No. 0 or no. 00 laryngoscope ETT blades | Valuable time can be lost trying to visualize the glottic opening if mistaken for a no. 1 blade |
| Curved no. 1 laryngoscope blades | Straight blades are preferred because of the following:<br>The epiglottis is picked up directly, not indirectly, by compressing the hyoepiglottic ligament in the vallecula<br>The tongue and mandibular anatomy are more easily elevated from the field of vision |
| 250-mL BMV | Cannot generate adequate tidal volumes |
| Cuffed ET tubes < 5.0 mm | If leak pressures are not monitored, ischemia of the tracheal mucosa may develop with the potential for scarring and stenosis |
| Oral airways < 50 mm | Unless appropriate size oral airways are used, they may act to increase, rather than relieve, obstruction |
| Any *other* equipment too small | Sizing is critical to function! |

Note: Only appropriate size is functional. Frequently, very small sizes are placed in the pediatric area without attention to appropriateness of size. This can greatly contribute to a failed airway outcome.

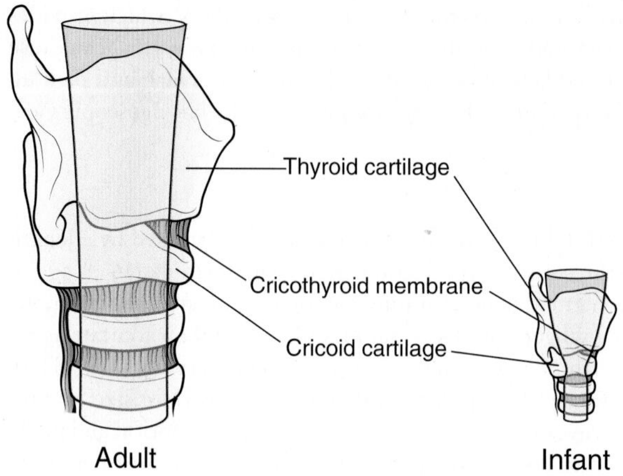


● **FIGURE 24-3. Airway Shape.** Note the position of the narrowest portion of the pediatric airway, which is at the cricoid ring, creating a funnel shape, versus the cylindrical shape seen in the adult, where the vocal cords form the narrowest portion. This is the rationale for using the uncuffed tube in the child; it fits snugly, unlike the cuffed tube used in the adult, which is inflated once the tube passes the cords to produce a snug fit. (Modified with permission from Cote CJ, Todres ID. The pediatric airway. In: Cote CJ, Ryan JF, Todres ID, et al, eds. *A Practice of Anesthesia for Infants and Children*. 2nd ed. Philadelphia, PA: WB Saunders; 1993.)

2. **Tube-securing devices**

An all too frequent complication following intubation is inadvertent extubation. ETTs must be secured at the mouth. Head and neck movement, particularly extension which translates into movement of the tube up and potentially out of the trachea, should be minimized. A cervical collar placed after intubation prevents flexion and extension and therefore can help prevent ETT dislodgement (**Fig. 24-4**). The ETT is traditionally secured by taping the tube to the cheek, although various commercial devices are also available.

3. **Oxygen masks**

The simple rebreather mask used for most patients provides a maximum of 35% to 60% oxygen and requires a flow rate of 6 to 10 L per minute. A non-rebreather mask can provide approximately 70% oxygen in children if a flow rate of 10 to 15 L per minute is used. For emergency airway

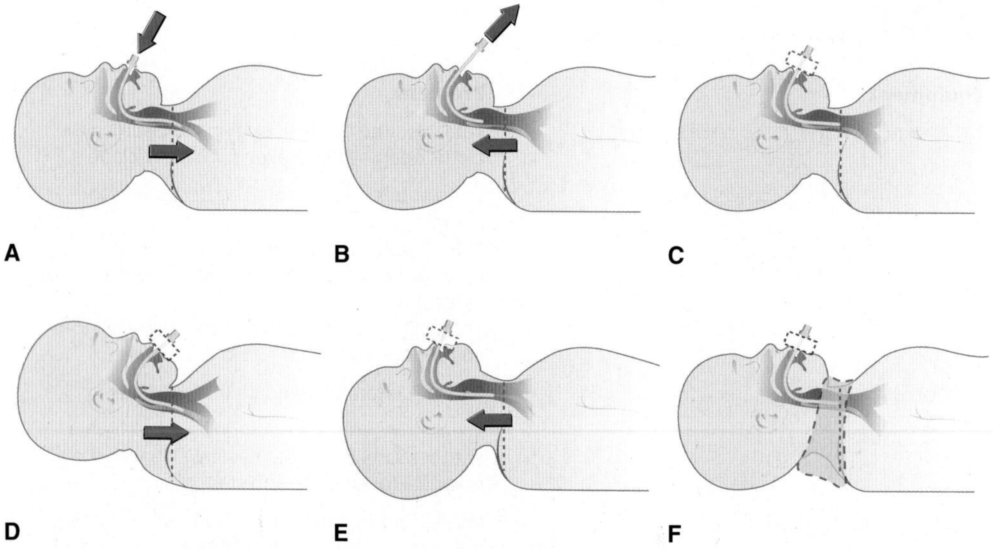


● **FIGURE 24-4. Securing the ET Tube. A:** Unsecured tube sliding in/down. **B:** Unsecured tube sliding out/up. **C:** Tube secured to prevent in/out, up/down movement. **D:** Secured tube moving down and in as head flexes. **E:** Secured tube moving up/out as head extends. **F:** Neck movement prevented by cervical collar, thus preventing tube movement in the trachea.

management, and particularly for preoxygenation for rapid sequence intubation (RSI), the pediatric non-rebreather mask is preferable. Adult non-rebreather masks can be used for older children, but are too large to be used for infants and small children and will entrain significant amounts of "room" air. Apneic oxygenation (see Chapter 5) should be considered in children (at a rate of 1 L per min per year of age) as a low-risk maneuver to prolong safe apnea time. Recent evidence suggests that, in adults, turning the oxygen flow rate to the "flush" rate of 40 to 70 L per minute (varies depending on the wall spigot) increases $FIO_2$ (>90%) and end-tidal oxygen measurements. This has not been studied in children, but may be reasonable to try if preoxygenation is difficult. Additionally, properly configured bag-mask systems (i.e., those that function as one-way inspiratory and expiratory valves and small dead space) are capable of delivering oxygen concentrations >90%, if correctly used. The spontaneously breathing patient opens the duck-billed inspiratory valve on inspiration, and on expiration, the expired volume with carbon dioxide ($CO_2$) pinches the duckbill valve closed and is vented through the expiratory valve into the atmosphere. Adult-type units tend not to be used in infants and small children because of dead space considerations and size-related awkwardness, leading some to prefer pediatric non-rebreather masks.

4. **Oral airways**

   Oral airways should only be used in children who are unconscious. In the conscious or semiconscious child, these airways can incite vomiting. Oral airways can be selected based on the Broselow tape measurement or can be approximated by selecting an oral airway that fits the distance from the angle of the mouth to the tragus of the ear.

5. **Nasopharyngeal airways**

   Nasopharyngeal airways are helpful in the obtunded but responsive child. The correctly sized nasopharyngeal airway is the largest one that comfortably fits in the naris but does not produce blanching of the nasal skin. The correct length is from the tip of the nose to the tragus of the ear and usually corresponds to the nasopharyngeal airway with the correct diameter. Care must be taken to suction these airways regularly to avoid blockage.

6. **Nasogastric tubes**

   BMV may lead to insufflation of the stomach, hindering full diaphragmatic excursion and preventing effective ventilation. A nasogastric (NG) tube should be placed soon after intubation to decompress the stomach in any patient who has undergone BMV and requires ongoing mechanical ventilation postintubation. Often in such patients, the abdomen is distended or tense, making the problem obvious, but other times it is difficult to identify the difference between this and the normally protuberant abdomen of the young child. Difficulty in ventilation that is felt to be related to reduced compliance should prompt the placement of an NG tube. Length-based systems identify the appropriate NG tube size.

7. **BMV equipment**

   For emergency airway management, the self-inflating bag is preferred by most over the anesthesia ventilation bag. These bag-mask units should have an oxygen reservoir so that at 10 to 15 L of oxygen flow, one can provide a $FIO_2$ of 90% to 95%. The smallest bag that should be used is 450 mL. Neonatal bags that are smaller (250 mL) do not provide effective tidal volume even for small infants. Many of the pediatric BMV devices have a positive-pressure relief (pop-off) valve. The pop-off valve may be set by the manufacturer to open at anywhere between 20 and 45 cm of water pressure (CWP), depending on whether the bag unit is intended for infants or small children (respectively) and is used to prevent barotrauma. Emergency airway management often requires higher peak airway pressures, so the bag should be configured without a pop-off valve or with a pop-off valve that can be closed. Practically, it is a good practice to store the BMV device with the pop-off valve closed so that initial attempts to ventilate the patient can achieve sufficient peak airway pressure to achieve ventilation. Chapter 25 discusses this issue in more detail and offers suggestions to prevent its occurrence.

8. **End-tidal $CO_2$ detectors**

   Colorimetric end-tidal $CO_2$ ($ETCO_2$) detectors are as useful in children as in adults. A pediatric size exists for children weighing <15 kg, while the adult model should be used for children weighing >15 kg. If an adult-sized $ETCO_2$ device is used inappropriately for a small child, there may be insufficient $CO_2$ volumes to cause the detector to change color,

TABLE 24-5 Alternatives for Airway Support

| | |
|---|---|
| BMV | May be the most reliable temporizing measure in children. Equipment selection, adjuncts, and good technique are essential |
| Orotracheal intubation (usually with RSI) | Still the procedure of choice for emergent airway in potential cervical spine injury and most other circumstances |
| Needle cricothyrotomy | Recommended as last resort in infants and children, but data lacking |
| Laryngeal mask | Viable alternative |
| Blind nasotracheal intubation | Not indicated for children younger than 10 y |
| GlideScope | Well studied in adults, a potential alternative in children |

resulting in a false-negative reading and removal of a correctly placed tube. Conversely, the resistance in a pediatric $ETCO_2$ detector may be sufficiently high to make ventilation difficult in a larger child.

9. **Airway alternatives** (Table 24-5)

Orotracheal intubation is the procedure of choice for pediatric emergency airway management including those patients with potential cervical spine injury where RSI with in-line manual stabilization is preferred. Nasotracheal intubation is relatively contraindicated in children.

Cricothyrotomy is the preferred emergency surgical airway in adults. The cricothyroid space emerges as one ages and is really only accessible after the age of 10 years. "Needle cricothyrotomy" in children younger than 10 years is the term used when one accesses the airway in a percutaneous manner in young children, even though it is recognized that the point of entry into the airway is often the trachea as opposed to the cricothyroid space.

Other devices that may be of use in failed airway management in young children are laryngeal mask airways (LMAs) and the GlideScope. LMAs are made for even newborns and young infants and may be useful as a temporizing measure when direct laryngoscopy proves difficult. The GlideScope is supplied in sizes appropriate for pediatric patients, although currently the penetration of this technology to all clinical settings has not occurred. These and other adjuncts are discussed in Chapter 25.

## INITIATION OF MECHANICAL VENTILATION

In emergency pediatrics, two modes of ventilation are used. Pressure-limited ventilation is the mode used for newborns and small infants, whereas volume-limited ventilation is used for older children and adults. One can arbitrarily set 10 kg as the weight below which pressure-limited ventilators should be used, although volume-limited ventilators have been used effectively in smaller children. Generally speaking, the younger the child is, the more rapid the ventilatory rate. The initial ventilatory rate in infants is typically set between 20 and 25 breaths per minute. Inspiratory:expiratory ratios are set at 1:2, and the typical peak inspiratory pressure at initiation of ventilation is between 15 and 20 CWP. These initial settings in a pressure-controlled ventilation mode will usually give a tidal volume of 8 to 12 mL per kg. These initial settings are adjusted according to subsequent clinical evaluation and chest rise. Positive end-expiratory pressure should also be set at 3 to 5 cm of water and $FIO_2$ at 1.0. The Broselow–Luten length-based system also provides guidance for approximate starting tidal volumes, ventilator rates, and inspiratory times.

**TABLE 24-6** Initiation of Mechanical Ventilation

| | | |
|---|---|---|
| **I.** Initial settings | | |
| Ventilator type | Pressure limited | Volume limited |
| Respiratory rate | 20–25/min | 12–20/min, by age |
| Positive end-expiratory pressure (cm $H_2O$) | 3–5 | 3–5 |
| $FIO_2$ | 1.0 (100%) | 1.0 (100%) |
| Inspiratory time | ≥0.6 s | ≥0.6 s |
| Inspiratory/expiratory ratio | 1:2 | 1:2 |
| Pressure/volume settings | For pressure ventilation, start with peak inspiratory pressure (PIP) of 15–20 cm $H_2O$. Assess chest rise and adjust to higher pressures as needed. For volume ventilation, start with tidal volumes of 8–12 mL/kg. Start at lower volumes and increase to a PIP of 20–30 cm $H_2O$. *These are initial setting guidelines only. Assess chest rise and adjust accordingly* | |
| **II.** Evaluate clinically and make adjustments | Most patients will be ventilated with volume-cycled ventilators. Poor chest rise, poor color, and decreased breath sounds require *higher* tidal volume. Check for pneumothorax or blocked tube. Ensure that tube size and position are optimal and leaks are not present. For patients ventilated with pressure-cycled ventilators, these findings may indicate the need to increase the PIP | |
| **III.** Laboratory information | Arterial blood gas should be performed approximately 10–15 min after settings are stabilized. Additional samples may be necessary after each ventilator adjustment, unless ventilatory status is monitored by $ETCO_2$ and $SpO_2$ | |

Once initial settings have been established, it is critical that the patient be quickly reevaluated and adjustments made, particularly as pulmonary compliance, airways resistance, and leak volumes change with time, precluding adequate ventilation with the initial settings of pressure-controlled ventilation. Clinical evaluation of ventilatory adequacy is more important than formulae to ensure adequate ventilation. Once adjustments are made and the patient appears clinically to be ventilated and oxygenating, blood gas determinations, or continuous pulse oximetry and $ETCO_2$ monitoring, should be used for confirmation and to guide additional adjustments (**Table 24-6** and **Box 24-2**).

## RSI TECHNIQUES FOR CHILDREN

The procedure of RSI in children is essentially the same as in adults, with a few important differences outlined as follows:

1. Preparation
   - Use resuscitation aids that address age- and size-related issues in drug dosing and equipment selection (e.g., Broselow–Luten tape).

BOX 24-2

**Emergency pediatric airway management–practical considerations.**

Anatomical

- Anticipate high anterior glottic opening
- Do not hyperextend the neck
- Uncuffed tubes are used in children younger than 8 years
- Use straight blades in young children

Physiologic

- Anticipate desaturation

Drug dosage and equipment selection

- Use length-based system. Do *not* use memory or do calculations
- NG tube is an important airway adjunct in infants
- Stock pediatric non-rebreather masks

Airway alternatives for failed or difficult airway

- Surgical cricothyrotomy–contraindicated until age 10 years
- Blind nasotracheal intubation–contraindicated until age 10 years
- Combitube–only if >4 ft tall
- Needle cricothyrotomy–acceptable

2. Preoxygenation
   - Be meticulous. Children desaturate more rapidly than adults do.
   - Consider apneic oxygenation as an adjunct to maximize safe apnea time.
3. Preintubation optimization
   - Weight-based isotonic fluid boluses or blood for hypotension. Maximize preoxygenation efforts. Consider atropine for infants <1 year of age.
4. Paralysis with induction
   - Induction agent selection as for adult: dose by length or weight.
   - SCh 2 mg per kg IV or rocuronium 1 mg per kg.
   - Anticipate desaturation; bag ventilate if oxygen saturation ($Spo_2$) is <90%.
5. Positioning with protection
   - Optional: apply Sellick maneuver.
6. Placement with proof
   - Confirm tube placement with $ETCO_2$ as for adult.
7. Postintubation management

   Ventilation guidelines have already been mentioned . In almost all cases, children who are intubated and mechanically ventilated should be sedated and paralyzed in the emergency department to prevent deleterious rises in intracranial or intrathoracic pressures and inadvertent ETT dislodgement.

## EVIDENCE

- **Is lack of experience in managing pediatric airways a major problem for Emergency Providers?** Since the inception of Emergency Medicine as a specialty, there has been a concern over the amount of training emergency medicine residents received in pediatrics.[1] The exposure to critically ill children has been lacking compared to the adult experience.[2,3] Introduction of the pneumococcal and *Haemophilus influenzae* vaccines, the change in sleep position which has reduced sudden infant death syndrome deaths, and the overall improvement in pediatric care have further reduced ED visits for acute respiratory events. A recent article from a large children's hospital with >90,000 ED visits a year demonstrated insufficient exposure to critical procedures, especially intubations.[4] Informal surveys from the *Difficult Airway Course: Emergency* reveal that emergency physician's experience and comfort with pediatric airways is woefully lacking. It is hoped that the focused education and training in the airway course, and other high-quality simulation programs, can bolster comfort levels.[5]

- **What are the particular barriers to successful airway management in children?** Time delay and cognitive errors are more common with pediatric emergency airway management.[6] Pediatric emergencies are complicated by the fact that children vary in size, creating logistical difficulties, especially with respect to drug dosing and equipment selection. This mental burden (or "cognitive load") can be reduced by the use of resuscitation aids which save time and reduce errors. A review analyzed the effect of these variables on the mental burden in the resuscitative process and demonstrated how resuscitation aids can help mitigate their effect.[7] Simulated emergency patient encounters have confirmed that the Broselow–Luten color-coded emergency system reduces time delay and errors by eliminating the cognitive burden associated with these situations.[8]

  To the extent that the process can be simplified (e.g., limiting the number of recommended medications, reducing the complexity and number of decisions required), time is freed up for critical thinking that can then be dedicated to the priorities of airway management. The management of children in extremis can be stressful, and as such, RSI should be kept simple and uncomplicated to reduce this stress.
- **Should atropine be used for RSI in children?** The evidence does not support the universal use of atropine in children; however, it is an issue that is difficult to definitively resolve based on current literature. Traditionally, atropine has been used to prevent the bradycardia associated with a single dose of SCh in children, a rare but serious event. A few recent studies failed to show a difference in response to SCh with or without atropine in children,[9,10] with similar numbers in the atropine- and nonatropine-treated groups developing transient, self-limited decreases in heart rate. The absence of evidence of benefit, however, should not be construed as "proof" when dealing with uncommon events. Atropine also has significant, but rare side effects including paradoxical bradycardia if incorrectly dosed.[11] Atropine may have a role when manipulating the airway of infants younger than 1 year because of their disproportionate predominance in vagal tone, coupled with a relatively greater dependency on heart rate for cardiac output.[12] However, most bradycardic episodes are because of hypoxia or are a transient, vagally mediated reflex response that resolves spontaneously. It is better to treat the hypoxia or the reflex if it occurs.

  In an effort to keep the process of RSI in children as simple as possible, we are not recommending the routine use of atropine. In special circumstances, such as with infants younger than 1 year (3, 4, and 5 kg, and pink or red zones on the Broselow–Luten tape and airway card), atropine can be considered optional.
- **SCh versus rocuronium as a paralytic in children—which is the preferred agent?** In the 1990s, the FDA warned against the use of SCh in children following case reports of hyperkalemic cardiac arrest following the administration of SCh to patients with undiagnosed neuromuscular disease. The pediatric anesthesia community at that time challenged the FDA decision on the basis of the risk versus benefit in patients requiring emergency intubation, leading to a modification of their position to a "caution." There is no body of evidence that specifically addresses the relative risks and benefits of SCh versus rocuronium in children to guide recommendations.

  Currently, SCh remains the agent of choice for emergency full-stomach intubations.[13,14] Although rocuronium is preferred in pediatrics by some practitioners, for simplicity's sake, we recommend SCh as first-line treatment for adults and children.
- **Are cuffed ETTs contraindicated in pediatric emergency airway management?** The issue of whether cuffed ETTs are safe or required in children younger than 8 to 10 years has

been debated for some time because of the anatomical and functional seal afforded by the subglottic area. Two studies have addressed this issue.[15,16] Deakers et al. studied 282 patients intubated in the operating room, emergency department, or ICU. In their observational prospective, nonrandomized study, they found no difference in postextubation stridor, the need for reintubation, or long-term upper airway complications. Khine et al.[16] compared the incidence of postextubation croup, inadequate ventilation, anesthetic gases leaking into the environment, and the requirement for a tube change resulting from air leak. In this study of children younger than 8 years, the authors found no difference in croup, more attempts at intubation with uncuffed tubes, less gas flow required with cuffed tubes, or less gas leakage into the environment.

Even though it may seem that the use of cuffed tubes in younger children does not result in any postextubation sequelae, it must be made clear that these studies monitored cuff inflation pressures, a practice that is uncommonly performed in emergency intubations. For this reason, it seems reasonable to recommend the use of uncuffed ETTs to avoid excessive tracheal mucosal pressure with the potential sequelae of scarring and stenosis. However, for some patients in whom high mean airway pressures are expected, such as those with acute respiratory diseases and asthma, the placement of a cuffed tube with the cuff initially deflated, and inflated if necessary, may be appropriate. The most recent Pediatric Advanced Life Support standards recommend cuffed tubes, but with the qualifier *only if leak pressures are monitored.*[17]

- **Why do children desaturate more quickly than adults with comparable degrees of preoxygenation?** An infant uses 6 mL of oxygen/kg/minute as compared with the adult who uses 3 mL/kg/minute. The FRC reduction in an apneic child is far greater than in the apneic adult. This is because of the differences in the elastic forces of the chest wall and the lung. In children, the chest wall is more compliant, and the lung elastic recoil is less than in adults. An analysis of these forces reveals that if they are brought into equilibrium as in the apneic patient, a value of FRC around 10% of total lung capacity is predicted instead of the observed value of slightly <40%. These same factors also reduce the FRC in the spontaneously breathing patient, albeit to a lesser degree. FRC is further reduced with the induction of anesthesia and by the supine position. The clinical implication of the decreased effective FRC combined with increased oxygen consumption is that the preoxygenated, paralyzed infant has a disproportionately smaller reservoir of intrapulmonary oxygen to draw on as compared with the adult. Pulmonary pathology in critically ill patients may further reduce the ability to preoxygenate. It is therefore critical that these factors be considered when preoxygenating a pediatric patient. BMV with cricoid pressure may be required to maintain oxygen saturation above 90% during RSI, especially if multiple attempts are required or the child has a disorder that compromises the ability to preoxygenate.[18,19]

## REFERENCES


1. Tamariz VP, Fuchs S, Baren JM, et al. Pediatric emergency medicine education in emergency medicine training programs. *Acad Emerg Med*. 2000;7(7):774–778.
2. Chen EH, Cho CS, Shofer FS, et al. Resident exposure to critical patients in the ED. *Pediatr Emerg Care*. 2007;11:774–778.
3. Miele NF. Inadequate exposure to pediatric patients in the ED. *Acad Emerg Med*. 2004;11(7):771–773.
4. Mittiga MR, Geis GL, Kerrey BT, et al. The spectrum and frequency of critical procedures in a pediatric emergency department: implications of a provider-level view. *Ann Emerg Med*. 2013;61(3):263–270.
5. Overly FL, Sudikoff SN, Shapiro MJ. High-fidelity medical simulation as an assessment tool for pediatric residents airway skills. *Pediatr Emerg Care*. 2007;1:11–15.
6. Oakley P. Inaccuracy and delay in decision making in pediatric resuscitation, and a proposed reference chart to reduce error. *Br Med J*. 1988;297:817–819.

7. Luten R, Wears R, Broselow J, et al. Managing the unique size related issues of pediatric resuscitation: reducing cognitive load with resuscitation aids. *Acad Emerg Med*. 2002;9:840–847.
8. Shah AN, Frush KS. Reduction in error severity associated with use of a pediatric medication dosing system: a crossover trial. Presented at the AAP 2001 National Conference and Exhibition, Section on Critical Care; October 2001; San Francisco, CA.
9. McAuliffe G, Bisonnette B, Boutin C. Should the routine use of atropine before succinylcholine in children be reconsidered? *Can J Anaesth*. 1995;42:724–729.
10. Fleming B, McCollough M, Henderson SO. Myth: atropine should be administered before succinylcholine for neonatal and pediatric intubation. *CJEM*. 2005;7:114–117.
11. Tsou CH, Chiang CE, Kao T, et al. Atropine-triggered idiopathic ventricular tachycardia in an asymptomatic pediatric patient. *Can J Anaesth*. 2004;51:856–857.
12. Rothrock SG, Pagane J. Pediatric rapid sequence intubation incidence of reflex bradycardia and effects of pretreatment with atropine. *Pediatr Emerg Care*. 2005;21:637–638.
13. Robinson AL, Jerwood DC, Stokes MA. Routine suxamethonium in children: a regional survey of current usage. *Anaesthesia*. 1996;51:874–878.
14. Weir PS. Anaesthesia for appendicectomy in childhood: a survey of practice in Northern Ireland. *Ulster Med J*. 1997;66:34–37.
15. Deakers TW, Reynolds G, Stretton M, et al. Cuffed endotracheal tubes in pediatric intensive care. *J Pediatr*. 1994;125:57–62.
16. Khine HH, Corddry DH, Kettrick RG, et al. Comparison of cuffed and uncuffed endotracheal tubes in young children during general anesthesia. *Anesthesiology*. 1997;86:627–631.
17. American Heart Association. Pediatric advanced life support. *Circulation*. 2005;112:IV-167–IV-187.
18. Agostoni E, Hyatt R: Static behavior of the respiratory system. In: *Handbook of Physiology. The Respiratory System*. Section III. Edited by Fishman A, Macklem P, Mead J, Geiger S. Bethesda, Maryland: American Physiological Society 1986,113:113–130.
19. Lumb A. Elastic forces and lung volumes. In: James E, ed. *Nunn's Applied Respiratory Physiology*. 5th ed. Oxford, England: Butterworth-Heineman; 2000:51–53.

Chapter 25

# Pediatric Airway Techniques

Robert C. Luten, Steven A. Godwin, and Nathan W. Mick

## INTRODUCTION

For the most part, the airway devices and techniques used in older children and adolescents are no different from those used in adults. The same cannot be said of small children (younger than 3 years) and infants (younger than 1 year), mostly related to two factors: the airway anatomy in these age groups is substantially different from the adult form, and some of the commonly used rescue devices are not available in pediatric sizes (e.g., Combitube, LMA Fastrach). We limit our discussion to those rescue devices that are available for the pediatric population *and* that have evidence of successful use in children.

Mastering these techniques is straightforward and necessary if one is to manage the emergent pediatric airway. The following discussion describes the appropriate use of the various airway modalities in pediatrics, with emphasis on age appropriateness.

## TECHNIQUES USED IN ALL CHILDREN

### Bag-Mask Ventilation and Endotracheal Intubation

Refer to Chapters 9 and 13 for a detailed description of bag-mask ventilation (BMV) and endotracheal intubation. As in adults, nasopharyngeal and oral airways are important adjuncts to BMV, especially in small children in whom the tongue is relatively large in relation to the volume of the oral cavity. Recommendations and the rationale for the use of specific equipment (curved or straight blades, cuffed vs. uncuffed tubes) are described in Chapter 24. Use of size-appropriate equipment for pediatric airway management is critical to success, even in the most experienced hands. Proper BMV technique is particularly important in pediatric patients because the indication for intervention is most often primarily related to a respiratory disorder, and the child is likely to be hypoxic. In addition, pediatric patients are subject to more rapid oxyhemoglobin desaturation, so that BMV with cricoid pressure (Sellick maneuver) applied to prevent gastric insufflation is frequently required during the preoxygenation and paralysis phases of rapid sequence intubation. Pediatric BMV requires smaller tidal volumes, higher rates, and size-specific equipment. The pediatric airway is particularly amenable to positive-pressure ventilation, even in the presence of upper airway obstruction (see Chapters 24 and 26).

## *Tips for Successful BMV Ventilation in Children*

Although BMV in the pediatric population fails infrequently, attention to detail remains critical to success: the mask seal must be adequate, the airway open, and the rate and volume of ventilation appropriate to the patient's age. Two errors of technique tend to occur. First, there is a tendency in the excitement of the situation to press the mask portion of the unit downward in an attempt to obtain a tight seal, resulting in neck flexion and upper airway obstruction. The head should be extended slightly rather than flexed, thereby relieving, rather than producing, obstruction caused by the tongue and the relaxed pharyngeal anatomy (**Fig. 25-1**).

Second, there is a tendency to bag at an excessive rate. The cadence for bagging should permit adequate time for exhalation (actually repeating the words "squeeze, release, release" is helpful to assure adequate cadence). Textbooks recommend faster rates for smaller children. From a practical point of view, however, this cadence can be used for all ages. Always place an oral airway in the unconscious child before ventilating with a bag and mask because the pediatric tongue is large relative to the size of the oropharynx and is more prone to obstruct the upper airway.

The positioning described in the previous paragraph is usually obtained while applying the one-handed, C-grip technique to the mask. The thumb and index finger support the mask from the bridge of the nose to the cleft of the chin, avoiding the eyes. The bony prominences of the chin are lifted up by the rest of the fingers, placing the head in mild extension to form the sniffing position. Care is taken to avoid pressure on the airway anteriorly to prevent collapsing and obstructing the pliable trachea.

The two-handed technique can also be used. While this technique is critical for successful rescue mask ventilation of adults, it may be selectively applied in small children. By opening the jaw slightly and pulling it forward, an obstruction may be relieved. The jaw can be moved further forward after opening the mouth slightly ("translating the mandible" forward; see Chapter 9), while using the thenar eminences of the palm to seal the mask on the face. The thenar grip is more effective at creating a uniform seal and minimizing leak around the margin of the mask. Once the mask is applied, a second provider squeezes the bag. If ventilation is not immediately facilitated with these maneuvers, positioning should be reassessed and a nasopharyngeal airway be placed to supplement the oropharyngeal airway.

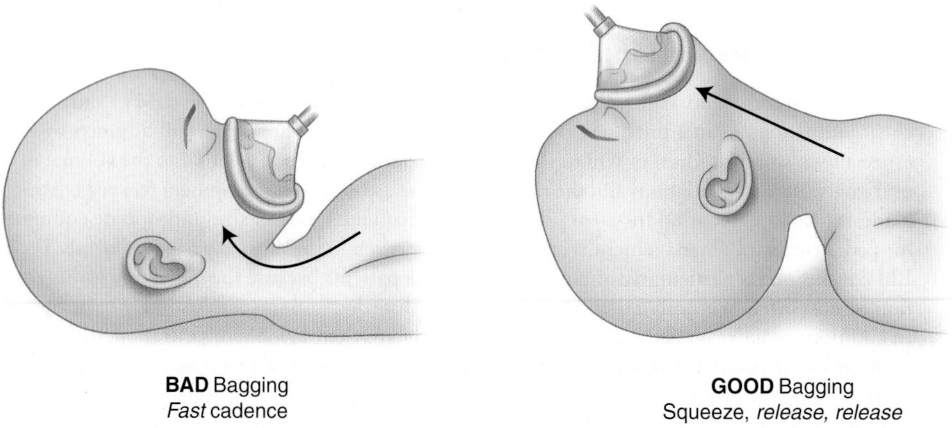


● **FIGURE 25-1. A:** *Bad* bagging. Fast cadence. **B:** *Good* bagging. Squeeze, release, release. Part A demonstrates the flexed position causing obstruction, whereas Part B demonstrates extended position which relieves obstruction.

## *Tips for Successful Endotracheal Intubation in Children*

### Preintubation

1. *Position correctly:* Proper patient positioning is key to prevent obstruction and provide optimal alignment of the axes of the airway. Optimal alignment of the laryngeal, pharyngeal, and oral axes in adults usually requires elevation of the occiput to flex the neck on the torso and extend the head at the atlanto-occipital joint. Because of the larger relative size of the occiput in small children, elevation of the occiput is usually unnecessary, and extension of the head may actually cause obstruction. Slight anterior displacement of the atlanto-occipital junction is all that is needed (i.e., pulling up on the chin to create the sniffing position). In small infants, elevation of the shoulders with a towel may be needed to counteract the effect of the large occiput that causes the head to flex forward on the chest. As a general rule, once correctly positioned, the external auditory canal should lie just anterior to the shoulders. Whether this position requires support beneath the occiput (older child/adult), the shoulders (small infant), or no support (small child) (**Fig. 25-2A**) can be determined using this rule of thumb. These are guidelines only, and each individual patient is different. A quick trial may be required to find the optimal position. **Figure 25-2B** demonstrates the most common position for intubating the small child, the so-called sniffing position, and how this is achieved in a child of this size.

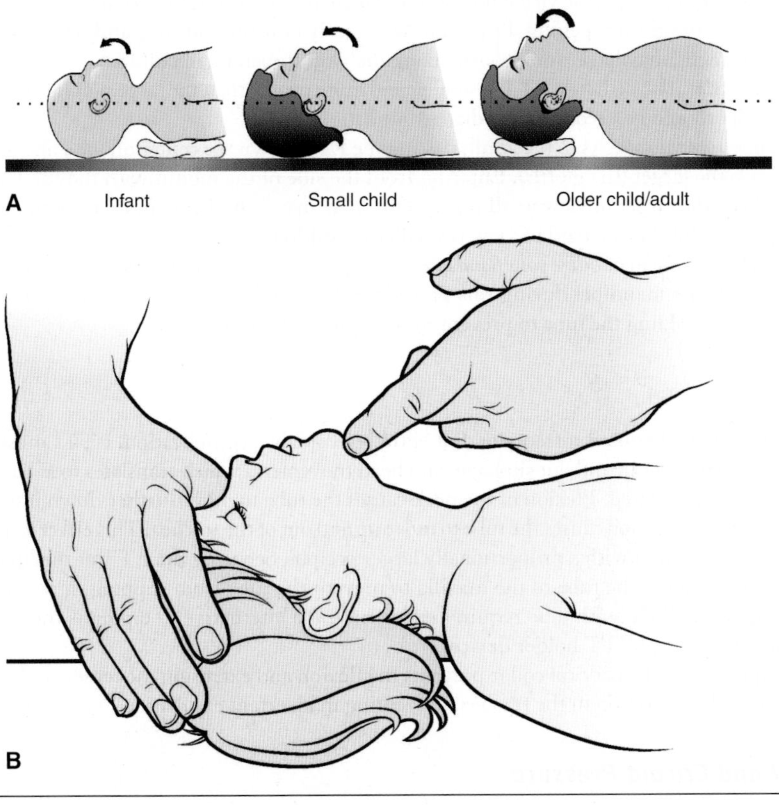


● **FIGURE 25-2. A:** Clinical determination of optimal airway alignment, using a line passing through the external auditory canal and anterior to the shoulder **B:** Application of the line to determine optimal position. In this small child, the occiput obviates the need for head support, yet the occiput is not so large as to require support of the shoulders. Note that a line traversing the external auditory canal will pass anterior to the shoulders. With only slight extension of the head on the atlanto-occipital joint, the sniffing position is achieved.

Even with optimal positioning, external manipulation of the airway (e.g., backward, upward [cephalad], and rightward pressure maneuver) may increase visualization of the glottis. This may be especially helpful in small children who have anterior airways and trauma patients who cannot be optimally aligned.

2. *Mark lip-to-tip distance with tape:* The endotracheal tube (ETT) has centimeter markings along its length. The lip-to-tip distance is the distance from the lip to a point half way between the vocal cords and the carina (i.e., midtrachea), which represents ideal positioning of the ETT in the trachea. Before a pediatric intubation, the ETT should be marked clearly with tape at the appropriate lip-to-tip distance. This will serve as a visual reminder to the intubator as to the correct ETT insertion depth for this patient.
3. *Always select one tube size larger and one tube size smaller than the predicted tube size:* Note all three tubes are taped at the same predicted lip-to-tip distance. The lip-to-tip distance is constant for a given patient and does not change if a smaller tube or larger tube is used. As a rule of thumb, three times the predicted ETT size is used to estimate the lip-to-tip distance; for example, for a 3.5-mm ETT, the lip-to-tip distance would be 10.5 cm. Should a smaller tube actually be used because of a traumatized, narrowed glottic opening, recalculation of the lip-to-tip distance using the smaller diameter would result in an incorrect distance.

### *Direct Laryngoscopy*

1. *Look up not deep:* The pediatric airway lies higher in the neck than the adult airway. When doing direct laryngoscopy, the visual line of sight angle must be adjusted so that the intubator can *look up* to see the glottic opening. Physicians who rarely intubate children, and who fail to make this adjustment, may have trouble visualizing the glottic opening in children.
2. *Use a stylet:* The pediatric ETT is smaller and more pliable than the larger adult tubes. Therefore, a stylet should be used for all pediatric intubations.
3. *Enter from the side:* As in the adult, passing the ETT down the center of one's line of sight obliterates the target (the glottis). Entering from the side of the mouth with the ETT permits one to keep the target in view at all times. This maneuver is probably more important in children than in adults as the field of view is smaller in children.
4. *Use the maxilla to stabilize your hand after passing the ETT:* The thumb of the right hand naturally contacts the mandible during this procedure. It should be stabilized and maintained in that position, holding the tube to prevent movement until it is secured.

### *Postintubation*

Inadvertent extubation is a frequent, but entirely avoidable, complication. ETTs must be secured at the lip to prevent in and out slippage, and head movement, which translates to ETT movement, must also be prevented. Flexion of the neck causes the tube to move further down into the airway, whereas neck extension causes the tube to move up and out of the trachea. This effect is most marked in the younger child with a proportionally larger occiput. Securing the ETT at the lip is traditionally done by taping the tube to the maxilla to prevent the tube from slipping in or out. Adequate securing of the ETT with tape requires experience. An alternative to taping is the application of various commercial ETT holder devices.

Application of a cervical collar prevents the flexion and extension movements of the neck and maintains ETT position in the trachea, preventing inadvertent extubation.

### *BMV and Cricoid Pressure*

Although the value of cricoid pressure in preventing aspiration during intubation is dubious, cricoid pressure prevents gastric insufflation with BMV, even with ventilation pressures >40 cm $H_2O$. This is especially important in infants, in whom gastric distention may compromise ventilation and increase the risk of aspiration.

### *Positive-Pressure Relief Valves ("Pop-Off" Valves)–The Good and The Bad*

A pop-off valve is designed to prevent the delivery of excessive pressure to the lower airway and limit the risk of barotrauma. These valves are incorporated in infant and pediatric resuscitation bags by most manufacturers. The relief valve opens at a preset peak airway pressure (varying from 20 to 45 cm water pressure, although most are set at 40 cm), limiting the peak pressure that can be delivered to the lungs. However, in the face of upper airway obstruction, increased airway resistance, or decreased pulmonary compliance, higher pressures may be required. In situations such as these, the operator should disable the valve.

In addition to the pop-off valve, many manufacturers incorporate manometers into the unit so that one can monitor peak airway pressures as they perform BMV. A leak at the site of the manometer port may interfere with one's ability to achieve airway pressures sufficient to effect adequate gas exchange.

Even though troubleshooting inadequate BMV starts with evaluating the adequacy of mask seal and assessing airway patency, the performance of a "leak test" immediately before beginning BMV will establish the status of the pop-off valve and test for a leak at the manometer site (or other parts of the unit). The leak test is performed by removing the mask from the bag, occluding the mask port with the palm of one hand, and squeezing the bag with the other hand. If the bag remains tight, no escape of gas, or "leak," has occurred. If the bag does not remain tight, gas is escaping from the system somewhere, most commonly from the pop-off valve or the manometer port, although other causes of the leak may be present. The pressure leakage from an open manometer port occurs immediately on compressing the bag as opposed to the open pop-off valve, which vents only once the preset pressure is exceeded. The amount of volume lost will vary, depending on the size of the leak. This test is also useful for screening adult bags for malfunctions and leaks. After a negative test (i.e., the bag remains tight with squeezing), the port occluding palm hand should be released, and the bag squeezed to confirm that gas escapes properly from the inspiratory limb of the bag.

## Laryngeal Mask Airways

The laryngeal mask airway (LMA) is a safe and effective airway management device for children undergoing general anesthesia and is considered a rescue option in the event of a failed airway in children and infants. Placement of the LMA in children is a relatively easily learned skill, particularly if the correct size is chosen. The LMA has also been used successfully in difficult pediatric airways and should be considered as an alternative device for emergency airway management in these patients (e.g., Pierre Robin deformity). As in the adult, difficult pediatric intubations have also been facilitated by the use of the LMA in combination with such devices as a flexible bronchoscope.

The LMA has a few important associated complications, which are especially prevalent in smaller infants, including partial airway obstruction by the epiglottis, loss of adequate seal with patient movement, and air leakage with positive-pressure ventilation. To avoid obstruction by the epiglottis in these younger children and infants, some authors have suggested a rotational placement technique in which the mask is inserted through the oral cavity "upside down" and then rotated 180° as it is advanced into the hypopharynx. The LMA is contraindicated in the pediatric patient or adult with intact protective airway reflexes, and, therefore, is not suitable for awake airway management unless the patient is adequately sedated and the airway is topically anesthetized. LMA use is also contraindicated if foreign body aspiration is present or suspected because it may aggravate an already desperate situation and it is unlikely to provide adequate ventilation and oxygenation because the obstruction is distal to the device. The LMA comes in multiple sizes to accommodate children from neonate to adolescent.

## Percutaneous Needle Cricothyrotomy or "Needle Cric"

Although virtually every textbook chapter, article, or lecture on pediatric airway management refers to the technique of needle cricothyrotomy as the recommended last-resort rescue procedure, there is little literature to support its use and safety. Few of the "experts" who write about needle cricothyrotomy have experience performing the procedure on live humans, but nevertheless, any clinician who manages pediatric emergencies as part of his or her practice must be familiar with the procedure and its indications, and must have the appropriate equipment readily accessible in the emergency department.

Needle cricothyrotomy is indicated as a life-saving, last-resort procedure in children younger than 10 years who present or progress to the "can't intubate, can't oxygenate" scenario and whose obstruction is proximal (cephalad) to glottic opening. The classic indication is epiglottitis where BMV and intubation are judged to have failed (although true failure of BMV is rare in epiglottitis, and failure is more often caused by a failure of technique than by a truly insurmountable obstruction). Other indications include facial trauma, angioedema, and other conditions that preclude access to the glottic opening from above. Needle cricothyrotomy is rarely helpful in patients who have aspirated a foreign body that cannot be visualized by direct laryngoscopy because these foreign bodies are usually in the lower airway. It would also be of questionable value in the patient with croup because the obstruction is subglottic. In these patients, the obstruction is more likely to be bypassed by an ETT introduced orally into the trachea with a stylet, than blindly by needle cricothyrotomy.

Various commercially available needles are also available for percutaneous needle cricothyrotomy (Table 25-1). The simplest equipment, appropriate for use in infants, consists of the following:

- 14G over-the-needle catheter
- 3.0-mm ETT adapter coupled with an IV extension set (These can be obtained commercially or constructed by cutting off 6 in of distal IV tubing and inserting a 2.5 m adapter into the opening; see **Fig. 25-3**.)
- 3- or 5-mL syringe

It is good practice to preassemble the kit, place it in a clear bag, seal the bag, and tape it in an accessible place in the resuscitation area.

## *Procedure*

Place the child in the supine position with the head extended over a towel under the shoulder. This forces the trachea anteriorly such that it is easily palpable and can be stabilized with two fingers of one hand. The key to success is strict immobilization of the trachea throughout the procedure. The following statement appears in many textbooks describing this procedure: "Carefully palpate the cricothyroid membrane." In reality, it is difficult to do this in an infant and is not essential. Indeed, in smaller children, it may be impossible to precisely locate the cricothyroid membrane, so the proximal trachea is utilized for access (hence the name percutaneous needle tracheostomy [PNT] vs. "needle cric"). The priority is an airway and provision of oxygen. Complications from inserting the catheter elsewhere into the trachea besides the cricothyroid membrane are addressed later. Consider the trachea as one would a large vein, and cannulate it with the catheter-over-needle device directed caudally at a 30° angle. Aspirate air to ensure tracheal entry and then slide the catheter gently forward while retracting the needle. Attach the 3.0-mm ETT adapter to the hub of the catheter and commence bag ventilation. The provider will note exaggerated resistance to bagging. This is normal and is related

**TABLE 25-1 Recommended Commercial Catheters**

These catheters are available commercially and can be used as an option:

*Jet ventilation catheter (Ravussin).* Sizes 13G and 14G, not the 16G catheter. Although listed as jet ventilation catheters, we recommend them only for use with BMV.

*6F Cook Emergency Transtracheal Airway Catheters.* They are available in two sizes, 5 and 7.5 cm. We only recommend the 5-cm catheter.

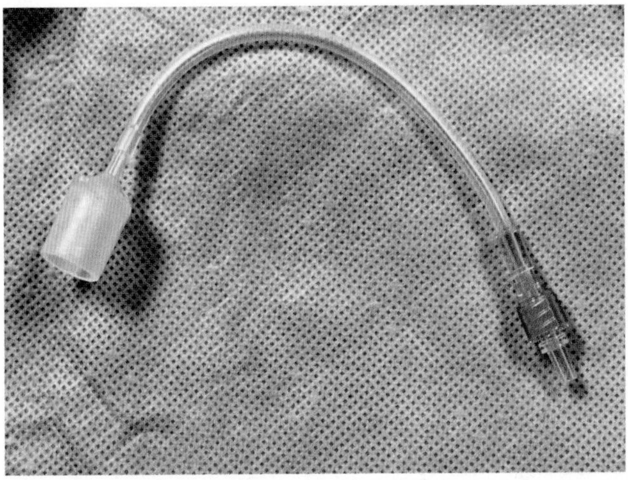

● **FIGURE 25-3. Components of a needle cric extension set.** This extension set is constructed by cutting off the terminal 6 in of standard IV tubing and inserting a 2.5 mm ETT adapter. The BVM is attached to the adapter at the proximal opening, and the distal end is inserted into the catheter that has been introduced into the trachea. This setup allows more freedom of movement during bag mask ventilation (BMV), with less concern for "kinking" or obstructing the catheter—a complication observed in animal studies when the bag was connected directly to the 3.0 ETT adapter.

to the small diameter of the catheter and the turbulence created by ventilating through it. It is not generally the result of a misplaced catheter or poor lung compliance secondary to pneumothorax. It is helpful to practice BMV through a catheter to experience the feel of this increased resistance. The operator must allow for full expiration through the patient's glottis and not through the catheter in order to prevent breath-stacking and barotrauma. This can be accomplished by watching for the chest to fall after inspiration.

The required pressures are well above the limits of the pop-off valve; therefore, it must be disabled in order to permit gas flow through the catheter. Jet ventilation has also been advocated in children; indeed, the terms "needle cric" and jet ventilation are frequently referred to in the literature as the procedure of choice. The reality is that the pressures generated by the classic jet ventilator are extremely high, both unnecessary and too dangerous as an adjunct for use with this procedure in children.

Ventilation with the percutaneous needle technique is said to be contraindicated in patients with complete upper airway obstruction. The reality is that the scenario of complete obstruction, implying no potential for egress of gas during ventilation, is extremely rare. Referring to the explanation of usual mechanism of obstruction (Chapter 26), one can see that the terminal events are respiratory arrest from closure of the airway secondary to negative patient breaths, which result in airway collapse. Once arrest occurs, negative patient breaths cease, and the airway relaxes and expands slightly. Also the negative patient breaths are replaced with positive-pressure ventilation, which may further expand the narrowed airway. Thus, egress of gas during ventilation is not an issue.

## TECHNIQUES USED IN ADOLESCENTS AND ADULTS

### Blind Nasotracheal Intubation

Nasotracheal intubation in children is uniformly discouraged and is frequently considered contraindicated. This recommendation is based on the fact that the sharp angle of the nasopharynx and pharyngotracheal axis in children precludes a reasonable likelihood of success with this technique when performed blindly. A second reason is that children are at increased risk for hemorrhage because of the preponderance of highly vascular and delicate adenoidal tissue. The direct visualization technique is, however, commonly used in small infants and children for chronic ventilator management in the intensive care unit setting. Using direct visualization with a laryngoscope once the ETT has passed into the oro- and hypopharynx, tracheal placement is aided with Magill forceps. However, this technique is not helpful in emergency airway management. In general, the technique of blind nasotracheal intubation, which is essentially the same as that described for adults, has few, if any, primary indications in pediatric emergency airway management, and, in any case, is not recommended for patients younger than 10 years.

## Combitube

The Combitube represents an excellent, easily learned rescue airway device that is available only for patients of height >48 in, so is of limited application in pediatric emergency airway-management.

## Surgical Cricothyrotomy

The cricothyroid membrane in small infants and children is minimally developed (**Fig. 25-4**). Surgical or cricothyrotome-based cricothyrotomy should not be attempted in children younger than 10 years of age because the size of the trachea and cricothyroid membrane precludes it. In children younger than 10 years, PNT with BMV is recommended. Note that our recommended limit of 10 years of age is not meant to be a rigid guideline. Various ages have been recommended as a cutoff for performing one procedure versus the other. For cricothyrotomy, it is really an issue of size. If the size of the patient's airway and cricothyroid membrane would permit performing a surgical cricothyrotomy, i.e., easily identifiable landmarks are present, then, regardless of age, it can be done. If not, then the needle technique should be performed. Cricothyrotomy using a commercially available kit (Pedia-Trake) has not been shown to be successful or even safe. **Box 25-1** summarizes recommendations for invasive airway procedures in children.

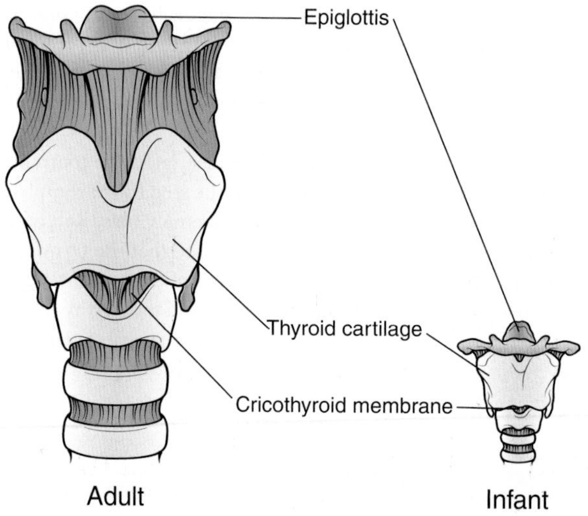


● **FIGURE 25-4. Cricothyroid Membrane.** Comparative size of the adult **(left)** versus pediatric **(right)** cricothyroid membrane. Note that not only is the larynx smaller, but the actual membrane is also proportionately smaller in comparison, involving one-fourth to one-third the anterior tracheal circumference versus two-thirds to three-fourths in the adult. This pediatric drawing is that of a toddler, which accommodates a 4.5-mm ETT.

**BOX 25-1**

## Summary recommendations for invasive airway procedures in children.

| | |
|---|---|
| **5 years** | |
| Percutaneous needle tracheostomy and bag ventilation | |
| **5–10 years** | |
| Percutaneous needle tracheostomy and bag ventilation[a] | |
| Percutaneous Seldinger technique and bag ventilation[b] | |
| **>10 years** | |
| Operator preference for various commercial kits | |
| Surgical cricothyrotomy | |

[a]There is less evidence to support this recommendation in this age group; however, it may be the only available option and should be converted to a more definitive airway.
[b]If the size of the cricothyroid membrane is sufficient.

## EVIDENCE

- **Does a needle cricothyrotomy with BMV in children provide sufficient oxygenation and ventilation to avoid hypoxia and hypercarbia?** The evidence surrounding pediatric needle cricothyrotomy is based on an animal study by Cote et al.[1] using a 30-kg dog model. Cote was able to demonstrate that dogs approximate in size to a 9- to 10-year-old child could be oxygenated through a 12G catheter and 3.0 ETT adapter with a bag for at least 1 hour (the study duration). Rises in $Paco_2$ levels were noted, but were not believed to be significant because children normally tolerate mild degrees of hypercarbia well.[1]

  One adult retrospective study reported that 48 patients were successfully oxygenated and ventilated using transtracheal ventilation through a 13G intratracheal catheter for up to 360 minutes. Transtracheal jet ventilation (TTJV) was used primarily in 47 of these patients, although 6 patients did receive conventional bagging measures until TTJV circuits could be initiated. During manual transtracheal ventilation, each patient demonstrated increases in $Paco_2$ on blood gases but maintained $Pao_2$ values >100 mm Hg.[2]
- **Should the LMA be considered as both a rescue device and an alternative airway in the management of difficult emergency pediatric airways?** Most of the literature regarding the use of LMAs in children has been compiled from the anesthesia experience in the operating room. Therefore, little information is available for the use of the LMA in the acute emergency setting. However, an observational study by Lopez-Gil et al.[3,4] has demonstrated that the skill for placement of the LMA could be rapidly learned by anesthesia residents with a low complication rate. Published case reports have demonstrated success of the LMA in the pediatric patient with difficult airways, including isolated severe retrognathia, Dandy-Walker syndrome, and Pierre Robin syndrome.[5,6]

  At least one prospective study reports a higher incidence of airway obstruction, higher ventilatory pressures, larger inspiratory leaks, and more complications in smaller children (those weighing <10 kg) with LMA use than in the older child. These authors recommend that the risk–benefit should be carefully weighed in younger children before using the LMA with paralysis and positive-pressure ventilation. Importantly, the success rate for placement of the LMA in this study that was performed in elective cases undergoing prolonged ventilation was high at 98%.[7] Although airway managers should be aware of these potential complications, this study is not generalizable to the emergency setting and should not deter providers from implementing this as a *rescue device* in infants or young children with failed airways, or as a planned approach to an infant or young child with an identified difficult airway. In the failed airway situation, the LMA may be a lifesaving bridge, providing effective oxygenation and ventilation until a definitive airway can be secured.

## REFERENCES


1. Cote CJ, Eavey RD, Todres ID, et al. Cricothyroid membrane puncture: oxygenation and ventilation in a dog model using an intravenous catheter. *Crit Care Med*. 1988;16:615–619.
2. Ravussin P, Freeman J. A new transtracheal catheter for ventilation and resuscitation. *Can Anaesth Soc J*. 1985;32:60–64.
3. Lopez-Gil M, Brimacombe J, Alvarez M. Safety and efficacy of the laryngeal mask airway: a prospective survey of 1,400 children. *Anaesthesia*. 1996;51:969–972.
4. Lopez-Gil M, Brimacombe J, Cebrian J, et al. Laryneal mask airway in pediatric practice: a prospective study of skill acquisition by anesthesia residents. *Anesthesiology*. 1996;84:807–811.
5. Selim M, Mowafi H, Al-Ghamdi A, et al. Intubation via LMA in pediatric patients with difficult airways. *Can J Anaesth*. 1999;46:891–893.
6. Stocks RM, Egerman R, Thompson JW, et al. Airway management of the severely retrognathic child: use of the laryngeal mask airway. *Ear Nose Throat J*. 2002;81:223–226.
7. Park C, Bahk JH, Ahn WS, et al. The laryngeal mask airway in infants and children. *Can J Anaesth*. 2001;48:413–417.

Chapter 26

# The Difficult Pediatric Airway

Joshua Nagler and Robert C. Luten

## OVERVIEW

Age-related anatomic and physiologic differences in the normal infant or small child can make airway management challenging. However, these differences can be anticipated and addressed in most pediatric patients as discussed in Chapter 24. The *difficult* pediatric airway, as in adults, is defined by historical or physical examination attributes that predict challenges with mask ventilation, laryngoscopy, or intubation. In the pediatric population, most of these cases result either from acute insults that modify normal airway anatomy or from known congenital abnormalities. Difficulty related to unpredictable anatomic abnormalities revealed only after unsuccessful attempts at airway management, resulting in a *failed* pediatric airway, is rare in children.

The approach to the emergent difficult airway in the adult patient is described in Chapters 2 and 3, which should be read before this chapter. The same concepts of anticipation and planning are also applicable in children. The use of rapid, easy-to-remember, and sensitive tools to identify patients with potential difficulty is paramount. Children differ from adults, however, with regard to which predictors of difficulty are most common (see Table 26-1). For example, age-dependent features (e.g., beards and age > 55 years) and progressive disease processes (e.g., cervical rheumatoid arthritis) are less applicable in children. However, using LEMON to prompt recognition of abnormal facial features and assessing for signs of obstructive airway disease will be of high yield (see Table 26-2).

**TABLE 26-1 A Sample Comparison of Pediatric and Adult Risk Factors**

A. Risk factors for adult difficult airway usually not present in infants and young children:
   1. Obesity
   2. Decreased neck mobility (excluding immobilization following trauma)
   3. Teeth abnormalities
   4. Temporomandibular joint problems
   5. Beards

B. Risk factors for pediatric difficult airway not present in adults:
   1. Small airway caliber susceptible to obstruction from edema or infection
   2. Discomfort secondary to dealing with age- and size-related variables
   3. Discomfort secondary to infrequency of patient encounters

TABLE 26-2 Key Features in Applying the LEMON Assessment in Children

| | |
|---|---|
| Look | ▪ Gestalt is the most important predictor of airway difficulty in children<br>▪ Presence of dysmorphic features is associated with abnormal airway anatomy and may predict difficulty<br>▪ Small mouth, large tongue, recessed chin, and major facial trauma are usually immediately apparent |
| Evaluate (3:3:2) | ▪ Has not been tested in children<br>▪ May be difficult to perform in an uncooperative child, or infant with a "pudgy" neck<br>▪ Gross assessment of mouth opening, jaw size, and larynx position may be utilized instead<br>▪ If 3:3:2 assessment is performed, use the child's, not the provider's fingers |
| Mallampati | ▪ Cooperation may be an issue<br>▪ Mixed data in children (see "Evidence" section) |
| Obstruction Obesity | ▪ Airway obstruction is a relatively frequent indication for airway management in children<br>▪ Second to the gestalt *Look*, assessing for obstruction is perhaps the most fruitful step in identifying difficulty airways in children<br>▪ A focused, disease-specific history and physical examination (voice change, drooling, stridor, and retractions) can accurately identify children with acute or chronic upper airway obstructive pathology<br>▪ Obesity is a growing epidemic in children, although the impact on the pediatric airway is less significant than in adults |
| Neck | ▪ Limited positioning in immobilized pediatric trauma patients is similar to that in adults<br>▪ Intrinsic cervical spine immobility from congenital abnormalities is very rare, and acquired conditions (e.g., ankylosing spondylitis and cervical rheumatoid arthritis) are essentially nonexistent in young children |

TABLE 26-3 General Approach to the Pediatric Airway Normal versus Difficult

The "Awake" Sedated look
The determination of whether a given patient has a normal or difficult airway is a subjective clinical decision that guides which equipment will need to be utilized to secure the airway. When the clinical assessment is uncertain, the clinician can administer 2 mg/kg of ketamine, which produces a state of dissociation while maintaining respiratory effort that allows the clinician to insert a laryngoscope and assess whether glottic opening visualization is feasible or not, thus guiding the appropriate method of intervention.

| | |
|---|---|
| **Anticipated "normal" airway** | |
| Condition | |
| Prerespiratory Failure | ▪ Non-rebreather<br>▪ Noninvasive ventilation |
| Respiratory Failure—Immediate and/or Transient | ▪ Bag-mask ventilation[a] |
| Respiratory Failure | ▪ Rapid sequence intubation<br>▪ Direct or video laryngoscopy |
| **Anticipated/unexpected "difficult" airway** | |
| Cannot Intubate, Can Ventilate[b] | ▪ Extraglottic device<br>▪ Video laryngoscopy |
| Cannot Intubate, Cannot Ventilate | ▪ "Surgical" airway (needle, Seldinger, or open) |

[a]May be useful as temporizing measure with airway obstruction
[b]May include dysmorphic features

The majority of children with difficult airways will present with recognizable disease processes or with known congenital abnormalities associated with airway difficulty. Therefore, this chapter will focus on these common etiologies of difficult pediatric airways and offer management strategies. Table 26-3 offers a general approach to the management of both normal and difficult pediatric airways.

## COMMON CAUSES OF DIFFICULT AIRWAYS IN CHILDREN

Causes of difficult airways in children can be categorized into four groups:

1. Acute infectious causes
2. Acute noninfectious causes
3. Congenital anomalies
4. No known abnormality, with unexpected difficulty

### Difficult Airways Secondary to Acute Infectious Causes

Examples of acute infectious processes that alter an otherwise normal anatomy include the following:

- Epiglottitis
- Croup
- Bacterial tracheitis
- Retropharyngeal abscess
- Ludwig's angina

Epiglottitis is the classic paradigm for an acute infectious process causing a difficult airway. Although disease incidence has declined dramatically since the introduction of the *Haemophilus influenzae* type b (Hib) vaccine, cases continue to be reported secondary to vaccine failures or alternative bacterial etiologies, most commonly gram-positive cocci. Progressive edema and swelling of the epiglottis and surrounding structures can quickly lead to proximal airway obstruction. Because the diagnosis is uncommon and the management is challenging, hospitals should promote protocols that allow emergency physicians, anesthesiologists, and surgical personnel to work quickly and collaboratively to construct an airway plan for any child with a concerning presentation. Agitating a child with epiglottitis can increase turbulent airflow and aggravate airway obstruction. Ideally airway evaluation and intervention should occur in the controlled setting of an operating room where equipment and staff are available for rigid bronchoscopy and surgical airway management as needed. However, if a child deteriorates, attempts at bag-mask ventilation (BMV), direct laryngoscopy, and endotracheal intubation may be necessary in the emergency department (ED). If these efforts are unsuccessful, needle cricothyrotomy (see Chapter 25) can be lifesaving. Epiglottitis represents a cardinal indication for an invasive airway, bypassing the proximal obstruction and allowing oxygenation and ventilation through the patent trachea.

Croup is a common reason for children to present to the ED with airway compromise. Although commonly grouped with epiglottitis, croup is a clinically distinct entity (see Table 26-4). Respiratory distress is common, as subglottic airway narrowing can have a profound effect on airway resistance on the smaller diameter trachea in children (see Table 26-5). However, croup patients are rarely toxic appearing. Fortunately, patients with croup respond well to nebulized epinephrine and steroids, and intubation is rarely required. If patients present in extremis or medical therapy fails, bagging may be difficult given the increased airway resistance; however, visualization during laryngoscopy is not usually affected.

Importantly, if a child with croup is ill enough to require intubation, a smaller endotracheal tube (ETT) should be used because the edematous subglottis will be narrowed and may not accommodate age- or length-predicted ETT size. It is important to remember, however, that the ETT insertion distance (i.e., lip-to-tip distance) is *not* affected despite using a smaller-sized tube. Therefore,

**TABLE 26-4** Management of the "Most Feared" Pediatric Airway Problems

| Disease | Pathology and Deterioration | Approach | FB Removal Maneuvers | BMV Two-Person Techniques | Intubation | Needle Cricothyrotomy |
|---|---|---|---|---|---|---|
| Epiglottitis | Rapidly progressing disease process affecting the supraglottic structures (epiglottis and aryepiglottic folds). Patients are usually ill-appearing, although they may be in minimal distress Decompensation can occur | Stable: observe → OR for defin airway Decompensation: BMV → intubation Failed Airway: needle cricothryoidotomy | Not indicated | Effective in *most* patients who deteriorate Technique: A two-handed seal, with another rescuer providing sufficient pressure to overcome the obstruction | Usually successful. Use tube size 1 mm smaller. Use stylet. Suction, visualize, press on chest, and look for bubble | The paradigm indication for needle cricothyrotomy *if* BMV and intubation are unsuccessful |
| | 1. When a patient is stimulated or manipulated, leading to dynamic airway obstruction | | | | | |
| | 2. As a result of progressive deterioration over time secondary to fatigue, although the respiratory arrest may occur precipitously | | | | | |

| | | | | | | |
|---|---|---|---|---|---|---|
| Croup | Slowly progressive (hours to days) disease process affecting the subglottic trachea, causing dynamic inspiratory augmented obstruction. Deterioration is usually progressive rather than sudden and related to respiratory muscle fatigue, although as in the case of epiglottis, the arrest may also occur precipitously | Stridor at rest: racemic epi and steroids<br>Persistent distress: ICU<br>Decompensation: BMV → Intubation | Not indicated | Effective. Positive pressure overcomes obstruction by acting as a stent. May require high pressures | Proximal airway normal; therefore, should not be problematic. Consider ETT one size smaller and use stylet | Not indicated because obstruction is distal to cricothyroid membrane |
| FB aspiration (see Chapter 27) | Patients with aspirated FBs have the potential for decompensation secondary to acute airway obstruction. The level of obstruction may vary from the hypopharynx, above or below the glottis, to the mainstem bronchus | Stable: observe → transfer for removal<br>Decompensation: FB removal maneuvers → Direct visualization and removal with Magill forceps → Intubation to force FB distally into mainstem bronchus | Indicated if *appropriate* (i.e., patient completely obstructs) | Should not be used before attempts to remove FB. May be obviated by intubation | Last resort in an effort to push FB distally into mainstem bronchus | Usually not indicated because FB will be distal to the obstruction if other efforts have failed |

FB, foreign body; BMV, bag-mask ventilation; OR, operating room; epi, epinephrine; ICU, intensive care unit; ETT, endotracheal tube.

TABLE 26-5 Effect of 1-mm Edema on Airway Resistance

| | Change in Cross-Sectional Area | Change in Resistance |
|---|---|---|
| Infant | 44% decrease | 200% increase |
| Adult | 25% decrease | 40% increase |

These figures reflect the quietly breathing infant or adult. If the child cries, the work of breathing is increased 32-fold. This underscores the principle of maintaining children in a quiet, nonthreatening, and comfortable environment during evaluation and in preparation for management.

although length-based references such as a Broselow–Luten tape to determine this distance will remain accurate, formulaic calculation based on the tube diameter (i.e., three times the ETT size) should be based on the predicted age-appropriate ETT size, not the downsized tube.

Bacterial tracheitis has become a leading cause of respiratory failure from acute upper airway infections. As in croup, inflammation in tracheitis is subglottic, although affected children tend to be older and are likely to be ill appearing. Airway management is similar to croup. Again, visualization is rarely compromised; however, a smaller ETT size should be used. Using a cuffed ETT has two advantages. First, it will allow for adjustments in cuff inflation volume to accommodate any air leak if the airway is less edematous than anticipated. Second, it will allow for higher airway pressures, if obstructive plaques in the distal airway were to produce higher airway resistance. It is important to recognize that the presence of such thick purulent secretions within the trachea will require vigilant monitoring for tube obstruction.

Retropharyngeal abscess rarely presents with airway compromise, although it is frequently included in the differential diagnosis of acute life-threatening upper airway obstruction. These patients most commonly present with odynophagia and neck stiffness. Lateral neck films reveal thickening of the retropharyngeal space. Most of these patients respond to antibiotics, although in some cases, drainage in the operating room is required. Rarely, if ever, is it necessary to actively manage the airway in the ED. If the obstruction is large enough to require emergent airway intervention, it is important to remember that an extraglottic device (EGD) may not be feasible, and alternative backup approaches should be considered.

Ludwig's angina is an exceedingly rare pediatric diagnosis and unlikely to require emergency airway management in the ED. If encountered, difficulty with displacement of the tongue into the inflamed submandibular space should be anticipated, and approaches other than direct laryngoscopy should be readily available.

## Difficult Airways Secondary to Noninfectious Processes

- Foreign body
- Burns
- Anaphylaxis and angioedema
- Trauma

Foreign body aspiration is perhaps the most feared pediatric airway problem. Therefore, the approach to the child with airway compromise from foreign body aspiration has earned a full discussion in Chapter 27.

Patients with upper airway burns or inhalational injuries can be identified by soot in the mouth, carbonaceous sputum, singed nasal hair, or facial burns. Caustic ingestions may show facial or oropharyngeal mucosal injury. If upper airway edema has already occurred, patients may have drooling, hoarseness, or frank stridor. In contrast to processes like croup that commonly improve with medical therapy, patients with significant mucosal injury or edema predictably worsen over time. Therefore, intubation should occur as early as possible as progressive edema will make visualization and tube passage dramatically more difficult over time (see Table 26-6). Succinylcholine

TABLE 26-6 **Timing of Intervention According to Anticipated Clinical Course**

**Expectant intervention group:** Intervene *only* if deterioration occurs:
1. Assemble subspecialty multidisciplinary team for definitive management:
   Foreign body
   Epiglottitis
2. Obtain subspecialty assistance if deterioration appears likely:
   Para-airway *diagnoses* (diseases such as retropharyngeal or peritonsillar abscess or Ludwig's angina that are usually stable on presentation and deterioration is uncommon)

**Early intervention group:** Intervene *early* (preventively):
Burns
Anaphylaxis: usually responds to medical treatment; anaphylactoid-like reactions such as angioedema respond less reliably to medical treatment
Trauma

may be used during rapid sequence intubation (RSI) as the risk of hyperkalemia from burns occurs after 3 to 5 days. Cuffed ETTs are recommended to accommodate the changes in airway edema over the natural course of recovery. EGDs may not pass easily, and therefore may be less reliable as rescue tools, so surgical airway equipment should be readily available.

Anaphylaxis and angioedema also cause progressive edema in the tongue, supraglottic structures, and the larynx. The goal is to always use aggressive medical therapy to limit progression. However, patients with compromised airways secondary to anaphylactic or anaphylactoid reactions (e.g., angioedema) who do not rapidly respond to medical treatment require early intervention. As with inhalation injuries, a backup airway management plan should be immediately available.

Trauma poses unique challenges in pediatric airway management. Facial trauma can impede an effective mask seal, limit mouth opening, or result in blood or secretions in the oropharynx, making visualization difficult. Avulsed teeth, blood, vomitus, or other foreign material can obstruct the airway. Expanding hematoma or displaced bony injuries can impede direct laryngoscopy. Primary neck trauma can distort anatomy or injure the larynx and trachea and risk complete airway compromise during intervention. Finally, the risk of cervical spine injury requires maintenance of immobilization, which affects the ability to position the patient for optimal visualization and intubation. Despite these challenges, the majority of pediatric trauma patients who require airway intervention will be managed with RSI and direct laryngoscopy for intubation. Video laryngoscopy, when available, is increasingly being used to improve visualization that may be otherwise compromised by cervical immobilization. Significant trauma may limit the utility of an EGD. Therefore, simultaneous preparation for a surgical airway should be performed as a backup airway plan.

## Difficult Airways Secondary to Congenital Anomalies

Patients with difficult airways secondary to congenital anomalies receive a disproportionate amount of attention in discussions of difficult airways in pediatrics. However, they are encountered much less frequently than the conditions described earlier. The literature concerning these patients usually describes elective situations, managed by experienced pediatric anesthesiology subspecialists in well-equipped operating rooms performed under controlled conditions. This information has limited relevance to the pediatric emergency airway management.

Often, patients with congenital anomalies presenting to the ED require intubation for reasons unrelated to their difficult airway (e.g., a child with Pierre Robin syndrome with respiratory failure secondary to asthma). The best approach for these patients, time permitting, is to obtain expert subspecialty assistance as early as possible and, as with all patients, to aggressively manage the medical condition to try to obviate the need for invasive airway management.

There are a range of anatomic abnormalities and named syndromes that predict difficulty with pediatric airway management. It is impractical and unnecessary to commit all to memory. Instead, common findings can be categorized into four groups, which can be identified using the LEMON assessment (see **Table 26-2**). These include a small chin (micrognathic mandible), a large tongue, a small or limited-opening mouth, and a neck that is either short or immobile.

The micrognathic mandible is the most common anatomical feature in the child, rendering intubation difficult. The small mandible reduces the available space (mandibular space) into which the tongue and submandibular tissue must be compressed with the laryngoscope blade to visualize the glottic opening (see **Fig. 26-1**). A significantly recessed (micrognathic) mandible can be recognized by drawing a line that touches the forehead and maxilla and continues inferiorly (**Fig. 26-2**). In a patient with grossly normal anatomy, the line also touches the tip of the chin. In the micrognathic patient, a gap between the line and the tip of the chin is observed. A relatively large tongue can have a similar effect, with limited room for displacement given its mass and resultant obstruction of the direct view of the glottis.

Similarly, a mouth that is small or does not open fully can make laryngoscopy difficult. The ability to place appropriately sized equipment into the oral cavity and to create a direct line of sight to the laryngeal structures can be compromised.

Restricted neck movement can also make it challenging to align the oral, pharyngeal, and tracheal axes, to permit direct visualization. A short neck exaggerates the acuity of the angle around the tongue toward the glottis, which can make laryngoscopy and/or passage of an ETT difficult.

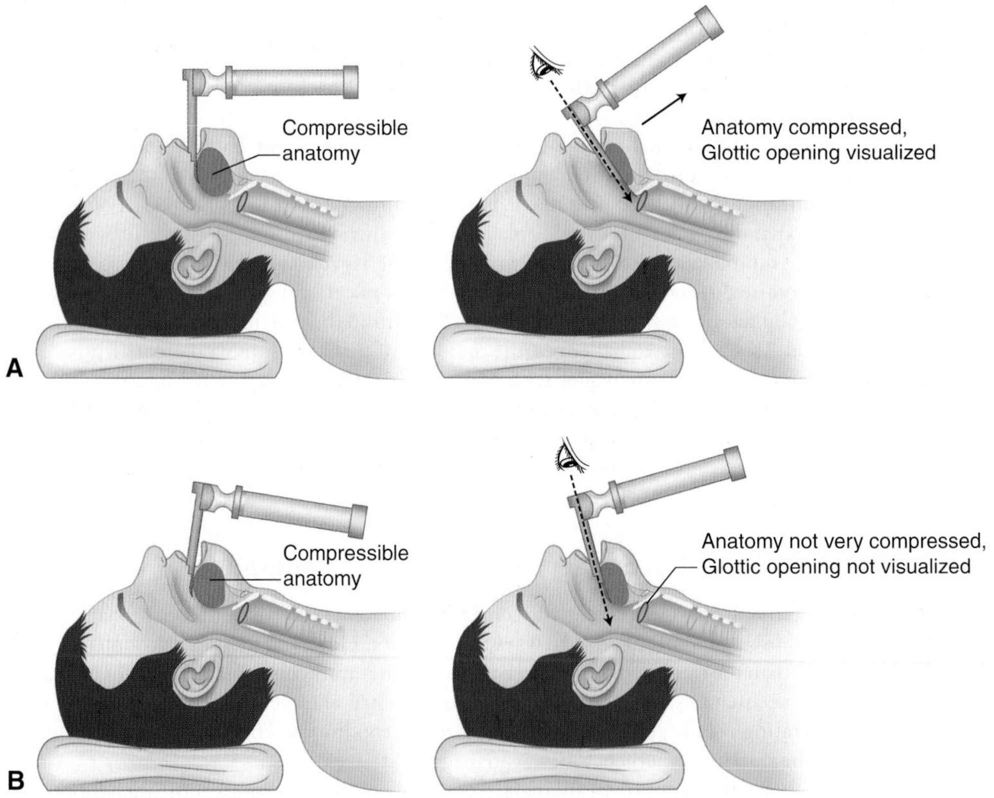


● **FIGURE 26-1. A:** A normal-sized mandible provides room for the tongue and associated tissue to be compressed into the mandibular space by the laryngoscope blade, allowing visualization of the glottic opening. **B:** A small mandible cannot easily accommodate the tongue, which therefore remains in the line of sight of the laryngoscopist.

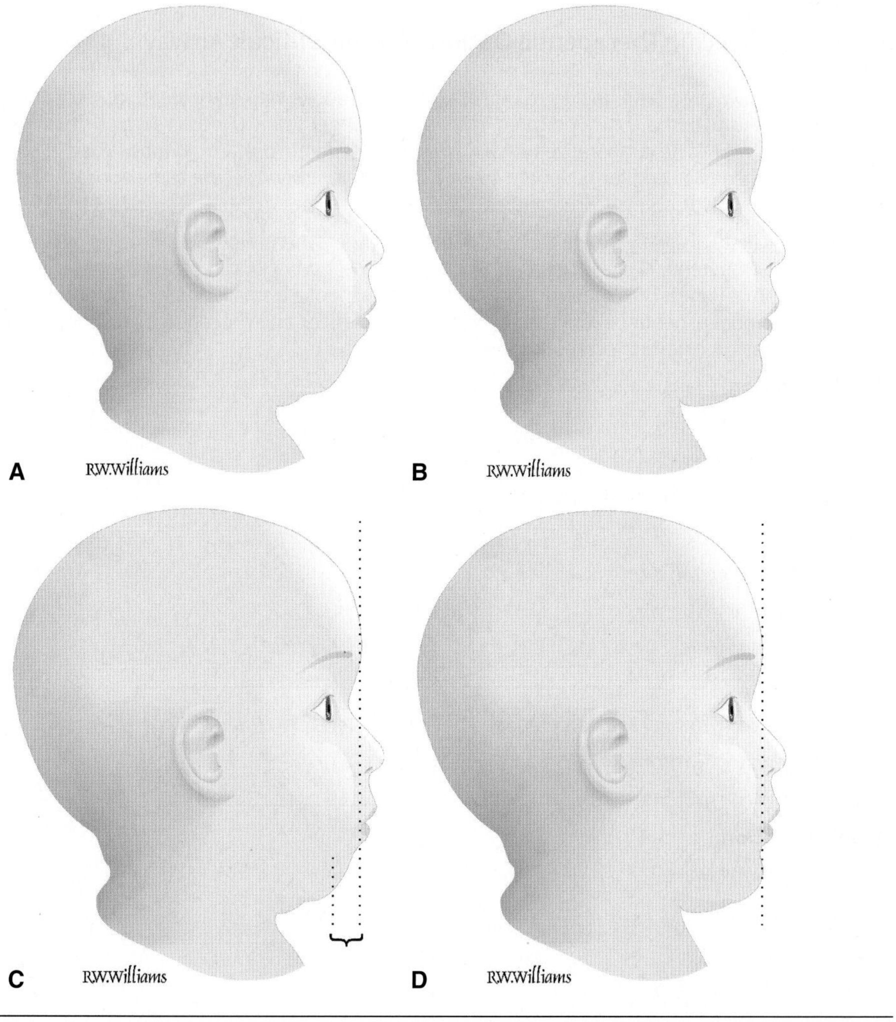


● **FIGURE 26-2.** It may not always be obvious that a given patient possesses a difficult airway. Micrognathia **(A)** may not be readily apparent unless compared to a normal child. **B:** In the normal patient, a line drawn from the forehead **(C)**, touching the anterior maxilla, will also touch the chin. **D:** Failure to do so indicates a degree of micrognathia. (©Extrapolated from Frankville D. *ASA Refresher Course*. Parkridge, IL: American Society of Anesthesiologists; 2001:126.)

In patients with known or newly identified anatomic abnormalities as described earlier, the difficult airway algorithm should be used. The airway approach in these patients might include an awake (sedated) look to assess the degree to which the mouth can be opened, the tongue can be displaced into the mandibular space, or the larynx can be viewed with limited neck positioning (**Table 26-3**). If the awake look suggests passage of an ETT is likely to be difficult and time permits, neuromuscular blockade and RSI should be avoided or postponed until backup strategies are in place. Other potential approaches are reviewed throughout this book, and summarized in **Table 26-7**.

For patients in extremis or in crash situations, the clinician is left with no other options than those used in other patients. Fortunately, even when difficulty is predicted, straightforward approaches such as BMV or endotracheal intubation are usually successful and should remain the mainstay of therapy.

TABLE 26-7 Specific Therapeutic Options for the Difficult Airway

| |
|---|
| The difficult airway algorithm applies to both children and adults with few exceptions; most notably, blind nasotracheal intubation is contraindicated in children younger than 10 y, as is surgical cricothyrotomy. Most children will not be cooperative with an awake, nonsedated look. Combitube, a useful adjunct in adults, is not manufactured for patients <48 in (122 cm) tall. Otherwise, the same approach and options are recommended for both children and adults. |
| There are a variety of airway devices for use in the pediatric patient. However, developing and maintaining competency is challenging with infrequent use, particularly in emergencies and by emergency practitioners. It is therefore probably best to choose a smaller number of options, but aim to gain the maximum experience with them. The following devices and procedures are listed according to appropriateness in different levels of clinical acuity |
| **Crash situation** |
| *Extraglottic devices* |
| Laryngeal mask airways |
| Combitube (>48 in [122 cm] tall) |
| King LT |
| *Endotracheal (ET) intubation* |
| Traditional laryngoscopy |
| Video laryngoscopy |
| *"Surgical" airway* |
| Needle cricothyrotomy aka percutaneous needle tracheostomy (<5+ y)[a] |
| Seldinger cricothyrotomy (>5 y) |
| Surgical cricothyrotomy (>10 y) |
| **Stable situation** |
| ET intubation (awake)[b] |
| ET intubation (RSI) |
| EGD |
| Fiber-optic intubation[b] |
| Blind nasotracheal intubation[b] |
| **Stable expectant management patients** |
| All EDs should have a plan in place for managing patients with disorders such as foreign body aspiration, epiglottitis, etc. This usually requires prior agreement of consultants willing to respond immediately to those emergencies |

[a]There are no published data to support the best means of ventilation in children following needle cricothyrotomy. Both transtracheal jet ventilation (TTJV) and BMV have been recommended. However, with no clear supporting data, and a high risk of barotraumas and complications related to TTJV, we suggest practitioners utilize BMV with conversion to a more definitive airway as soon as possible. If a cricothyrotomy catheter has been placed (by Seldinger or surgical technique) BMV should be used.

[b]Rarely performed in pediatrics, greatest success in adolescents and adults.

## No Known Abnormality, with Unexpected Difficulty

Perhaps the greatest fear for most practitioners is to encounter unexpected difficulty after initiating airway management in a child *without* recognized congenital or acquired abnormalities. Based on data from large anesthesia registries, the incidence of *unanticipated* difficult intubation is vanishingly low, a reflection of the infrequency of difficult airways, as well as the ability of practitioners to use systematic strategies to effectively identify those patients with difficulty in advance. The management approaches for the *unexpected* pediatric difficult airway are similar to those for the expected difficult airway (see Table 26-3).

## TIMING THE INTERVENTION

As is the case for adults, the patients' anticipated clinical course becomes a key determinant in deciding whether to actively intervene in the airway or to observe the patient for possible deterioration. Table 26-6 groups disorders from both infectious and noninfectious causes according to timing of intervention based on anticipated clinical course. The expectant intervention group represents patients in whom the safest course of action may be a period of close observation, during which preparation is rapidly undertaken for definitive management were it to be required. In these children, evidence of clinical deterioration during observation will prompt active airway management in the ED. Alternatively, medical management may stabilize the patient such that invasive airway management can be avoided, or allow sufficient time for transfer to a controlled environment such as the operating room, and/or the recruitment of a multidisciplinary team with expertise in the management of difficult airways. Treatment in less than ideal conditions may lead to untoward outcomes.

The signs and symptoms of impending airway obstruction in children will guide the approach to the early intervention group. These disorders, if left to expectant treatment, have a greater potential for deterioration. An example, as discussed earlier, is the burn or caustic ingestion patient with early signs of voice change. This symptom may herald deterioration, although the degree and pace of progression cannot be predicted. However, it must be assumed that progression to the point of obstruction is possible, in which case intubation will be extremely difficult if not impossible. For this reason, intervention earlier rather than later is recommended. Patients with compromised airways secondary to anaphylactic or anaphylactoid reactions (e.g., angioedema) who do not respond immediately to medical treatment similarly require early intervention.

## SUMMARY

- Effective pediatric airway management is focused on anticipating and planning for difficulties.
- The systematic approach to identify the difficult airway in adults can also be used in children. In general, looking for obvious abnormalities (L of LEMON) and evaluating for upper airway obstruction (O) are the highest yield features of the LEMON assessment, when applied to children.
- Most difficult pediatric airways are related to acute infectious or traumatic alterations to otherwise normal anatomy. Known congenital abnormalities are uncommon, and unexpected difficulty in children is very rare.
- Pattern recognition is important to the appropriate management of the common presentations of acute infectious and noninfectious compromise airway emergencies.
- Management of children with difficult airways should follow the difficult airway algorithm, just as with adults. The vast majority of patients will still be managed with RSI and direct laryngoscopy.

## EVIDENCE

- **What is the incidence of difficult and failed airways in children?** Although definitions and contexts vary, pediatric data demonstrate the rarity of difficult airways in children. Using a database of nearly 9,000 children being endotracheally intubated *in the operating room* at a tertiary care children's hospital where referral bias predicts more complex patients, the incidence of difficult airways was just 0.42%.[1] Importantly, even for those with difficult airways, there were no mask ventilation failures or need for surgical airways in this study. More recent data from over 11,000 pediatric general anesthesia cases found an overall incidence of difficulty laryngoscopy of just over 1%, although the rate climbed to nearly 5% in children less than 1 year of age.[2] A recent report of more than 1,000 pediatric ED intubations (age < 15 years) revealed a first-attempt success rate of 83% and an ultimate success rate of 99.5%. There were no reported surgical airway procedures.[3]

- **What techniques are used to intubate children in the ED?** The NEAR III registry reported on 1,053 pediatric intubations over a 10-year period. RSI was used in 81% of encounters.[3] Etomidate and succinylcholine were the most commonly used induction and neuromuscular blocking agents employed (78% and 67%, respectively). Direct laryngoscopes were used most often, in 94% of encounters, although their use was decreasing (whereas video laryngoscope use was increasing) toward the end of the study. EGD use was rare (only two encounters), and no surgical airways were recorded.
- **How reliable is the Mallampati scoring system in children?** The concept of evaluating the size of a child's tongue relative to his/her oral cavity remains important, although the data regarding the predictive value of Mallampati scoring are limited in pediatrics. Children, particularly those below school-age, are unlikely to cooperate with testing. A "modified" approach is to use a tongue blade to facilitate mouth opening and maximal tongue excursion. The original study in pediatrics included 476 patients, ranging from newborns to 16 years of age. The predictive sensitivity of Mallampati testing was only 0.162. Importantly, of 16 patients with a poor view on laryngoscopy, 12 (75%) had Mallampati class 1 or 2 airways and therefore were not predicted to be difficult.[4] A more recent study did show that in children with Mallampati scores of 3 and 4, the incidence of difficult laryngoscopy was 6.4%, versus 0.4% for those with Mallampati 1 or 2.[2] Given the mixed data and the challenges of performing this examination, Mallampati testing is not often performed during emergent airway management in pediatrics.
- **Have clinical tools to predict difficult airways in children been validated?** The predictive merits of individual anthropomorphic measurements (e.g., hyomandibular, thyromental, mandibular, and interdental lengths) and systematic clinical evaluation are largely confined to adults and have not been well tested in children. One recent study confirmed that during bedside assessment, micrognathia (reported as frontal plane to chin distance) as shown in **Figure 26-2** is the best predictor of difficult laryngoscopy, particularly in younger children.[5] These limited data along with logic and anecdotal experience support that global assessment for features that might predict airway difficulty is important and should be routinely performed.

## REFERENCES

1. Tong DC, Beus J, Litman RS. The children's hospital of philadelphia difficult airway registry. *Anesthesiology*. 2007;107:A1637.
2. Heinrich S, Birkholz T, Ihmsen H, et al. Incidence and predictors of difficult laryngoscopy in 11,219 pediatric anesthesia procedures. *Paediatr Anaesth*. 2012;22:729–736.
3. Pallin DJ, Dwyer RC, Walls RM, et al. Techniques and trends, success rates, and adverse events in emergency department pediatric intubations: a report from the National Emergency Airway Registry. *Ann Emerg Med*. 2016;67(5):610–615.
4. Kopp VJ, Bailey A, Calhoun PE, et al. Utility of the Mallampati classification for predicting difficult intubation in pediatric patients. *Anesthesiology*. 1995;83:A1147.
5. Mansano AM, Módolo NSP, Silva L, et al. Bedside tests to predict laryngoscopic difficulty in pediatric patients. *Int J Pediatr Otorhinolaryngol*. 2016;83:63–68.

Chapter 27

# Foreign Body in the Pediatric Airway

Robert C. Luten and Joshua Nagler

## BACKGROUND

Foreign body aspiration (FBA) is a common cause of morbidity and mortality in children. Thousands of children are seen in emergency departments each year for choking-related episodes, and choking is a leading cause of death in young children. The age group most at risk is 1 to 3 years of age. These children may choke on food substances given their incomplete dentition, immature swallowing coordination, and tendency toward distraction during meals. In addition, infants and toddlers are newly adapted to walking and have a tendency to put everything in their mouths. This increases their risk of unwitnessed choking events. Older children more commonly aspirate things such as pins and pen caps, which they are holding in their mouths.

## PRESENTATION

Children who have aspirated foreign material may present acutely following a *witnessed or reported* event. Families commonly report a choking or gagging episode. Such an event, followed by sudden onset of coughing with unilateral wheezing or decreased aeration, represents the classic diagnostic triad for FBA in the mainstem or lower bronchi. When the foreign body becomes lodged more proximally, partial upper airway obstruction can lead to hoarseness or stridor. Complete obstruction of the trachea or larynx can occur either from mechanical blockage or from induced laryngospasm. The mortality with complete laryngeal obstruction approaches 50%.

Many children have *unwitnessed or unreported* aspiration events. Infants are preverbal, and young children may not recognize the need to tell their parents. Alternatively, if immediate symptoms resolve, caregivers may not recognize the significance of the event unless a provider directly asks about recent choking episodes. As a result, respiratory symptoms may be incorrectly attributed to illnesses such as asthma or croup. Subsequent recurrent pulmonary infections may lead to the delayed diagnosis of chronic FBA. This can occur weeks to months after the aspiration event.

For the purpose of this chapter, we will focus only on acute airway management in the context of known or suspected FBA.

## TECHNIQUE

The approach to the management of FBA will differ depending on whether the obstruction is partial or complete, and the child's level of consciousness.

### Partial Airway Obstruction

Children with FBA who have the ability to cough, cry, or speak are demonstrating adequate air exchange, and by definition have incomplete airway obstruction. Beyond infancy, children will naturally hold themselves in a position that maximizes airway patency. In addition, they possess a reflexive cough, which is the most effective means of clearing the airway. These patients, therefore, should be managed "expectantly." That is, no attempts at relief maneuvers should be attempted to avoid dislodgement of the foreign body to a location that worsens the degree of obstruction.

Resources should be summoned to facilitate removal in the operating room setting whenever possible. If an operating room or pediatric expert resources are unavailable, an alternative plan must be initiated. Appropriately sized equipment should be gathered for foreign body removal, as well as for more definitive airway management in the event that the child progresses to complete airway obstruction (discussed below).

Attempts at removal of the foreign body for children with partial airway obstruction are rarely performed in the emergency department. Children are unlikely to cooperate with efforts to remove an airway foreign body even with effective topical anesthesia. Furthermore, unintentionally placing a laryngoscope blade too deeply in small children will risk placing direct pressure on the foreign body, which can further obstruct the airway. Therefore, in most cases, the child should be allowed to continue to attempt to clear the foreign body reflexively as long as possible, or until an operating room is available. Only when the patient is showing signs of tiring or progression toward complete obstruction should attempts at removal be made. In such circumstances, sedation with ketamine titrated intravenously (1 to 2 mg per kg IV) to effect if possible (or 4 mg per kg IM if not) reliably produces dissociative sedation while maintaining respiratory drive and airway reflexes. Once sedated, the laryngoscope is inserted methodically, while the provider maintains anatomic visualization attempting to identify any supraglottic foreign body.

If the patient progresses to complete obstruction, either because of unavoidable progression or as a result of attempts at removal, immediate intervention is required.

### Complete Airway Obstruction

The loss of the ability to phonate in an awake child with a suspected FBA indicates complete airway obstruction. Chest wall movement will persist with attempted respiratory efforts; however, no sounds will be heard on inspiration or expiration. Conscious children will appear scared, although infants will not reliably place their hands to their neck to signify choking as older children or adults will. Instead, they will often raise clenched fists above their heads with eyes wide open as an expression of distress.

Pediatric basic life support techniques should be used immediately in the conscious patient with complete airway obstruction from FBA. The goal is to generate intrathoracic pressure to expel the foreign body from the airway. In infants, this is most safely attempted with the child in a head down position, using repeated cycles of back blows and chest compressions, five per cycle. Subdiaphragmatic abdominal thrusts (the Heimlich maneuver) are not recommended in infants because of the risk of accidental injury to the relatively large liver protruding beneath the costal margin. In children older than 1 year, the Heimlich maneuver is recommended, just as with adults. These initial maneuvers should be repeated until either the foreign body is expelled or the patient becomes unresponsive.

There is no role for attempting instrumentation to remove the foreign body in a conscious child who will not cooperate with removal. With complete obstruction of the airway, rapid oxygen desaturation will render the patient unconscious within 1 or 2 minutes, at which point attempts at removal can be made. For the child who presents unconscious, the oropharynx should first be examined for a visible foreign body. If something is seen, it should be removed directly.

If no foreign material is seen, a blind oropharyngeal finger sweep should *not* be performed. In the emergency department, the immediate maneuver is direct laryngoscopy for possible foreign body visualization and removal. This is exactly analogous to the adult patient (see Chapter 41). The administration of a neuromuscular blocking agent is not indicated for the initial attempt. Only if children have a clenched mouth or other signs of muscle activity will it be necessary to use a rapid-onset neuromuscular blocking agent. If the foreign body can be identified under direct laryngoscopy, it should be removed using Magill or alligator forceps, or other available instruments. Care must be taken to avoid advancing the foreign body to a position where it becomes more tightly lodged or to a location where it is no longer retrievable. Similarly, organic material may be friable, and although rapid resolution of complete obstruction is the immediate goal, care should be taken when possible to grasp gently to avoid creating smaller fragments that can fall deeper into the tracheobronchial tree.

If the foreign body cannot be retrieved during laryngoscopy or expelled by blind maneuvers, attempts should be made to advance the foreign material distally into either mainstem bronchus using an endotracheal tube. First, the standard "lip-to-tip" distance should be identified using the Broselow–Luten tape, Airway Card mobile device app, or other formulas. It may be helpful to tape or mark this distance on the endotracheal tube. A stylet should be used. The child should then be intubated, with the endotracheal tube (stylet in situ) advanced as deeply as possible. The obstructing material will be pushed down the trachea, past the carina, and into a mainstem bronchus, most often the right based on a shallower take-off angle. The tube should then be withdrawn back to the standard "lip-to-tip" distance previously marked on the tube. The foreign material will now be completely obstructing one bronchus, with effective ventilation through the other, effectively moving from complete obstruction to single lung ventilation (see **Fig. 27-1**). If there is improved ventilation but high resistance following this maneuver, soft material such as food substances may have become lodged within the endotracheal tube tip, preventing easy passage of air. If this occurs, replacement of the endotracheal tube, using the appropriate insertion depth, provides the most effective means to ventilate the patient through the patent mainstem bronchi.

A percutaneous approach (e.g., needle cricothyrotomy) is rarely indicated in FBA. Details of this approach are provided in Chapter 25. Needle cricothyrotomy will only be successful if the needle entry site is distal to the obstruction (e.g., a foreign body just below the vocal cords at the cricoid ring). If the foreign body cannot be visualized during attempts at direct laryngoscopy, it is unlikely that a percutaneous approach will be distal to the object, rendering the procedure ineffective. Ventilation strategies following percutaneous airway techniques are reviewed in Chapter 25. In patients with complete airway obstruction, it is important to remember that no air can exit through the glottis into the pharynx. The only means for exhalation is through the narrow lumen of the catheter; therefore, the risk of barotrauma increases following each delivered breath.

Both forced intubation and needle cricothyrotomy are temporizing measures designed to reestablish some degree of oxygenation and ventilation. When successful, the patient can then be taken to the operating room for removal of the foreign body with a bronchoscope or by thoracotomy as needed.

An overview of the stepwise approach to managing FBA in children is presented in **Figure 27-2**. The same for adults is seen in Figure 41-1.

## TIPS AND PEARLS

1. Many aspiration events in children are unwitnessed, and young children are incapable of verbalizing what has happened. Consider aspiration in any infant/toddler with acute onset of respiratory distress.
2. The safest removal of a foreign body from a pediatric airway occurs in the operating room. Recruit necessary personnel and resources as early as possible.
3. Reflexive cough is likely to be the most successful mechanism for clearing a foreign body from a partially obstructed airway. Avoid interfering with an alert child who is sitting in a position of comfort and coughing.

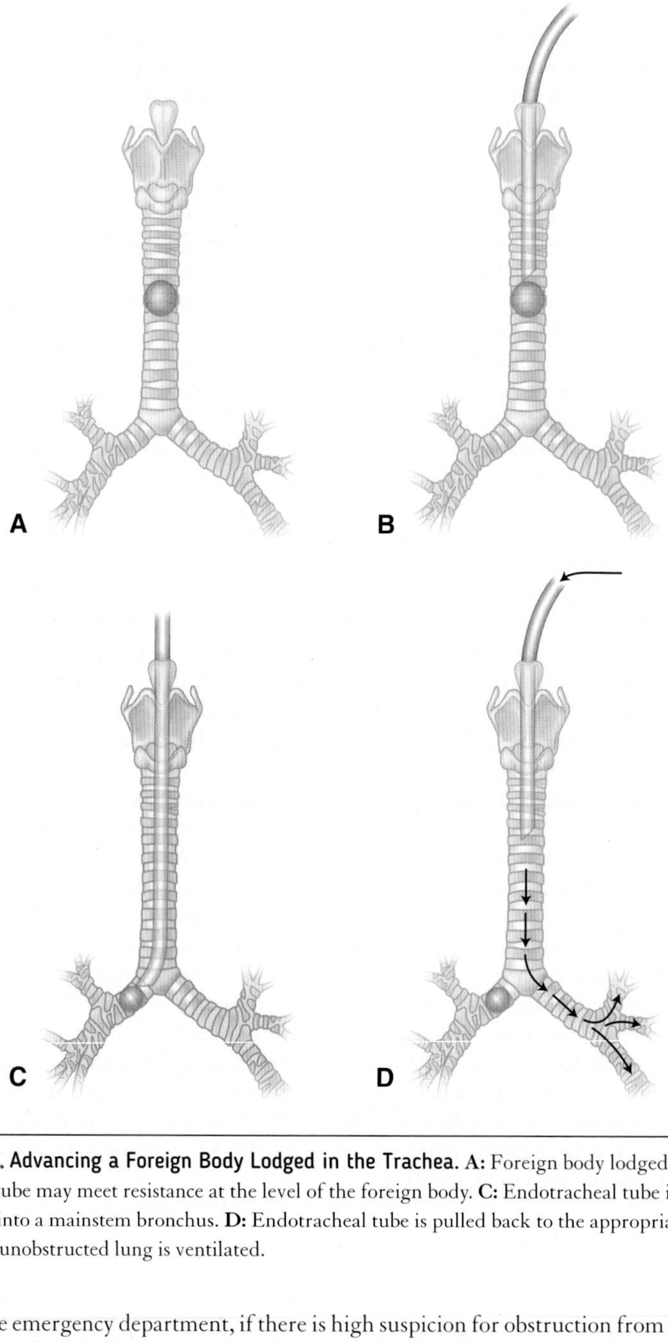


● **FIGURE 27-1. Advancing a Foreign Body Lodged in the Trachea.** **A:** Foreign body lodged in the trachea. **B:** Endotracheal tube may meet resistance at the level of the foreign body. **C:** Endotracheal tube is advanced to push the foreign body into a mainstem bronchus. **D:** Endotracheal tube is pulled back to the appropriate "lip-to-tip" distance, and the unobstructed lung is ventilated.

4. In the emergency department, if there is high suspicion for obstruction from FBA, direct laryngoscopy for possible direct removal should be attempted before positive-pressure breaths to avoid advancing the foreign body to an unreachable position. If equipment is not immediately available, bag-mask ventilation may stent open the airway and allow small amounts of oxygen around the foreign material to support oxygenation until attempts at laryngoscopy for visualization and removal are made, or intubation to advance the foreign material can be performed (see **Fig. 27.3**).
5. Avoid the Heimlich maneuver in children <1 year of age to prevent inadvertent injury to the liver.
6. Needle cricothyrotomy is unlikely to be successful in any child in whom the foreign body cannot be visualized above or immediately below the glottis, and therefore should not be attempted in these patients.

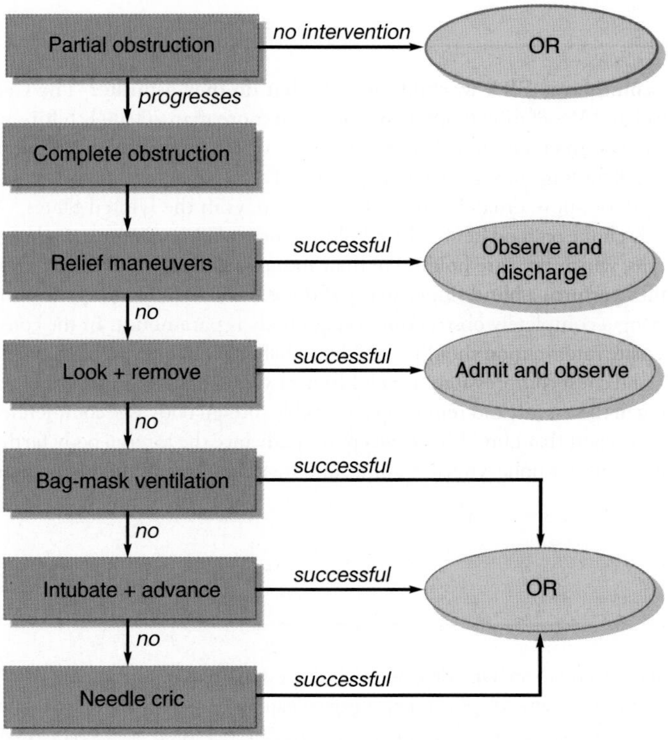


● **FIGURE 27-2.** Stepwise approach for the management of an aspirated foreign body.

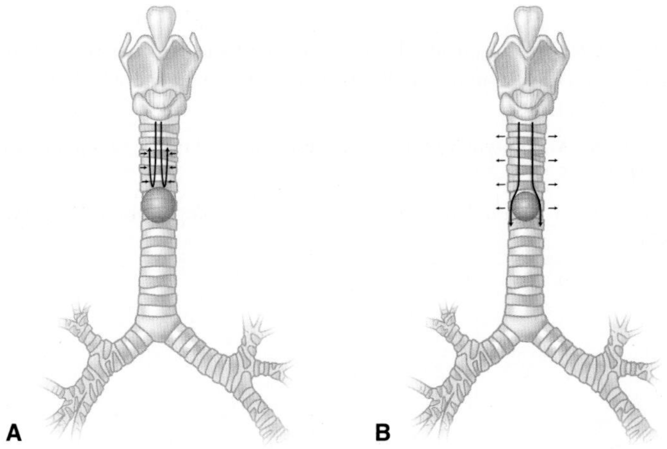


● **FIGURE 27-3. A:** With spontaneous respiratory effort, lower pressure in the airway pulls the walls inward, tightening the seal preventing airflow past the foreign body. **B:** With positive-pressure ventilation, the walls of the airway are pushed outward and a small amount of airflow around the foreign body may be possible, serving to temporize oxygenation until definitive management is possible.

## EVIDENCE

- **How common is FBA in children and what do they aspirate?** The Centers for Disease Control and Prevention (CDC) estimates that more than 200,000 children under 10 years of age are seen in emergency departments each year for nonfatal, unintentional foreign body injuries including choking-related episodes.[1] Data suggest that choking on food alone causes the death of approximately one child every 5 days in the United States.[2] Younger children typically choke on food items; older children more commonly aspirate things such as pins and pen caps, which they are holding in their mouths, although variability exists by country.[3,4]
- **Should I perform a blind finger sweep if there is concern for complete obstruction?** Rapidly removing a completely obstructing foreign body is paramount. In the conscious patient, the immediate intervention should be the Heimlich maneuver (for children >1 year old) or back blows and chest compressions (for children <1 year old).[5] If the victim becomes unresponsive, looking in the mouth and removing any visible foreign body is recommended. Data from case reports suggest that blind finger sweeps may advance the foreign body farther into the airway and may cause oropharyngeal trauma, and therefore should not be performed.[5–7]

## REFERENCES

1. United States Centers for Disease Control and Prevention. Ten leading causes of death and injury. Available at http://www.cdc.gov/injury/wisqars/leadingcauses.html. Accessed January 2, 2016.
2. Committee on Injury, Violence, and Poisoning Prevention. Prevention of choking among children. *Pediatrics*. 2010;125(3):601–607.
3. Chapin MM, Rochette LM, Annest JL, et al. Nonfatal choking on food among children 14 years or younger in the United States, 2001–2009. *Pediatrics*. 2013;132(2):275–278.
4. Singh H, Parakh A. Tracheobronchial foreign body aspiration in children. *Clin Pediatr (Phila)*. 2014;53(5):415–419.
5. Berg MD, Schexnayder SM, Chameides L, et al. Pediatric basic life support: 2010 American Heart Association Guidelines Cardiopulmonary Resuscitation and Emergency Cardiovascular Care. *Pediatrics*. 2010;126:e1345–e1360.
6. Hartrey R, Bingham RM. Pharyngeal trauma as a result of blind finger sweeps in the choking child. *J Accid Emerg Med*. 1995;12:52–54.
7. Vunda A, Vandertuin L. Nasopharyngeal foreign body folloing a blind finger sweep. *J Pediatr*. 2012;160(2):353.

# Section VII

# EMS Airway Management

Chapter 28

# Introduction to EMS Airway Management

Frederick H. Ellinger Jr, Michael Keller, and Darren A. Braude

## THE CLINICAL CHALLENGE

The prehospital setting presents unique challenges to all patient care, not the least of which is airway management. The patient's disease process is often undifferentiated, resources and equipment may be more limited than in the hospital setting, and there may be issues of patient access, lighting, adverse weather, confined space, turbulence or road vibration, and safety of the provider among others. When these factors are taken in aggregate, it is unreasonable to expect that out-of-hospital airway management will look identical to in-hospital airway management. Furthermore, airway management will not look the same in any two emergency medical services (EMS) systems owing to differences in provider levels of training, scope of practice, medical direction, treatment guidelines, transport times, equipment, and availability of backup, including air medical transport.

Despite these challenges, the core concepts of emergency airway management are the same in the prehospital and hospital environments: maintaining oxygenation and ventilation while mitigating complications. The airway algorithms are fundamentally equivalent; however, as we will discuss in the following chapters, accommodations need to be made when specific equipment or skills are not available. If oxygenation cannot be maintained via bag-mask ventilation (BMV) and the patient cannot be intubated, it does not matter whether it is because rapid sequence intubation (RSI) is not within the scope of practice or because RSI was attempted and unsuccessful; the airway has failed, and urgent placement of an extraglottic device (EGD) or cricothyrotomy is indicated regardless of the environment.

The prehospital setting is often unforgiving and may even be considered "error prone." These risks may be offset by careful planning, continuing education, use of algorithms and checklists, quality oversight, and strong medical director involvement. System administrators, medical directors, educators, and providers must all be committed to rigorous evaluation of the care delivered, patient outcomes, and the latest literature and how it applies to that system's practice.

## APPROACH TO THE AIRWAY

EMS airway management must focus on rapid assessment and simultaneous interventions. The goals are optimization of oxygenation and ventilation with minimization of complications such as aspiration, while facilitating extrication and transport, and performing any other critical treatments that may be indicated. In general, the least-invasive and time-consuming interventions that achieve the stated goals are preferable. Given the inherent limitations of the prehospital environment, the goals are not necessarily to achieve definitive airway management. For example:

- A 55-year-old presents for an exacerbation of left-sided congestive heart failure with pulmonary edema, resulting in respiratory distress and hypoxemia to 75%. The primary issue is oxygenation. If supplemental oxygen delivery in a position of comfort does not rapidly correct the problem, then administration of sublingual nitroglycerin and titration of continuous positive airway pressure (CPAP) along with initiation of transport are appropriate in most EMS systems. Administration of diuretics, nitroglycerin infusions, and intubation, if necessary, may usually be deferred to the hospital unless transport times are prolonged.
- A 14-year-old female thrown from a horse initially presents with a Glasgow Coma Scale (GCS) of 13, and a flight crew is dispatched. While transporting the patient, her mental status deteriorates with a noted rise in blood pressure and drop in respirations. Because of the confined space of the aircraft, the flight crew elects to perform a Rapid Sequence Airway (RSA) procedure with placement of an EGD rather than RSI. The patient receives analgesia, the ventilator is placed and titrated to maintain normal $ETCO_2$, a gastric tube is inserted and attached to suction, and oxygen is titrated down until the saturation just falls below 100%. On arrival to the ED, the patient is taken directly to the CT scanner, an epidural hematoma is detected, and the EGD is exchanged for an endotracheal tube using a flexible endoscope while awaiting arrival of the neurosurgeon. The best possible outcome for the patient has been ensured without definitive airway management in the field.
- A 27-year-old male with multisystem blunt trauma presents with GCS of 11, a systolic blood pressure of 90, and a saturation of 85%. The first actions are to maintain spinal motion restriction, roll the patient to clear the airway, apply supplemental oxygen, assess for tension pneumothorax, and start an IV for fluid administration, all while moving towards the hospital. As long as the provider addresses hypotension and hypoxemia, avoids hyperventilation, and makes reasonable attempts to prevent aspiration (or further aspiration), the goals have been met even though the airway has not been secured. If the provider has time, the airway is not predicted to be anatomically difficult outside of cervical precautions, and medication-facilitated airway management (MFAM) is available, then it should be considered. However, as discussed later, the evidence of benefit is limited while the potential for harm is real if the patient is allowed to become hypoxemic, hypotensive, hypocarbic, or hyperoxic.

In each of these cases, the providers focused on the most efficient means of establishing oxygenation and ventilation, and minimizing complications, not on any particular procedure. Invasive airway management, including MFAM, has a role in prehospital care as long as it is done carefully and judiciously with close supervision and medical oversight. It is our belief that care for each patient should be individualized based on the presenting clinical condition and anticipated clinical course, transport time, predicted difficulties, and the provider's experience and scope of practice. It is critical to keep in mind that many studies and reviews have failed to demonstrate improved patient outcome from prehospital endotracheal intubation, and several have demonstrated worse outcomes (see Evidence section).

The indications for prehospital intubation are the same as for hospital-based care, with appropriate consideration of resource constraints, transport mode and time, and the option to provide less-invasive, temporizing care while transporting to the hospital. The Universal and Main Emergency Airway Algorithms are applicable for prehospital providers recognizing that those providers not performing MFAM will primarily function in the Crash and Failed Airway Algorithms. In addition, the primary question for EMS providers is not whether the patient "needs intubation" but whether they need any form of invasive airway management before arrival at the hospital. The application of the Difficult and Failed Airway Algorithms to prehospital care is discussed in Chapter 30.

## LEVELS OF TRAINING AND SCOPE OF AIRWAY PRACTICE

Generally speaking, the different levels of training and scope of practice for prehospital providers in the United States are defined by the National Highway Traffic Safety Administration (NHTSA) in both their National EMS Scope of Practice Model (February 2007) and National Emergency Medical Services Education Standards (January 2009) documents. These provide the scope of practice and individual psychomotor skills for each level of prehospital provider. Both the scope of practice document and the education standards outline the individual credential levels as follows:

- Emergency Medical Responder (EMR)
- Emergency Medical Technician (EMT)
- Advanced Emergency Medical Technician (AEMT)
- Paramedic

Many states have chosen to adopt these credentialing terms, whereas others have not, preferring older terms such as First Responder, EMT-Basic, and EMT-Intermediate. In an even more confusing approach, some states have chosen to adopt the national document terminology; yet their scope of practice privileges differs greatly from the published psychomotor skillset. For the purposes of this publication, the authors will attempt to describe national scope of practice skillset and education standards as most widely accepted in clinical practice in the United States, recognizing that international practice may be very different, especially because many such systems may be primarily physician-based.

Both the EMR and EMT are categorized as Basic Life Support (BLS) providers. These providers' psychomotor airway skillset is limited to foreign body removal with external techniques, supplemental oxygen delivery, positioning, BMV, and the use of oropharyngeal (OPA) and nasopharyngeal (NPA) airways. It is worth noting that the NHTSA papers recommend OPA only for the EMR and both OPA and NPA for the EMT level, whereas most states do not limit the use of NPAs from EMR personnel.

In another example of where individual states and accepted clinical practice differ from government documents, the NHTSA National EMS Scope of Practice Model and the National Emergency Medical Services Educational Standards do not recommend the use of extraglottic devices at the AEMT and Paramedic levels, which is not consistent with most clinical practice in the United States. Many states even allow the use of extraglottic devices for EMT's.

The National Association of State EMS Officials published the National Model EMS Clinical Guidelines in October 2014. This evidence-based document does not differentiate between BLS and Advanced Life Support (ALS) providers with respect to airway management, but rather the guidelines simply approach clinical recommendations in a stepwise fashion. That is, begin with least-invasive maneuvers (BMV, Non-invasive Positive Pressure Ventilation (NIPPV)), and progress in complexity (EGD and endotracheal intubation) until optimal airway management is achieved.

The NHTSA documents recognize the Paramedic as the highest credentialed prehospital provider in the United States. These publications recognize and recommend the highest level of airway management skills for the paramedic, including endotracheal intubation and surgical cricothyrotomy. All of the 50 States in the United States allow paramedics to perform oral tracheal intubation, but internationally this is not always the case. There is even wider variability in whether cricothyrotomy is permitted and via which method—surgical or percutaneous transtracheal ventilation (PTV). In addition, MFAM is extremely controversial in EMS, and many jurisdictions do not allow paramedics to use medications to facilitate airway management.

Other areas of prehospital medical practice include the Prehospital Registered Nurse, Critical Care Paramedic, Certified Flight Paramedic, or Certified Flight Registered Nurse. The U.S. federal documents do not address these credentials or distinctions, but many states either encourage or require providers to have these types of specialty training or certifications to perform advanced airway management skills such MFAM in the out-of-hospital environment.

## MECHANISMS FOR MAINTENANCE OF AIRWAY COMPETENCY

Unfortunately, it has become harder for training programs to make supervised live intubations available because of a variety of issues including an overload of learners in the surgical suites, less intubation procedures being performed in the surgical environment, and concerns of liability. Overall, we believe there is great value to spending time with an experienced anesthesia or emergency medicine provider, but not just for intubations. There is equal or greater value, in our opinion, to supervised BMV and

EGD placement as well as the intellectual discussions that often ensue. Anesthesia and emergency medicine providers are therefore strongly encouraged to help provide initial and ongoing learning opportunities for EMS providers in their catchment areas. Because it is extremely rare for EMR, EMT, and AEMT students to get time in the OR, it must be recognized that they may be at a disadvantage when initially providing care in the field and will require close supervision and mentorship.

It is incumbent on each provider, agency, and system to set standards that ensure patient safety and optimize success. Checklists have been used in many healthcare and non-healthcare settings and should be strongly considered for out-of-hospital airway management. A sample checklist is shown in **Figure 28-1**.

## AIRWAY CHECKLISTS

### PREPARATION

**OXYGENATE**

- ☐ NRB at highest flow possible
- ☐ $SpO_2$ < 93%? Consider CPAP, BMV, DSI or RSA
- ☐ Place patient on stretcher
- ☐ Medical: sniffing/ramped Trauma: reverse Trendelenburg unless low BP
- ☐ Nasal cannula at 5–15 lpm (5 for peds < 1 year)

**RESUSCITATE**

- ☐ Fluids/blood
- ☐ Vasopressors

**ANTICIPATE**

- ☐ Assess difficulty — ROMAN, RODS, SMART, LEMONS
- ☐ Determine and announce Plan A, Plan B and Plan C
  - ☐ Prepare Equipment
    - ☐ BP cuff opposite $SpO_2$ probe and IV
    - ☐ Oral and nasal airways
    - ☐ Bag and mask with PEEP valve
    - ☐ Suction
    - ☐ Laryngoscope
    - ☐ ET tube with correct stylet shape (DL = straight to cuff)
    - ☐ Bougie
    - ☐ EGD and cricothyroidotomy kit
    - ☐ Capnography
    - ☐ Ventilator
  - ☐ Prepare Medications
    - ☐ Pretreatment
    - ☐ Induction
    - ☐ Paralysis
    - ☐ Analgesia and sedation
- ☐ Assign tasks: c-spine/jaw thrust, ELM, ventilation, watch $SpO_2$

the difficult airway course™ EMS

● **FIGURE 28-1.**

## AIRWAY CHECKLISTS

### RSI/RSA PROCEDURE

- ☐ Verbalize Time out!
  - ☐ Is this still a good plan?
  - ☐ Who is watching $SpO_2$ & general well being of patient?
  - ☐ Is everyone ready?
    - ☐ Will we need to do PPV?
- ☐ Give pretreatment if indicated and wait 3 minutes
- ☐ Push induction agent and <u>immediately</u> push paralytic
- ☐ Positive pressure ventilation if indicated
- ☐ Wait 45–60 seconds after the paralytic to start the procedure
- ☐ Pass ET tube or EGD
- ☐ Move to plan B and plan C as needed
- ☐ Confirm with $ETCO_2$ and lung sounds
- ☐ Go to post-RSI/RSA checklist

### POST RSI/RSA

- ☐ Secure tube
- ☐ Replace cervical collar if indicated
- ☐ Continuous capnography
- ☐ Place ventilator
- ☐ Analgesia and sedation
- ☐ Check Plateau pressure and PIP — adjust vent as needed
- ☐ Gastric tube
- ☐ Titrate $FiO_2$ down as appropriate for condition
- ☐ Adjust PEEP to maintain goal $SpO_2$
- ☐ Titrate minute ventilation to keep $ETCO_2$ at goal

thairwaysite.com



the difficult airway course™ EMS

● **FIGURE 28-1.** *(continued)*

## EVIDENCE

- **How successful is out-of-hospital airway management, and what is the current scope of practice?** Intubation success varies greatly based on provider skillset and volume. Data from more than 8,400 prehospital intubations in the National EMS Information System (NEMSIS) revealed that the overall intubation success rate was 77%, and successful use of an alternate airway device was 87%.[1] In head-injured patients, data suggest that airway management success and patient outcome depends on EMS system and provider experience.[2–7] Guidelines published by the NHTSA in both their National EMS Scope of Practice Model and National Emergency Medical Services Education Standards documents define the range of airway maneuvers from BMV to MFAM to surgical techniques for the most skilled prehospital providers.[8,9] The most recent recommendations by The National Association of State EMS Officials published in 2014 recommend a stepwise escalation that begins with least-invasive maneuvers and progress in complexity until optimal airway management is achieved.[10]

- **What experience and training is recommended for prehospital providers?** Although the best method to attain initial airway training is not clearly delineated in the existing literature, it is clear that a sufficient number of procedures are required to attain proficiency. One study of EMS trainees has shown that it takes 15 intubations to achieve a 90% chance of success in the controlled OR environment, but even 30 intubations does not predict 90% success in the challenging prehospital environment.[11] Although some oversight bodies such as the Committee of the Accreditation of Education Programs for the EMS professions (CoAEMSP) allow students to learn from any combination of live patients, high-fidelity simulations, low-fidelity simulations, or cadaver labs, other oversight agencies and bodies require paramedic students to perform a minimum number of supervised live intubations.[12] Although initial training is essential for competence, ongoing skill maintenance is challenging in the prehospital arena. Once licensed and working, opportunities for intubation skill maintenance are often limited owing to the increased use of NIPPV and EGDs as well as the increased number of providers working clinically resulting in skill dilution.[13] Intubation outcomes in patients suffering from out-of-hospital cardiac arrest correlate with the number of intubations that the treating paramedic had performed in the previous 5 years.[14] As a result, many agencies set requirements for a minimum numbers of encounters and success, often relying on low-fidelity simulation. The Committee on Accreditation of Medical Transport Systems (CAMTS) requires one adult, pediatric, and infant intubations (and all agency carried EGD's) per quarter, or a total of 12 intubations per year, all of which may be simulated.[15] Despite this mandate, a 2014 study of almost 5,000 intubations by air medical crews primarily using RSI demonstrated a first-pass success of less than 80% and an overall success of 92%.[16] This suggests that the standards may be insufficient to maintain competence. It is incumbent on each provider, agency, and system to set standards that ensure patient safety and optimizes success.
- **Should checklists be used for prehospital airway management?** The challenges of the prehospital environment described earlier can make procedure completion difficult and error prone, particularly during complex, high-intensity skills such as MFAM or stressful scenarios such as failed airways. In general aviation, human factors account for up to 82% of accidents.[17] We do not know the full extent of human error involved in EMS-related morbidity and mortality, but a recent simulation-based study of pediatric resuscitation by EMS providers confirmed a very high error rate during a simulated, prehospital, pediatric cardiopulmonary arrest.[18] It is safe to assume from the available data that critical and preventable errors are occurring in prehospital airway management. We know that human factors play an important role in both skill and decision making, and therefore, EMS systems must look for ways to identify and mitigate error. Learning from the aviation industry, in-hospital medical professionals have begun to embrace the use of procedural checklists, and there is good evidence that this can reduce both technical and cognitive errors.[19] Our recommendation is that EMS administrators, Medical Directors, and providers should embrace the use of checklists particularly for high-risk, low-frequency, or complex skills such as MFAM. Any checklist utilized needs to be relevant and useful. Checklists for airway procedures such as MFAM should address patient preparation, equipment, drugs, and team variables.[20] The authors of this chapter would recommend reading *The Checklist Manifesto: How to Get Things Right* by Atul Gawande.[21].

## REFERENCES


1. Wang HE, Mann NC, Mears G, et al. Out-of-hospital airway management in the United States. *Resuscitation*. 2011;82(4):378–385.
2. Cudnik MT, Newgard CD, Daya M, et al. The impact of rapid sequence intubation on trauma patient mortality in attempted prehospital intubation. *J Emerg Med*. 2010;38(2):175–181.
3. Bossers SM, Schwarte LA, Loer SA, et al. Experience in prehospital endotracheal intubation significantly influences mortality of patients with severe traumatic brain injury: a systematic review and meta-analysis. *PLoS One*. 2015;10(10):e0141034.
4. Sobuwa S, Hartzenberg HB, Geduld H, et al. Outcomes following prehospital airway management in severe traumatic brain injury. *S Afr Med J*. 2013;103(9):644–646.
5. Karamanos E, Talving P, Skiada D, et al. Is prehospital endotracheal intubation associated with improved outcomes in isolated severe head injury? A matched cohort analysis. *Prehosp Disaster Med*. 2014;29(1):32–36.
6. Hussmann B, Lefering R, Waydhas C, et al. Prehospital intubation of the moderately injured patient: a cause of morbidity? A matched-pairs analysis of 1,200 patients from the DGU Trauma Registry. *Crit Care*. 2011;15(5):R207.
7. Davis DP, Stern J, Sise MJ, et al. A follow-up analysis of factors associated with head-injury mortality after paramedic rapid sequence intubation. *J Trauma*. 2005;59(2):486–490.
8. National Highway Traffic Safety Administration. National EMS Scope of Practice Model. http://www.ems.gov/education/EMSScope.pdf. 2007.
9. National Highway Traffic Safety Administration. National Emergency Medical Services Education Standards. http://www.ems.gov/pdf/811077a.pdf. 2009.
10. National Association of State EMS Officials. National Model EMS Guidelines. https://nasemso.org/Projects/ModelEMSClinicalGuidelines/documents/National-Model-EMS-Clinical-Guidelines-23Oct2014.pdf. 2014.
11. Wang HE, Seitz SR, Hostler D, et al. Defining the learning curve for paramedic student endotracheal intubation. *Prehosp Emerg Care*. 2005;9(2):156–162.
12. Committee on Accreditation of Educational Programs for the Emergency Medical Services Professions. Airway Management Recommendation. http://coaemsp.org/Documents/Airway-Recommendation-10-2013.pdf.
13. Pouliot RC. Failed prehospital tracheal intubation: a matter of skill dilution? *Anesth Analg*. 2010;110(5):1507–1508; author reply 1509.
14. Wang HE, Balasubramani GK, Cook LJ, et al. Out-of-hospital endotracheal intubation experience and patient outcomes. *Ann Emerg Med*. 2010;55(6):527.e526–537.e526.
15. Commission on Accreditation of Medical Transport Systems. Tenth edition accreditation standards of the Commission on Accreditation of Medical Transport Systems. http://www.camts.org/10th_Edition_Standards_For_Website.pdf. 2015.
16. Brown CA, Cox K, Hurwitz S, et al. 4,871 emergency airway encounters by air medical providers: a report of the air transport emergency airway management (NEAR VI: "A-TEAM") project. *West J Emerg Med*. 2014;15(2):188–193.
17. US Department of Transportation, Federal Aviation Administration. A human error approach to aviation accident analysis: the Human Factors Analysis and Classification System. DOT/FAA/AM-00/7. https://www.nifc.gov/fireInfo/fireInfo_documents/humanfactors_classAnly.pdf. 2000.
18. Lammers RL, Willoughby-Byrwa M, Fales WD. Errors and error-producing conditions during a simulated, prehospital, pediatric cardiopulmonary arrest. *Simul Healthc*. 2014;9(3):174–183.

19. Haynes AB, Weiser TG, Berry WR, et al. A surgical safety checklist to reduce morbidity and mortality in a global population. *N Engl J Med*. 2009;360(5):491–499.

20. Cook T, Woodall N, Harper J, et al. Major complications of airway management in the UK: results of the Fourth National Audit Project of the Royal College of Anaesthetists and the Difficult Airway Society. Part 2: intensive care and emergency departments. *Br J Anaesth*. 2011;106(5):632–642.

21. Gawande, A. *The Checklist Manifesto: How to Get Things Right*. New York, NY: Metropolitan Books; 2010.

Chapter 29

# Techniques in EMS Airway Management

Kevin Franklin, Darren A. Braude, and Michael G. Gonzalez

## THE CLINICAL CHALLENGE

Airway management in the prehospital environment is fraught with challenges. Many of these same challenges may be encountered when airway management is required in nontraditional locations within the hospital. This chapter focuses on unique management techniques and variations of traditional techniques designed to overcome these challenges.

### Location and Environmental Factors

When possible, patients should be moved to a secure, private, warm, well-lit, and spacious environment prior to airway management. This might be best achieved simply by moving a patient in cardiac arrest from a small bathroom to the living room, or might require moving a patient from the roadside into the back of an ambulance. Certain scenarios may require management of the patient in situ: if they are entrapped, if the need for airway management is immediate, if there is no more optimal place close by, or if it is otherwise unsafe to attempt movement. In these circumstances, rescuers should limit airway procedures to only those that are absolutely necessary; this may include only basic airway management until care can be rendered safely.

### Patient Positioning for Airway Management

Proper patient positioning can often be exceedingly challenging in the prehospital setting. Prehospital patients are frequently found on the floor, recumbent on soft surfaces, or entrapped. These unique positions may make it difficult to obtain optimal positioning for preoxygenation and airway interventions. Providers often handicap themselves by trying to manage the patient in the position in which they are found rather than taking a brief period to achieve better positioning, which can be beneficial for the provider and patient.

Whenever possible, patients found on the floor or other suboptimal position should be moved to a stretcher before airway management (**Fig. 29-1**). This practice has the advantage of improving airway management and avoids having to move the patient onto the stretcher while intubated, which could result in tube dislodgement. For patients with cardiac arrest, it may not be feasible or desirable to place the patient on the stretcher. In such cases, towels may be placed behind the head to

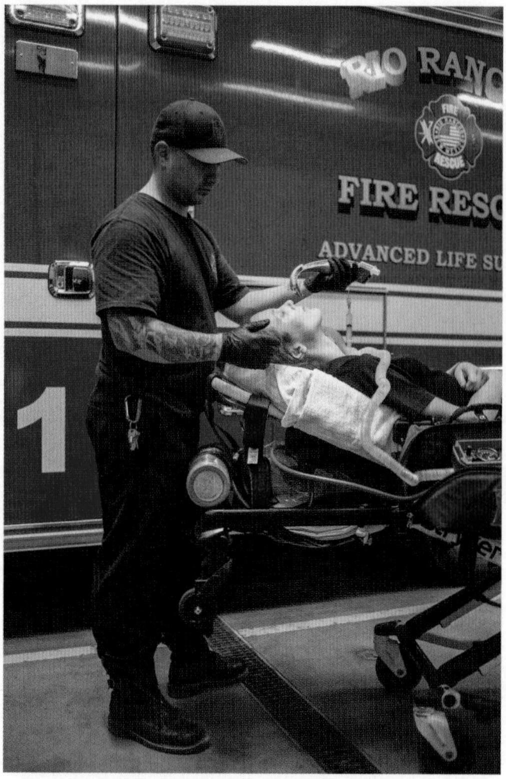


● **FIGURE 29-1.** Placing the patient on the EMS stretcher and lifting it up allows for intubation to occur at an optimal height.

achieve the classic sniffing position; towels may also be improvised with a small piece of emergency medical services (EMS) equipment or patient belongings (**Fig. 29-2**). Even more challenging is trying to create a ramped position for an obese patient on the ground, because this requires more padding and can interfere with chest compressions. Ideally, the obese, supine patient without cardiac arrest should be moved to the stretcher and positioned as shown in **Figure 29-3**.

For the obese, supine patient with cardiac arrest, the best possible sniffing position should be achieved while continuing chest compressions. If these maneuvers do not create an adequate laryngoscopic view, ventilation should be attempted via an extraglottic device (EGD). If the patient cannot be adequately ventilated with an EGD, two providers can replicate a ramped position by grasping the patient's outstretched arms from the front and pulling them into position (**Fig. 29-4**). This procedure should only be maintained for a few seconds, but because cardiopulmonary resuscitation (CPR) must be interrupted in order to perform the maneuver, longer periods are not recommended.

## Bag-Mask Ventilation

Although bag-mask ventilation (BMV) is a fundamental airway skill taught to EMS providers at all levels starting at the Emergency Medical Responder level, it can be very difficult to perform in the prehospital setting for a variety of complex reasons. Patients often present with multiple predictors of difficulty based on the ROMAN mnemonic (see Chapter 2), access and positioning may not be optimal, personnel may be limited, and, perhaps most importantly, the procedure is often relegated to the least-experienced provider. Strategies to mitigate these issues include emphasizing optimal technique (proper positioning, use of appropriate airway adjuncts, using two-person and two-handed technique), use of a transport ventilator to free up hands, and assigning a senior person to perform or supervise this critical skill (**Fig. 29-5**).

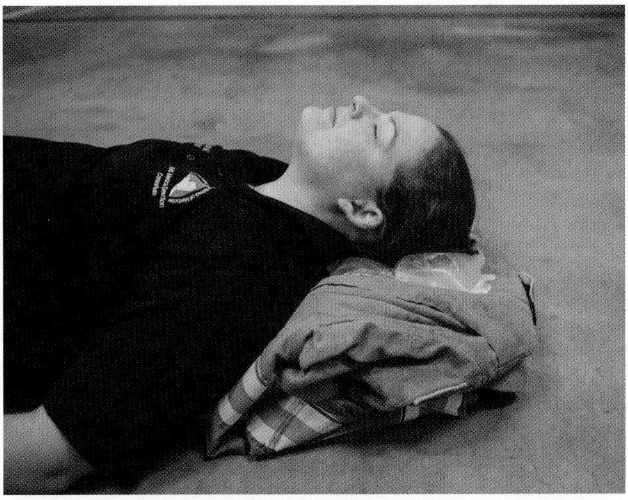

● **FIGURE 29-2.** Achieving sniffing position with improvised supplies, in this case firefighter bunker gear and IV bags.

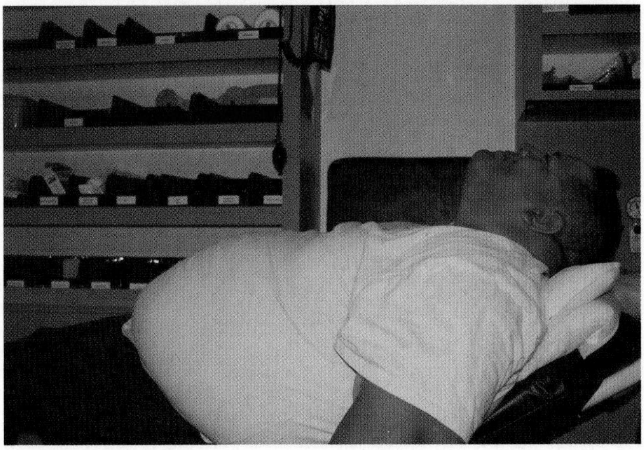

● **FIGURE 29-3.** Achieving a ramped position for an obese patient using a combination of padding and elevation of the head of the stretcher.

When difficulty is encountered with achieving an adequate mask seal, early consideration should be given to bypassing these anatomic difficulties with an EGD. EMS providers who are forced to provide one-person BMV without benefit of a ventilator might also consider use of the NuMask, which may be helpful.

## *Noninvasive Positive Pressure Ventilation*

One of the most significant advances in EMS over the last decade has been the widespread adoption of Noninvasive Positive Pressure Ventilation (NIPPV), typically continuous positive airway pressure (CPAP); in some jurisdictions, CPAP has been extended to the Emergency Medical Technician (EMT) level. Numerous products are now available to provide CPAP in the prehospital setting, from simple single-use devices to complex ventilators. In systems without medication-facilitated airway management (MFAM), CPAP is most commonly used as a bridge to facilitate transport to the hospital, because the only other options in the conscious yet distressed hypoxemic patient are

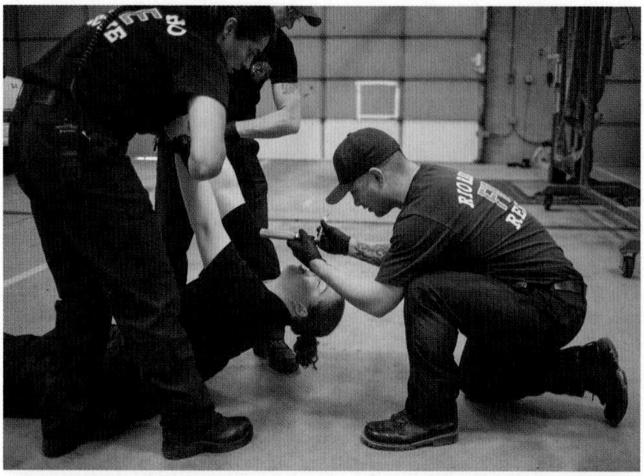

● **FIGURE 29-4.** Assistants lifting a patient's arms to demonstrate how to quickly and briefly position an obese patient lying on the ground for intubation without having to build a ramp.

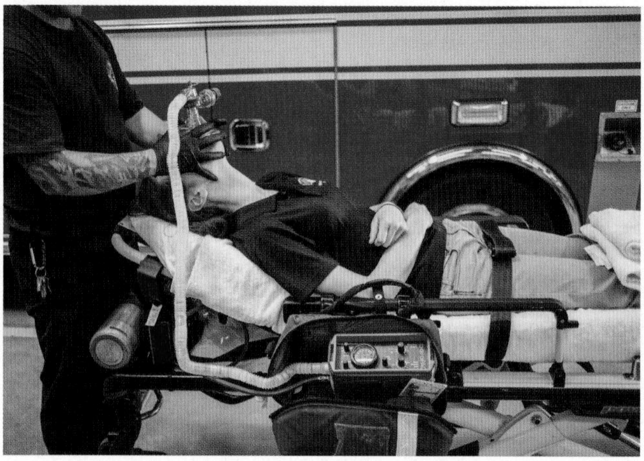

● **FIGURE 29-5.** Use of a simple transport ventilator to free up hands so that one provider may use both hands to achieve an optimal mask seal.

either blind nasotracheal intubation (BNTI) or assisted respirations with BMV, both of which are often poorly tolerated. In MFAM systems, CPAP is also used as a preoxygenation strategy and as an alternative to intubation in patients where intubation is predicted to be difficult, where the need for positive pressure respiratory support is predicted to be short, or in those patients in need of ventilatory support but with a "Do Not Intubate" order. Interestingly, despite our own positive anecdotes, the evidence behind prehospital CPAP is mixed (see Chapter 31).

The greatest barrier to applying CPAP in the prehospital setting is having to coach a hypoxemic, hypercarbic, and anxious patient in a loud and chaotic environment to wear the requisite tight-fitting mask. It is important for the provider to display gentle persistence and a calm confident demeanor—even if they have little actual experience with the procedure. It is helpful to make eye contact and tell the patient "This will help you breathe" while having them help hold the mask on their face until they can feel the benefit. Ideally, one provider will be dedicated to coaching the patient through the first several minutes of use; the person chosen for this "coaching" task does not have to be the most experienced airway manager, but they must be able to work effectively with the patient.

One area of controversy discussed in Chapter 31 is the use of CPAP in patients with altered mental status. It is our opinion that altered mental status (AMS) should be considered a relative but not absolute contraindication, and the pros and cons should be weighed in each individual case. Clearly, a patient with Glasgow coma scale (GCS) of 3 and poor respiratory effort needs BMV. Conversely, a somnolent and confused hypercarbic or hypoxemic patient who can remain seated may be a very reasonable CPAP candidate when EMS crews can provide vigilant one-on-one observation at all times during transport. It also makes sense to employ CPAP liberally, despite AMS, for preoxygenation. If, for example, a crew of two or three is rapidly setting up for MFAM in a spontaneously breathing but unconscious patient, tying up one crew member to assist respirations may not be an optimal use of resources.

Another unique prehospital challenge in the use of NIPPV is the availability of oxygen and compressed gases. There is wide variability among commercially available devices, requiring extra attention for rescuers who may be inexperienced. EMS personnel must have appropriate training and expertise to determine the rate of oxygen consumption with their particular NIPPV device, and must be able to calculate the amount of gas, and consequently, time that remains. One tool available to assist in this process is a table that cross-references flow rate and compressed gas pressure to time (see **Table 29-1**).

## Endotracheal Intubation

General intubation techniques, as well as preoxygenation, are covered extensively elsewhere in this text. The decision-making process surrounding intubation in the prehospital setting is discussed separately in Chapter 28. Primarily, when access is limited or patients cannot be optimally positioned, responders should have a low threshold for use of an EGD, at least until the patient can be moved to a location that is more conducive to definitive airway management.

One potential situation involves the seated and entrapped patient (e.g., entrapped driver in vehicle) who requires invasive airway management. When intubation is clearly indicated for such patients, a common approach is face-to-face laryngoscopy (**Fig. 29-6**). This technique can be extremely challenging as the normal anatomic relationships encountered in direct laryngoscopy are reversed, and the psychomotor skills involved in placing an endotracheal tube have to be altered. Video laryngoscopy offers a significant advantage when a face-to-face intubation is required (see Evidence section). Another option, when access above the patient is available, is for the intubator to stand behind and over the patient, allowing space to lean over and perform laryngoscopy in a more familiar orientation (**Fig. 29-7**).

**TABLE 29-1** **Oxygen Consumption Table for Portable D Cylinder**

| D Tank Duration (minutes) | | Oxygen Tank Pressure (psi) | | | | | | |
|---|---|---|---|---|---|---|---|---|
| | | 2000 | 1750 | 1500 | 1250 | 1000 | 750 | 500 |
| Flow Rate (L/mm) | 6 | 53 | 46 | 40 | 33 | 26 | 20 | 13 |
| | 10 | 32 | 28 | 24 | 20 | 16 | 12 | 8 |
| | 12 | 26 | 23 | 20 | 16 | 13 | 10 | 6 |
| | 15 | 21 | 18 | 16 | 13 | 10 | 8 | 5 |
| | 20 | 16 | 14 | 12 | 10 | 8 | 6 | 4 |
| | 25 | 12 | 11 | 9 | 8 | 6 | 4 | 3 |
| | 30 | 10 | 9 | 8 | 6 | 5 | 4 | 2 |
| | 35 | 9 | 8 | 6 | 5 | 4 | 3 | 2 |
| | 40 | 8 | 7 | 6 | 5 | 4 | 3 | 2 |
| | 45 | 7 | 6 | 5 | 4 | 3 | 2 | 1 |
| | 50 | 6 | 5 | 4 | 4 | 3 | 2 | 1 |
| | 55 | 5 | 5 | 4 | 3 | 2 | 2 | 1 |
| | 60 | 5 | 4 | 4 | 3 | 2 | 2 | 1 |

Note: None

| Color Scale |
|---|
| > 60 minutes |
| 45-59 minutes |
| 21-44 minutes |
| 10-20 minutes |
| < 10 minutes |

Courtesy of West Michigan Air Care.

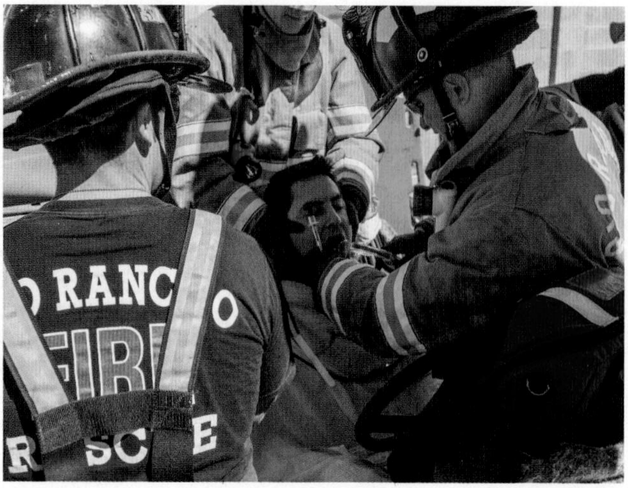


● **FIGURE 29-6.** Video laryngoscopy with the intubator positioned in front of, or face-to-face with, the entrapped patient.

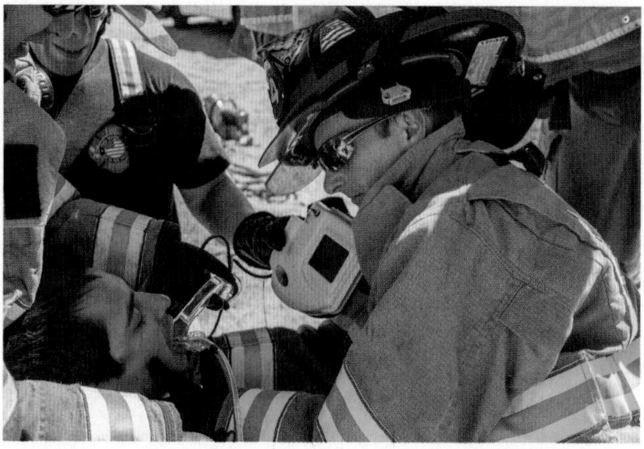

● **FIGURE 29-7.** Video laryngoscopy with the intubator positioned behind and above the entrapped patient.

There are numerous positioning options for intubating a patient who is supine on the floor/ground, including sitting, straddling, kneeling, and lying prone or in a left lateral orientation (**Fig. 29-8A–C**). There is insufficient evidence to recommend one position over another. It is best, as discussed earlier, to reposition or elevate the patient whenever possible prior to intubation rather than attempting the procedure with the patient on the ground. Several tips for proper positioning and achieving a ramped position for obese patients are discussed earlier.

If the posterior cartilages cannot be visualized on initial attempt—despite external laryngeal manipulation and the jaw thrust maneuver—and great force is required to maintain the view, intubation will be difficult or impossible. An option in this situation, especially when the intubator has limited upper arm strength, is a two-person approach (**Fig. 29-9**). In this maneuver, a trained assistant reaches over the patient from an inferior position of mechanical advantage and carefully takes control of the laryngoscope handle from the primary intubator with two hands. The primary intubator can then direct minor blade movements, if necessary, although in our experience this optimizes the view enough that this is not usually required.

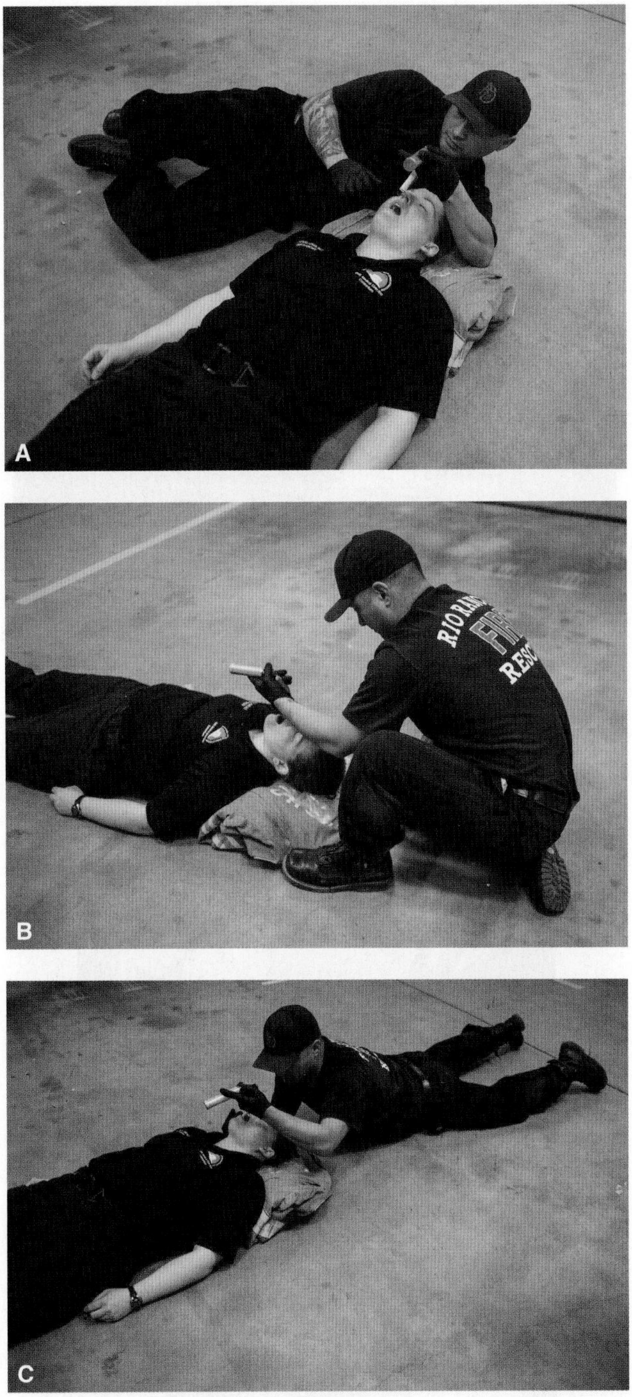


● **FIGURE 29-8.** A–C: The left lateral, prone, and kneeling positions for intubating a supine patient on the ground or floor. Note that the prone and left-lateral positions are more difficult when the patient is placed into a sniffing or ramped position.

Intubation in direct sunlight or bright ambient light can be very difficult, particularly with video technology. If intubation must be attempted in these conditions, the intubator may consider placing a blanket over themselves and the patient's head or enlist other personnel to provide shade with their bodies or clothing such as a turnout coat (**Fig. 29-10**).

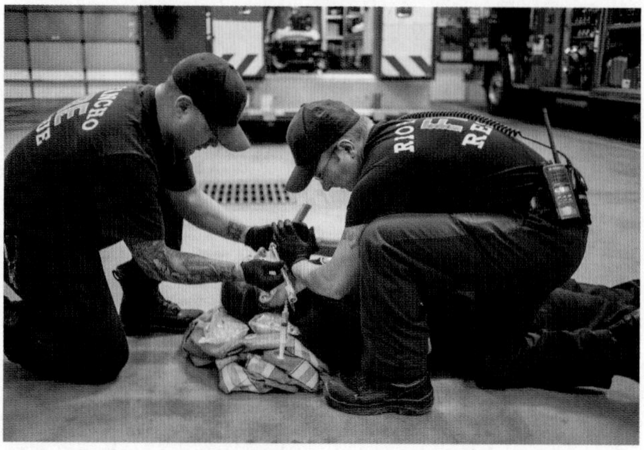

● **FIGURE 29-9.** Two-person direct laryngoscopy with an assistant providing lift along the axis of the handle from a position of mechanical advantage (after the intubator has appropriately placed the blade) while the intubator provides ongoing direction and passes the tube.

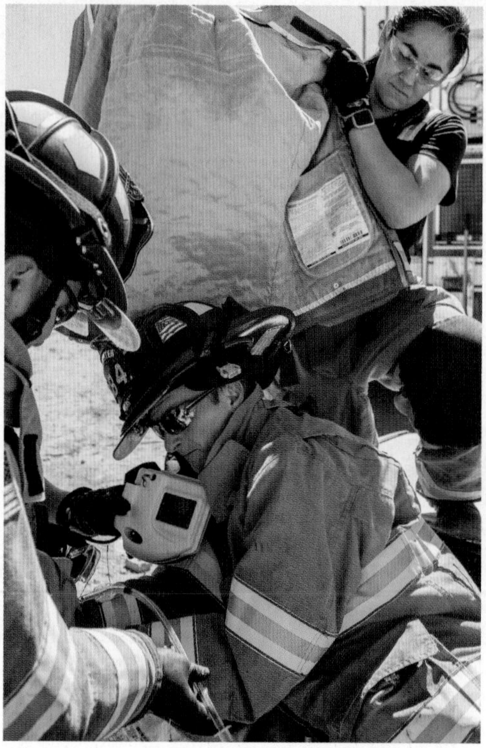

● **FIGURE 29-10.** A provider uses a turnout coat to provide shade during laryngoscopy to prevent bright light from affecting the view in the mouth or of the video screen.

Because patients undergoing emergency airway management are at high risk for regurgitation and aspiration, it is important to have suction equipment immediately available. This is another reason why it is often preferable to manage the patient in the ambulance, aircraft, or hospital. In addition, because most portable suctions do not have the capacity to manage massive emesis, consider having two units available and always be prepared to roll the patient.

### *Blind Nasotracheal Intubation*

Over the past two decades, the use of BNTI during airway management in the hospital and many prehospital settings has largely been replaced by NIPPV, MFAM, or visualized nasal intubation using flexible endoscopy. In addition, ICUs uniformly exchange these tubes as soon as they arrive and discourage their placement. However, BNTI remains within the paramedic scope of practice in many areas because either MFAM is not within scope of practice, or options for awake oral or visualized nasal intubation to manage the predicted difficult airway are limited by equipment and expertise. Unfortunately, it should be noted that success rates for BNTI are lower than those for rapid sequence intubation (RSI), even when it was commonly performed, and complications are generally higher (see Chapter 18). This is especially true as the opportunity for skill maintenance by observing or performing the procedure in the hospital setting has become virtually nonexistent. Many experienced EMS educators have never performed the procedure. If EMS providers are going to continue to perform this technique, they should review and simulate the procedure regularly, carry endotracheal tubes intended for nasal intubation, weigh risks, benefits and alternatives carefully, and always have a backup plan available.

## Cricothyrotomy

The various roles for a prehospital cricothyrotomy are discussed in Chapter 30, and most commonly include the following: (1) Backup technique when BMV fails to provide critical oxygenation, and EGD placement or intubation is not possible such as in the hypoxemic trauma patient with trismus in a non-MFAM system, and (2) Backup technique after failed intubation when EGD placement has also failed or is predicted to fail. Difficult airway management is generally predictable, and failed airways occur less often when an appropriate airway assessment is undertaken *before* airway management begins. Occasionally, unanticipated difficulties may lead to a failed airway and require immediate intervention. It is therefore imperative that paramedics always have appropriate equipment for emergency cricothyrotomy available and consider that option early.

Mostly, surgical airways are performed too late to be lifesaving; once the patient has experienced cardiac arrest from respiratory failure it is much harder to resuscitate. In the setting of MFAM, providers should palpate the neck anatomy as part of their routine airway assessment and preparation, even if it is not predicted to be necessary. The controversy surrounding the choice of surgical and less-invasive cricothyrotomy techniques is discussed in Chapter 31. Our preference is for the bougie-aided surgical approach using a scalpel, bougie, and 6-0 cuffed endotracheal or tracheostomy tube (see Chapter 19). The classic surgical technique calls for use of a scalpel, tracheal hook, Trousseau dilator, and tracheostomy tube, most of which are not available to EMS providers.

### *Medication-Facilitated Airway Management*

This is a complex procedure performed in very sick or injured patients. When performed under less-than-ideal conditions, the potential for adverse events goes up significantly. Those agencies that perform prehospital MFAM need to have initial training and a system for ongoing skill maintenance to stay proficient. Teams should also look for system-level solutions to increase operator efficiency and mitigate risk. Some examples include the use of carefully labeled and standardized syringes for different classes of medications (see **Fig. 29-11**).

Because MFAM is a team effort and there may only be one or more crew members on scene, it is important to train the first responding personnel as assistants. This is a major component of

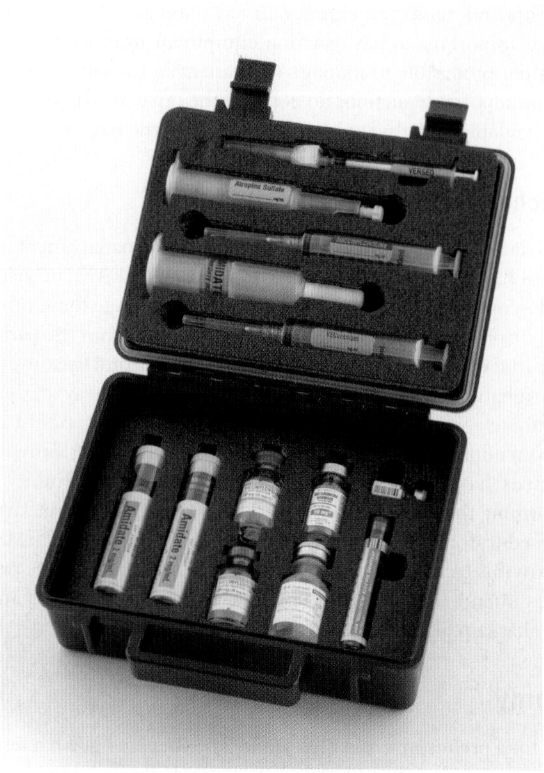


● **FIGURE 29-11.** This custom kit from Chinook Medical Gear, Inc. has all the medications for airway management labeled, organized, and highly visible.

the First Airway "Fundamentals of Airway Management" course for Basic Life Support (BLS) and Intermediate Life Support (ILS) providers. These providers may be trained to assist with external laryngeal manipulation, in-line cervical spine stabilization with jaw thrust, passing tubes over a bougie, and monitoring saturations. It is also helpful to train first responders to provide advanced life support (ALS) providers with the estimated patient weight prior to their arrival, which allows medications to be drawn up and the ventilator prepared. Because the most common patient to undergo prehospital MFAM is the adult male with trauma, the ventilator can be set up at the beginning of the shift for this hypothetical patient to minimize the need for adjustments. It is also imperative to ensure that all equipment is functional and in its appropriate location prior to use.

## Verification of Airway Management Procedures

It is imperative that all invasive airway procedures be confirmed objectively, with capnography serving as the gold-standard technique, as unrecognized esophageal intubations can occur when capnography is not performed. Hopefully all EMS systems have this technology available, but just because it is available it does not mean it always gets used. Even in the OR, where patients are intubated all day long, under much more ideal conditions, capnographic confirmation is assessed 100% of the time. This should also be the standard in prehospital care. Ignoring or disbelieving capnography results and continuing to ventilate through a displaced device can be a critical mistake. When in doubt, pull the device and go back to BMV. On the contrary, when saturations are slow to improve, or are dropping, but capnography reveals a normal waveform, trust the tube and look for other causes of hypoxemia.

There may be situations where capnography is unavailable or not functioning and the tube must be confirmed by other objective means. The most readily available alternative is a bougie, which can be placed through an established endotracheal tube to assess for palpable tracheal rings or a "hold-up" at a mainstem bronchus. Another alternative is an esophageal detector device, which uses suction to assess tube location. In the case of an esophageal intubation, the esophageal detector device will collapse the esophagus, impeding airflow and restricting the reinflation of the inflatable bulb or syringe. If the endotracheal tube is correctly positioned in the trachea, the bulb will quickly reinflate after being squeezed.

## Managing the Intubated Patient

Once an invasive device is placed in the prehospital setting (either EGD or endotracheal tube), careful attention must be given to prevent dislodgement. EGDs are more forgiving than an ETT or cricothyrotomy, but even these devices should be carefully secured using appropriate equipment. Methods used to achieve this are the same in the prehospital and hospital settings. One additional consideration is the use of a cervical collar in medical patients, particularly in pediatrics, to prevent head extension and subsequent tube movement. Although this has been very popular in some jurisdictions, a competing concern is the potential impairment of cerebral blood flow. Another reason is that the patient will undergo unnecessary imaging procedures because the "message" will get lost in multiple patient hand-offs, and subsequent providers will assume that a cervical injury was suspected. Generally, we do not routinely recommend this technique but prefer securing the device well in the mouth. If services elect to immobilize the cervical spine to prevent tube dislodgement, this should be decided at the system level and be communicated clearly at the time of transfer of care to the hospital.

Overventilation is extremely harmful to many patients regardless of the type of advanced airway placed. Hyperoxia can also be harmful. The optimal way to prevent overventilation is with the use of a mechanical ventilator. Numerous ventilators are now available for prehospital use, ranging from simple devices that allow only for adjustment of rate and volume to complex critical care transport devices that are nearly as sophisticated as ICU ventilators. Many of these will also allow for the titration of oxygen concentration. We recommend that ventilators always be used in the setting of MFAM, including both RSI and rapid sequence airway. When available, these devices may also be used for mask ventilation and during cardiac arrest management.

## Tips and Pearls

- Move patients to a stretcher prior to airway management.
- In the absence of cervical spine precautions, use whatever is available to achieve a sniffing or ramped position.
- Have an experienced person perform or supervise BMV rather than delegating to the junior most provider. Consider using an EGD in the event of difficult mask seal despite a two-handed and two-provider technique.
- Display gentle persistence and a calm confident manner when coaching a patient to tolerate CPAP. Consider having them hold the mask themselves.
- It may be appropriate to utilize CPAP in selected cases of altered mental status with close one-on-one monitoring.
- A bougie can help with a challenging cricothyrotomy.
- Train assistants in advance to help during MFAM.
- All invasive airways should be confirmed objectively with $ETCO_2$. When the $ETCO_2$ cannot be detected or drops precipitously, remove the device and resume BMV.
- A transport ventilator should be used for all MFAM.

Chapter 30

# Difficult and Failed Airway Management in EMS

Jan L. Eichel, Mary Beth Skarote, and Darren A. Braude

## THE PREHOSPITAL CHALLENGE

As discussed in Chapter 29, the prehospital environment presents an array of unique challenges to the prehospital provider including, but not limited to, noise, bright sunlight or darkness, temperature extremes, patient access issues, and challenges in patient positioning. Taken in sum, it is clear that all airway management in the prehospital setting should be treated as difficult, although careful evaluation for specific features predicting difficulty is still warranted to allow any modifiable factors to be addressed and to make a comprehensive informed decision about whether, and how, to proceed. Experience would suggest that errors in prehospital medication-facilitated airway management (MFAM) are more often errors in decision making than errors in performance of purely technical skills, often related to a failure to anticipate difficulty.

## PREDICTION OF THE DIFFICULT AIRWAY IN THE PREHOSPITAL SETTING

The anatomic and physiologic factors governing the prediction of difficult intubation, difficult bag-mask ventilation (BMV), difficult extraglottic airway placement and ventilation, and difficult performance of a cricothyroidotomy are all discussed at length in Chapter 2, and for the most part apply equally well in the prehospital setting. In emergency medical services (EMS), however, we modify the LEMON mnemonic to become LEMONS with the "S" standing for Situation. Situational factors to consider include immediate hazards, personnel and equipment resources and limitations, environmental considerations, limitations in patient access and positioning, planned mode of transportation, and transport time. For example, an edentulous thin patient with no anatomic predictors of difficulty may become very difficult to manage when trapped in a vehicle at night with an ambient temperature of 20°F and snow. Physiologic factors contributing to difficulty are also paramount in the prehospital setting just as they are in the hospital. The patient's oxygen saturation, after attempts at optimal preoxygenation, will be a major determinant of the time available for laryngoscopy before it becomes necessary to abort. When time is limited, many borderline laryngoscopy and intubation cases become impossible. In other words, preoxygenation creates reserve and reserve creates time, which in turn results in greater intubation success. Careful evaluation for anatomic, physiologic, and situational factors that may cause airway difficulty allow the provider to make informed decisions and establish an optimal primary backup and rescue airway plan.

## THE PREHOSPITAL CONUNDRUM

Although basic airway measures can never wait, prehospital providers have the unique option to defer advanced airway management until arrival at an emergency department (ED). Therefore, predictive factors must be placed into a more complicated decision algorithm that not only includes questions such as "Does this patient need advanced airway management?" but also "Does this patient need advanced airway management right now?" and "Is this patient better served by airway management now or delaying until arrival at the hospital or arrival of additional providers such as a critical care transport team?" These questions must be asked before rushing a patient off the scene into a moving ambulance to avoid critical airway compromise during transport. In addition, some patients, such as those with inhalation injury or anaphylaxis, may have better outcomes if managed aggressively early, when they have more reserve and/or before their disease process progresses. Given these factors, the decision to embark on invasive airway management is complex.

### When Is it Better to Wait?

Although this question should be asked with every emergency airway encounter, it is particularly important in the prehospital setting. Consider, for example, the following two cases, each with an anticipated 10-minute transport time to an appropriate receiving facility:

- A 40-year-old, 80-kg man with sudden collapse, new left hemiparesis, Glasgow Coma Scale of 6, marked hypertension, no swallowing reflex, normal respiratory pattern with $O_2$ saturations of 99%, nasal end-tidal $CO_2$ of 40, and severe ankylosing spondylitis.
- A 40-year-old, 80-kg man extricated from a house fire, with stridor, $O_2$ saturations of 70% despite mask ventilation, and evidence of upper airway burns.

Both patients have clear indications for securing the airway, although the decision process for the prehospital airway manager, particularly with respect to urgency, should be quite different. In the first case, if the patient is not deteriorating further, assessment of risks and potential benefits suggest it would be best to defer intubation to the ED, where a more formal and controlled rapid sequence intubation (RSI), augmented by difficult and failed airway tools, can be performed. In addition, alternate management options (such as awake techniques) for this predicted difficult airway are available and easier to perform in a hospital setting. In this case, the difficulty is related to a chronic condition, one that is unlikely to become more difficult if intubation is delayed until hospital arrival. The patient's oxygenation and ventilation status is adequate, and although the patient is clearly at risk for aspiration, this is a theoretical risk or it may have already occurred. Training must emphasize that having the ability to perform a procedure, especially to prevent a complication that may or may not occur, does not always equate with the need to perform the procedure. The provider and system medical directors and administrators must be wary of the *technical imperative*—that operators generally will perform an authorized procedure more often than it is required or indicated. In fact, there is growing evidence that in certain situations, prehospital intubation may not improve outcomes and may even lead to worse outcomes (see Evidence section, Chapter 28).

In the second case, the provider is forced to actively manage the airway despite predicted difficulty with laryngoscopy. Even a brief delay, such as a 10-minute transport, allows time for further deterioration and hypoxemic damage, increasing the threat to the patient and making intubation progressively more difficult. If the provider is authorized to perform MFAM, the decision to intubate here is clear on the basis of "Forced to Act" (see Chapter 2). The non-MFAM ALS provider may be forced to perform a cricothyroidotomy. Thus, both the nature and the "stability" of the difficult airway become key factors in the "intubate-vs.-transport" decision. This has been previously identified as "context sensitive" airway management.

## APPLYING THE EMS DIFFICULT AIRWAY ALGORITHM FOR MFAM PRACTITIONERS

The EMS difficult airway algorithm is modeled after the ED difficult airway algorithm and incorporates both predicted difficult airways and experienced difficult airway situations encountered in the prehospital environment, with modification as necessary to consider transport times, local protocols, preference, and medical direction (**Fig. 30-1**). The first step is to call for help when

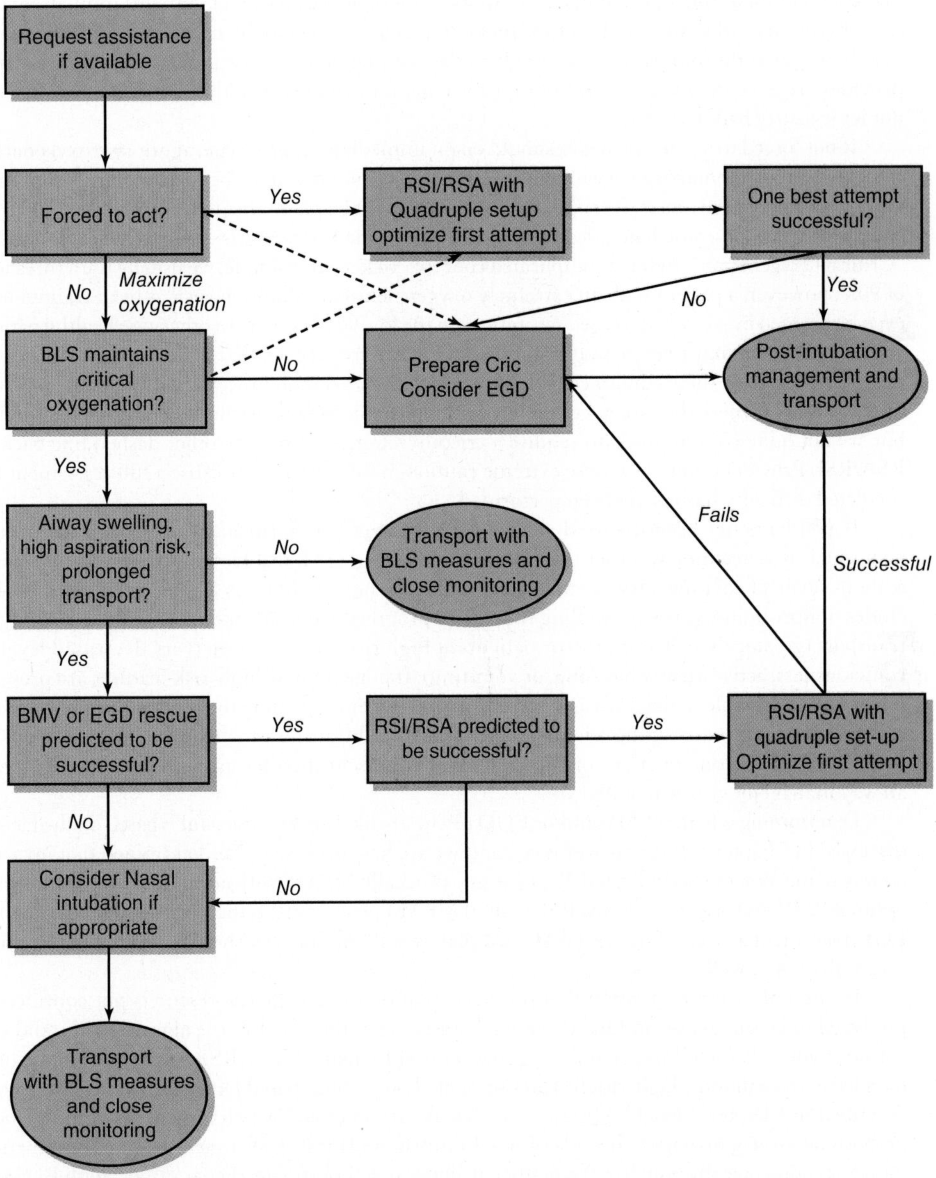


● **FIGURE 30-1. The EMS Difficult Airway Algorithm.** See discussion of the Difficult Airway Algorithm in Chapter 3 for explanation. RSI, rapid sequence intubation or other medication-assisted intubation technique; PIM, postintubation management; EGD, extraglottic device; ILMA, intubating laryngeal mask airway; VL, video laryngoscopy; BNTI, blind nasal tracheal intubation.

available from a second paramedic unit, a supervisor, or a critical care unit. Critical Care Transport providers managing patients at outlying hospitals should not overlook any providers that might be available in the facility.

The next step is to determine if you are *forced to act* (see Chapter 2). Essentially, this means you have determined that the patient is likely to die or suffer severe disability if nothing is done in the next few minutes, and you therefore prepare to undertake a single attempt at RSI or rapid sequence airway (RSA; the techniques with the highest odds of success) in a patient that you would otherwise try to avoid paralyzing because of high-risk difficult airway features. In such a situation, you should be simultaneously preparing for any potentially appropriate route of management including optimal mask ventilation, extraglottic airway placement, intubation, *and* cricothyrotomy—the quadruple setup. In some rare cases, it may be necessary to move immediately to a cricothyrotomy, represented by a dashed line on the algorithm. It is imperative that providers reserve the *forced-to-act* concept for true, immediately life-threatening situations and not let it justify bad decisions.

If not forced to act, the provider should begin immediate, appropriate, aggressive oxygenation measures, supplemental oxygen, and mask ventilation or Noninvasive Positive Pressure Ventilation and assess their effectiveness. If critical oxygenation cannot be maintained, the provider should consider preparing for immediate cricothyrotomy and consider extraglottic device (EGD) placement. "Critical Oxygenation" itself is a complicated concept. To keep this simple, we usually use a threshold of 90%; however, a patient with an extremely oxygen-sensitive condition such as head trauma may even be harmed by sustained oxygen saturations in the low 90s, whereas an otherwise healthy patient with bronchiolitis may tolerate saturations in the low 80s for an extended period. The sophisticated provider will factor these clinical considerations into their decision process. Some patients may fall into a gray area where they are not considered so hypoxemic to fall into the "forced-to-act" situation but are not quite compromised to require a cricothyrotomy—hence the other dashed line back to RSA/RSI. Providers should exercise extreme caution in this situation, because a full assessment for predicted difficulty has not yet been performed.

If you have not been diverted at the "forced-to-act" or "Critical Oxygenation" steps, the next step is to determine whether there are particular high-risk features to tip the risk-to-benefit scale in favor of invasive airway management even when saturations are maintained. This includes nonprecipitous airway swelling that could progress, especially if coupled with a prolonged transport (greater than 30 minutes) or patients at high risk for aspiration (very decreased level of consciousness, active airway bleeding, or vomiting). If none of these high-risk features are present, it is usually advisable to defer invasive airway management, continue the basic life support (BLS) measures that are maintaining adequate saturations, and transport to an appropriate facility. On the other hand, if one or more of these features is present, further assessment of difficulty in airway management is warranted.

Determining whether BMV and/or EGD rescue are likely to be successful is based on the factors discussed in Chapter 2. If the answer is yes, and we are here because it was determined that invasive airway management was indicated, the next step is usually MFAM with additional preparations for optimal BMV and cricothyrotomy. If the initial MFAM plan was RSI, then you should be ready for EGD placement as well. If the initial MFAM plan was RSA, then you should consider being ready for intubation as well.

In the unfortunate situation that mask ventilation or extraglottic rescue is not confidently predicted to be successful, and by the very fact of being at this point in the algorithm you did not consider yourself forced to act and oxygenation is sufficient, RSI or RSA would not be recommended even with some high-risk features present. The hospital-based Difficult Airway Algorithm described in Chapter 2 would now move to "awake techniques," which are not available to most prehospital airway managers, outside of nasal intubation. If it is determined that nasal intubation (blind or endoscopically visualized) is neither available nor appropriate, then transport with BLS and close monitoring are appropriate. If at any point the provider feels they are forced to act by clinical changes or oxygenation status deteriorates, the provider reenters the algorithm from the top. Those providers that do have other awake procedures within their scope of practice, such as certain critical care transport teams, would refer to the algorithm in Chapter 2.

## THE DIFFICULT AIRWAY FOR THE NON-MFAM PROVIDER

For the provider that does not have the option for MFAM, most invasive airway management is performed for cardiac arrest or advanced respiratory failure. The point of predicting difficulty in these situations is not to decide whether to "burn bridges" or not with administration of a neuromuscular blocking agent (NMBA) but rather to prepare quickly for the anticipated difficulty and consider early usage of EGDs and cricothyrotomy. These providers operate primarily in the EMS Crash Airway Algorithm (with the exception of NMBA use). In some circumstances, the Difficult Airway Algorithm may still be appropriate, although any branch point that leads to RSI/RSA would not be an option.

## THE FAILED AIRWAY IN EMS

The definitions of the prehospital failed airway are the same as those presented in Chapter 2 for the hospital environment: failure to maintain critical oxygenation whether an intubation attempt has occurred or not and failure to intubate after three attempts even if oxygenation is adequate. Therefore, a failed *attempt* does not always equate to a failed *airway*. Because it is the oxygenation status that often distinguishes a failed attempt from a failed airway, it is critical that the EMS airway manager focus on meticulous pre- and peri-intubation oxygenation strategies and be ready to employ optimal BMV as discussed in Chapter 9 as soon as an attempt fails.

In the event of a failed intubation attempt, assess oxygenation and what was visualized. If the saturation is ≤93% or dropping, perform optimal BMV, and prepare for a failed airway. If oxygenation can be corrected and the epiglottis was visualized initially, an additional attempt may be appropriate. If the epiglottis was not visualized, it may be appropriate to move to an EGD or cricothyrotomy. Try to ascertain what happened on the first attempt, and make appropriate corrective action; it is rarely productive to repeat the exact same process. Consider using a bougie, repositioning the head and neck, external laryngeal manipulation (ELM), a change in device and/or blade size, or a change in intubator.

In the prehospital setting, it is particularly important to focus on first-attempt success and consider moving to an EGD or cricothyrotomy after only one or two unsuccessful intubation attempts to minimize the risk of complications as well as to limit time spent on the scene. As a result of this imperative, combined with the infrequent performance of procedures and the unique challenges of the prehospital environment, failed airways should be considered inevitable despite optimal technique. It might be better to think of these as "missed airways"—analogous to a missed approach in aviation jargon—to avoid the negative connotation of failure.

Failed airway algorithms have traditionally been based around two dichotomous clinical situations: cannot intubate, can oxygenate *(have time) and* cannot intubate, and cannot oxygenate (*have no time)*. The former is managed with devices and techniques not typically available in the prehospital setting, whereas the latter is primarily managed with a cricothyrotomy. The primary focus should be on maintaining or improving oxygenation to allow for safe transport to definitive care, and as such, these two situations may practically be lumped together. This allows for a very simplified approach to any failed airway: Consider an EGD, and prepare for cricothyroidotomy, preferably surgical if within scope of practice. Therefore, a completely failed airway algorithm is not necessary and just adds complexity to what should have been a very simple and rapid decision process.

As our EGD choices and experience grow, it is much more common for these devices to be placed first, and they will usually maintain oxygenation and ventilation until arrival at the hospital. In the event that an EGD is not predicted to be successful based on the RODS assessment, it is reasonable to move directly to cricothyrotomy. Although cricothyrotomy in the field is and should be a rare event, providers must not be afraid to perform the procedure when indicated and should do so as soon as possible.

Although resources are often limited in the field, the use of a second, experienced provider cannot be underestimated, particularly in MFAM and/or when the airway is identified as difficult.

The additional operator should serve as a "second opinion" for checks and balances to make sure the decision to proceed is valid. They may then assist the primary airway manager with ELM, jaw thrust, and bougie as indicated but should be particularly focused on preparations for a failed airway including, in cases of great difficulty, having an EGD out and ready and the neck prepped for a cricothyrotomy. The second provider may also be extremely helpful for watching saturations and helping the intubator, who is focused on their task, recognize when the attempt or the airway has failed.

## TIPS AND PEARLS

- Even under optimal conditions, all prehospital airways should be considered difficult, and contingency plans should be made in advance regarding the airway devices.
- LEMON(*S*) accounts for situational factors that often arise in prehospital care.
- EMS providers must not only consider if a patient needs invasive airway management but also whether that management may be safely deferred to the hospital. However, in situations of rapid airway deterioration or critical hypoxemia, crews should stay in place and fix the problem rather than trying to rush to the hospital.
- In the prehospital environment, the use of two advanced providers for any medication-facilitated airway is recommended. In the event of predicted or experienced difficulty, additional help should be summonsed when available.
- Be wary of the technical imperative.
- Always consider the airway in the context of the situation and the particular patient. It is impossible to have a "one-size-fits-all" approach.
- Do not hesitate to move to an EGD or cricothyroidotomy if oxygenation cannot be maintained by other means.
- Avoid the use of NMBAs or potent sedative agents unless you are confident you can provide effective gas exchange or are *forced to act*.
- Slow down, take a methodical approach, and communicate. Success lies with the team. Planning even in crash intubation is vital. Making proper use of your partner and others may mean the difference between success and failure.

## EVIDENCE

- **Is there any evidence that experienced prehospital providers perform better than less experienced ones?** There is, and it is related specifically to the number of airways managed. Wang et al.[1] found that greater numbers of intubations per practitioner increased success rates. Perhaps the more important finding in this study, however, was that as the experience level of the practitioner increased, the numbers of intubations performed decreased. The implication is that more experience permitted practitioners to use alternative methods, perhaps, because they were able to predict intubation difficulty. Garza et al.[2] found that paramedics frequently operate under poor environmental conditions and encounter significant distractions while attempting to perform endotracheal intubation. Endotracheal intubation is a complex and difficult procedure that requires substantial training, medical oversight, and quality management to maintain clinical proficiency.[3]
- **Is there evidence that the endotracheal tube introducer or the gum elastic bougie (GEB) enhances intubation success rates in EMS?** Evidence specific to EMS does not exist. However, there is ample evidence that success rates and time to intubate are enhanced by this simple device in the hands of anesthesiologists and emergency physicians.[4,5]
- **How common is the difficult and failed airway in EMS, and is an algorithmic approach beneficial?** Studies of prehospital endotracheal intubation have reported failed intubation rates from 3.4% to 25%.[6,7] It is this variation that has called into question the advisability

of prehospital care personnel performing endotracheal intubation in general, and RSI in particular. We know that airway management in the emergency prehospital setting is more difficult than that in the operating room. In a prospective study of more than 2,500 patients, a simple algorithm of endotracheal tube introducer (or GEB), intubating laryngeal mask airway (ILMA), and cricothyrotomy were adopted, and 160 difficult airways were successfully managed.[7] Being prepared with an algorithmic plan and simple tools for the difficult airway is proven beneficial in the prehospital emergency setting.

## REFERENCES


1. Wang HE, Abo BN, Lave JR, et al. How would minimum experience standards affects the distribution of out-of-hospital endotracheal intubations? *Ann Emerg Med*. 2007;50:246–252.
2. Garza AG, Gratton MC, McElroy J, et al. Environmental factors encountered during out-of-hospital intubation attempts. *Prehosp Emerg Care*. 2008;12:286–289.
3. Emergency medical services: clinical practice and systems oversight. In: Cone D, Brice JH, Delbridge TH, et al, eds. *Clinical Aspects of EMS*. Vol 1. 2nd ed; 2015.
4. Tomek S. Bougie it! The gum elastic bougie is a viable adjunct for the difficult endotracheal intubation. *EMS World*. 2011;40(1):26–30, 32.
5. Hung O, Murphy MF. *Management of the Difficult and Failed Airway*. New York, NY: McGraw Hill Medical; 2012.
6. Bassam B, Kane I, MacKeil-White K, et al. Difficult airways, difficult physiology and difficult technology: respiratory treatment of the special needs children. *Clin Pediatr Emerg Med*. 2012;13:81–90.
7. Combes X, Jabre P, Margenet A, et al. Unanticipated difficult airway management in the prehospital emergency setting: prospective validation of an algorithm. *Anesthesiology*. 2011;114:105–110.

Chapter 31

# Controversies in EMS Airway Management

Jeff Birrer, Ken Davis, and Darren A. Braude

## INTRODUCTION

Although airway management has been a fundamental part of emergency medical services (EMS) for many decades, there remain areas of controversy that deserve focused attention. By the very nature of being considered controversial, it is presumed that there is insufficient evidence to make definitive recommendations. In contrast to other chapters where the pertinent evidence is summarized at the end, we will do our best to consider the available evidence and our experiences, as we discuss each topic, to provide balanced guidance.

## SKILL TRAINING AND MAINTENANCE

Human factor study has shown that in high-stress, high-risk, low-frequency procedures, we will sink to our level of training rather than rise to the occasion. Confounding this, there is no consistent standard for initial EMS airway training, particularly with regards to how many intubations a paramedic student should complete and whether all need to be live. Research in the operating room demonstrates little improvement in success or decrease in complications during the first 13 intubation attempts by paramedic students with significant improvement between the 14th and 30th intubations, and by the 30th intubation most students were achieving 90% first-pass success in a controlled environment.[1]

Turning research into standards, the U.S. Committee on Accreditation of Education Programs for the Emergency Medical Services Professional (CoAEMSP) recommends a combination of a minimum of 50 "airway encounters" across all age ranges, with 100% success in 20 consecutive encounters.[2] They state that airway management "may be accomplished utilizing any combination of live patients, high-fidelity simulations, low-fidelity simulations, or cadaver labs." Although discouraged, it is possible for a paramedic student to complete initial training without a single live intubation. On the other hand, the Provence of Alberta, Canada, requires 10 intubations in a simulated setting and 15 on live patients in a clinical practicum.[3] Throughout the world, there is variability with regards to initial training requirements that depend on number of learners and availability of operating room time. It is our belief that simulators are excellent for developing muscle memory in optimal technique as well as the sequencing of medication-facilitated airway management (MFAM), but a variety of live or cadaver tissue is necessary to become comfortable with human diversity. It seems reasonable that the more live intubations a student performs the more successful they will become, but there is little research to support this assumption.

There is even less consensus on recommendations for skill maintenance. There are several studies demonstrating that even with targeted training, skills degrade with time.[4] Most importantly, there is a study that correlates patient outcome to the number of airway procedures performed by the treating provider in the previous 5 years; as a result, many agencies set minimum numbers of encounters and success requirements, often relying on low-fidelity simulation.[5] The Commission on Accreditation of Medical Transport Systems (CAMTS) requires three adult, pediatric, and infant intubations per quarter, or a total of 36 intubations per year, all of which may be simulated.[6] Despite this mandate, a 2014 study of almost 5,000 intubations by air medical crews primarily using rapid sequence intubation (RSI) demonstrated a first-pass success of less than 80% and an overall success of 92%.[7] This suggests that the standards may be insufficient to maintain competence. It is incumbent on each provider, agency, and system to set their own standard that ensures patient safety and optimizes success.

## PEDIATRICS

Prehospital pediatric intubations are exceedingly uncommon, and success rates are less than that for adults. One large air medical study found that only 5% of intubation cases were for patients above or below 14 years of age.[7] A ground-based study in a large metropolitan area that allows MFAM recently reported only 299 pediatric intubation in 6.3 years, with a first-pass success of 66% overall, 53% for infants, and 56% for children with cardiac arrest.[8] This system reports that an average paramedic student performs six pediatric intubations during training, which we suspect far exceeds the national average, yet still performs poorly on pediatric intubation. At the same time there is high-quality evidence from a large, randomized, controlled trial that pediatric patients do just as well with simple bag-mask ventilation (BMV) as they do with endotracheal intubation (ETI).[9] There are now numerous extraglottic devices (EGDs) available for pediatric patients, providing another option to endotracheal intubation. This has led some jurisdictions to remove pediatric intubation from the scope of practice or protocols in favor of BMV or EGDs. Each patient is unique, and firm recommendations cannot be made at this point; however, it seems reasonable for prehospital providers to rely on solid rescue mask ventilation skills or EGD use in lieu of tracheal intubation. EMS systems that continue to perform pediatric intubation, and especially pediatric MFAM, should carefully track their success, complications, and outcomes, and must have processes in place to ensure patient safety.

## ATTEMPTS

Many EMS Quality Assurance programs and publications report overall success for prehospital intubation without a breakdown of the number of attempts it required to successfully place an endotracheal tube in the trachea. There is evidence from the hospital setting that complications increase significantly with each successive attempt. For instance, there is a marked increase in complications including cardiac arrest, with three or more attempts at intubation compared with fewer than three attempts.[10] Another group reported that complications increased from 14.2% on the first attempt to 63.6% with more than three attempts.[11] Bodily et al.[12] demonstrated an increase in hypoxemia with more than a single intubation attempt. Taken together, it is clear that when intubating critically ill and injured patients in the prehospital setting the focus should be on first-attempt success rather than overall success.

The obvious implication of this mindset is that providers must set themselves, and the patient, up for success on the first attempt using all the techniques discussed in this text. We must simultaneously be ready, both mentally and physically, to move quickly to an alternative technique. There may be patients for whom intubation is clearly preferred to BMV or an EGD, such as those with massive obesity or upper airway pathology. In these cases, providers may consider the relative risks and benefits of a second or third attempt but only if there is something that can be changed to increase the chance of success on the subsequent attempt such as position, device, technique, or intubator.

## NIPPV

Although Noninvasive Positive Pressure Ventilation (NIPPV) has become commonplace in most EMS systems, it is often restricted to paramedics. Given that this technology is very simple to employ using disposable devices, and can be used to manage a wide range of hypoxemic conditions, and this device is used routinely by patients at home, we believe this technology should be included in BLS and ILS scopes of practice. However, acquiring new skills and learning new equipment, even one as simple as continuous positive airway pressure (CPAP), requires adding hours to training programs, which can spread resources thin and limit the number of providers being trained, especially in volunteer systems.

Altered mental status (AMS) was traditionally considered an absolute contraindication to NIPPV because the patient may have to remove the mask in the event of vomiting or, at a minimum, alert a provider that he/she is about to vomit. It is our opinion that AMS should be considered a relative contraindication, and the pros and cons should be weighed in each individual case. Clearly, a patient with Glasgow comas scale (GCS) of 3 and poor respiratory effort needs rescue mask ventilation. On the hand, a slightly sleepy or confused patient with hypercarbia or hypoxemia who can remain seated may be a very reasonable CPAP candidate when EMS crews can provide vigilant one-on-one observation at all times during transport. It also makes sense to employ CPAP liberally, despite AMS, for preoxygenation. If, for example, a crew of two or three is trying to quickly set up for MFAM in a spontaneously breathing but unconscious patient, tying up one crew member to assist respirations may not be an optimal use of resources.

Another area of controversy with NIPPV is its use in conditions other than congestive heart failure and asthma/chronic obstructive pulmonary disease, such as pneumonia. Some sources state that pneumonia is a contraindication owing to the potential for increasing the risk of bacteremia from the translocation of bacteria into the bloodstream. Other sources state that NIPPV is a good temporary treatment option for suspected pneumonia with hypoxemia in the prehospital setting.[13] Generally, pending further evidence, we believe the risks from both hypoxemia refractory to simple supplemental oxygen as well as the risks of prehospital MFAM outweigh the small potential risk of bacteremia from the short-term use of NIPPV.

## SEDATION-FACILITATED INTUBATION

Given the obvious risks of chemical paralysis, many EMS systems and medical directors are enticed by the notion of facilitating intubation with a strong sedative agent, such as midazolam, without concurrent use of a neuromuscular blocking agent. This technique may be termed sedation-facilitated intubation (SFI) to distinguish it from RSI. Unfortunately, this well-intended approach has a lower success rate and higher potential for complications than RSI. The National Emergency Airway Registry data shows that RSI has a first-pass success rate of 83% in all patients, adult and pediatric, versus 76% for SFI.[14] As intubation on the first attempt minimizes complications, this is particularly germane. A prehospital trial comparing etomidate and midazolam for SFI reported an overall success rate of only 76%, gagging in up to 65% of the patients, and vomiting in up to 13%.[15] One concern with SFI is the risk of vomiting in an obtunded patient who is aware enough to have a preserved gag reflex but not awake enough to protect against aspiration. Case series in aeromedical services have found a 92% success rate with RSI compared with 25% when only etomidate was used.[16]

Best available evidence suggests that SFI is inferior to RSI. If the system medical director does not believe that RSI can be safely employed, it would be better to avoid MFAM altogether or consider rapid sequence airway (RSA). Ketamine may represent a unique agent because of preservation of airway reflexes, and we await evidence to ascertain if this represents a safer variant of SFI in the prehospital setting.

## RSA AND DSI

RSA employs the same preparation and sequence of medications as RSI, with the planned immediate placement of an EGD without any prior attempt at intubation. Because EGDs can generally be placed much quicker and with a much higher first-attempt success compared with tracheal intubation, RSA has the potential to decrease hypoxemia and other complications of multiple intubation attempts.[17] The newest generation of EGDs also offer more protection against aspiration than earlier devices.[18] At this point, publications on RSA are limited to case reports, small case series, and simulator trials, but the technique is currently utilized by some ground and air services.[18] Until further evidence becomes available, RSA is a reasonable option for local systems and medical directors to consider weighing the risks and benefits, in particular local success rates and complications, with intubation.

Delayed sequence intubation (DSI) involves providing "procedural sedation" to facilitate the "procedure" of preoxygenation in a patient who is hypoxic, combative, and unable to comply with oxygenation efforts. DSI has been described as administering a dissociative dose of ketamine (1.0 mg per kg IV) that is unlikely to negatively affect respiratory drive or airway reflexes but will allow for adequate preoxygenation with a facemask or NIPPV. Once oxygenation improves the sequence is resumed and a paralytic agent administered to facilitate intubation. This technique has been shown to be effective in a small multicenter case series involving highly skilled airway managers in the hospital setting and should be undertaken with caution.[19] Sedating critically ill patients who are on the cusp of decompensation may result in further respiratory compromise or even arrest, and because of the small numbers of patients in the existing literature, the true rate of complications is not known at this time. If DSI is employed, the airway manager must be prepared to definitively manage the airway should respiratory status worsen after the administration of any sedative agent. Although there are anecdotal reports of this technique being used by some EMS agencies - and is something we personally use in our practice - the routine use of DSI cannot be strongly recommended at this time without further study.

## DIRECT VERSUS VIDEO AND OPTICAL LARYNGOSCOPY

Video laryngoscopy (VL) is an evolving technology that has failed to permeate into the prehospital arena driven in large part by the upfront cost of most devices. There are no large prehospital studies comparing success rates, complications, and/or outcomes between direct laryngoscopy (DL) and VL, and its potential for EMS use must be extrapolated from hospital data. There is overwhelming evidence that shows that the novice or infrequent operator will obtain a better view of the glottis with VL compared to DL, and some evidence that this leads to a higher first-pass success rate. However, this sometimes comes at the cost of longer time to tube passage when compared to DL.[20] One trial showed that first-pass success improved from 44% to 74% with introduction of the King Vision; however, the improved rate is still suboptimal.[21] Another study from a busy urban EMS system with a long experience using VL still reports poor first-pass success in pediatrics.[22]

One concern for the use of prehospital VL is the high prevalence of secretions, blood, and/or emesis that might obscure image acquisition. Interestingly, a recent ED study of trauma patients found that VL had a higher success rate than DL, suggesting that blood and emesis may not actually be a major concern.[23] In another study from the national emergency airway registry (NEAR) registry, adult patients intubated with gastrointestinal bleeding had similar first-attempt success rates with VL and DL.[24] Regardless, when using VL, it is important to have suction available and to suction before blade insertion.

It is clear that VL is an exciting and emerging technology that has the potential to transform prehospital airway management. However, VL should not be seen as the panacea for poor first-pass intubation rates but may be part of a comprehensive program, especially as more affordable choices become available. Systems often adopt VL without a full appreciation for the differences in technique compared with DL and the need for initial and ongoing training and practice. Given the existing data, many EMS systems, especially those that do not utilize MFAM, may elect to focus training time on optimizing BMV and EGD placement rather than introducing VL.

## CRICOTHYROTOMY

Prehospital cricothyrotomy (PC) is a very infrequent procedure occurring in less than 2% of airway encounters in most studies but up to 10% in one air medical study.[25] Cricothyrotomy is generally performed in the sickest of patients, typically after failed attempts at intubation, who have progressed to the "cannot intubate-cannot oxygenate" scenario. Techniques available include an "open" or "surgical" approach with or without bougie assistance, needle cricothyrotomy, and various hybrid "percutaneous" or "minimally invasive" approaches. A prehospital meta-analysis found a remarkably higher success rate for surgical compared to needle cricothyrotomies.[26] The fourth National Audit Project study of major airway complications during anesthesia in Great Britain found a 60% failure rate for less-invasive techniques and concluded that "anesthetists should be trained to perform a surgical airway." Other studies have also demonstrated higher complications in the less-invasive approaches, which may seem counterintuitive.[27]

There is a wide range of EMS practice across jurisdictions, recognizing that surgical airways are generally restricted to patients above 10 years of age. Based on our experience and the available evidence, we recommend that all paramedics be trained and allowed to perform surgical airways in the appropriate age group and circumstances as dictated by local medical direction.

A recent analysis of the national EMS information system (NEMSIS) database revealed only 47 prehospital pediatric needle cricothyrotomy procedures across 40 states in 1 year. Success rates and outcomes are not available, but it is unlikely that all were successful or that all patients had survivable conditions from the outset. In a recent report of pediatric ED intubations from NEAR, there was not a single reported pediatric surgical airway in more than a 1,000 pediatric airway encounters.[28] Therefore, the incidence of cases in which pediatric needle cric is going to be lifesaving is remarkably low. Local medical directors and administrators need to decide on a case-by-case basis if continued training in pediatric needle cricothyrotomy is justifiable.

## VENTILATORS

A landmark paper from San Diego found that head-injured patients who underwent prehospital RSI but arrived at the hospital via ground EMS did worse than those who arrived via helicopter, even when controlling for transport time.[29] It subsequently became apparent that the difference was capnography and ventilators; the flight crews routinely used this combination to maintain normal $ETCO_2$, which in turn has been tied to outcome in this population. Although it is theoretically possible to titrate $ETCO_2$ with capnography and a self-inflating bag for ventilation, this is very challenging in the prehospital environment when providers have multiple distractions, and often the least experienced provider is tasked with bagging. There is also compelling evidence that certain patient populations such as traumatic brain injury and post-cardiac arrest patients are very susceptible to injury from hyperoxia, and it is hard to titrate oxygen delivery without a ventilator.[30] We strongly recommend ventilators always be used in the setting of MFAM, including both RSI and RSA, and be used for all patients with invasive airways when available. Ventilators also have a potential role during mask ventilation and for management of out-of-hospital cardiac arrest.

## CAPNOGRAPHY

It is clear that continuous, waveform capnography can confirm appropriate endotracheal tube position and immediately detect dislodgement, in addition to guiding and troubleshooting ventilator management. There is also strong evidence that EMS systems not using capnography will have an unacceptable rate of undetected esophageal tube placements.[31] Therefore, continuous capnography should be considered a mandatory part of any intubation program, whether medication-facilitated or not. Capnography is also a useful adjunct with extraglottic devices and BMV and many EMS systems are now utilizing nasal detectors for spontaneously breathing patients.

## MEDICATION-FACILITATED AIRWAY MANAGEMENT

MFAM remains one of the most controversial areas in all of EMS owing to concerns about safety and data suggesting the same if not better outcomes when BMV is performed instead. Although it is true that MFAM makes difficult intubation easier, it does not make impossible intubation possible, and it is unclear whether it improves patient outcomes. Because MFAM is employed, by definition, in patients who are spontaneously breathing—albeit it may be ineffective breathing—the risk of taking away the patient's intrinsic respiratory drive and being unable to replace it is real. Not every system will be able to implement, support, or sustain a quality MFAM program. The MFAM program should not be considered a requirement for any or all providers; some systems limit participation to senior paramedics or special operations staff.

Systems that elect to include MFAM in their scope of practice must weigh the evidence as well as local factors such as transport times, volumes, and success rates. Any system considering or employing prehospital MFAM should have engaged and supportive medical oversight and a supportive local medical community including anesthesiologists willing and able to provide opportunities for skill maintenance in the OR. A robust initial training program that is adequate to ensure success, a continuous quality improvement process including 100% chart review for every procedure, the maturity to focus on first-pass success, and the commitment to utilize EGDs would be best. In addition, a budget sufficient for continuous capnography, transport ventilators, and consideration of VL technology would make prehospital MFAM the safest for patients.

In summary, prehospital airway management including its success, adverse events, techniques, and scope of practice is changing. Further research is required before additional recommendations can be made.

## REFERENCES

1. Mulcaster J, Mills J, Hung O, et al. Laryngoscopic intubation. *Anesthesiology*. 2003;98(1):23–27.
2. CoAEMSP. Airway Management Recommendation. 2016. http://coaemsp.org/Documents/Airway-Recommendation-10-2013.pdf. Accessed February 28, 2016.
3. Alberta College of Paramedics. Position Statement - Intubation Education Requirements. http://www.collegeofparamedics.org/wp-content/uploads/2016/04/intubation_statement_feb_4_2014__2_.pdf.
4. Davis D, Heister R, Poste J, et al. Ventilation patterns in patients with severe traumatic brain injury following paramedic rapid sequence intubation. *Neurocrit Care*. 2005;2(2):165–171.
5. Wang H, Yealy D. Out-of-hospital endotracheal intubation: where are we? *Ann Emerg Med*. 2006;47(6):532–541.
6. CAMTS. 10th edition standards – Final. 2016. http://www.camts.org/10th_Edition_Standards_Complete.pdf. Accessed February 28, 2016.
7. Brown C III, Cox K, Hurwitz S, et al. 4,871 emergency airway encounters by air medical providers: a report of the air transport emergency airway management (NEAR VI: "A-TEAM") project. *West J Emerg Med*. 2014;15(2):188–193.
8. Prekker M, Delgado F, Shin J, et al. Pediatric intubation by paramedics in a large emergency medical services system: process, challenges, and outcomes. *Ann Emerg Med*. 2016;67(1):20–29.
9. Gauche M, Lewis R, Stratton S, et al. Effect of out-of-hospital pediatric endotracheal intubation on survival and neurological outcome: a controlled clinical trial. *Survey Anesthesiol*. 2000;44(5):289–290.
10. Mort T. Emergency tracheal intubation: complications associated with repeated laryngoscopic attempts. *Anesth Analg*. 2004;99:607–613.

11. Sakles J, Chiu S, Mosier J, et al. The importance of first pass success when performing orotracheal intubation in the emergency department. *Acad Emerg Med*. 2013;20(1):71–78.

12. Bodily J, Webb H, Weiss S, et al. Incidence and duration of continuously measured oxygen desaturation during emergency department intubation. *Ann Emerg Med*. 2016;67(3):389–395.

13. Belenguer-Muncharaz A, Reig-Valero R, Altaba-Tena S, et al. Noninvasive mechanical ventilation in severe pneumonia due to H1N1 virus. *Med Intensiva (English Edition)*. 2011;35(8):470–477.

14. Brown CA III, Bair AE, Pallin DJ, et al. Techniques, success, and adverse events of emergency department adult intubations. *Ann Emerg Med*. 2015;65(4):363–370.

15. Jacoby J, Heller M, Nicholas J, et al. Etomidate versus midazolam for out-of-hospital intubation: a prospective, randomized trial. *Ann Emerg Med*. 2006;47(6):525–530.

16. Bozeman W, Young S. Etomidate as a sole agent for endotracheal intubation in the prehospital air medical setting. *Air Med J*. 2002;21(4):32–37.

17. Bercker S, Schmidbauer W, Volk T, et al. A comparison of seal in seven supraglottic airway devices using a cadaver model of elevated esophageal pressure. *Anesth Analg*. 2008;106(2):445–448.

18. Braude D, Richards M. Rapid Sequence Airway (RSA) – a novel approach to prehospital airway management. *Prehosp Emerg Care*. 2007;11(2):250–252.

19. Weingart S, Trueger N, Wong N, et al. Delayed sequence intubation: a prospective observational study. *Ann Emerg Med*. 2015;65(4):349–355.

20. Sakles J, Javedani P, Chase E, et al. The use of a video laryngoscope by emergency medicine residents is associated with a reduction in esophageal intubations in the emergency department. *Acad Emerg Med*. 2015;22(6):700–707.

21. Jarvis J, McClure S, Johns D. EMS intubation improves with king vision video laryngoscopy. *Prehosp Emerg Care*. 2015;19(4):482–489.

22. Prekker M, Delgado F, Shin J, et al. Pediatric intubation by paramedics in a large emergency medical services system: process, challenges, and outcomes. *Ann Emerg Med*. 2016;67(1):20–29.

23. Sakles J, Patanwala A, Mosier J, et al. Comparison of video laryngoscopy to direct laryngoscopy for intubation of patients with difficult airway characteristics in the emergency department. *Intern Emerg Med*. 2013;9(1):93–98.

24. Carlson JN, Crofts J, Walls RM, et al. Direct versus video laryngoscopy for intubating adult patients with gastrointestinal bleeding. *West J Emerg Med*. 2015;16(7):1052–1056.

25. Bair A, Panacek E, Wisner D, et al. Cricothyrotomy: a 5-year experience at one institution. *J Emerg Med*. 2003;24(2):151–156.

26. Hubble M, Wilfong D, Brown L, et al. A meta-analysis of prehospital airway control techniques part ii: alternative airway devices and cricothyrotomy success rates. *Prehosp Emerg Care*. 2010;14(4):515–530.

27. Schober P, Hegemann M, Schwarte L, et al. Emergency cricothyrotomy – a comparative study of different techniques in human cadavers. *Resuscitation*. 2009;80(2):204–209.

28. Pallin DJ, Dwyer RC, Walls RM, et al. Techniques and trends, success rates, and adverse events in emergency department pediatric intubations: a report from the National Emergency Airway Registry. *Ann Emerg Med*. 2016;67(5):610–615.

29. Davis D, Stern J, Sise M, et al. A follow-up analysis of factors associated with head-injury mortality after paramedic rapid sequence intubation. *J Trauma*. 2005;59(2):486–490.

30. Kilgannon J, Roberts B, Jones A, et al. Arterial blood pressure and neurologic outcome after resuscitation from cardiac arrest. *Crit Care Med*. 2014;42(9):2083–2091.

31. Silvestri S, Ralls G, Krauss B, et al. The effectiveness of out-of-hospital use of continuous end-tidal carbon dioxide monitoring on the rate of unrecognized misplaced intubation within a regional emergency medical services system. *Ann Emerg Med*. 2005;45(5):497–503.

# Section VIII

# Special Clinical Circumstances

Chapter 32

# The Unstable Patient: Cardiopulmonary Optimization for Emergency Airway Management

Jarrod M. Mosier, Alan C. Heffner, and John C. Sakles

## THE CLINICAL CHALLENGE

The primary goal of airway management is to maintain airway patency and support systemic oxygenation and effective ventilation in patients who cannot sustain these vital functions on their own. Unlike elective intubation in the operating room, intubation in critical illness is often performed because cardiorespiratory physiology is disturbed. As such, these patients are particularly vulnerable to the adverse consequences of apnea and hemodynamic changes associated with induction and positive-pressure ventilation. Furthermore, failure to maintain oxygenation and ventilation during airway management leaves patients at risk of hemodynamic deterioration and cardiac arrest.

In the context of the unstable patient, the emergency airway manager is faced with patients who are hemodynamically compromised or cannot maintain adequate gas exchange prior to intubation. These patients are particularly vulnerable to rapid decompensation during and after the procedure. This chapter will focus on techniques to decrease the risk of deterioration during intubation of the unstable patient. A clear understanding of pertinent principles and physiology helps to optimize the peri-intubation period.

## OPTIMIZATION FOR FIRST LARYNGOSCOPY ATTEMPT SUCCESS

Airway management of the critically ill patient is a high-risk situation. Determining the need for, and timing of, intubation requires balancing respiratory and cardiovascular considerations in these fragile patients. The airway manager should optimize conditions to achieve first-pass success, because prolonged or repeated attempts with laryngoscopy are associated with increased risk of adverse events. **Box 32-1** summarizes important practical issues and modifications required for safe airway management of unstable critically ill patients.

BOX 32-1

**Considerations and modifications necessary for unstable patients.**

- Hemodynamic monitoring and optimizing preintubation status
  - Review current hemodynamic status for high-risk features
    - Hypotension, SI ≥ 0.8, pulmonary hypertension, RV failure, pericardial effusion
  - Establish monitoring for precipitous hemodynamic decline
    - Consider invasive, continuous arterial monitoring for high-risk patients
  - Confirm adequate IV access for rapid fluid boluses and/or vasopressor infusion
  - Empiric fluid loading prior to airway management (i.e., 20 mL per kg crystalloid) in absence of fluid overload or RV failure
  - When appropriate, delay intubation to improve hemodynamic status
  - Initiation or immediate availability of vasopressor support to treat or avoid hypotension
- Preoxygenation
  - Suboptimal preoxygenation resulting from high systemic oxygen extraction, ineffective spontaneous breathing, shunt physiology, or equipment limitations
  - Rapid desaturation limiting period of apneic normoxia for laryngoscopy
  - Preoxygenation with positive pressure should be considered. If unavailable, standard NRB plus standard nasal cannula up to the flush flow rate should be used
- RSI and drug use
  - Greater untoward cardiovascular effects of RSI drugs
  - Need for reduced dose sedative-hypnotic agent
  - Slower onset of action of RSI drugs
  - Awake intubation is an option in some patients
- Postintubation management
  - Expected ventilatory requirement should guide intubation plan. Patients with very high minute ventilation may require awake intubation to control their own respiratory drive
  - Lung-protective ventilation (≤7 mL per kg IBW) for all patients
  - Avoid dynamic hyperinflation and auto-PEEP
  - Low-dose titrated analgesia and sedation

## Timing of Airway Management

Unstable patients add complexity to the airway management plan. The very procedure intended to secure the airway and improve gas exchange may contribute to patient deterioration when the traditional "A-B-Cs" of resuscitation are rigidly pursued. Prioritization of immediate airway management versus preintubation support is a common clinical dilemma. Three main considerations may assist with the decision:

- **What is the reversibility and severity of respiratory compromise?**
  Knowledge of the underlying pathophysiology inciting respiratory compromise is critical for determining the best course of action. As an example, acute cardiogenic pulmonary edema with reversible precipitants (i.e., uncontrolled hypertension or volume overload) often responds to aggressive medical therapy in minutes, averting the need for intubation. In contrast, hypoxemia due to pneumonia or acute respiratory distress syndrome (ARDS) does not reverse

rapidly, and consideration of early intubation is prudent to avoid worsening gas exchange and preintubation conditions. Severe intrapulmonary shunt physiology that accompanies these conditions also contributes to difficult preoxygenation. These patients are at high risk of rapid desaturation during intubation, which can lead to cardiovascular collapse prior to successful endotracheal tube placement.

Noninvasive positive-pressure ventilation (NIPPV) and high-flow nasal cannula (HFNC) are effective methods of managing acute respiratory failure in many patients. However, it is vital to identify patients who are failing these modalities and require tracheal intubation. Sustained high $F_{IO_2}$ requirement (>75%) to maintain oxygen saturation ($Sp_{O_2}$) > 92% indicates severe intrapulmonary shunt, and intubation should be strongly considered in the absence of immediate reversibility. Delaying intubation until manifestation of refractory hypoxemia is associated with a high incidence of peri-intubation complications and adverse outcomes.

Acute respiratory failure due to obstructive lung diseases, such as asthma or chronic obstructive pulmonary disease (COPD), often responds to noninvasive ventilation. Mechanical ventilation of the patient with severe obstructive lung physiology is complicated, and intubation is often reserved as a last resort after unequivocal failure of NIPPV and medical support. However, these patients require vigilant monitoring to recognize the early signs of deterioration that help avoid delayed intubation in the setting of severe hypercapneic acidosis.

Patients with ventilatory failure due to a metabolic acidosis present different management considerations. In patients with a metabolic demand that outstrips their ability to compensate because of shock (e.g., sepsis), the metabolic acidosis is often best improved by early intubation to reduce the respiratory work of breathing and oxygen consumption by the respiratory muscles. However, when the metabolic demand outstrips compensatory capability because of organic acid formation, such as diabetic ketoacidosis or salicylate toxicity, maintaining and supporting spontaneous respiration to avoid intubation, given the patient's ability to protect their airway, is the best course of action. This is due to the physical limitations of the mechanical ventilator in meeting the ventilatory requirements required to compensate for the metabolic acidosis that will not improve with offloading of respiratory muscle work.

- **What is the current cardiovascular status and risk of peri-intubation deterioration?**

Cardiovascular shock is the final common pathway for many life-threatening diseases. Preintubation hemodynamic instability increases the likelihood of severe complications, including cardiac arrest, during or following intubation. Postintubation hypotension (PIH) complicates up to 25% of emergency intubations and is strongly associated with adverse outcomes including death. Rapid sequence intubation (RSI) and mechanical ventilation can have a substantial negative impact on the already fragile cardiopulmonary status. Structured assessment of cardiovascular status coupled with preinduction hemodynamic preparation are important facets of emergency airway management.

Work of breathing can be substantial and is often underestimated. Patients in shock may expend up to 20% or more of the cardiac output on ventilation, and intubation of patients who are failing cardiovascular resuscitation is frequently advocated to allow redistribution of blood flow to other vital organs. The cause of shock is an important consideration in the decision and timing of intubation in shocked patients. Effects of positive-pressure ventilation on cardiac function vary depending on the underlying cardiovascular state. Positive intrathoracic pressure reduces transmural cardiac pressure and thereby reduces left ventricular afterload. This impact may improve the performance of severe left ventricular dysfunction. In contrast, patients with normal or mildly reduced function suffer greater impact because of impedance of venous return. Prioritizing early fluid resuscitation and use of vasopressor support to maintain systemic pressure and venous return during induction sympatholysis is important for these patients, especially those with prominent vasodilation (i.e., sepsis, cirrhosis, and anaphylaxis).

In contrast to vasodilated shock and left heart disease, induction and mechanical ventilation can precipitate cardiovascular collapse in other forms of shock. Decompensated right heart failure is very sensitive to the increase in pulmonary vascular resistance that is normally induced by mechanical ventilation. Patients with cardiac tamponade preserve venous return via intense peripheral vasoconstriction. Loss of sympathetic tone with induction and initiation of mechanical ventilation are associated with cardiovascular collapse and arrest in patients with both of these conditions, and delaying intubation for effective therapies (including emergency pericardial drainage) is prioritized over early intubation. Bedside echocardiography can be a useful tool when evaluating the hemodynamic profile of a critically ill patient and to predict the hemodynamic response to intubation.

Most of the critically ill patients present in *compensated* shock with a narrow pulse pressure but sustained normotension. Episodic or sustained hypotension characterizing *uncompensated* shock is a late sign of hypoperfusion that develops when physiologic mechanisms to maintain normal perfusion pressure are overwhelmed. Mean arterial pressure (MAP) < 65 mm Hg, systolic blood pressure (SBP) < 90 mm Hg, or MAP > 20 mm Hg below baseline are important signs even in the absence of overt clinical hypoperfusion. Peri-intubation cardiac arrest rates complicated up to 15% of patients undergoing emergency intubation in the context of hypotensive shock. Efforts should focus to establish improved hemodynamic stability prior to induction of patients in shock unless immediate intubation is absolutely required.

Unfortunately, SBP is an imperfect single indicator of cardiovascular status, and normal or elevated blood pressure should not be interpreted as an unequivocal sign of adequate perfusion. Shock index (SI), calculated as HR/SBP, is a simple marker of cardiac efficiency that helps identify vulnerable patients despite deceptively normal blood pressure. Elevated SI is associated with cardiovascular deterioration across a range of clinical conditions including emergency intubation. Preintubation SI ≥ 0.8 independently forewarns of peri-intubation hemodynamic deterioration. However, one-third of patients develop peri-intubation deterioration below this threshold, and all patients undergoing emergency intubation should be considered at risk.

Inadequately oxygenated patients are at extremely high risk of desaturation during intubation, which increases the risk of hemodynamic decompensation. Medications and positive-pressure ventilation may also reduce cardiovascular performance and precipitate irreversible decompensation. Both must be titrated carefully to the patient's cardiovascular status.

Inadequate spontaneous breathing is a late sequela of shock. Respiratory failure in patients with shock, particularly sudden hypoventilation (i.e., bradypnea or apnea), often signifies impending cardiac arrest and requires immediate attention. Prompt respiratory support is indicated but must be coordinated with immediate cardiovascular support. Less severely ill patients may benefit from supplemental oxygen or bag-valve-mask support to optimize preoxygenation, whereas improvement of cardiovascular status is gained through administration of crystalloid and vasopressor support.

- **What is the anticipated clinical course?**

  Many critically ill patients demonstrate a biphasic course wherein early resuscitation slows the spiral of shock and organ dysfunction, only to be followed by deterioration hours later. In most instances, hypotension and malperfusion are improved but not entirely reversed by initial therapy. Tissue edema stemming from volume resuscitation, the progression of end-organ dysfunction (including acute lung injury), cumulative work of breathing, and metabolic debt combine to exhaust physiologic reserve leading to respiratory failure minutes or hours following initial "successful" resuscitation. Frequent reassessment of critically ill patients is required, with particular attention to respiratory status. Increasing the respiratory work or oxygen requirement signals worsening of acute lung injury. Hemodynamic status may also subtly, but progressively, deteriorate, indicated by malperfusion or escalating vasopressor support. Intubation should occur early when this downward cycle is identified, rather than wait for overt cardiovascular or respiratory failure.

## Preoxygenation Considerations in the Unstable Patient

Optimizing preoxygenation is more difficult in critically ill patients. Ineffective spontaneous ventilation, decreased pulmonary and systemic perfusion, high systemic oxygen extraction, shunt physiology, and equipment limitations all compromise preoxygenation. Although saturated hemoglobin accounts for the majority of blood oxygen content, systemic oxygenation is regulated (and limited) by cardiac performance. Even with optimal preoxygenation, the rate of desaturation is dependent on cardiovascular status and systemic oxygen extraction. The clinical repercussion is a marked reduction in the period of apneic normoxia to complete intubation. Hypercapnia during intubation also has the potential to exacerbate acidemia, further increasing this risk.

Standard methods of preoxygenation are often inadequate in critically ill patients. Preoxygenation with a non-rebreather (NRB) mask for 3 minutes or eight vital capacity breaths is extrapolated from data in the operating room, where NRB masks create a tight seal and patients are on a closed circuit. Outside of the operating room, NRB masks are rigid, poor fitting without a seal, and rely on filling an attached reservoir with oxygen to increase $F_{IO_2}$ close to 100%. Without the mask seal, room air is entrained around the mask and dilutes the oxygen content provided from the reservoir. High minute ventilation can also easily outstrip oxygen flow, resulting in NRB preoxygenation approximating 50% to 65% $F_{IO_2}$. When oxygen flow is increased to the "flush flow" rate of 40 to 70 L per minute, an $F_{IO_2}$ of nearly100% can be maintained with a standard NRB mask. In addition, patients with shunt physiology exhibit hypoxemia refractory to increased $F_{IO_2}$. For these reasons, preoxygenation with NIPPV is advocated to provide higher $F_{IO_2}$ (via high flow rate to meet demand and tight-fitting mask) and promote alveolar recruitment with positive end-expiratory pressure (PEEP). Newer HFNC devices that provide heated and humidified oxygen at flow rates of 30 to 70 L per minute are useful for preoxygenation in patients who cannot tolerate NIPPV. Approximately 1 cm $H_2O$ pressure of PEEP is estimated for every 10 L per minute of HFNC flow, but correlation with PEEP of NIPPV is unclear. Data comparing HFNC devices to standard methods of preoxygenation in critically ill patients have been mixed. Lastly, low-dose inhaled vasodilators such as inhaled nitric oxide or inhaled prostaglandins may decrease ventilation–perfusion mismatch and improve preoxygenation.

Oxygen provided to the upper airway during the apneic period may prolong the safe duration of apnea during laryngoscopy. Continuous oxygen extraction by the pulmonary circulation during apnea creates a gradient by which oxygen delivered to the upper airway diffuses into alveoli. Data on apneic oxygenation in critically ill patients are mixed. However, this low-cost intervention is minimally disruptive during emergency airway management and is advocated in high-risk population.

Systemic oxygenation during intubation is critical. Hypodynamic cardiovascular performance results in significant lag in peripheral $Sp_{O_2}$ compared to central arterial oxygenation. The delay is exacerbated by signal averaging of pulse oximetry (see Chapter 8) and accentuated during hypoxia (i.e., starting at the inflection point of the oxyhemoglobin dissociation curve). During acute arterial desaturation, the repercussion of this delay is that central arterial oxygenation can lag the peripheral $Sp_{O_2}$ monitor output for up to 60 to 90 seconds. Conversely, $Sp_{O_2}$ response may be disconcertingly delayed following successful intubation and 100% oxygen delivery following intubation. Forehead and ear probes are closer to the heart and respond more quickly than distal extremity probes. Forehead reflectance probes are often preferred in critically ill patients for this reason, and they provide more reliable signal detection during hypotension. Limited detection of cutaneous arterial pulsatility generally reduces accuracy of pulse oximetry with SBP $< 80$ mm Hg.

## Hemodynamic Optimization

Most critically ill patients have a disturbance in volume balance, exaggerating the response to induction agents and positive intrathoracic pressure. These volume balance disturbances are precipitated by volume depletion (e.g., hemorrhagic shock), volume overload (e.g., nephrogenic pulmonary edema), vascular compliance abnormalities (e.g., decreased systemic vascular resistance in sepsis), or cardiac dysfunction (cardiogenic pulmonary edema, right ventricular (RV) failure). A thoughtful approach to resuscitation is necessary to guide targeted therapies specifically at the underlying pathophysiology.

Adequate intravenous access should be established to allow for aggressive resuscitation. Second, determination of volume responsiveness should be performed. There are several dynamic assessments of volume responsiveness available to determine if a patient's cardiac output is likely to respond to a fluid challenge. Although most patients will respond to an empiric fluid challenge, assessment of volume responsiveness should be performed in unstable patients to avoid the untoward effects of volume overload. In patients who have been fluid resuscitated, or are not responsive on dynamic assessment, vasopressor support should be initiated. For patients who are unstable prior to intubation, continuous infusions are preferred over bolus infusions. In patients who are at high risk of PIH, vasopressors should be prepared and readied for rapid initiation.

Given the risk associated with intubation of patients in hemodynamic crisis, close hemodynamic monitoring is indicated. Continuous cardiac monitoring with frequent noninvasive blood pressure recording at least every 3 to 5 minutes should be performed in the peri-intubation period. Continuous monitoring should be considered during the preintubation period to facilitate monitoring of high-risk patients. Regardless of the measurement tool, it should be remembered that blood pressure is not equivalent to blood flow (i.e., cardiac output and oxygen delivery). Progressive bradycardia not associated with hypoxia or laryngoscopy is a frequent sign of severe shock and impending cardiac arrest.

## Induction

Drugs commonly used for intubation can be a double-edged sword in the critically ill. They facilitate intubation but can have severe adverse cardiovascular consequences including precipitation of shock and cardiac arrest. Patients with reduced physiologic reserve because of hypovolemia, vasodilation, or abnormal cardiac function are at higher risk of adverse events during airway management. Patients with hypotensive shock represent the extreme example. Most shock states are associated with high sympathetic tone, which serves a compensatory mechanism to maintain critical cardiac output.

Induction agents induce potent sympatholysis and attenuate reflex sympathetic discharge during laryngeal manipulation. Opioids, often given as a preintubation sympatholytic agent to patients with hypertensive emergencies, are contraindicated in patients with compromised cardiovascular status including compensated shock. Any drug that extinguishes endogenous catecholamine response, including sedative-hypnotic agents and neuroleptics, can have similar deleterious impact. Reduction of endogenous sympathetic tone leads to venous and arterial vasodilation with decreased venous return and hypotension. Some anesthetic agents also induce direct myocardial depression.

Drug choice must be considered carefully. Even at reduced doses, sedative-hypnotic induction obliterates endogenous catecholamines with subsequent arterial and venous vasodilation. The reduced pressure gradient for venous return induced by systemic venodilation is compounded by positive intrathoracic pressure upon initiation of mechanical breathing. In some critically ill patients, awake intubation with preservation of spontaneous respiration is the best course of action because of predicted difficulty either with intubation or with mechanical ventilation after intubation. Sedative induction drugs exhibit similar sympatholysis but are essential for facilitation of RSI. Adverse cardiovascular effects are both agent- and dose-dependent. Commonly recommended doses are based on patients with normal hemodynamics and cardiovascular reserve and therefore can be hazardous to critically ill patients. Frank hypotension or compensated shock requires a dose reduction of one-half to one-third of the standard dose. Reasonable sedation and amnesia is ensured with the recommended agents, particularly with proper management of sedation and analgesia in the immediate postintubation period.

Cardiovascular effects vary with sedative-hypnotic agent. Etomidate and ketamine are widely regarded as the most hemodynamically stable induction agents; however, despite their improved cardiovascular effects, both etomidate and ketamine require dose adjustment for administration to shocked patients (e.g., etomidate 0.1 to 0.15 mg per kg or ketamine 0.5 to 0.75 mg per kg). It is better to err on the side of too little rather than too much. Airway managers should anticipate delay in drug onset resulting from dose adjustment and the prolonged circulation time.

Neuromuscular blocking agents (NMBAs) pose little hemodynamic risk and should be dosed normally. Succinylcholine and rocuronium are both hemodynamically stable NMBAs. In patients with identified difficult airway attributes, awake intubation using a flexible endoscope, facilitated by topical anesthesia and limited (or no) sedation, addresses the difficult airway and also avoids the potential hypotension of induction agents. Intubation with succinylcholine alone is unusual but might be required for the obtunded patient with severe shock or impending cardiac arrest who necessitated muscular relaxation for intubation and is unable to tolerate a small dose of induction agent. Intubation without any medications is reserved for arrested or moribund patients (see Chapter 8). However, neither of these situations obviates the need for attention to safe ventilation to minimize the negative cardiovascular impact of positive-pressure breathing.

## Postintubation Management

### Mechanical Ventilation

Following intubation, positive-pressure ventilation should be initiated with caution. Positive intrathoracic pressure limits venous return to the right heart, which is accentuated during hypovolemia. Pathologic states of tension pneumothorax and auto-PEEP exacerbate intrathoracic pressure and negative hemodynamic effects. Although most clinicians recognize the risk associated with tension pneumothorax, dynamic hyperinflation is much more common. Intentional or inadvertent hyperventilation leads to dynamic hyperinflation if expiratory time limits complete tidal volume (TV) elimination. Dynamic hyperinflation results in retained intrathoracic volume, which ultimately results in positive intrathoracic pressure known as auto-PEEP and impedes venous return. The risk of dynamic hyperinflation is increased with obstructive lung disease, but any patient can develop auto-PEEP under positive-pressure breathing. Unrecognized auto-PEEP can lead to irreversible hypotension and cardiac arrest.

Immediately after intubation, hyperventilation with an inappropriately high rate and TV is particularly common during manual bag ventilation. This is a vulnerable period given the simultaneous action of induction anesthesia. Recognize that most resuscitation bags have 1,500 mL reservoirs and require single-hand ventilation to provide TV approximating 500 mL. Similarly, rapid reexpansion of the bag following breath delivery is not a cue for the next breath, and a clock second hand or counting cadence should be used to ensure that the rate is not excessive. The airway manager needs to be particularly attentive to the risk of manual hyperventilation when other staff provide this support. Specific instruction is required regarding both volume (extent of bag squeeze) and rate (counting cadence, such as "1, 2, 3, 4, 5, breath, 1, 2, 3, 4, 5, breath. . ."). That sufficient time is allowed for complete expiration can be ascertained by simply listening to the patient's chest during ventilation. The chest should be quiet, representing completion of expiratory airflow, before initiation of the subsequent breath. Interrogation of the ventilator time-flow graphics to confirm return to zero flow at the completion of each breath cycle is a more sophisticated analysis of the same issue.

Mechanical ventilation strategy depends mainly on the underlying pathophysiology. Lung-protective ventilation should be provided with TV $\leq$ 7 mL per kg of ideal body weight (IBW) for all patients. See Chapter 7.

### Postintubation Sedation

Postintubation sedation holds the same potential to induce sympatholysis-related hypotension as induction agents. The first priority is patient comfort and patient-ventilator synchrony. Sedation requirements are frequently overestimated, and analgesia and hypnotics should be titrated to patient condition. Although many prefer benzodiazepines (e.g., lorazepam and midazolam) to propofol because of perceived hypotension risk, appropriately titrated dose of the selected agent is likely most important. Intermittent or continuous opioid infusions are a growing first choice for postintubation sedation. In the absence of painful invasive procedures, light sedation that maintains patient tolerance of tracheal intubation is preferred over deeper sedation, which may worsen hypotension or increase vasopressor requirements. Despite its favorable hemodynamic properties, etomidate should not be used for postintubation sedation because of the risk for severe adrenal suppression.

PIH is a common clinical situation but should not be interpreted as an innocuous consequence of intubation. PIH occurs in one-quarter of normotensive patients undergoing emergency intubation and is severe (SBP $<$ 70 mm Hg) in up to 10% of cases. PIH is independently associated with increased risk of in-hospital death. Whether PIH directly contributes to worse outcome or merely represents a high-risk marker of severe disease is unclear. In either case, the risk associated with PIH warrants an early and organized hemodynamic resuscitation response similar to systemic hypotension (uncompensated shock) unrelated to airway management.

## SUMMARY

The ultimate goal with airway management is to maintain adequate systemic oxygenation, ventilation, and perfusion. Unstable patients have altered physiology that makes this goal complicated. Although intubation is an essential part of the resuscitation of a critically ill patient, preintubation management, the intubation technique, medications, and postintubation mechanical ventilation strategy impact peri-intubation hemodynamics that are associated with patient outcomes (**Box 32-2**). Careful planning, coordinated resuscitation, and peri-intubation management seek to optimize safe intubation and outcomes.

BOX 32-2

**Strategies to optimize intubation in unstable patient situations.**

| | Preoxygenation | Hemodynamic Optimization | Induction | Postintubation Management | Comments |
|---|---|---|---|---|---|
| Hypovolemic shock | ▪ Facemask + Nasal cannula<br>▪ HFNC<br>▪ Positive pressure likely to worsen hypotension until fluid resuscitation performed | ▪ Rapid fluid boluses<br>▪ Early transfusions when necessary<br>▪ Large bore IV access | ▪ Hemodynamically neutral sedative<br>▪ RSI | ▪ Lung-protective ventilation<br>▪ Avoid auto-PEEP | ▪ Fluid boluses preferred over vasopressors given high systemic vascular resistance (SVR) state |
| Septic shock | ▪ Facemask + Nasal cannula<br>▪ HFNC<br>▪ NIPPV if pneumonia/ARDS | ▪ Empiric fluid resuscitation<br>▪ Dynamic assessment of volume responsiveness<br>▪ Fluids if responsive<br>▪ Norepinephrine infusion | ▪ Hemodynamically neutral sedative at decreased doses<br>▪ RSI | ▪ Lung-protective ventilation<br>▪ Avoid auto-PEEP | ▪ Hemodynamic profile is variable based on stage of sepsis and underlying etiology |
| Right ventricular failure | ▪ Facemask + Nasal cannula<br>▪ HFNC<br>▪ NIPPV with low PEEP | ▪ Bedside ultrasound assessment of RV function<br>▪ Gentle fluids<br>▪ Early vasopressor infusions<br>▪ Pulmonary vasodilators | ▪ Hemodynamically neutral sedatives | ▪ Low mean airway pressure<br>▪ Prevent atelectasis, hypoxemia, and hypercapnea | |

| | | | | | |
|---|---|---|---|---|---|
| Cardiac tamponade | ■ Facemask + Nasal cannula<br>■ HFNC<br>■ NIPPV likely to worsen hypotension | ■ Fluid resuscitation<br>■ Delay intubation for priority of pericardiocentesis when possible | ■ Hemodynamically neutral sedative at decreased doses<br>■ RSI | ■ Aggressive fluid resuscitation<br>■ Pericardiocentesis | |
| Severe metabolic acidemia (MA) | ■ Facemask + Nasal cannula<br>■ HFNC<br>■ NIPPV | ■ Appropriate balanced or alkalinizing intravenous fluid (IVF) resuscitation to avoid worsening MA<br>■ Insulin drip if DKA<br>■ Consider early hemodialysis for toxic associated MA | ■ Avoid neuromuscular blocking agents if high minute ventilation (>30 L/min) due to limits with mechanical ventilation | ■ Recognize need to provide respiratory compensation for MA<br>■ Match preintubation minute ventilation<br>■ Patient-ventilator synchrony | |
| Hypoxemic respiratory failure | ■ NIPPV preferred<br>■ HFNC<br>■ Facemask + nasal cannula | ■ Dynamic assessment of volume responsiveness<br>■ Limit unnecessary IVF<br>■ Norepinephrine infusion | ■ Hemodynamically neutral sedative<br>■ RSI | ■ Lung-protective ventilation<br>■ Continuous paralytics<br>■ High PEEP if refractory hypoxemia | Many patients with ARDS and septic shock have cardiac dysfunction. Thus, assessment of volume responsiveness should be performed |

## EVIDENCE

- **Who is likely to develop peri-intubation hypotension?** In a retrospective cohort study of all patients intubated in an urban emergency department over a 1-year period, a preintubation SI of $\geq$0.8 had a sensitivity of 67% and specificity of 80% for PIH.[1] Similarly, a preintubation SI $>$ 0.90 has an odds ratio of 3.17 (95% CI, 1.36 to 7.73) of developing PIH for patients intubated in the intensive care unit.[2] Although preintubation SI is useful, one-third of patients with a normal SI developed PIH.
- **What is the evidence for hemodynamic complications with intubation?** PIH is reported in nearly half of patients intubated in the ICU.[3] Severe cardiovascular collapse was recently reported in 30% of patients in an analysis of 1,400 consecutive intubations in 42 ICUs.[4] Peri-intubation hypotension not only increases the immediate risk of death with intubation but also increases the risk of in-hospital mortality, longer ICU stays, and prolonged mechanical ventilation.[5–7]
- **Is there any evidence to recommend the best method of preoxygenation?** In a prospective study of 42 consecutive intubations, Mort showed that best efforts to achieve optimal facemask preoxygenation in critically ill patients were effective in less than 20% of patients.[8] He repeated the study and doubled the preoxygenation time from 4 to 8 minutes, with no significant difference in efficacy.[9] A randomized controlled trial showed that NIPPV significantly improved preoxygenation compared to facemask preoxygenation in critically ill ICU patients.[10] Evidence on HFNC use is mixed. Two randomized controlled trials show no significant difference in desaturation rates, whereas one observational study shows benefit in the ICU.[11–13]

## REFERENCES


1. Heffner AC, Swords DS, Nussbaum ML, et al. Predictors of the complication of postintubation hypotension during emergency airway management. *J Crit Care.* 2012;27:587–593.
2. Trivedi S, Demirci O, Arteaga G, et al. Evaluation of preintubation shock index and modified shock index as predictors of postintubation hypotension and other short-term outcomes. *J Crit Care.* 2015;30:861.e1–867.e1.
3. Simpson GD, Ross MJ, McKeown DW, et al. Tracheal intubation in the critically ill: a multi-centre national study of practice and complications. *Br J Anaesth.* 2012;108:792–799.
4. Perbet S, De Jong A, Delmas J, et al. Incidence of and risk factors for severe cardiovascular collapse after endotracheal intubation in the ICU: a multicenter observational study. *Crit Care.* 2015;19:257.
5. Green RS, Edwards J, Sabri E, et al. Evaluation of the incidence, risk factors, and impact on patient outcomes of postintubation hemodynamic instability. *CJEM.* 2012;14:74–82.
6. Green RS, Turgeon AF, McIntyre LA, et al. Postintubation hypotension in intensive care unit patients: a multicenter cohort study. *J Crit Care.* 2015;30:1055–1060.
7. Heffner AC, Swords D, Kline JA, et al. The frequency and significance of postintubation hypotension during emergency airway management. *J Crit Care.* 2012;27:417.e9–417.e13.
8. Mort TC. Preoxygenation in critically ill patients requiring emergency tracheal intubation. *Crit Care Med.* 2005;33:2672–2675.
9. Mort TC, Waberski BH, Clive J. Extending the preoxygenation period from 4 to 8 mins in critically ill patients undergoing emergency intubation. *Crit Care Med.* 2009;37:68–71.
10. Baillard C, Fosse JP, Sebbane M, et al. Noninvasive ventilation improves preoxygenation before intubation of hypoxic patients. *Am J Respir Crit Care Med.* 2006;174:171–177.

11. Semler MW, Janz DR, Lentz RJ, et al; FELLOW Investigators; the Pragmatic Critical Care Research Group. Randomized trial of apneic oxygenation during endotracheal intubation of the critically ill. *Am J Respir Crit Care Med.* 2016;193:273–280.
12. Vourc'h M, Asfar P, Volteau C, et al. High-flow nasal cannula oxygen during endotracheal intubation in hypoxemic patients: a randomized controlled clinical trial. *Intensive Care Med.* 2015;41:1538–1548.
13. Miguel-Montanes R, Hajage D, Messika J, et al. Use of high-flow nasal cannula oxygen therapy to prevent desaturation during tracheal intubation of intensive care patients with mild-to-moderate hypoxemia. *Crit Care Med.* 2015;43:574–583.

# Chapter 33

# The Trauma Patient

Michael A. Gibbs, Ali S. Raja, and Michael G. Gonzalez

## THE CLINICAL CHALLENGE

Effective airway management is a cornerstone of resuscitation of the critically injured patient. Although the nature and timing of airway intervention is influenced by assessment and prioritized management of multiple injuries, the fundamental principles of trauma airway management are no different than those applied to management of the airway in other complex medical situations. A consistent approach and a reproducible thought process will maximize success.

The requirement for intubation in a trauma patient depends on myriad factors that reach well beyond the airway. The indications for intubation, discussed in Chapter 1, include failure of the patient's ability to maintain or protect the airway (as in traumatic coma). In such cases, the need for intubation is clear. Failure of ventilation or oxygenation is less common. The former is often related to intoxicants, head injury, or direct chest injury, such as pneumothorax or hemothorax. The latter may arise not only from direct chest trauma but also from pulmonary edema caused by diffuse capillary injury in the lung from shock ("shock lung"), or acute respiratory distress syndrome. One of the most common indications for intubation in trauma, however, is also the most challenging. This is the "anticipated clinical course" indication, wherein multiple injuries, need for imaging, hemodynamic instability, need for painful procedures or surgery, likelihood of deterioration, combative behavior, and other considerations lead to a decision to intubate—even though the airway itself, oxygenation, and ventilation are all adequate.

In the National Emergency Airway Registry (NEAR) database, the most common indication for intubation was traumatic head injury, accounting for 12% of all intubations—medical or traumatic.

## APPROACH TO THE AIRWAY

Although many trauma intubations turn out to be straightforward, all should be considered at least potentially difficult. A targeted patient assessment should be performed with the aim of answering two fundamental questions. First: Will the procedure be difficult? Systematic use of the difficult airway mnemonics (Chapter 2) will help answer this question. Second: Will physiology suffer? This question prompts the clinician to anticipate predictable changes in physiology that may occur before, during, or immediately following intubation, as a result of the injuries present, the procedure itself, or the patient's premorbid condition. Focusing on preintubation cardiopulmonary optimization (Chapter 20) will help mitigate adverse hemodynamic consequences of rapid sequence intubation (RSI).

## Assessment of Difficulty

Application of the difficult airway mnemonics (LEMON, ROMAN, SMART, and RODS) allows the clinician to rapidly identify the difficult airway at the bedside. It is worth noting that the LEMON mnemonic, originally published in the first edition of this manual, in 2000, is recommended as the airway assessment tool of choice in the current (ninth) version of advanced trauma life support (ATLS). The mnemonics are provided in detail in Chapter 2 but are adapted here specifically for airway management in the acutely injured patient:

1. *L*: Look externally. Injury to the face, mouth, or neck may distort anatomy or limit access, making the process of intubation difficult or impossible. Robust mask seal may be impaired by facial hair, external bleeding, preexisting physiognomy, or anatomic disruption (RO*M*AN). Injury to the anterior neck, such as by a clothesline mechanism or hematoma, may confound successful cricothyrotomy (S*M*ART) or extraglottic device (EGD) placement (RO*D*S).
2. *E*: Evaluate 3-3-2. In blunt trauma, the cervical spine is immobilized, and a cervical collar is usually in place at the time that the airway decisions must be made. While a cervical collar is not particularly effective at limiting cervical spine movement during intubation, it does greatly impair mouth opening, limiting both laryngoscopy and insertion of an EGD (*R*ODS). The front portion of the collar should be opened to facilitate the primary survey and removed entirely during intubation, or cricothyrotomy, with manual in-line cervical stabilization maintained. Other injuries, such as mandibular fractures, may either facilitate or impair oral access, and mouth opening should be assessed as carefully as possible.
3. *M*: Mallampati. The trauma patient is rarely able to cooperate with a formal Mallampati assessment, but the airway manager should at least attempt to gently open the patient's mouth as widely as possible and inspect the oral cavity for access, using a tongue or laryngoscope blade on the anterior portion of the tongue to gently flatten it and estimate oral access. At this time, potential hemorrhage or disruption of the upper airway may also be evident (RO*D*S). It is important to refrain from "checking the gag reflex" during mouth opening, because this adds no useful information and may precipitate vomiting.
4. *O*: Obstruction, Obesity. Obstruction, usually by hemorrhage or hematoma, can interfere with laryngoscopy, bag and mask ventilation (R*O*MAN), or EGD placement (R*O*DS). Obesity in the trauma patient presents the same challenges as for the nontrauma patient.
5. *N*: Neck mobility. All patients suffering blunt trauma require in-line stabilization of the cervical spine during airway management. By definition, in-line stabilization significantly impairs the ability to place the patient in the sniffing position, and as a result, direct visualization of the glottis will be predictably difficult. When in-line stabilization is required, other measures to improve glottic visualization such as optimal external laryngeal manipulation (OELM) or the use of video laryngoscopy should be used. Rescue devices (e.g., bougie, EGD, and surgical airway equipment) should be prepared as part of the overall airway management plan. Two areas of controversy are related to the need for spinal immobilization in patients suffering cranial gunshot wounds and those suffering penetrating wounds to the neck. In the former group, there is sound evidence that the amount of force delivered by a gunshot wound to the head or face in and of itself is insufficient to fracture the spine. In both groups, decision making should be guided by the neurologic examination. Simply stated, a normal neurologic examination is an indication that the neck can be gently moved to optimize visualization of the airway. A neurologic deficit suggestive of cervical spinal cord injury mandates in-line stabilization.

## Special Clinical Considerations

The trauma airway is one of the most challenging clinical circumstances in emergency care. It requires knowledge of a panoply of techniques, guided by a reproducible approach (the airway algorithms), sound judgment, and technical expertise. In this section, we describe the considerations unique to several high-risk trauma airway scenarios (see Table 33-1).

TABLE 33-1 The "ABCs" of the Trauma Airway

| | |
|---|---|
| A | ■ Is there an injury to the Airway? |
| B | ■ Is there traumatic Brain injury? |
| C | ■ Is there a significant Chest injury? |
| | ■ Is there a risk of Cervical spine injury? |
| S | ■ Is the patient in Shock? |

### A–Injury to the Airway

Here, the very condition that mandates intubation may also render it much more difficult and prone to failure. Direct airway injury may be the result of the following:

- Maxillofacial trauma
- Blunt or penetrating anterior neck trauma
- Smoke inhalation

In cases of distorted anatomy caused by traumatic injury, the approach must minimize the potential for catastrophic deterioration. Airway disruption may be marginal or significant, real or potential. In either case, the guiding principle is to secure the threatened airway early, while more options are preserved and the patient's stability permits a more deliberate approach. Careful decisions guided by the airway algorithms will need to be made about the use (or not) of neuromuscular blockade, the primary method of airway management, and the airway rescue plan. The importance of mobilizing resources (equipment and personnel), strong leadership, and effective communication with the entire team cannot be overemphasized.

As for any other anatomically distorted airway, application of the difficult airway algorithm will often lead to a decision to perform an awake intubation. In patients with signs of significant airway compromise (e.g., stridor, respiratory distress, and voice distortion), both the urgency of the intubation and the risk of using neuromuscular blockade are high. When symptoms are more modest, there is more time to plan and execute an airway intervention, but in neither case is delay advisable. The patient's oxygenation should be assessed (i.e., "is there time?"), and it should be determined if RSI is advisable, likely under a double setup, even though the airway is difficult (see Chapter 3). This will depend on the clinician's confidence about the likelihood of success of oxygenation using a bag and mask or an EGD, and intubation by direct or video laryngoscopy. Often, an airway not amenable to direct laryngoscopy (DL) can be managed using a video laryngoscope. In rare circumstances, a precipitous deterioration invokes the "forced to act" RSI principle (Chapter 3). In this circumstance, the need for immediate airway control outweighs the patient's difficult airway attributes and permits a "one best attempt," using neuromuscular blockade, with immediate recourse to a surgical rescue should that one attempt fail. When time permits and the airway is not obscured by blood, the best approach often is awake intubation using a flexible endoscope technique with sedation and topical anesthesia (see Chapter 16). This permits both examination of the airway and careful navigation through the injured area, even when the airway itself has been violated. This is especially true if a tracheal injury is suspected, because no other method of intubation allows the airway to be visualized both above and below the glottis. When the airway is disrupted, the endotracheal tube used should be as small as is reasonable to maximize the likelihood of success and to minimize the likelihood of additional airway injury.

Smoke inhalation can present on a spectrum from mild exposure to complete airway obstruction and death. The initial assessment should be designed to identify the presence or absence of high-risk historical features (e.g., closed space fire) and physical findings (e.g., singed nasal hairs, perinasal or perioral soot, carbon deposits on the tongue, hoarse voice, and carbonaceous sputum). When evidence of significant smoke inhalation is present, direct examination of the airway, often with intubation, is important. This is best done with topical anesthesia and token amounts of sedation (if required) using either a flexible endoscope or video laryngoscope. Both the devices permit evaluation of the airway and immediate progression to intubation, if indicated. Supraglottic edema is an indication for intubation, even if the edema is mild, because progression can be both rapid and occult. Observation in lieu of airway examination can be hazardous because the airway edema can worsen significantly without any external evidence, and by the time the severity of the situation is apparent, intubation is both required immediately and extremely difficult or impossible. If examination of the upper airway identifies that the injury is confined to the mouth and nose, and the supraglottic area is spared (normal), then intubation can safely be deferred, with subsequent examination at the discretion of the operator. If it is unclear whether edema is present, it is useful to periodically perform a repeated upper airway examination (e.g., 30 to 60 minutes), even if symptoms or signs do not develop or worsen.

## B–Traumatic Brain Injury

In the NEAR studies, head injury is the most common indication for emergency department (ED) trauma airway management. Traumatic brain injury (TBI) is the number one cause of injury-related death worldwide. The principles of management of the patient with TBI and elevated intracranial pressure are discussed in more detail in Chapter 34.

When neurologic status is altered, by TBI or spinal injury or both, a rapid but thorough neurologic examination is important before any intubation attempt is undertaken, so that baseline neurologic status is documented to guide subsequent assessments and therapeutic decisions. Airway management decisions in the patient with severe TBI are centered on the prevention of secondary injury, that is, minimizing the magnitude and duration of hypoxia or hypotension. Secondary injury is the term applied when the insult to the injured brain is worsened by hypoxia, hypotension, or both.

Concrete steps can be taken to reduce the risk of secondary injury before, during, and after airway management:

**First**—Bring the principles of secondary brain injury prevention to the field. Emergency medical service providers should be educated and equipped to begin volume resuscitation and oxygen therapy before the patient arrives in the ED. Maintenance of adequate perfusion pressure (mean arterial blood pressure) and oxyhemoglobin saturation are the keys.

**Second**—Operators should focus on preintubation optimization and adequate brain perfusion before intubation. Appropriate volume replacement with normal saline solution, blood products, or both may mitigate or prevent hypotension. Selecting a hemodynamically stable and neuroprotective induction agent, such as etomidate, can further offset adverse hemodynamic consequences of RSI drugs and positive-pressure ventilation.

**Third**—Make wise decisions regarding RSI medications. Hemodynamically stable and neuroprotective induction agents, such as etomidate, are preferred. The dose should be reduced from 0.3 mg/kg to 0.15 mg/kg in the face of compensated or decompensated hypovolemic shock. Drugs that can precipitate hypotension (propofol, midazolam) should be avoided unless other options are unavailable. If the patient is severely compromised, ketamine is the agent of choice. The dose of ketamine is reduced to 0.5 mg/kg if the patient is in shock. Fentanyl, often used to optimize a *hypertensive* patient with presumed elevated intracranial pressure (ICP), is relatively contraindicated in polytrauma patients with marginal or low blood pressure even in the face of concomitant head injury.

**Fourth**—Avoid hyperventilation. Earlier thought to be a basic tool in the management of severe TBI, the use of hyperventilation is now known to lead to poorer outcomes. There is no question that hyperventilation transiently reduces ICP. It does so, however, by reducing central nervous system (CNS) perfusion, violating the central tenant of secondary injury prevention.

## C–Cervical Spine Injury

Severely injured blunt trauma patients are assumed to have sustained cervical spine injury until proven otherwise and require in-line stabilization during airway management. Although in-line stabilization is believed to help protect against spinal cord injury during intubation, it can create several problems as well. Intoxicated or head-injured patients typically become agitated and difficult to control when strapped down on a backboard. Physical and chemical restraint may be required. Aspiration is a significant risk in the supine patient with TBI or if they are vomiting. In the supine position, ventilation may be impaired, particularly for obese patients, and chest injury may make matters even worse. High-flow oxygen should be provided to all patients, and suction must be immediately available.

The practice of obtaining a cross-table lateral cervical spine X-ray before intubation is extinct. This single view, even if technically perfect, has a sensitivity of <80% and is inadequate to exclude injury. The intubation itself should be performed as gently as possible, ideally using a video laryngoscope and in-line cervical stabilization. Use of OELM will improve visualization of the glottis during DL without compromising spine stabilization. Both the preintubation neurologic status of the patient and the fact that in-line stabilization was used should be clearly documented in the medical record.

Video laryngoscopy is superior to standard laryngoscopy when airway management is performed with the neck is maintained in neutral position. Better views of the glottis are achieved in less time, and intubation success rates are higher. Traditional flexible endoscopic intubation remains a valuable tool in the patient with cervical spine trauma. Recent fluoroscopic studies comparing cervical motion during standard laryngoscopy, video laryngoscopy, and flexible fiberoptic intubation demonstrate that the flexible endoscopic approach is associated with the least amount of cervical displacement. Translating this information into clinical practice, video laryngoscopy appears to be the best approach for the majority of at-risk blunt trauma patients requiring cervical immobilization. Flexible endoscopic intubation should be considered in patients with known or strongly suspected unstable cervical spine fractures, or in those with coexisting anterior neck injuries with distorted anatomy, provided sufficient time, appropriate equipment, and expertise are available.

### *C–Chest Trauma*

Blunt and penetrating chest trauma and produce injuries that are extremely relevant to the airway management process. Pneumothorax, hemothorax, flail chest, pulmonary contusion, or open chest wounds all impair ventilation and oxygenation. Preoxygenation may be difficult or impossible, and rapid desaturation following paralysis is the rule. The postintubation delivery of positive-pressure ventilation may convert a simple pneumothorax to a tension pneumothorax. When a pneumothorax is known or suspected, a single provider should perform needle decompression before intubation when feasible. During resuscitations by a trauma team, formal tube thoracostomy can often occur simultaneously with intubation efforts provided RSI is planned and the patient is fully induced.

Penetrating chest wounds with the potential to cause cardiac injury deserve special mention. Acute traumatic pericardial tamponade is a rapidly progressive and highly lethal condition. In the setting of tamponade physiology, cardiac output becomes preload dependent. For this reason, cardiovascular collapse can occur following administration of induction agents or use of positive-pressure ventilation. If available, a bedside ultrasound should be performed early in the resuscitation. If pericardial tamponade is detected, it should be relieved before the intubation or immediately following intubation whenever possible. If urgent intubation is required and a cardiac wound is known or suspected, volume infusion is important to increase cardiac preload. The dose of induction agent (ketamine or etomidate) should be substantially reduced in this setting (e.g., 50%) perhaps opting for "amnesia over anesthesia" particularly for the patient in extremis.

### *S–Shock*

Shock in the patient with multiple injuries can be broadly classified as hemorrhagic or nonhemorrhagic (e.g., tension pneumothorax, pericardial tamponade, myocardial contusion, or spinal shock). A targeted physical examination and selective bedside testing (chest X-ray, pelvic X-ray, and e-FAST) will help identify the cause(s). As the causes of shock are elucidated and addressed, airway management decisions must consider the erosion of hemodynamic reserve in these patients. Common decisions include the following:

- Should the patient be intubated now, or is there time for physiologic optimization?
- How does the patient's hemodynamic status influence the choice and dose of the induction agent?

Although there is no simple answer to these fundamental questions, the central tenet here is: The more hemodynamically unstable, the more important it is to resuscitate before intubation to mitigate the potential adverse hemodynamic effects of RSI drugs.

Patients in "compensated shock" can appear deceptively stable. The presence or absence of shock should never be simplistically equated with the presence or absence of a blood pressure reading of <90 mm Hg. Because of adaptive postinjury responses, relatively normal blood pressure is often maintained despite significant hypoperfusion. Hypotension is typically a late finding indicative of significant decompensation. The operator must select the induction agent (and its dose) and determine the rate, timing, and quantity of resuscitative fluid or blood products in the context of the patient's overall circulatory status and response to resuscitation, rather than be guided only by a systolic blood pressure.

Table 33-2 provides summary guidance on how to anticipate and manage changes in physiology during airway management. See Chapters 20 and 32 for a detailed discussion of both preintubation optimization and airway management in the unstable patient.

# TECHNIQUE

## Paralysis versus Rapid Tranquilization of the Combative Trauma Patient

The combative trauma patient presents a series of conflicting problems. The potential causes of combative behavior are numerous and include head injury, drug or ethanol intoxication, preexisting medical conditions (e.g., diabetes), hypoxemia, shock, anxiety, psychiatric disease, and others. The priority is to rapidly control the patient so that potentially life-threatening causes can be identified and corrected, and the risk of injury to medical providers is minimized. Controversy exists as to whether such patients ought to undergo rapid tranquilization with a neuroleptic agent or sedative, or whether immediate intubation with neuromuscular blockade is appropriate. Rapid tranquilization using haloperidol is well established as a safe and effective means for gaining control of the combative trauma patient who cannot be settled by other means. Haloperidol can be used intravenously in 5- to 10-mg increments every 5 minutes until a sufficient clinical response is achieved. The decision to use rapid tranquilization rather than RSI with neuromuscular blockade depends on the nature of the patient's presentation and injuries. If intubation is required based on the patient's injuries and vital signs, independent of the combative behavior, then immediate intubation is indicated. If, however, the patient is presenting primarily with control problems and does not appear to have injuries that would mandate intubation, then rapid tranquilization is appropriate. In many situations, the decision will not be clear-cut, and judgment will be required. Control of the patient is an essential step in overall management.

## RSI of the Trauma Patient

Except when consideration of the patient's injuries argues otherwise, RSI is the preferred method of airway management for the majority of injured patients. The potential for difficulty or failure is inherent in trauma airway management, and formulation of a backup (rescue) plan is a key part of preparing for the airway interventions.

As in other critically ill patients, the universal, difficult, and failed airway algorithms will guide the clinician in navigating the multitude of unique clinical scenarios that may arise in the injured patient (see Chapter 3). Familiarity with the algorithms and with the drugs and techniques of RSI, and alternative airway techniques, will maximize the likelihood of a positive outcome.

TABLE 33-2 **Anticipating Changes in Physiology during Trauma Airway Management**

| Clinical Scenario | Challenge | Considerations |
|---|---|---|
| **Airway injury** | | |
| ▪ Facial/neck trauma | ▪ Will intubation be difficult? | ▪ Rapid sequence intubation (RSI) versus an awake technique?<br>▪ Identify rescue device(s)<br>▪ Prepare for surgical airway |
| ▪ Smoke inhalation | ▪ Will intubation be difficult?<br>▪ Will there be airway edema?<br>▪ Will lung injury limit reserve? | ▪ RSI versus an awake technique?<br>▪ Supraglottic rescue device may not work<br>▪ Prepare for surgical airway<br>▪ Have a smaller endotracheal tube ready<br>▪ Anticipate rapid desaturation |
| **Brain and cervical spine injury** | | |
| ▪ Brain injury and multisystem trauma with hemodynamic compromise | ▪ Will blood pressure (and central nervous system perfusion) fall further during induction? | ▪ Optimize preload<br>▪ Reduce dose of etomidate or ketamine<br>▪ Avoid other induction agents |
| ▪ Cervical spine | ▪ Is there a risk of spinal cord injury during intubation? | ▪ Blunt trauma patients are presumed to have this risk until proven otherwise<br>▪ Maintain in-line stabilization<br>▪ Use of video laryngoscopy or flexible endoscopy if available |
| | ▪ Will in-line stabilization impair visualization of the airway? | ▪ Use the optimal external laryngeal manipulation during direct laryngoscopy (DL)<br>▪ Video laryngoscopy is superior to DL |
| **Chest injury** | | |
| ▪ Blunt | ▪ Is there a pneumothorax or hemothorax?<br>▪ Will drugs or positive-pressure ventilation precipitate cardiovascular collapse?<br>▪ Will chest injury limit reserve? | ▪ Consider needle chest decompression<br>▪ Optimize preload<br>▪ Ketamine or reduced dose etomidate for induction<br>▪ Anticipate rapid desaturation |
| ▪ Penetrating | ▪ Is there a pneumothorax or pericardial tamponade?<br>▪ Will drugs or positive-pressure ventilation precipitate cardiovascular collapse?<br>▪ Will chest injury limit reserve? | ▪ Consider needle chest decompression<br>▪ Optimize preload<br>▪ Ketamine or reduced dose etomidate for induction<br>▪ Anticipate rapid desaturation |
| ▪ Shock | ▪ Will drugs or positive-pressure ventilation precipitate cardiovascular collapse? | ▪ Optimize preload<br>▪ Ketamine or reduced dose etomidate for induction |

### Choice of Neuromuscular Blocking Agent

Succinylcholine (SCh) and rocuronium are both excellent choices for RSI in the trauma patient. SCh is highly desirable because of its rapid, reliable onset and brief duration of action. The latter permits earlier neurologic reassessment in head-injured patients. Although spinal cord injury, extensive burns, and severe crush injuries are risk factors for SCh-induced hyperkalemia, the receptor upregulation that can lead to hyperkalemia takes a few days to develop and is not a clinical concern in the acute setting. SCh is contraindicated in these patients beginning 3-5 days post injury and extending for 6 months or until the burns are healed. In these patients, rocuronium is a suitable replacement.

Suspected elevation of ICP is not a contraindication to SCh. SCh-induced fasciculations have been implicated in producing elevation of ICP in the patient with TBI, and in the past using a defasciculating dose of a nondepolarizer was recommended. This rise in ICP is not thought to be clinically significant, and defasciculation is neither needed nor recommended.

### Choice of Induction Agent

In most circumstances, etomidate is the drug of choice for patients with trauma, because of its rapid onset, hemodynamic stability, favorable effect on cerebral metabolic oxygen demand, and the extensive experience with its use. However, despite its reputation for hemodynamic stability, etomidate can aggravate hemodynamic status in susceptible patients, leading to the recommendation to reduce the induction dose to 0.15 mg per kg in these patients. The transient depression of steroid synthesis by etomidate has not been shown to adversely affect outcome in patients with hemodynamic shock (see Chapters 21 and 32).

Ketamine may be the best induction agent for patients in compensated or decompensated shock. However, because ketamine may increase blood pressure in normotensive or hypertensive patients, such as patients with isolated severe head injury, etomidate is probably the preferable agent in these patients. Induction agent selection is summarized in Table 33-3.

## THE FAILED AIRWAY

The failed airway is managed according to the failed airway algorithm. The LEMON-, ROMAN-, RODS-, and SMART-guided evaluations during the preintubation assessment are intended to minimize the risk of encountering a failed airway. Cricothyrotomy equipment for a "double setup" should always be readily available.

**TABLE 33-3 Rapid Sequence Intubation Sedative Induction Agent Selection in the Trauma Patient**

| Clinical Scenario | First Choice | Alternatives |
|---|---|---|
| **No brain injury** | | |
| Hemodynamically stable | Etomidate | Propofol, Midazolam |
| Shock | Ketamine | Etomidate[a] |
| **Brain injury** | | |
| Hemodynamically stable | Etomidate | Propofol |
| Shock | Etomidate[a] | Ketamine[a,b] |
| Profound shock | Ketamine[a] | None |

[a]In the presence of shock, reduce the dose by 25% to 50%.
[b]Hemodynamic considerations outweigh intracranial pressure controversy.

## TIPS AND PEARLS

1. Airway management of the patient with multiple injuries follows the same general principles as any other patient. The primary challenge for the intubator is to resist distraction by the patient's external injuries, combative behavior, or the anxiety that accompanies care of the severely injured trauma victim.
2. Resist the temptation to simply observe the patient with upper airway injury or smoke inhalation. Delay can lead to disaster. Examine the upper airway periodically with a flexible endoscope passed nasally.
3. Consider early intubation for potentially unstable patients who are to be moved out of the ED for diagnostic studies or transported to another facility.
4. There is substantial and increasing evidence that video laryngoscopy is superior to DL for airway management in the ED. This is especially true in those requiring in-line cervical stabilization. Clinicians who manage trauma patients on a regular basis must give serious consideration to routine incorporation of video laryngoscopy. Hyperangulated video laryngoscopes may be better at glottic visualization than those that are traditionally shaped in patients with cervical collars.
5. The hemodynamically compromised trauma patient may be much more severely injured than is apparent. Young patients, in particular, can preserve a reasonably "normal" blood pressure in the face of significant hemorrhage. Occult instability may be suddenly unmasked by the administration of sedative agents or positive-pressure ventilation. If the need for intubation is not immediate, cardiopulmonary optimization should be undertaken to mitigate the adverse hemodynamic consequences of RSI.

## EVIDENCE

- **Are there large studies of intubated trauma patients?** Dunham et al.[1] performed a comprehensive, evidence-based literature overview (demographics, airway management techniques, and success rates) of trauma patients requiring emergency airway management. Although most of these patients were critically ill, the degree of injury was highly variable; the mean injury severity score was 29 (range 17 to 54), and the mean Glasgow Coma Scale was 6.5 (range 3 to 15). On average, 41% of patients died (range 2% to 100%). In the recently published report from the NEAR, 31% of patients were victims of injury, and the vast majority were managed by emergency physicians using RSI.[2] In a recent Japanese airway registry study in which 723 intubated patients with trauma were reviewed, cricothyrotomy was required in 2.2% of patients. It is almost always used as a rescue technique, and when performed, it had a high success rate and low rate of adverse events.[3]
- **Has inadequate or inappropriate airway management been linked to preventable death?** A study evaluating 51 preventable deaths at a large regional trauma center in Los Angeles found that only one death (1.9%) was directly attributable to failure to manage the airway in the ED.[4] Although encouraging, it should not diminish the appreciation that trauma airways are high risk and that developing and maintaining skills necessary for trauma airway management is a priority.[5–7]
- **Does hyperventilation worsen outcomes in patients with severe TBI?** Davis et al.[8] examined the impact of prehospital ventilation strategies on outcomes in 890 intubated head injury patients in San Diego County. By protocol, arterial blood gases were obtained upon ED arrival. Hyperventilation was defined as a $P_{CO_2} < 30$ mm Hg, and hypoventilation as a $P_{CO_2} > 49$ mm Hg. Patients with a $P_{CO_2}$ of 30 to 49 mm Hg had lower mortality and better neurologic outcomes. Warner et al.[9] conducted a similar prospective assessment of 576 intubated TBI patients in Seattle. These authors defined severe hypocapnea as an arrival $P_{CO_2} < 30$ mm Hg, and severe hypercapnea as an arrival $P_{CO_2} > 45$ mm Hg. Targeted ventilation was defined as an arrival $P_{CO_2}$ between 30 and 35 mm Hg. The rate of severe hypocapnea (i.e., hyperventilation) was 18%. Patients in the targeted ventilation range were less likely to die than those

who were hyperventilated (odds ratio, 0.57; 95% confidence interval, 0.33 to 0.99). The most recent guidelines published by the Brain Trauma Foundation discourage "routine" hyperventilation and restrict use to a very narrow segment of patients with unequivocal evidence of herniation (i.e., blown pupil or motor posturing) for which mannitol therapy has failed.[10]

- **Is video laryngoscopy superior to DL in trauma patients who are at risk for cervical or head injury?** In a prospective study of 198 NEAR patients, 26% of which were injured, Brown et al.[11] demonstrated superior visualization of the glottis using a Storz Video Macintosh Laryngoscope compared with standard laryngoscopy. In a simulation study assessing intubation success rates with in-line stabilization, Takahashi et al.[12] demonstrated that intubation with the Airway Scope (AWS) was more effective than DL (success rates 100% AWS; 93% DL). Three recent studies have compared cervical motion with DL, video laryngoscopy, and flexible endoscopic intubation in healthy human volunteers.[13–15] Cervical motion was examined using fluoroscopy. The results demonstrated more cervical motion with DL than with video laryngoscopy and the least amount of cervical motion with flexible endoscopic intubation. Yeatts et al.[16] reported on 623 head-injured patients randomized to intubation with either GlideScope (GVL) or DL. The GVL group was observed to have higher rates of hypoxia (50% vs. 24%) and death (30% vs. 14%), proposed to be from longer average (9 seconds) intubation attempts with GVL. However, the study had significant methodological problems including very high rates (nearly 1/3) of randomization dropout owing to "operator preference," poor preoxygenation techniques, and variability in postintubation care, making the result both hard to interpret and hard to believe.
- **Is etomidate safe in trauma patients?** In a single-center study, Hildreth et al.[17] confirmed transient suppression of the adrenal response to exogenous adrenocorticotrophic hormone and questioned the safety of etomidate in trauma patients, claiming such outcomes increased ventilator time, hospital length of stay, ICU days, and the requirement for blood products. The study was poorly designed, failing to control for key clinical variables among many other fatal flaws. There is no credible evidence that use of etomidate in trauma patients, including those in shock, is risky. On the contrary, etomidate's ability to preserve hemodynamic status makes it an excellent agent for use in trauma.
- **Is ketamine safe in patients with TBI?** A 2014 review of this topic by Zeiler et al.[18] concluded that the historical bias against the use of ketamine in patients with TBI is not evidence-based. On the contrary, they found that ketamine is an attractive alternative in the hemodynamically unstable trauma patient. In the past, ketamine had been largely ignored because of the concern of increasing ICP; however, it is in fact safe for use in trauma patients and may actually decrease ICP.

## REFERENCES


1. Dunham CM, Barraco RD, Clark DE, et al. Guidelines for emergency tracheal intubation immediately after traumatic injury. *J Trauma*. 2003;55(1):162–179.
2. Brown CA, Bair AE, Pallin DJ, et al; NEAR III Investigators. Techniques, success, and adverse events of emergency department adult intubations. *Ann Emerg Med*. 2015;65(4):363.e1–370.e1.
3. Nakao S, Kimura A, Hagiwara Y, et al. Trauma airway management in emergency departments: a multicentre, prospective, observational study in Japan. *BMJ Open*. 2015;5(2):e006623.
4. Teixeira PGR, Inaba K, Hadjizacharia P, et al. Preventable or potentially preventable mortality at a mature trauma center. *J Trauma*. 2007;63(6):1338–1346; discussion 1346–7.
5. Kortbeek JB, Al Turki SA, Ali J, et al. Advanced trauma life support, 8th edition, the evidence for change. *J Trauma*. 2008;64(6):1638–1650.
6. Horton CL, Brown CA, Raja AS. Trauma airway management. *J Emerg Med*. 2014;46(6):814–820.

7. American College of Surgeons Committee on Trauma. *Advanced Trauma Life Support for Doctors, Student Course Manual*. 9th ed. Chicago: American College of Surgeons; 2012.

8. Davis DP, Idris AH, Sise MJ, et al. Early ventilation and outcome in patients with moderate to severe traumatic brain injury. *Crit Care Med*. 2006;34(4):1202–1208.

9. Warner KJ, Cuschieri J, Copass MK, et al. The impact of prehospital ventilation on outcome after severe traumatic brain injury. *J Trauma*. 2007;62(6):1330–1336; discussion 1336–8.

10. Brain Trauma Foundation; American Association of Neurological Surgeons; Congress of Neurological Surgeons; Joint Section on Neurotrauma and Critical Care; AANS/CNS; Bratton SL, Chestnut RM, Ghajar J, et al. Guidelines for the management of severe traumatic brain injury. I. Blood pressure and oxygenation. *J Neurotrauma*. 2007;24 suppl 1:S7–S13.

11. Brown CA, Bair AE, Pallin DJ, et al; National Emergency Airway Registry (NEAR) Investigators. Improved glottic exposure with the Video Macintosh Laryngoscope in adult emergency department tracheal intubations. *Ann Emerg Med*. 2010;56(2):83–88.

12. Takahashi K, Morimura N, Sakamoto T, et al. Comparison of the Airway Scope and Macintosh laryngoscope with in-line cervical stabilization by the semisolid neck collar: manikin study. *J Trauma*. 2010;68(2):363–366.

13. Hirabayashi Y, Fujita A, Seo N, et al. Cervical spine movement during laryngoscopy using the Airway Scope compared with the Macintosh laryngoscope. *Anaesthesia*. 2007;62(10):1050–1055.

14. Maruyama K, Yamada T, Kawakami R, et al. Upper cervical spine movement during intubation: fluoroscopic comparison of the AirWay Scope, McCoy laryngoscope, and Macintosh laryngoscope. *Br J Anaesth*. 2008;100(1):120–124.

15. Wong DM, Prabhu A, Chakraborty S, et al. Cervical spine motion during flexible bronchoscopy compared with the Lo-Pro GlideScope. *Br J Anaesth*. 2009;102(3):424–430.

16. Yeatts DJ, Dutton RP, Hu PF, et al. Effect of video laryngoscopy on trauma patient survival: a randomized controlled trial. *J Trauma Acute Care Surg*. 2013;75:212–219.

17. Hildreth AN, Mejia VA, Maxwell RA, et al. Adrenal suppression following a single dose of etomidate for rapid sequence induction: a prospective randomized study. *J Trauma*. 2008;65(3):573–579.

18. Zeiler FA, Teitelbaum J, West M, et al. The ketamine effect on ICP in traumatic brain injury. *Neurocrit Care*. 2014;21(1):163–173.

# Chapter 34

# Elevated ICP and HTN Emergencies

Bret P. Nelson and Andy S. Jagoda

## THE CLINICAL CHALLENGE

Elevated intracranial pressure (ICP) poses a direct threat to the viability and function of the brain by limiting blood flow and oxygen delivery. In head trauma, elevated ICP has been clearly associated with worse outcomes. The problems associated with elevated ICP may be compounded by many of the techniques and drugs used in airway management, because they may cause further elevations of ICP. In addition, victims of multiple traumas may present with hypotension, thus limiting the choice of agents and techniques available. This chapter provides the basis for an understanding of the problems of increased ICP and the optimal methods of airway management in this patient group.

When increased ICP occurs as a result of an injury or medical catastrophe, the brain's ability to regulate blood flow (autoregulation) over a range of blood pressures is often lost. In general, ICP is maintained through a mean arterial pressure (MAP) range of 80 to 180 mm Hg. Elevation in ICP often is a sign that autoregulation has been lost. In this setting, excessively high or excessively low blood pressure could aggravate brain injury by promoting cerebral edema or ischemia. Hypotension, even for a very brief period, is especially harmful. Hypotension and hypoxia have been shown to be independent predictors of mortality and morbidity in patients with traumatic brain injury (TBI).

Cerebral perfusion pressure (CPP) is the driving force for blood flow to the brain. It is measured by the difference between MAP and ICP, expressed as the formula:

$$\text{CPP} = \text{MAP} - \text{ICP}$$

It is clear from this formula that excessive decreases in MAP, as might occur during rapid sequence intubation (RSI), would decrease CPP and contribute to cerebral ischemia. Conversely, increases in MAP, if not accompanied by equivalent increases in ICP, may be beneficial because of the increase in the driving pressure for oxygenation of brain tissue. It is generally recommended that the ICP be maintained $<20$ mm Hg, the MAP between 100 and 110 mm Hg, and the CPP near 70 mm Hg. There are a number of confounding elements that may increase ICP during airway management.

## Reflex Sympathetic Response to Laryngoscopy

The reflex sympathetic response to laryngoscopy (RSRL) is stimulated by the rich sensory innervation of the supraglottic larynx. Use of the laryngoscope, and particularly the attempted placement of an endotracheal tube, results in a significant afferent discharge that increases sympathetic activity to the cardiovascular system mediated through direct neuronal activity and release of catecholamines. More prolonged or aggressive attempts at laryngoscopy and intubation result in greater sympathetic nervous system stimulation. This catecholamine surge leads to increased heart rate and blood pressure, which significantly enhances cerebral blood flow (CBF) at the apparent expense of the systemic circulation. These hemodynamic changes may contribute to increased ICP, particularly if autoregulation is impaired; therefore, it is desirable to mitigate this RSRL. Gentle intubation techniques (including the use of experienced operators and video laryngoscopy devices) that minimize airway stimulation and pharmacologic adjuncts (e.g., $\beta$-blockade and synthetic opioids) have been studied to accomplish this mitigation.

Evidence is mixed regarding the use of lidocaine to blunt the hemodynamic response to laryngoscopy. Studies in patients without cardiovascular disease have failed to show effect. Other studies have shown variable results with respect to hemodynamic protection, with some appearing to demonstrate benefit and others showing none. As a result, lidocaine is not recommended, currently, for the mitigation of the RSRL associated with emergency intubation.

The short-acting $\beta$-blocker esmolol, in contrast, has consistently demonstrated the ability to control both heart rate and blood pressure responses to intubation. A dose of 2 mg per kg given 3 minutes before intubation has been shown to be effective. Unfortunately, administration of $\beta$-blocking agents in emergency situations may be problematic for several reasons. Even a short-acting agent, such as esmolol, may exacerbate hypotension in a trauma patient, or confound interpretation of a decrease in the blood pressure immediately following intubation. For these reasons, although esmolol is consistent and reliable for mitigation of RSRL in elective anesthesia, it is generally not used for this purpose for emergency intubation.

Fentanyl at doses of 3 to 5 μg per kg has also been shown to attenuate the RSRL associated with intubation. Although a full sympathetic blocking dose of fentanyl is 9 to 13 μg per kg, the recommended dose of fentanyl for physiologic optimization during emergency RSI is 3 μg per kg and should be administered as a single dose over 60 seconds. This technique permits effective mitigation of the RSRL, with greatly reduced chances of apnea or hypoventilation before sedation and paralysis (see Chapter 20).

Several studies have investigated the potential advantages of flexible endoscopic intubation over direct laryngoscopy, working on the premise that these techniques minimize tracheal stimulation and thus the RSRL. Results of these studies are mixed and do not permit any conclusions recommending one technique over the other. In a controlled operating room setting, the insertion of the endotracheal tube into the trachea is more stimulating than a routine laryngoscopy.

At present, based on the best available evidence, it seems advisable to administer 3 μg per kg of fentanyl intravenously (IV) 3 minutes before administration of the induction and neuromuscular blocking agents (NMBAs) to mitigate the RSRL for patients who may be intolerant to spikes in heart rate, vascular sheer forces, or ICP. Fentanyl should not be administered to patients with incipient or actual hypotension or to those who are dependent on sympathetic drive to maintain an adequate blood pressure for cerebral perfusion. In such cases, the ensuing hypotension may cause further central nervous system injury. In addition to pharmacologic maneuvers to reduce RSRL, intubation should be performed in the gentlest manner possible, limiting both the time and intensity of laryngoscopy.

## Reflex ICP Response to Laryngoscopy

Laryngoscopy may also increase the ICP by a direct reflex mechanism not mediated by sympathetic stimulation of the blood pressure or heart rate. The details of this reflex are poorly understood. Insertion of the laryngoscope or endotracheal tube may, therefore, further elevate ICP, even if the RSRL is blunted. Although it would be desirable to blunt this ICP response to laryngoscopy in patients at risk for having elevated ICP, literature related to the use of lidocaine for this purpose is mixed, at best. Given how specific the timing and dosage of lidocaine needed to be even in studies where an effect was shown, and how cognitive and staff resources could be used maximizing patients' safety in other ways prior to intubation (such as optimizing hemodynamics, improving preoxygenation, etc.), we no longer recommend lidocaine as a pretreatment medication in an attempt to blunt this response or for any other purpose during emergency airway management.

### ICP Response to Neuromuscular Blockade

Succinylcholine (SCh) itself may be capable of causing a mild and transient increase in ICP. Studies have shown that this increase is temporally related to the presence of fasciculations in the patient but is not the result of synchronized muscular activity leading to increased venous pressure. Rather, there appears to be a complex reflex mechanism originating in the muscle spindle and ultimately resulting in an elevation of ICP. One recent study challenged the claim that SCh causes an elevation of ICP, and SCh remains a commonly used NMBA for management of patients with elevated ICP because of its rapid onset and short duration. Although we recommended in earlier editions of this manual the routine use of a defasciculating agent when SCh is administered to a patient with elevated ICP, we no longer advocate this practice. There is insufficient evidence to support the use of a defasciculating agent, and it adds unnecessary complexity.

Neuromuscular blockade with nondepolarizing agents such as rocuronium is becoming more common, and recent registry data suggests nearly half of all emergency RSIs are now performed with rocuronium. At doses of 1.0 to 1.2 mg per kg, ideal intubating conditions at 60 seconds are similar to SCh. Because rocuronium does not carry a risk of elevating ICP and is not associated with hyperkalemia, it is a viable option for neuromuscular blockade in brain injury. One important note is that the duration of paralysis with rocuronium is much longer than that with SCh (about 1 hour at 1 mg per kg) and is dose-dependent. If a shorter duration of paralysis is desirable, SCh should be considered.

### Choice of Induction Agent

When managing the patient with potential brain injury, it is important to choose an induction agent that will not adversely affect CPP. Ideally, one would like to choose an induction agent that is capable of improving or maintaining CPP and providing some cerebral protective effect by decreasing the basal metabolic rate of oxygen utilization of the brain ($CMRO_2$). This effect can be likened to decreasing myocardial oxygen demand in the ischemic heart. Etomidate is a short-acting imidazole derivative that exhibits this beneficial cerebroprotective profile with the added benefit of hemodynamic stability. In fact, etomidate is the most hemodynamically stable of all commonly used induction agents except ketamine (see Chapter 21). Its ability to decrease $CMRO_2$ and ICP and its remarkable hemodynamic stability make it the drug of choice for patients with elevated ICP.

In the past, ketamine has been avoided in patients with known elevations in ICP because of the belief that it may elevate the ICP further. Several case series in spontaneously breathing patients with known cerebral spinal fluid (CSF) outflow obstructions, which contained no control groups, formed the basis for this concern. The evidence regarding this phenomenon is mixed, however, and more recent data suggests that ketamine is safe for use in head injury (discussed in Chapter 21). Ketamine may in fact increase cerebral perfusion. In patients with elevated ICP and hypotension, ketamine's superior hemodynamic stability, on balance, argue for its use. In the hypertensive patient, etomidate is preferred owing to the possibility that ketamine can increase MAP.

## APPROACH TO THE AIRWAY

RSI is the preferred method for patients with suspected elevated ICP because it provides protection against the reflex responses to laryngoscopy and rises in ICP. The presence of coma should not be interpreted as an indication to proceed without pharmacologic agents or to administer only a NMBA

BOX 34-1

**Doses for lidocaine, succinylcholine, and etomidate are mg not mcg.**

| Time | Action |
|---|---|
| Zero minus 10+ min | **P**reparation |
| Zero minus 10+ min | **P**reoxygenation |
| Zero minus 10+ min | **P**re-Intubation Optimization<br>Fentanyl 3 μg/kg (over 1 min if not hypotensive) |
| Zero | **P**aralysis with induction:<br>Etomidate 0.3 mg/kg IV<br>Or<br>Ketamine 1.5 mg/kg IV<br>SCh 1.5 mg/kg IV<br>Or<br>Rocuronium 1 mg/kg IV |
| Zero plus 30 s | **P**ositioning |
| Zero plus 45 s | **P**lacement with proof: intubate, confirm placement |
| Zero plus 60 s | **P**ostintubation management |

without a sedative induction drug. Although the patient may seem unresponsive, laryngoscopy and intubation will provoke the reflexes described previously if appropriate sympatholytic and induction agents are not used. Following appropriate assessment and preparation, as described in Chapters 2 and 20, the sequence in **Box 34-1** is recommended for patients with elevated ICP.

## INITIATING MECHANICAL VENTILATION

Mechanical ventilation in the patient with elevated ICP should be predicated on three principles: (1) optimal oxygenation, (2) normocapnia, and (3) avoidance of ventilation mechanics (e.g., positive end-expiratory pressure, high peak inspiratory pressure) that would increase venous congestion in the brain.

Although there never was a scientific basis for the use of "therapeutic" hyperventilation, it was widely and enthusiastically adopted. The Brain Trauma Foundation Guidelines for the Management of Severe TBI recommend that prophylactic hyperventilation should be avoided and that patients with severe TBI be ventilated in such a way as to target the lower limits of normocapnia ($Paco_2$ of 35 to 40 mm Hg). A similar approach seems prudent in patients with medical causes of elevations of ICP (e.g., cerebral hemorrhage).

Although there is no outcome evidence supporting its use or demonstrating any benefit, hyperventilation to a $Paco_2$ of 30 mm Hg still may have a limited role as a temporizing measure in patients demonstrating clinical signs of herniation (blown pupil or decerebrate posturing) unresponsive to appropriate interventions using osmotic agents, cerebrospinal fluid drainage, or both. This should be initiated only with continuous capnography to guide ventilation efforts and avoid harmful sequelae of excessive hypocapnia. In addition, advanced neuromonitoring for cerebral ischemia should be considered. Normal initial physiologic ventilation parameters are described in Chapter 7. Initial inspired fraction of oxygen ($Fio_2$) should be 1.0 (100%). $Fio_2$ can later be decreased according to pulse oximetry, as long as 100% oxygen saturation is maintained. Carbon dioxide tension can be followed with arterial blood gases or, preferably, continuous capnography, the first assessment of which should occur approximately 10 minutes after initiation of steady-state mechanical ventilation. To permit early and frequent neurologic examinations (e.g., by a neurosurgeon to decide whether there is sufficient persisting neurologic functioning to warrant an attempt at surgical evacuation of a massive subdural hematoma), long-term sedation is best accomplished by using a propofol infusion, which can be terminated as needed with prompt patient recovery. Deep sedation is desired, however, to permit effective controlled mechanical ventilation and other necessary interventions while mitigating the stimulating effects of the tube in the trachea and eliminating any possibility of the patient coughing or bucking. Propofol is not an analgesic, and an opioid analgesic, such as fentanyl, is used to improve endotracheal tube tolerance and reduce stimulation and responsiveness.

## TIPS AND PEARLS

- RSI clearly is the desired method for tracheal intubation in patients with suspected elevation of ICP. The technique allows control of various adverse effects and optimal control of ventilation after intubation. However, the use of neuromuscular blockade in patients with potential neurologic deficit carries the responsibility of performing a detailed neurologic evaluation on the patient before initiation of neuromuscular blockade. The patient's ability to interact with the surroundings, spontaneous motor movement, response to deep pain, response to voice, localization, pupillary reflexes, and other pertinent neurologic details must be assessed carefully before administration of neuromuscular blockade. The careful recording of these findings will be invaluable for the ongoing evaluation of the patient.
- If the patient's intrinsic ventilatory drive is severely compromised by head injury or concomitant injuries, positive-pressure ventilation with bag and mask may be required throughout the intubation sequence. In such circumstances, one is trading off the increased risk of aspiration against the hazard of inadequate oxygenation and rising $Paco_2$ during the intubation sequence. When such a tradeoff arises, it should be resolved in favor of oxygenation over the risk of aspiration.

## EVIDENCE

Evidence-based recommendations depend on a careful analysis of the methodology used in the studies reviewed and an understanding of the outcome measure, which must be sound to make the study clinically relevant. In this light, it becomes challenging to make evidence-based recommendations regarding airway management in the patient with a brain injury, as is the case in many other areas of airway management. Regarding methodology, most of the studies of the effect of interventions discussed in this chapter were performed on stable patients in the operating room setting; others were performed on deeply anesthetized patients in the intensive care unit during tracheal suctioning. It is difficult to extrapolate the findings in these patient groups to critical patients undergoing emergency intubation. In addition, the timing and dosing of pharmacologic interventions varied significantly, making it difficult to compare one study with another. There is only one randomized double-blind interventional study identified that was performed in the emergency department (ED) on patients with head injury.[1] This prospective double-blind study found that esmolol and lidocaine had similar efficacy in attenuating the hemodynamic response to intubation of patients with isolated head injury.

Regarding outcome, there is no study in the literature that compares airway interventions with a functional outcome measure, that is, disability or death. Rises in heart rate, blood pressure, and ICP are the commonly measured parameters comparing one technique or pharmacologic intervention with another because these affect CPP. However, there is no evidence that these are valid surrogates for more meaningful outcome measures such as disability, nor is there evidence that transient rises in any of the previously mentioned measures have any meaningful impact on morbidity or mortality.

Based on the foregoing, there is no evidence that the interventions presented in this chapter do harm, and pending more direct evidence, it does seem intuitive that minimizing adverse changes in ICP, blood pressure, and heart rate would likely contribute to maximizing good outcomes.

- **Is physiologic optimization indicated for patients with elevated ICP?** Sympatholysis is an option, as part of physiologic optimization, during RSI for patients being intubated with cerebrovascular or cardiovascular hypertensive emergencies. The choices of sympatholytic agents include fentanyl and esmolol. Lidocaine and defasciculating agents are no longer recommended based on poor evidence and inconsistent results. Evidence for the use of fentanyl at a dose of 3 mg per kg IV, 3 minutes before induction, is discussed in Chapter 20. Fentanyl is known to blunt the reflex sympathetic response to upper airway manipulation, mitigating the extent of catecholamine release and, therefore, rise in MAP.

  Esmolol has been studied as a medication to blunt the RSRL through its $\beta$-blocking properties and was previously found to control heart rate and blood pressure better than fentanyl, although no recent high-quality studies in emergency populations have provided new information. Dexmedetomidine and remifentanil are newer agents that have a role in the OR for controlling perioperative hypertension, although these are uncommon drugs in the ED.[2] There is some controversy, but no evidence, whether the increase in ICP caused by SCh is clinically significant, and whether a defasciculating dose of a competitive NMBA is capable of mitigating this response. We no longer recommend the use of a defasciculating dose (one-tenth of the paralyzing dose) of a competitive NMBA before SCh is given. Based on the best evidence available at this time, the following recommendations can be made regarding the pharmacologic mitigation of exacerbations of elevated ICP or blood pressure during emergency intubation:
  - Administration of Lidocaine, 1.5 mg per kg, 3 minutes before airway manipulation is no longer recommended.
  - In patients without compensated or decompensated shock, administer fentanyl, 3 µg per kg, 3 minutes before airway manipulation in order to mitigate increases in ICP from RSRL. If there is insufficient time or a concern that blood pressure will drop after administration, then fentanyl should not be given.
  - When patients with elevated ICP are paralyzed with SCh, use of a defasciculating dose of a nondepolarizing paralytic agent is no longer recommended.
  - Esmolol is an effective agent in mitigating rises in ICP from RSRL; however, because of its potential to cause or aggravate hypotension, especially in patients with hypovolemia, it is not recommended for routine use in emergency intubation.
- **Is hyperventilation ($ETCO_2$ 30 to 35 mm Hg) recommended in the management of the TBI patient with suspected elevated ICP?** Hyperventilation can be defined as a $Paco_2 < 35$ or an $ETCO_2 < 30$ to 35; the correlation between the two measures is generally good in patients who are normotensive. It causes vasoconstriction and thus reduces ICP. Unfortunately, hyperventilation will also cause a reduction in CBF. Because CBF is reduced following TBI, hyperventilation poses a risk of exacerbating ischemia.

  Despite observations that hyperventilation reverses the clinical signs of herniation, there is no evidence that hyperventilation improves outcomes possibly offset by the deleterious impact on CBF.[3] In an observational study, 59 adult severe TBI patients who required RSI for intubation were matched to 177 historical nonintubated controls. The study used $ETCO_2$ monitoring and found an association between hypocapnia and mortality, and a statistically significant association between ventilatory rate and $ETCO_2$.[4,5] Both the lowest and final $ETCO_2$ readings were associated with increased mortality versus matched controls. Another retrospective study of 65 brain trauma patients with a Glasgow Coma Scale of 8 found that patients who were normocarbic on initial assessment had an in-hospital mortality of 15%.[6] In contrast, patients with hypercarbia had a mortality of 61%, and hypocarbia was associated with a mortality of 77%. These studies contribute to the growing body of evidence arguing against hyperventilation under any circumstance in TBI patients, and this is likely analogous to patients with medically caused elevated ICP.

- **Is ketamine safe for use as an induction agent in patients with suspected elevated ICP?** A systematic review of the effect of ketamine on intracranial and CPP found mild mixed effects on ICP but no adverse effect of CPP or neurologic outcomes across ten trials including 953 adults.[7] The authors concluded based on available evidence that ketamine is unlikely to elevate ICP in any meaningful way. There is a clear need for a well-controlled comparative study using a meaningful outcome measure to determine which, if any, of these interventions will decrease morbidity or mortality in patients with elevated ICP undergoing emergency RSI. Pending such a study, which will likely never be done because of logistical challenges, the approach outlined in Box 34-1 seems rational. Management of the patient at risk for elevated ICP should primarily ensure cerebral perfusion and oxygenation.
  - Hyperventilation ($ETCO_2 < 30$ to 35) should be carefully avoided in patients with medical intracranial catastrophe or TBI who do not demonstrate signs of increased ICP ("blown pupil" or extensor posturing) that is refractory to osmotic agents, CSF drainage, or both. Even in this circumstance, there is no solid evidence to support its use, and so operator judgment prevails.
  - There is no evidence that hyperventilation improves outcome in patients with elevated ICP, and there is some evidence that it causes harm. If hyperventilation is considered, it should only be used briefly, as a temporizing measure, in the management of patients exhibiting signs of herniation who have failed to respond to osmotic agents.
  - Intubated patients with TBI should have continuous $ETCO_2$ monitoring in order to avoid inadvertent hypocapnia ($ETCO_2 < 35$).

## REFERENCES


1. Levitt M, Dresden G. The efficacy of esmolol versus lidocaine to attenuate the hemodynamic response to intubation in isolated head trauma patients. *Acad Emerg Med*. 2001;8:19–24.
2. Lee KH, Kim H, Kim HT, et al. Comparison of desmedetomidine and remifentanil for attentuation of hemodynamic responses to laryngoscopy and tracheal intubation. *Korean J Anesthesiol*. 2012;63(2):124–129.
3. Brain Trauma Foundation. Guidelines for the management of severe traumatic brain injury, third edition. *J Neurotrauma*. 2007;24(suppl 1):S1–S108.
4. Davis DP, Dunford JV, Poste JC, et al. The impact of hypoxia and hyperventilation on outcome after paramedic rapid sequence intubation of severely head-injured patients. *J Trauma*. 2004;57:1–10.
5. Davis DP, Dunford JV, Ochs M, et al. The use of quantitative end-tidal capnometry to avoid inadvertent severe hyperventilation in patients with head injury after paramedic rapid sequence-intubation. *J Trauma*. 2004;56:808–814.
6. Dumont TM, Agostino JV, Rughani AI, et al. Inappropriate prehospital ventilation in severe-traumatic brain injury increases in-hospital mortality. *J Neurotrauma*. 2010;27:1233–1241.
7. Cohen L, Athaide V, Wickham ME, et al. The effect of ketamine on intracranial and cerebral perfusion pressure and health outcomes: a systematic review. *Ann Emerg Med*. 2015;65(1):43–51.

# Chapter 35

# Reactive Airways Disease

Bret P. Nelson and Andy S. Jagoda

## THE CLINICAL CHALLENGE

There are a number of confounders that make airway management of the patient with asthma or chronic obstructive pulmonary disease (COPD) challenging. These patients are often hypoxic, desaturate quickly, and can be hemodynamically unstable. Unlike many other clinical conditions, intubation itself does not resolve the primary problem, which is obstruction of the small, distal airways. The actual intubation may be the easiest part of the resuscitative sequence, because postintubation ventilation may be extremely difficult with persistent or worsening respiratory acidosis, barotrauma, or hypotension caused by high intrathoracic pressures with diminished venous return. Thus, the decision to intubate must be made carefully, and the appropriate technique must be chosen to facilitate the best possible outcome.

Severe asthma often presents one of the most difficult airway management cases encountered in the emergency department. Diaphoresis is a particularly ominous sign, and the diaphoretic asthmatic patient who cannot speak full sentences, appears anxious, or is sitting upright and leaning forward to augment the inspiratory effort must not be left unattended until stabilized.

Standard initial management of acute severe asthma exacerbation includes reversal of dynamic bronchospasm using continuous $\beta_2$-agonist nebulization therapy (Albuterol 10 to 15 mg per hour) and anticholinergic nebulization therapy (ipratropium bromide 0.5 mg every 20 minutes for three doses). Although the benefit is not immediate, oral or intravenous (IV) steroids are indicated for the treatment of the inflammatory component. If the patient is severely bronchospastic and cannot comply with a nebulized treatment, intramuscular epinephrine or terbutaline 0.25 to 0.5 mg is beneficial. For severe, refractory asthma, administration of IV magnesium sulfate 2 g in adults and 25 to 75 mg per kg (up to a maximum of 2 g) in children may be of benefit, although evidence supporting this is mixed. The addition of inhaled or IV anticholinergic agents (atropine or glycopyrrolate), titrated doses of IV ketamine, or inhalational helium/oxygen mixture is controversial but also may be considered in severe cases (**Fig. 35-1**).

In COPD, much of the obstruction is fixed, comorbidity (especially cardiovascular disease) plays a greater role, and the prognosis (even with short-term mechanical ventilation) is worse. In the patient with COPD, anticholinergic therapy may be as important as $\beta_2$-agonist therapy. Steroids are again important to attenuate underlying inflammation. As is the case for many asthma patients, it is progression of fatigue, not worsening bronchospasm, that leads to respiratory failure and arrest. The intubated COPD patient may have a prolonged, difficult course, and weaning from the ventilator is not assured. Therefore, unless the patient's condition forces early or immediate intubation,

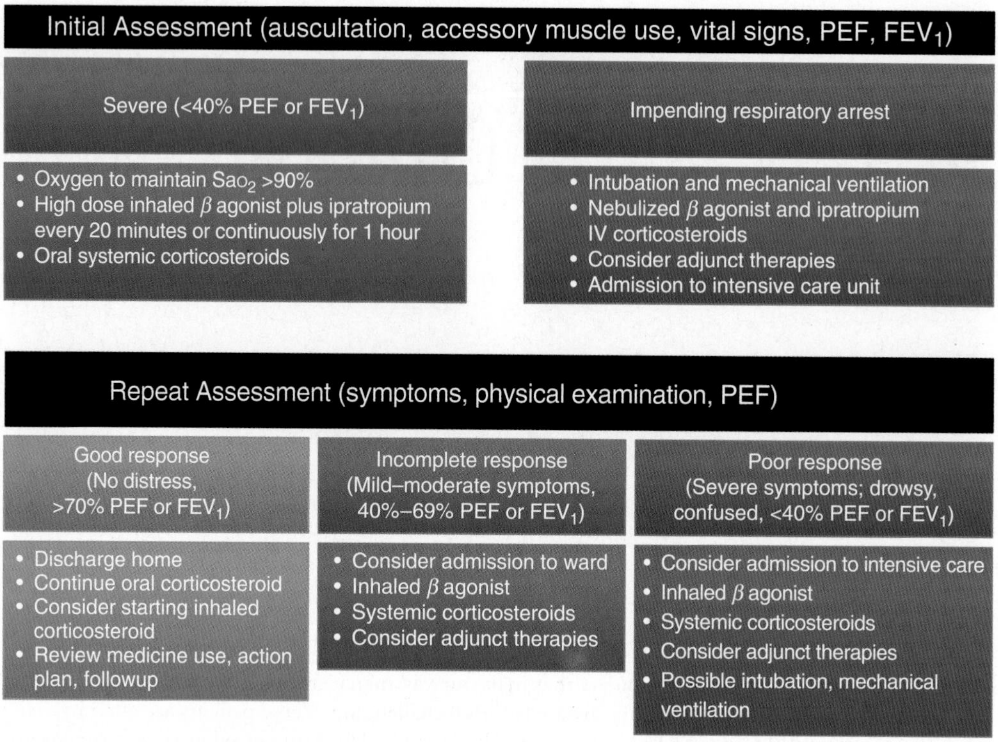
Initial Assessment (auscultation, accessory muscle use, vital signs, PEF, $FEV_1$)
Severe (<40% PEF or $FEV_1$)
Impending respiratory arrest
• Oxygen to maintain $Sao_2$ >90%
• High dose inhaled β agonist plus ipratropium every 20 minutes or continuously for 1 hour
• Oral systemic corticosteroids
• Intubation and mechanical ventilation
• Nebulized β agonist and ipratropium IV corticosteroids
• Consider adjunct therapies
• Admission to intensive care unit
Repeat Assessment (symptoms, physical examination, PEF)
Good response (No distress, >70% PEF or $FEV_1$)
Incomplete response (Mild–moderate symptoms, 40%–69% PEF or $FEV_1$)
Poor response (Severe symptoms; drowsy, confused, <40% PEF or $FEV_1$)
• Discharge home
• Continue oral corticosteroid
• Consider starting inhaled corticosteroid
• Review medicine use, action plan, followup
• Consider admission to ward
• Inhaled β agonist
• Systemic corticosteroids
• Consider adjunct therapies
• Consider admission to intensive care
• Inhaled β agonist
• Systemic corticosteroids
• Consider adjunct therapies
• Possible intubation, mechanical ventilation

● **FIGURE 35-1.** Approach to the patient with severe asthma exacerbation. (Adapted from National Heart, Lung, and Blood Institute, National Institutes of Health, National Asthma Education and Prevention Program. *Expert Panel Report 3 (EPR-3): Guidelines for the Diagnosis and Management of Asthma—Summary Report 2007.*

a trial of noninvasive ventilation is recommended. Noninvasive ventilation (bilevel positive airway pressure [BL-PAP] is of proven value in certain COPD patients and may help avoid intubation (see Chapter 6). As for the asthmatic patient, mechanical ventilation after intubation in COPD is notoriously difficult to manage. Ventilation pressures often are high, and breath stacking (automatic positive end-expiratory pressure [auto-PEEP]) is common, even with excellent ventilator management. Increased intrathoracic pressures induced by mechanical ventilation, combined with volume depletion from the patient's work of breathing before intubation, coexisting cardiovascular disease, and hemodynamic changes related to decreased sympathetic tone after intubation makes the peri-intubation period highly dynamic and unstable. Ventilator management is discussed in the following section.

## APPROACH TO THE AIRWAY

Despite this vast array of noninvasive medical treatment modalities, 1% to 3% of acute severe asthma exacerbations will require intubation. These patients are usually fatigued and have reduced functional residual capacity; so it may be challenging to preoxygenate them optimally, and rapid desaturation must be anticipated. Because most of these patients have been struggling to breathe against severe resistance, usually for hours, they have little if any residual physical reserve, and mechanical ventilation will be required. In fact, the need for mechanical ventilation is the indication for tracheal intubation; the airway itself is almost invariably patent and protected. This fact argues strongly for rapid sequence intubation (RSI), which often is the preferred method even if a difficult airway is identified on preintubation assessment (the "forced to act" scenario; see Chapters 2 and 3). If the patient has a difficult airway, the operator might plan intubation even earlier than for the nondifficult patient, in an attempt to have the best conditions and greatest amount of time possible for an awake technique.

### Technique

The single most important tenet in managing the status asthmaticus patient who requires intubation is to take total control of the airway as expeditiously as possible. Patients typically adopt an upright posture as their respiratory status worsens; this position should be maintained as much as possible during the preintubation period. Preoxygenation should be achieved to the greatest extent possible (see Chapters 5 and 20). Noninvasive ventilation may be considered as a means of increasing $F_{IO_2}$ during this phase while decreasing work of breathing. The RSI drugs chosen should be administered with the patient in their position of comfort, often sitting upright. As the patient loses consciousness, the patient should be placed supine, the head and neck should be positioned, and laryngoscopy and intubation should be performed, preferably with an 8.0- to 9.0-mm endotracheal tube (ETT) to decrease ventilator resistance and facilitate pulmonary toilette.

### Drug Dosing and Administration

Ketamine is the induction agent of choice in the asthmatic patient because it stimulates the release of catecholamines and also has a direct bronchial smooth muscle relaxing effect that may be important in this clinical setting. Ketamine 1.5 mg per kg IV is given immediately before the administration of 1.5 mg per kg of succinylcholine or 1.0 to 1.2 mg per kg of rocuronium. If ketamine is not available, etomidate may be used. Other induction agents (such as propofol or midazolam) are options but may predispose these patients to hypotension in the setting of hypovolemia and increased intrathoracic pressure changes. In COPD patients with concomitant cardiovascular disease, etomidate may be preferred to avoid the catecholamine stimulation of ketamine.

## POSTINTUBATION MANAGEMENT

After the patient is successfully intubated and proper tube position has been confirmed, sedation and analgesia are titrated according to a sedation scale (see Chapter 20). Neuromuscular blockade may be required during the first few hours of mechanical ventilation to prevent asynchronous respirations, promote total relaxation of fatigued respiratory muscles, decrease the production of carbon dioxide, and allow optimal ventilator settings. Often, however, these same goals are achieved using a proper balance of sedation and analgesia. Prolonged neuromuscular blockade is not required and may worsen the patient's overall course of management. Intravenous epinephrine drips can be initiated in the most severe cases. Meticulous ventilator management is critical in achieving the best patient outcome. Additional ketamine, as well as continuous in-line albuterol and other pharmacologic adjuncts, may also be given.

### Mechanical Ventilation

All asthmatic patients have obstructed small airways and dynamic alveolar hyperinflation with varying amounts of end-expiratory intra-alveolar gas and pressure (auto-PEEP or intrinsic PEEP). Elevations in auto-PEEP increase the risk for baro/volutrauma. Reversal of airflow obstruction and decompression of end-expiratory filled alveoli are the primary goals of early mechanical ventilation in the asthmatic patient. The former requires prompt administration of IV steroids and continuous in-line nebulization with $\beta_2$-agonists until reversal is objectively measured (decrease in peak and plateau airway pressures) or unacceptable side effects are produced. Safe, uncomplicated alveolar decompression requires prolonged expiratory time (inspiration/expiration [I/E] ratio of 1:4 to 1:5), which is achieved by using smaller tidal volumes than usual, with a high-inspiratory flow (IF) rate to shorten the inspiratory cycle time, permitting a longer expiratory phase. A general discussion of ventilation parameters can be found in Chapter 7.

The initial goal of ventilator therapy in the asthmatic patient is to improve arterial oxygen tension to adequate levels without inflicting barotrauma on the lungs or increasing auto-PEEP. Initial tidal volume should be reduced to 6 to 8 mL per kg to avoid barotrauma and air trapping. The speed at which a mechanical breath is delivered in liters per minute, typically 60 L per minute, is called the inspiratory flow rate (IFR). In asthma, the initial IFR should be increased to 80 to 100 L per minute with a decelerating flow pattern. Pressure control is preferred to volume control because of the lower risk of barotrauma. If volume control is used, the operator should select the flow waveform to use ramp (decelerating) instead of square (constant). The ventilation rate should be determined in conjunction with the tidal volume. An initial rate of 8 to 10 breaths per minute (bpm) with a high IFR promotes a prolonged expiratory phase that allows sufficient time for alveolar decompression. It is acceptable to permit the maintenance or gradual development of hypercapnia through reduced minute ventilation (the product of tidal volume and ventilatory rate) in the asthma or COPD patient, because this approach reduces peak inspiratory pressure (PIP) and thus minimizes the potential for barotrauma. High intrathoracic pressure may compromise cardiac output and produce hypotension; therefore, it is to be avoided.

The highest measured pressure at peak inspiration is the PIP. The patient's lungs, chest wall, ETT, ventilatory circuit, ventilator, and mucus plugs all contribute to the PIP. This reading has an inconsistent predictive value for baro/volutrauma but ideally should be kept under 50 cm $H_2O$. A sudden rise in PIP should be interpreted as indicating tube blockage, mucous plugging, or pneumothorax until proven otherwise. A sudden, dramatic fall in PIP may indicate extubation.

The measured intra-alveolar pressure during a 0.2- to 0.4-second end-inspiratory pause is referred to as the *plateau pressure* ($P_{plat}$). Values <30 cm $H_2O$ are the best and are not usually associated with baro/volutrauma. Measurement and trending of $P_{plat}$ is an excellent objective tool to confirm optimal ventilator settings and the patient's response, as well as the reversal of airflow obstruction. If initial ventilator settings disclose a $P_{plat}$ of more than 30 cm $H_2O$, consider lowering minute ventilation and increasing IF, both of which will prolong expiratory time and attenuate hyperinflation. If $P_{plat}$ is unavailable, PIP may be used as a surrogate.

Most status asthmaticus patients who require intubation are hypercapnic. The concept of controlled hypoventilation (permissive hypercapnia) promotes *gradual* development (over 3 to 4 hours) and maintenance of hypercapnia ($Pco_2$ up to 90 mm Hg) and acidemia (pH as low as 7.2). This treatment is done primarily to decrease the risk of ventilator-related lung injury and prevent hemodynamic compromise as a result of increasing intrathoracic pressure from auto-PEEP or intrinsic PEEP. Permissive hypercapnia is usually accomplished by reducing minute ventilation, increasing IF rate to 80 to 120 L per minute. Optimal sedation and analgesia are required, with some patients also requiring neuromuscular blockade, to tolerate these settings. Permissive hypercapnia may be instrumental in promoting prolonged expiratory times and reducing auto-PEEP.

## Summary for Initial Ventilator Settings

1. Determine the patient's ideal body weight.
2. Set a tidal volume of 6 to 8 mL per kg with $Fio_2$ of 1.0 (100% oxygen).
3. Set a respiratory rate of 8 to 10 bpm.
4. Set an I/E ratio of 1:4 to 1:5. Pressure control is preferred. If using pressure control, the I/E ratio is adjusted directly by the I/E ratio parameter or by adjusting the inspiratory time parameter. If using volume control, the I/E ratio can be adjusted by increasing the peak flow rate, and the ramp inspiratory waveform should be selected. Peak IF can be as high as 80 to 100 L per minute.
5. Measure and maintain the plateau pressure at <30 cm $H_2O$; try to keep PIP at <50 cm $H_2O$.
6. Focus on the oxygenation and pulmonary pressures initially. If necessary, allow maintenance or gradual development of hypercapnia to avoid high plateau pressures and increasing auto-PEEP.

7. Ensure continuous sedation and analgesia with propofol or a benzodiazepine along with a nonhistamine-releasing opioid, such as fentanyl.
8. Consider paralysis with a nondepolarizing muscle relaxant if it is difficult to achieve ventilation goals.
9. Continue in-line $\beta_2$-agonist therapy and additional pharmacologic adjunctive treatment based on the severity of the patient's illness and objective response to treatment.

## Complications of Mechanical Ventilation

Two of the more common complications seen in mechanically ventilated asthmatic patients are lung injury (baro/volutrauma) and hypotension. Lung injury is exemplified by tension pneumothorax. In those patients without tension pneumothorax, hypotension is usually related to either absolute volume depletion or relative hypovolemia caused by decreased venous return from increasing auto-PEEP and intrathoracic pressure. The inherent risks of developing either one of these complications are directly related to the degree of pulmonary hyperinflation. Of the two, hypotension occurs much more frequently than tension pneumothorax. Most asthmatic patients will have intravascular volume depletion because of the increased work of breathing, decreased oral intake following the onset of asthma exacerbation, and generalized increased metabolic state. It is appropriate for these reasons to infuse empirically 1 to 2 L of normal saline (NS) either before the initiation of RSI or early during mechanical ventilation.

Pneumothorax and volume depletion are two common and important conditions to consider. Pneumothorax can reliably be excluded with the aid of a physical examination, point-of-care ultrasound, or chest X-ray. Alternatively, a trial of hypoventilation (apnea test) may be used to distinguish tension pneumothorax from volume depletion. The patient is disconnected from the ventilator and allowed to be apneic up to 1 minute as long as adequate oxygenation is ensured by pulse oximetry. In volume depletion, the mean intrathoracic pressure will decline quickly, blood pressure should begin to increase, pulse pressure will widen, and pulse rate will decline within 30 to 60 seconds. With high amounts of auto-PEEP, reductions in tidal volume and increases in IF and I/E times will be required to reduce intrathoracic pressures. If auto-PEEP is not an issue, then an empiric volume infusion of 500 mL NS should be instituted and may be repeated based on the patient's response to the additional volume. With tension pneumothorax, cardiopulmonary stability will not correct during the apnea time. If physical examination fails to identify the culprit lung, immediate insertion of bilateral chest tubes is indicated. Reassessment of ventilatory pressure settings will be required thereafter. The initial ventilator settings and potential ventilator complications of the asthma patient are shared by the COPD patient.

# EVIDENCE

- **Does lidocaine improve clinical outcomes when patients with status asthmaticus are intubated?** Lidocaine was previously recommended to attenuate the bronchospastic response to intubation and ETT placement in patients with reactive airway disease. However, there are no studies that have demonstrated that premedicating with IV lidocaine during RSI changes outcomes in severe asthma or improves pulmonary mechanics after, particularly if the patient has been treated with $\beta$-agonsists. Administering lidocaine may result in adverse cardiovascular effects and complicates RSI by adding an additional step, increasing the chance of a dosing error or allergic reaction. We no longer recommend the routine use of lidocaine during emergency airway management.
- **Do inhaled anticholinergics improve outcomes in acute reactive airways disease when compared with inhaled $\beta$-agonists alone?** The bronchodilatory effects of anticholinergic agents are well known, but there has been controversy over whether these agents act synergistically with $\beta$-agonists in the setting of acute bronchospasm. A meta-analysis of 32 randomized controlled trials, involving more than 3,500 patients, concluded that there is a modest benefit when it

is used in conjunction with *β*-agonists.[1] The use of inhaled anticholinergics was associated with reduced hospital admissions in adults and children, as well as improved spirometric parameters within 2 hours of treatment. For severe asthma exacerbations, the number needed to treat to prevent one admission was 7 for adults and 14 for children. The meta-analysis recommended the use of inhaled ipratropium bromide, because the benefit appears to outweigh any risks. In addition, pooled data suggest that multiple doses convey more benefit than single-dose regimens. A recent prospective, double-blind, randomized controlled trial examined the benefit of adding continuous nebulized ipratropium bromide to a continuous albuterol nebulization.[2] In this study, the addition of ipratropium bromide was not found to improve peak expiratory flow rate (PEFR) or admission rates compared with albuterol alone in a total of 62 enrolled patients. In COPD, it is well known that maintenance anticholinergic agents are helpful; however, in acute exacerbations, it remains unclear. A Cochrane Database review summarized four studies comparing inhaled albuterol with ipratropium bromide in the setting of acute COPD exacerbation.[3] Pooled data from these studies (129 total patients) demonstrated no difference in $FEV_1$ at 1 hour or 24 hours between the albuterol and ipratropium bromide groups. The addition of ipratropium bromide to albuterol did not yield any benefit over albuterol alone. Despite this relative paucity of evidence, the American Thoracic Society and European Respiratory Society the Global Initiative for Chronic Obstructive Lung Disease advocate the use of inhaled ipratropium in acute COPD exacerbations.[4] Thus, based on available evidence, anticholinergic agents should be used in severe acute asthmatic patients as standard therapy and should be considered in the treatment of acute COPD exacerbations, especially when little improvement is seen with *β*-agonists alone.

- **Does the use of IV magnesium improve outcomes in patients with acute asthma?** Magnesium plays a role in smooth muscle relaxation, and recent research has focused on the role of this medication in alleviating bronchospasm. A meta-analysis of magnesium sulfate use in 1,669 patients demonstrated efficacy of IV magnesium (used in 15 studies) but not nebulized delivery (used in nine studies).[5] In both children, IV magnesium is associated with reduced hospital admissions and improved pulmonary function in both children and adults. There is no good evidence that magnesium decreases the need for intubation. Based on these data, IV magnesium therapy should be considered as adjunctive therapy for severe asthma or in patients unresponsive to initial therapy.
- **Are there noninvasive ventilatory strategies that may improve attempts at preoxygenation in acute asthma?** Noninvasive positive-pressure ventilation (NIPPV) has been used successfully to decrease the work of breathing and to preoxygenate patients; however, agitation and delirium can confound attempts to preoxygenate in severe cases. A recent multicenter prospective observational study described the technique of *delayed sequence intubation* (DSI), which could be employed in patients whose delirium or agitation prevents optimal preoxygenation via facemask or NIPPV.[6] In DSI, a dissociative dose of ketamine is administered to allow preoxygenation. In this prospective study of 62 patients, mean oxygen saturation increased after DSI (90% to 99%), and no adverse effects were noted even in high-risk patients. Although data from this study are promising, lack of randomization, direct comparison to RSI, and small sample size preclude making a recommendation for its routine use.
- **Is there a role for heliox in the management of acute asthma exacerbations?** In obstructive lung disease with bronchospasm, increased turbulent flow through proximal airways decreases airflow and may contribute to increased work of breathing. Heliox, with a lower density than air–oxygen mixtures, has been believed to decrease turbulent flow and could increase carriage of nebulized medications to distal airways. A Cochrane review of 10 trials (including 544 asthma patients) concluded that heliox may be beneficial in patients unresponsive to initial therapy.[7] Another systematic review examined controlled studies of acute asthma and COPD exacerbations.[8] For asthma, heliox-driven nebulizers improved PEFR in pooled data from two studies. No differences in admission rates were found. Heliox was found in a single study to improve PEFR when used as a breathing gas in intubated asthmatics. In another study of 132 nonintubated asthmatics receiving heliox-driven nebulization or air-driven nebulization,

there was an increased $FEV_1$ in the heliox-driven group, but only in patients with severe disease (baseline $FEV_1 \leq 50\%$).[9] At this time, there is insufficient evidence of outcome benefit to justify the cost and complexity of routine heliox administration.

- **Is IV ketamine of benefit in severe asthma?** Theoretically, ketamine is a logical choice in managing the airway of the severe asthmatic because it increases circulating catecholamines, is a direct smooth muscle dilator, inhibits vagal outflow, and does not cause histamine release. However, there are no good controlled studies demonstrating the benefit of IV ketamine in the management of the nonintubated asthmatic patients. Case reports of marked improvement in pulmonary function with ketamine have driven its popularity, but no randomized studies have been performed to demonstrate ketamine's superiority over other agents. Recently, a double-blind, placebo-controlled study randomized 33 pediatric asthma patients to ketamine infusion (0.2 mg per kg bolus, followed by 0.5 mg per hour for 2 hours) and 35 patients to placebo.[10] Each group also received albuterol, ipratropium bromide, and glucocorticoids. No significant difference in pulmonary index scores (consisting of respiratory rate, wheeze, I/E ratio, accessory muscle use, and oxygen saturation) was found between the two groups. No difference in hospitalization rate was noted. At the present time, based on its mechanism of action and safety profile, ketamine appears to be the best agent available for RSI in the asthmatic. In the absence of ketamine, other agents may be used. There is insufficient evidence to support the use of IV ketamine as adjunctive therapy in nonintubated or ventilated patients.

## REFERENCES


1. Rodrigo GJ, Castro-Rodriguez JA. Anticholinergics in the treatment of children and adults with acute asthma: a systematic review with meta-analysis. *Thorax*. 2005;60:740–746.
2. Salo D, Tuel M, Lavery R, et al. A randomized, clinical trial comparing the efficacy of continuous nebulized albuterol (15 mg) versus continuous nebulized albuterol (15 mg) plus ipratropium bromide (2 mg) for the treatment of asthma. *J Emerg Med*. 2006;31(4):371–376.
3. McCrory DC, Brown CD. Anticholinergic bronchodilators versus $beta_2$-sympathomimetic agents for acute exacerbations of chronic obstructive pulmonary disease. *Cochrane Database Syst Rev*. 2003;(1):CD003900.
4. Global Initiative for Chronic Obstructive Lung Disease. Global strategy for diagnosis, management and prevention of COPD.
5. Mohammed S, Goodacre S. Intravenous and nebulised magnesium sulphate for acute asthma: systematic review and meta-analysis. *Emerg Med J*. 2007;24:823–830.
6. Weingart SD, Trueger NS, Wong N, et al. Delayed sequence intubation: a prospective observational study. *Ann Emerg Med*. 2015;65(4):349.
7. Rodrigo G, Pollack C, Rodrigo C, et al. Heliox for nonintubated acute asthma patients. *Cochrane Database Syst Rev*. 2006;(4):CD002884.
8. Colebourn CL, Barber V, Young JD. Use of helium-oxygen mixture in adult patients presenting with exacerbations of asthma and chronic obstructive pulmonary disease: a systematic review. *Anaesthesia*. 2007;62:34–42.
9. El-Khatib MF, Jamaleddine G, Kanj N, et al. Effect of heliox- and air-driven nebulized bronchodilator therapy on lung function in patients with asthma. *Lung*. 2014;192(3):377–383.
10. Allen JY, Macias CG. The efficacy of ketamine in pediatric emergency department patients who present with acute severe asthma. *Ann Emerg Med*. 2005;46(1):43–50.

# Chapter 36

# Distorted Airways and Acute Upper Airway Obstruction

Ali S. Raja and Erik G. Laurin

## THE CLINICAL CHALLENGE

The *upper airway* refers to that portion of the airway anatomy that extends from the lips and nares down to the first tracheal ring. The first portion of the upper airway is redundant: a nasal pathway and an oral pathway. However, at the level of the oropharynx, the two pathways merge, and this redundancy is lost. The most common life-threatening causes of acute upper airway distortion and obstruction occur in the region of this common channel, and they are typically laryngeal. In addition, disorders of the base of the tongue and the pharynx can cause obstruction (**Box 36-1**). This chapter deals with problems that distort or obstruct the upper airway. Foreign bodies in the upper airway are addressed in Chapters 27 and 41.

**BOX 36-1**

**Causes of upper airway obstruction.**

A. *Infectious*
   a. Viral and bacterial laryngotracheobronchitis (e.g., croup)
   b. Parapharyngeal and retropharyngeal abscesses
   c. Lingual tonsillitis (a lingual tonsil is a rare but real congenital anomaly and a well-recognized cause of failed intubation)
   d. Infections, hematomas, or abscesses of the tongue or floor of the mouth (e.g., Ludwig angina)
   e. Epiglottitis (also known as supraglottitis)

B. *Neoplastic*
   a. Laryngeal carcinomas
   b. Hypopharyngeal and lingual (tongue) carcinomas

(*continued*)

BOX 36-1

**Causes of upper airway obstruction. (continued)**

C. *Physical and chemical agents*
  a. Foreign bodies
  b. Thermal injuries (heat and cold)
  c. Caustic injuries (acids and alkalis)
  d. Inhaled toxins
D. *Allergic/idiopathic:* including ACEI-induced angioedema
E. *Traumatic:* blunt and penetrating neck and upper airway trauma

## APPROACH TO THE AIRWAY

The signs of upper airway distortion and obstruction may be occult or subtle. Life-threatening deterioration may occur suddenly and unexpectedly. Seemingly innocuous interventions, such as small doses of sedative hypnotic agents to alleviate anxiety or the use of topical local anesthetic agents, may precipitate sudden and total airway obstruction. Rescue devices may not be successful and may even be contraindicated in some circumstances. The goal in patients with upper airway obstruction or distorted upper airway anatomy is to manage the airway in a rapid yet controlled fashion before complete airway obstruction occurs.

### When Should an Intervention Be Performed?

Chapter 1 deals with the important question of when to intubate. If airway obstruction is severe, progressive, or imminent, then immediate action (often "*forced-to-act*" rapid sequence intubation [RSI] or cricothyrotomy) is required without further consideration of transferring the patient to another venue (e.g., the operating room or another hospital). It is critical to recognize patients who require an inevitable surgical airway and to perform the procedure without delay, as valuable time is often used up trying other methods to obtain airway control. Failing an indication for an *immediate* intervention, the question becomes more nuanced: What is the expected clinical course?

Penetrating wounds to the neck and airway are notoriously unpredictable (see Chapter 33). Some experts advocate for securing the airway regardless of warning signs, whereas others advocate expectant observation. There are substantial problems with the latter strategy. The first is that the patient often remains relatively asymptomatic until they suddenly and unexpectedly develop total obstruction, resulting in an airway (and patient) that cannot be rescued. The second is that unless a flexible endoscope is used, the observer is only able to see the anterior portion of the airway and not the posterior and inferior parts where the obstruction will likely occur. In other words, when not using a flexible endoscope, one sees only "the tip of the iceberg."

The time course of the airway threat is also important. All other things being equal, a patient who presents with airway swelling, such as angioedema, which has developed over 8 to 12 hours, is at substantially less risk for sudden obstruction than a similar patient where the same degree of swelling has developed over 30 minutes. Overall, for any condition in which the obstruction may be rapidly progressive, silent, and unobservable externally (e.g., angioedema, vascular injuries in the neck, and epiglottitis), acting earlier rather than later to secure the airway is the most prudent course.

There are four cardinal signs of acute upper airway obstruction:

- "Hot potato" voice: The muffled voice one often hears in patients with mononucleosis and very large tonsils

- Difficulty in swallowing secretions, either because of pain or obstruction: The patient is typically sitting up, leaning forward, and spitting or drooling secretions
- Stridor
- Dyspnea

The first two signs do not necessarily suggest that total upper airway obstruction is imminent; however, stridor and dyspnea do. The patient presenting with stridor has already lost at least 50% of the airway caliber and requires immediate intervention. In the case of children younger than 8 to 10 years with croup, medical therapy may suffice. In older children and adults, the presence of stridor may necessitate a surgical airway or, at least, intubation using a double setup. This technique uses an awake attempt from above, ideally using a flexible endoscope, with the capability (prepared in advance) to rapidly move to a surgical airway if needed. Properly performed bag-mask ventilation (BMV) will often be successful in cases with soft tissue obstructions (including laryngospasm) but generally will not overcome a fixed obstruction (such as extrinsic compression of the airway by a hematoma) and, in any case, should not be considered more than just a temporizing maneuver.

## What Options Exist If the Airway Deteriorates or Obstruction Occurs?

The key considerations here are as follows:

- *Will rescue BMV be possible?* Will a mask seal be possible to achieve, or is the lower face disrupted? Has a penetrating neck wound entered the airway, rendering it incompetent to high airway pressures? As discussed in Chapter 9, the bag and mask devices most commonly used in resuscitation settings are capable of generating 50 to 100 cm of water pressure in the upper airway, provided that they do not have positive-pressure relief valves and that an adequate mask seal can be obtained. Pediatric and neonatal devices often incorporate positive-pressure relief valves that easily can be deactivated (if needed). This degree of positive pressure often is sufficient to overcome the moderate degree of upper airway obstruction caused by redundant tissue (e.g., in the obese), edematous tissue (e.g., in angioedema, croup, and epiglottitis), or laryngospasm. However, lesions that are hard and fixed, such as hematomas, abscesses, cancers, and foreign bodies, produce an obstruction that cannot be reliably overcome with BMV, even with high upper airway pressures.
- *Where is the airway problem?* If the lesion is at the level of the face or oro/nasopharynx, and orotracheal intubation is judged to be impossible (for whatever reason), an extraglottic rescue device (such as a laryngeal mask airway or King LT) may be considered if there is oral access. If the lesion is at or immediately above the level of the glottis, an extraglottic device (EGD) may not be effective, and intubation (if the obstruction can be bypassed) or cricothyrotomy (if it cannot) are required. If the lesion is below the vocal cords, cricothyrotomy will not bypass the obstruction, and an entirely different strategy is used (see Chapters 27 and 41).

## What Are the Advantages and Risks of an Awake Technique?

In most instances, unless the patient is in crisis or deteriorating rapidly, awake examination using a flexible endoscope is the best approach. The endoscopic examination allows both assessment of the airway and, if indicated, intubation (see Chapters 16 and 23). Alternatively, awake laryngoscopy can be performed using a video or conventional laryngoscope. If adequate glottic visualization is achieved by direct or video laryngoscopy, intubation is performed. If visualization is suboptimal, but the epiglottis can be seen and is in the midline, orotracheal intubation using RSI is often feasible, especially with a bougie, unless the working diagnosis is a primary laryngeal disorder. On rare occasions, however, the airway may be more difficult to visualize after induction and paralysis or may have deteriorated abruptly between the awake examination and administration of RSI drugs. For these reasons, RSI drugs should be drawn up before the awake laryngoscopy is performed, with intubation often best performed at the time of the initial examination rather than after the delay needed to withdraw the laryngoscope to subsequently perform RSI. If the lesion is suspected to be at the laryngeal level, complete visualization of the larynx and, particularly the glottis, is important (e.g., flexible endoscopic visualization).

### Is RSI Reasonable?

If one is confident that orotracheal intubation is possible and highly confident that the patient can be successfully ventilated using BMV or EGD, then it is reasonable to proceed with RSI (e.g., early in the course of a penetrating neck injury). A double setup with readiness for an immediate surgical airway is advisable. The decision to proceed with RSI versus an awake examination or primary cricothyrotomy is a matter of clinical judgment. A patient with early upper airway injury (e.g., inhalation of products of combustion) is often easily intubated via the oral route (absent preexisting difficult airway markers), provided this is done before bleeding from the injury and airway swelling are allowed to progress. The key determinant is the clinician's confidence that intubation likely will succeed and, if not, that oxygenation through BMV or EGD (or by cricothyrotomy) will be timely and successful.

The challenges of patients presenting with upper airway obstruction underscore the importance of possessing alternative airway devices, such as a flexible endoscope and a video laryngoscope, in addition to a conventional laryngoscope and bougie. Patients with upper airway obstructions in whom direct laryngoscopy likely would be impossible, such as severe angioedema, may be successfully intubated with a narrow profile video laryngoscope (e.g., a GlideScope) and are often reasonably straightforward candidates for flexible endoscopic intubation. The latter device essentially transforms an impossible intubation into a challenging but a very achievable one.

## TIPS AND PEARLS

- Be reluctant to transfer patients with suspected acute upper airway obstruction and unsecured airways, even short distances. With rare exception, it is almost always prudent to secure the airway of a patient with significant acute penetrating neck injury or blunt laryngeal trauma (examples of "dynamic" upper airway obstruction) before transport.
- Angioedema of the upper airway is a potentially dangerous and unpredictable condition, particularly when it has occurred over a short period of time. External examination of the lips, tongue, and pharynx may reveal little of what is going on at the level of the airway. Intervention earlier rather than later is the most prudent course of action. Usually, flexible endoscopy will provide definitive information and serve as a conduit for intubation, if indicated.
- The patient with acute upper airway obstruction, a disrupted airway, or a distorted airway who *can* protect and maintain the airway and *can* maintain oxygenation and ventilation should always be considered a *difficult airway*, and the difficult airway algorithm should be used.
- The patient with upper airway obstruction, a disrupted airway, or a distorted airway who *cannot* maintain oxygenation or ventilation should be considered a *failed airway*, and the failed airway algorithm should be used.
- Blind airway management techniques (e.g., blind nasotracheal intubation) in patients with upper airway obstruction or distorted anatomy are contraindicated and should not be attempted.
- BMV alone cannot be relied on to rescue an airway, particularly if the obstruction is caused by a fixed lesion.
- RSI is usually contraindicated unless the operator is forced to attempt a "one-best-shot" intubation attempt invoking the *forced-to-act* principle (see Chapter 3), the awake look is reassuring, or the operator judges that RSI is likely to be successful and a backup plan (double setup) is in place.
- Be prepared for a cricothyrotomy before performing an awake laryngoscopy, recognizing that manipulation of an irritated upper airway, administration of a sedative agent, or application of a topical anesthetic may precipitate total obstruction.

## EVIDENCE

- **What evidence guides emergency management of patients with acute upper airway obstruction?** The evidence regarding the emergency management of the patient with an airway that is potentially or actually disrupted, distorted, or obstructed is essentially anecdotal. Most of the information dealing with the topic comes either from the surgical or anesthesia literature: primarily small series or case reports. A recent report from the National Emergency Airway Registry revealed that approximately 1% of all adult emergency airway encounters are managed with a flexible endoscope, most often employed in the setting of airway obstruction.[1] There are no controlled studies comparing intervention with expectant observation.
- **How commonly does angiotensin-converting enzyme inhibitor (ACEI)–induced angioedema require intubation?** The clinical course of ACEI-induced angioedema is extremely unpredictable. Life-threatening presentations requiring airway interventions are reported in up to 20% of these patients, and 0% to 22.2% will require intubation.[2,3] One study found that intubation with video or fiberoptic laryngoscopy were equally successful (although videolaryngoscopy was faster).[4] The clinical course of angioedema, especially ACEI-induced, is unpredictable. Patients not requiring intubation should be observed in the emergency department (ED), an ED Observation Unit, or an inpatient setting. The optimal duration of observation is not known, and recommendations vary. Patients presenting <12 hours after onset of angioedema should probably be observed for at least 6 hours (longer for more severe cases). Patients presenting more than 12 hours after onset should be observed until there is confidence that no further progression is occurring.
- **Is it true that application of topical anesthetic agents to a distorted airway can trigger total airway obstruction?** There are no studies related to this topic, but most experienced airway managers have seen it, and there is at least one published case report.[5] Although the mechanism by which this occurs is a matter of speculation, it is a real phenomenon, and caution should be exercised in the setting of preexisting airway obstruction when topical anesthesia and instrumentation of the airway is contemplated. Rescue strategies should be planned in advance, and the examination should occur in a setting where quick rescue can be executed if complete obstruction occurs.

## REFERENCES


1. Brown CA 3rd, Bair AE, Pallin DJ, et al. Techniques, success, and adverse events of emergency department adult intubations. *Ann Emerg Med*. 2015;65(4):363–370.
2. Kostis JB, Kim HJ, Rusnak J, et al. Incidence and characteristics of angioedema associated with enalapril. *Arch Intern Med*. 2005;165(14):1637–1642.
3. Moellman JJ, Bernstein JA, Lindsell C, et al. A consensus parameter for the evaluation and management of angioedema in the emergency department. *Acad Emerg Med*. 2014;21(4):469–484.
4. Wood A, Choromanski D, Orlewicz M. Intubation of patients with angioedema: a retrospective study of different methods over three year period. *Int J Crit Illn Inj Sci*. 2013;3(2):108–112.
5. Ho AMH, Chung DC, To EWH, et al. Total airway obstruction during local anesthesia in a non-sedated patient with a compromised airway. *Can J Anaesth*. 2004;51(8):838–841.

Chapter 37

# The Pregnant Patient

Richard D. Zane and Cheryl Lynn Horton

## THE CLINICAL CHALLENGE

The physiologic and anatomic changes associated with pregnancy may pose challenges to all facets of airway management including oxygenation, ventilation, and securing the airway. Along with many physiologic changes, late-term pregnancy also presents unique difficulties related to the airway. In fact, complications related to airway management in the parturient patient are the most significant cause of anesthetic-related maternal mortality. Pregnancy changes the patient's anatomy and physiology in a variety of distinct ways:

- *Oxygen reserve and depletion:* There is an approximately 20% reduction in expiratory reserve volume, residual volume, and functional residual capacity (FRC) and an increased maternal basal metabolic rate and oxygen demand by the fetal unit. These changes lead to more rapid desaturation during apnea (approximately 3 minutes compared to 6-8 minutes for the normal nonpregnant adult) and are further exacerbated in the obese pregnant patient.
- *Physiologic hyperventilation:* Progesterone increases the ventilatory drive and leads to hyperventilation. Maternal minute ventilation increases early in pregnancy largely because of an increase in tidal volume. This results in alteration of "normal" blood gas parameters, which must be considered when managing mechanical ventilation. Maternal $Paco_2$ falls to approximately 32 mm Hg, which is associated with a compensatory decrease in bicarbonate from 26 to 22 mEq per L in order to maintain a normal maternal pH. Mechanical ventilation must provide some degree of hyperventilation in order to maintain maternal pH. A reasonable approach is to increase the minute ventilation by approximately 20% for the pregnant woman in the first trimester, increasing to 40% by term.
- *Cardiopulmonary compromise in late pregnancy:* In the late stages of pregnancy when the patient is placed supine, the effects of the gravid uterus on the diaphragm and, occasionally, increased breast size on the chest wall further decrease the FRC. In addition to decreasing FRC, supine positioning in the late second and third trimester of pregnancy can result in aortocaval compression by the gravid uterus. This significantly reduces blood return to the heart, impairing maternal and fetal perfusion. This can be mitigated to a certain degree by placing the patient in the left lateral decubitus position.
- *Effects on laryngoscopy and bag-mask ventilation (BMV):* Pregnancy also can affect laryngoscopy and BMV. Weight gain, greater resistance to chest expansion by abdominal contents, and increased breast size may make BMV difficult in a manner analogous to that seen with

an obese patient. Enlarged breast size can also make insertion of a laryngoscope more difficult. The effects of estrogen and increased blood volume contribute to mucosal edema of the nasal passages and pharynx, causing airway tissues to become redundant, friable, and more prone to bleeding, especially with airway manipulation. This mucosal edema can also lead to dynamic distortion of the airway structures and difficulty both in identifying structures and in passing the endotracheal tube through the upper airway to the glottis. This upper airway distortion can be worsened by preeclampsia, active labor with pushing, and the infusion of large volumes of crystalloid fluids. Vascular engorgement also leads to a decrease in luminal size in the trachea, requiring a smaller than expected endotracheal tube (6.5 to 7 on average). The engorged upper airway tissues also can make BMV more difficult.

- *Increased propensity for aspiration:* As pregnancy progresses, gastric acid secretion increases, causing a decrease in maternal gastric pH as well as an increase in gastrin levels, a reduction in gastric activity, and an increase in gastric emptying time that can result in an increase in resting gastric volume. Gastroesophageal sphincter tone is also reduced in pregnancy. Enlargement of the uterus increases the pressure exerted on the stomach, which combined with a reduction in gastroesophageal sphincter tone, increases the risk of reflux. A "full stomach" should always be a concern in these patients. Administration of neuromuscular blockade will exacerbate this further by causing a loss of supporting abdominal muscle tone. These normal changes in gastrointestinal physiology start early in the second trimester, but become most problematic in the mid- to late second and third trimesters.
- *Effects on neuromuscular blocking agents:* Maternal plasma cholinesterase activity is reduced by 25%; however, this does not result in any significant effects on elimination, half-life, or duration of effect of succinylcholine. Pregnancy, however, does result in enhanced sensitivity to the aminosteroid muscle relaxants such as vecuronium and rocuronium, which may prolong their effect.

## APPROACH TO THE AIRWAY

In early pregnancy, fluid and FRC changes predominate, but the airway itself is unchanged. As pregnancy progresses, difficulty in both intubation and BMV should be anticipated. Nevertheless, the approach to airway management in the pregnant patient is no different from that of any other emergent intubation, except for consideration of the unique features of pregnancy described in The Clinical Challenge section, which may create airway difficulty beyond the sixth month of pregnancy.

Key issues to consider for airway management in these patients are as follows:

1. Anatomically, think of the third trimester pregnant patient as analogous to an obese patient, and use the difficult airway algorithm. If careful assessment using the LEMON, ROMAN, RODS, and SMART mnemonics (see Chapter 2) indicates that rapid sequence intubation (RSI) is reasonable, have backup devices readily at hand, and anticipate more rapid oxyhemoglobin desaturation than for the nonpregnant patient.
2. If flexible endoscopic intubation is the chosen method, avoid the nasal route in favor of the oral. The mucosa may be engorged, edematous, and friable, and nasotracheal intubation is more likely to lead to mucosal damage and bleeding.
3. Preoxygenate fully, using at least eight vital capacity breaths or 3 minutes of breathing 100% oxygen; as FRC is reduced, oxygen consumption is increased, and apnea leads to desaturation more rapidly. This is best provided with the patient in an upright position while passively breathing through either a bag and mask apparatus or a non-rebreather (NRB) facemask with oxygen delivered at the "flush flow rate" (see Chapter 5) of 40 to 70 L per minute. Passive oxygenation during the apneic phase, using nasal cannula at 5 to 15 L per minute flow, should be used routinely if possible. Although neither have been studied in term pregnant women, they significantly delay desaturation in obese patients who have similar physiologic aberrations.

4. All opioids and induction agents may reduce maternal blood flow to the placenta and, therefore, blood flow to the fetus. These agents also cross the placental barrier. Because muscle relaxants are quaternary ammonium salts and are fully ionized, they do not readily cross the placenta. Antihypertensive agents such as metoprolol, labetalol, and esmolol cross the placenta and carry a risk of inducing fetal bradycardia. In the context of emergent airway management, however, maternal well-being supersedes the potential for fetal exposure. When these agents are administered and delivery of the fetus is imminent, the caregiver charged with the management of the neonate immediately after delivery should be fully briefed regarding the agents administered to the mother.
5. Although there is no hard evidence in support the use of the "Sellick maneuver," it is widely used and recommended in pregnant patients, however, because of the gastrointestinal changes described previously. We consider the maneuver optional, but if it is to be used, the person tasked with applying it should be trained and skilled in the application of cricoid pressure.
6. Although rescue airway devices, such as the laryngeal mask airway (LMA), intubating LMA, and the King airway, may be used in the event of a failed intubation similar to the nonpregnant patient, the enhanced risk of aspiration in the nonfasted pregnant patient creates additional urgency for definitive airway control. The successful placement of one of these extraglottic rescue devices may achieve adequate gas exchange, giving the provider additional time to secure a definitive airway and avoid a surgical airway. Nonetheless, as the term pregnant patient may rapidly desaturate, cricothyrotomy should not be delayed when intubation fails and adequate oxygenation cannot be maintained using a bag and mask or an extraglottic device (EGD).

## Recommended Intubation Sequence

### *Preparation*

A detailed difficult airway examination, including LEMON, ROMAN, RODS, and SMART, should always be performed before making a decision regarding the appropriateness of RSI. Even if other markers of difficult laryngoscopy are not present, obesity, enlarged breasts, and physiologic airway edema can nevertheless complicate the ability to successfully secure the airway of the pregnant patient. By default, even in the absence of typical predictors of a potentially difficult airway, the difficult airway algorithm should be used for patients in late-term pregnancy. As with the nonpregnant patient, if the intubator does not have confidence that oxygenation (by BMV or EGD) and intubation will be successful, an awake, sedated technique with topical anesthesia is used, such as flexible endoscopy, video laryngoscopy, or awake direct laryngoscopy.

Assemble your airway equipment both for immediate management and for potential rescue of a failed airway. Be sure to include a selection of smaller-sized endotracheal tubes with stylets loaded; a bougie, short-handle laryngoscope if direct laryngoscopy will be attempted; and, if available, a rescue device with which you are familiar and equipment for a surgical airway.

### *Preoxygenation*

Preoxygenate fully using eight vital capacity breaths or 3 minutes with 100% oxygen (see earlier). Use left lateral decubitus positioning when in the supine position to avoid aortocaval compression; tilt the abdomen slightly to the left with a wedge or pillow under the right hip to displace the gravid uterus from the inferior vena cava.

### *Preintubation Optimization*

Similar to the nonpregnant patient, ensure optimal hemodynamics with fluid resuscitation and blood, if indicated. Hypotensive patients in late pregnancy should be placed in the left lateral decubitus position. Severe preeclampsia or eclampsia should be treated primarily with magnesium sulfate; however, fentanyl can also be used to mitigate hypertensive responses.

### Paralysis with Sedation

Agent selection is as for the nonpregnant patient. Unless contraindicated, succinylcholine is recommended for paralysis in a dose of 1.5 mg per kg. If succinylcholine is contraindicated, a nondepolarizing agent, ideally rocuronium 1 mg per kg, should be administered, despite the risk of prolonged effect after administration. The choice of induction agent is dictated by maternal hemodynamic condition as in the nonpregnant patient. There is no evidence to support the use of one particular induction agent in pregnancy.

### Positioning

Intubation success can be significantly enhanced with proper positioning before administration of induction agents. For the obese parturient patient or one with excessive breast tissue, placing a roll, a pillow vertically between the shoulder blades moves the glottic structures forward and assists in displacing the breasts away from the neck. Positioning of the occiput is equally important because too much extension of the neck can move the glottic structures anteriorly and impede visualization. Placing a pad or folded sheet under the patient's head to bring it into a neutral position may eliminate this. A head up position (20° to 30°) can help with ventilation both in the spontaneously breathing patient and when positive-pressure ventilation is required. Cricoid pressure intuitively may be more important in the pregnant patient, but evidence supporting its routine use is scant. If cricoid pressure is used and glottic visualization is difficult, release the glottic pressure to improve glottic view and allow the intubator to perform external laryngeal manipulation if desired.

### Placement with Proof

As with the nonpregnant patient, tube placement must be confirmed by detection of end-tidal carbon dioxide in addition to physical examination no matter how certain the operator is that the trachea has been successfully intubated.

## Management of the Failed Intubation

As with any patient for whom emergent intubation is required, unanticipated difficulty can be encountered despite a careful difficult airway assessment. In the pregnant patient, the approach needs to be modified slightly to accommodate the anticipated physiologic changes imposed by pregnancy. Primarily, this is driven by the rapidity with which the mother desaturates and the commonly encountered airway edema and friability. We recommend reducing the number of attempts at laryngoscopy before moving to the failed airway algorithm from three to two in the pregnant patient, unless success on the third attempt is believed to be highly likely. Even though maintaining oxygenation and ventilation is important for all patients, it is paramount in the pregnant patient, who has reduced physiologic reserve. In this circumstance, one should always choose a rescue device with which he or she is most facile and has the most experience. Properly performed, two-handed, two-person BMV may buy time to allow an alternative to cricothyrotomy. Nevertheless, one needs to be prepared to go to surgical airway if the rescue device is not able to provide adequate ventilation. Keep in mind that upper airway edema is a common cause of inability to both visualize the glottic structures and ventilate with BMV or supraglottic devices, making insertion of appropriately sized or even oversized airways of even greater importance. Resistance to diaphragmatic excursion by the uterus and the weight of the gravid breast on the chest will further impede successful ventilation, which may be mitigated by placing the patient in a reverse Trendelenburg position to cause the abdominal contents to shift caudally.

## Postintubation Management

Pregnancy is associated with an increased metabolic rate, which requires increasing minute ventilation as the pregnancy progresses. At term, this translates into a 30% to 50% increase in minute ventilation. Arterial blood gases or pulse oximetry and end-tidal carbon dioxide monitoring will aid in adjusting the ventilation parameters. Modest adjustments of both rate (start at 12 to 14 per minute) and tidal volume (start at 12 mL per kg) should meet the ventilatory need. If ventilation pressures are high, placing the patient in reverse Trendelenberg and left lateral decubitus position to move the abdominal contents down off the diaphragm may bring some improvement. In addition, tidal volume can be reduced somewhat and the respiratory rate increased.

## SUMMARY

Late-term pregnancy induces changes that affect almost every aspect of airway management. Classification of the late-term pregnant patient as a difficult airway, use of the difficult airway algorithm, and consideration of rapid oxyhemoglobin desaturation and the technical challenges of laryngoscopy and BMV will help the operator develop a cogent plan, including rescue from intubation failure.

## TIPS AND PEARLS

- Proper positioning of the pregnant patient including placing the head slightly up with a roll between the shoulders and good support under the occiput before induction and attempting intubation may improve success.
- Anticipate rapid desaturation. Robust preoxygenation using flush flow rate oxygen through a NRB mask and apneic nasal oxygen during RSI will prolong the period of safe apnea.
- Supraglottic edema is a common cause for failure to secure the airway in the pregnant patient; therefore, a smaller (6.5 to 7 mm ID) endotracheal tube may be required.
- Although not specifically studied in the pregnant patient to date, it is likely that video laryngoscopy offers substantial advantages for glottic visualization and intubation when compared with direct laryngoscopy.
- As for the nonpregnant patient, cricoid pressure is optional. In the event of difficult laryngoscopy, or a failed airway requiring a rescue EGD, releasing cricoid pressure may improve success at placement.
- When choosing pharmacologic agents to facilitate intubation, the general rule of thumb is "if it benefits the mother in the acute setting, it will ultimately benefit the fetus."

## EVIDENCE

- **Which EGD is best for the pregnant patient?** There are no randomized studies comparing the various rescue airway devices in pregnant patients. There are, however, a number of case reports, case series, and observational studies detailing the use of the LMA Classic, LMA ProSeal, LMA Supreme, LMA Fastrach, King laryngeal tube, and Combitube. Naturally, these reports largely focus on the positive outcomes when these devices are used, so the risks and benefits of each are difficult to discern. None of these devices provide complete protection against aspiration, which remains a significant concern in the airway management of the pregnant patient. The addition of a second lumen for passing an oral gastric tube as found in the King laryngeal tube, LMA Supreme, and the LMA ProSeal may offer at least a conduit for stomach contents to exit if regurgitation occurs. The LMA ProSeal also has an airway cuff that seals at higher pressures than a classic LMA allowing for higher ventilatory pressures, a finding constant across a wide range of body mass index scores. Compared with a classic LMA, these features may be advantageous in the pregnant population. Both the Combitube and the laryngeal tube have a lumen/balloon that can provide some barrier to regurgitation; however, experience with both devices in obstetrics is limited. Although the LMA ProSeal, LMA Supreme, King laryngeal tube, and Combitube may offer some advantage against the risk of aspiration, they cannot be used to secure definitive endotracheal intubation as can the intubating LMA. Currently, the intubating LMA is probably the best choice as a rescue device in the pregnant patient because it can be used as both a rescue device and an intubation device. Nonetheless, the choice of rescue device should be influenced by operator experience and device availability.[1–7]

- **What is the rate of failed intubations in obstetrics and has it improved with recent advances in difficult airway management?** There is variability and controversy regarding the exact rate of failed intubations in the pregnant patient reported in the Anesthesia literature, but according to closed claim analysis it is 1 in 250 to 1 in 300[8]; however, a recent review of the literature dating back to 1970 found the incidence to be 1 in 390.[9] Several studies have found these rates to be declining, with the overall rate of general anesthesia in obstetrics decreasing over time. A cross-sectional study of obstetric complications extracted from the 1998 to 2005 Nationwide Inpatient Sample of Healthcare Cost and Utilization Project found a decrease of >40% in rates of severe complications of anesthesia including airway problems.[10,11] Several studies of obstetric anesthesia claims for injuries also found improved safety, with a decrease in respiratory complications from 24% to 4% and a decrease in claims from inadequate oxygenation/ventilation or aspiration of gastric contents and esophageal intubations.[12,13] A third study found the rate of difficult intubations in a 20-year cohort analysis of 2,633 patients to be 4.7% and failed intubations to be 0.8%, and these rates remained stable over the 20 years reviewed.[14] These studies suggest significant risks are associated with airway management in obstetrical patients and that these rates have been stable or declining in incidence. One recent retrospective study evaluated 180 obstetric intubations over a three-year period and found 157 of 163 direct laryngoscopy intubations and 18 of 18 video laryngoscopy intubations were successful in the first attempt. The one failed direct laryngoscopy intubation was rescued using a video laryngoscope.[15] It is highly recommended to anticipate and recognize the difficult airway in pregnancy and to follow difficult airway algorithms with a few well-chosen devices considering the anatomic and physiologic changes occurring in pregnancy. It is also recommended to maintain ongoing training and education in this area.[16]

## REFERENCES


1. Gaiser R. Physiologic changes of pregnancy. In: Chestnut DH, ed. *Obstetric Anesthesia: Principles and Practice*. 4th ed. Philadelphia, PA: Mosby; 2009:15–36.
2. Goldszmidt E. Principles and practices of obstetric airway management. *Anesthesiol Clin*. 2008;26(1):109–125.
3. Vasdev GM, Harrison BA, Keegan MT, et al. Management of the difficult and failed airway in obstetric anesthesia. *J Anesth*. 2008;22(1):38–48.
4. Zand F, Amini A. Use of the laryngeal tube-S for airway management and prevention of aspiration after a failed tracheal intubation in a parturient. *Anesthesiology*. 2005;102:481–483.
5. Halaseh BK, Sukkar ZF, Hassan LH, et al. The use of ProSeal laryngeal mask airway in caesarean section—experience in 3000 cases. *Anaesth Intensive Care*. 2010;38(6):1023–1028.
6. Zamora JE, Saha TK. Combitube rescue for Cesarean delivery followed by ninth and twelfth cranial nerve dysfunction. *Can J Anaesth*. 2008;55(11):779–784.
7. Yao WY, Li SY, Sng BL, et al. The LMA Supreme in 700 parturients undergoing Cesarean delivery: an observational study. *Can J Anaesth*. 2012;59(7):648–654.
8. McDonnell NJ, Paech MJ, Clavisi OM, et al; ANZCA Trials Group. Difficult and failed intubation in obstetric anaesthesia: an observational study of airway management and complications associated with general anaesthesia for caesarean section. *Int J Obstet Anesth*. 2008;17:292–297.
9. Kinsella SM, Winton AL, Mushambi MC, et al. Failed tracheal intubation during obstetric general anaesthesia: a literature review. *Int J Obstet Anesth*. 2015;24(4)356–374.
10. Kuklina EV, Meikle SF, Jamieson DJ, et al. Severe obstetric morbidity in the United States: 1998–2005. *Obstet Gynecol*. 2009;113:293–299.

11. Mhyre JM. What's new in obstetric anesthesia in 2009? An update on maternal patient safety. *Anesth Analg*. 2010;111:1480–1487.
12. Davies JM, Posner KL, Lee LA, et al. Liability associated with obstetric anesthesia: a closed claims analysis. *Anesthesiology*. 2009;110:131–139.
13. Kuczkowski KM, Reisner LS, Benumof JL. Airway problems and new solutions for the obstetric patient. *J Clin Anesth*. 2010;15:552–563.
14. McKeen DM, George RB, O'Connell CM, et al. Difficult and failed intubation: incident rates and maternal, obstetrical, and anesthetic predictors. *Can J Anaesth*. 2011;58:514–524.
15. Aziz MF, Kim D, Mako J, et al. A retrospective study of the performance of video laryngoscopy in the obstetric unit. *Anesth Analg*. 2012;115(4):904–906.
16. Biro P. Difficult intubation in pregnancy. *Curr Opin Anaesthesiol*. 2011;24(3):249–254.

# Chapter 38

# The Patient with Prolonged Seizure Activity

Stephen Bush and Cheryl Lynn Horton

## THE CLINICAL CHALLENGE

A general discussion of the diagnosis and treatment of seizure disorder is beyond the scope of this book. This chapter focuses on the considerations of airway management in the seizure patient. In the simple, self-limited, generalized seizure, airway management is directed at termination of the seizure and prevention of hypoxia from airway obstruction. Paralysis and intubation should be considered when decline despite supplemental oxygen or when typical first-line measures fail to terminate the seizure in a reasonable time. For the simple seizure, basic airway maneuvers, expectant observation (most seizures end spontaneously), supplemental high-flow oxygen, and vigilance are usually all that is necessary. Airway protection from aspiration is rarely required in the simple, self-limited seizure because the uncoordinated motor activity precludes coordinated expulsion of gastric contents.

Determining when to proceed from supportive measures to intubation is the main clinical challenge. The Epilepsy Foundation has revised its definition of *status epilepticus* as follows: Any continuous seizure activity for 5 or more minutes or multiple seizures without recovery to a baseline neurologic condition. The rationale for 5 minutes (previously 30) was that the majority of non–status-related seizures are much shorter in duration, typically 2 to 3 minutes. The brain's compensatory mechanisms to prevent neuronal damage rely on adequate oxygenation and cerebral blood flow are often compromised well before 30 minutes, particularly in patients with underlying illness. Evidence also suggests that with longer seizure duration, pharmacologic therapies become less effective. The mortality rate for status epilepticus is >20% and also increases with duration of seizure activity. Therefore, intubation should be undertaken early as a part of overall supportive therapy in cases where the seizure is not promptly terminated by anticonvulsant medications. The absolute and relative indications for intubation in the seizing patient are listed in **Box 38-1**.

BOX 38-1

**Indications for endotracheal intubation for the seizing patient.**

**Absolute indications**

1. Hypoxemia ($Spo_2 < 90\%$) secondary to hypoventilation or airway obstruction
2. Treatment of underlying etiology (e.g., intracranial bleed with elevated ICP)
3. Prolonged seizure refractory to anticonvulsants (to prevent accumulating metabolic debt [acidosis and rhabdomyolysis])
4. Generalized convulsive status epilepticus

**Relative indications**

1. Prophylaxis for the respiratory depressant effect of large doses of anticonvulsants (e.g., benzodiazepines and barbiturates)
2. Termination of seizure activity to facilitate diagnostic workup (e.g., CT scanning)
3. Airway protection in prolonged seizures

## APPROACH TO THE AIRWAY

### Self-Limited Seizure

Most seizures terminate rapidly, either spontaneously or in response to medication, and require only supportive measures. Positioning the patient on his or her side, providing oxygen by face mask, suctioning secretions and blood carefully, and occasionally using the jaw thrust to relieve obstruction are usually all that is necessary to prevent hypoxia and aspiration. Bite blocks should not be placed in the mouths of seizing patients. They are not indicated and will only serve to increase the likelihood of injury. Attempts to ventilate during a seizure are usually ineffective and rarely necessary.

### Prolonged Seizure Activity

Although most self-limited seizures do not require intubation, several indications exist for intubation in the prolonged seizure. Extensive generalized motor activity will eventually cause hypoxia, hypotension, significant acidosis, rhabdomyolysis, hypoglycemia, and hyperthermia. Respiratory depression may result from high doses or combinations of anticonvulsants. Hypoxia despite supplemental high-flow oxygen, is an indication for immediate intubation.

No clear guideline specifically defines the duration of seizure activity requiring intubation. A good rule of thumb is that patients with seizures lasting <5 minutes with evidence of hypoxemia (central cyanosis or pulse oximetry readings <90% despite supplemental oxygen and clearly inadequate respirations) or patients with seizures lasting beyond 5 minutes despite appropriate anticonvulsant therapy should be considered for intubation. Generally, when first-line (benzodiazepine) anticonvulsants fail to terminate grand mal seizure activity, rapid sequence intubation (RSI) is indicated. Phosphenytoin, which has a relatively short loading time, may be initiated as a second-line agent before intubation, if time allows. Other second-line anticonvulsants (phenytoin and phenobarbital) require at least 20 minutes for a loading dose; therefore, at the time of initiation, intubation is advisable. The initiation of a propofol or phenobarbital infusion may also be an indication for intubation because of their respiratory depressant effects. Both agents act synergistically with benzodiazepines, which increases the likelihood of apnea and the need for airway management.

## TECHNIQUE

RSI is the method of choice in the seizing patient. In addition to its technical superiority, RSI ends all motor activity, allowing the body to begin to correct the metabolic debt. However, cessation of motor activity while the patient is paralyzed does not represent termination of the seizure, and effective loading doses of appropriate anticonvulsants (e.g., phenytoin) are required immediately after intubation. The recommended technique for the seizure patient is described in **Box 38-2**.

Standard RSI technique is appropriate in the seizing patient with the following modifications:

1. *Preoxygenation*: Preoxygenation may be suboptimal because of uncoordinated respiratory effort; therefore, pulse oximetry is critical. After giving succinylcholine, the patient may desaturate to <90% before complete relaxation and thus may require oxygenation using a bag and mask apparatus and 100% oxygen before attempts at intubation and continuous passive oxygenation by nasal cannula at 5 to 15 L per minute throughout the intubation sequence.
2. *Paralysis with induction:* Etomidate is a good induction agent if there is associated hypotension. Etomidate may raise the seizure threshold (and therefore inhibit seizure activity) in generalized seizures. Ketamine has been shown to be effective at terminating status epilepticus and at reducing the need for intubation in children. Propofol has also been used as an induction agent in this setting at a dose of 1.5 mg per kg. Little data exist on propofol as an induction agent in patients with seizures; however, there is evidence that it provides rapid suppression of seizure activity after a bolus and infusion and has been used in refractory status epilepticus. Midazolam is an alternative, but the dosage reduction required in a hemodynamically compromised patient means it functions poorly as an induction agent. It is not known whether midazolam offers

**BOX 38-2**

### RSI for patients with prolonged seizure activity.

| Time | Action |
|---|---|
| Zero minus 10+ min | Preparation |
| Zero minus 10+ min | Preoxygenation |
| Zero minus 10+ min | Preintubation optimization |
| Zero | Paralysis with induction |
| | Ketamine 1.5 mg/kg *or* etomidate 0.3 mg/kg *or* propofol 1.5–2 mg/kg or midazolam 0.3 mg/kg |
| | Succinylcholine 1.5 mg/kg |
| Zero plus 30 s | Protection and positioning |
| Zero plus 45 s | Placement with proof |
| Zero plus 60 s | Postintubation management |
| | Midazolam drip 0.05–0.2 mg/kg/h IV |
| | Or |
| | Propofol drip, 1–5 mg/kg/h IV |
| | Vecuronium 0.1 mg/kg IV (but sedation is preferable to paralysis) |
| | EEG monitoring if patient has ongoing paralysis |
| | Increased respiratory rate if significant acidosis present |

any additional anticonvulsant activity in a setting in which benzodiazepine seizure therapy has already been maximized. The full induction dose of midazolam is 0.3 mg per kg, but this often is reduced to 0.1 to 0.2 mg per kg for status epilepticus patients to prevent hemodynamic compromise, particularly because most patients have already received benzodiazepine therapy. Succinylcholine is recommended for neuromuscular blockade in this setting because of its very short duration of action. An intubating dose of rocuronium will result in paralysis for roughly an hour and thus will prevent the clinician from knowing if there is ongoing seizure activity without continuous electroencephalogram (EEG) monitoring.

3. *Postintubation management:* There are three additional considerations with respect to postintubation management.
   - Prolonged, deep sedation with an agent that suppresses seizures is desirable for the first hour after intubation to facilitate investigations (e.g., CT scan) and to allow acidosis to correct with controlled ventilation. Propofol infusion permits rapid reversal of sedation, which allows repeated or ongoing assessment of seizure activity and neurologic status, so often used for this purpose.
   - Long-term neuromuscular blockade should be avoided, if at all possible; however, if it is used, it should be accompanied by adequate doses of a sedation agent and continuous EEG monitoring, if available. Continuous bedside EEG monitoring, if available, should be initiated in the paralyzed patient to assess for ongoing seizure activity. If this is not immediately available, motor paralysis should be allowed to wear off before repeat dosing, to evaluate the effectiveness of anticonvulsant therapy. Effective sedation with a convulsive suppressant such as a propofol or midazolam infusion is preferable to motor paralysis.
   - If elevated intracranial pressure (ICP), head injury, known CNS pathology, or suspected meningitis is present, the elevated ICP intubation technique should be used (see Chapter 34).

## Drugs and Dosages

1. Preintubation seizure management
   - Lorazepam 0.1 mg per kg intravenously (IV) up to 2 mg per minute

     *or*
   - Diazepam 0.1 to 0.3 mg per kg IV up to 5 mg per minute or 0.5 mg per kg per rectum

     *or*
   - Midazolam 0.1 to 0.3 mg per kg IV up to 5 mg per minute

     THEN
   - Phosphenytoin 20 mg per kg (as milligrams of phenytoin equivalent)
2. Induction agents
   - Etomidate 0.3 mg per kg

     *or*
   - Propofol 1.5 to 2 mg per kg

     *or*
   - Ketamine 1.5 mg per kg
3. Postintubation sedation and therapy
   - Midazolam 0.05 to 0.2 mg/kg/hour IV infusion

     *or*
   - Propofol 1 to 5 mg/kg/hour IV infusion

# TIPS AND PEARLS

1. Check early to ensure that hypoglycemia is not the cause of the seizure. Perform a bedside glucose measurement or administer IV dextrose solution in all cases. Similarly, check for hyponatremia.
2. Even in the difficult airway, RSI is generally preferred for airway management in the actively seizing patient because any technique without neuromuscular blockade is unlikely to succeed.

Some difficult airway assessment may be challenging (e.g., mouth opening for the 3-3-2 rule or the Mallampati assessment). Airway difficulty, therefore, often is a judgment call. If the operator presumes that the intubation will be difficult, a double setup should be used.

3. The paralyzed patient may continue to seize, possibly causing neurologic injury despite the lack of motor activity. Administer effective doses of long-acting anticonvulsants, and use benzodiazepines for long-term sedation. Avoid long-term paralysis, if possible. If a long-acting neuromuscular blocking agent is used, arrange continuous EEG monitoring.
4. Prolonged seizure activity almost always represents a significant change in seizure pattern for the patient. A careful search for an underlying cause, including a head CT scan, is indicated.

## EVIDENCE

- **Which induction is best?** Although lorazepam and diazepam are the prototypical agents for termination of acute seizure activity, there are no data on the ideal agent as an induction agent in status epilepticus. Etomidate, propofol, and midazolam are all acceptable options. Ketamine has been shown to be effective at terminating status epilepticus, especially in children, and would be a good fourth option.[1–4]
- **Midazolam, propofol, or pentobarbital for postintubation therapy?** For postintubation care, the patient should be sedated using a drug that not only provides amnesia and anxiolysis but also optimizes antiepileptic therapy. Benzodiazepines have all these properties and are readily available in the acute care setting. Midazolam is preferred over diazepam and lorazepam as a continuous IV infusion because of its shorter half-life, water solubility, hemodynamic stability, and greater clinical experience in refractory status epilepticus.

  Midazolam and propofol are preferred first-line agents although no prospective randomized trial exists comparing these therapies directly. Despite the popularity of propofol for refractory seizure management in the ICU setting, there is little experience in the emergency setting, and the ICU studies are too small to draw any conclusions.[5,6] The recommended dosing for propofol is 1 to 2 mg per kg IV bolus (or induction) followed by a 1 to 5 mg/kg/hour infusion. Higher sustained doses have been associated with a propofol infusion syndrome.

## REFERENCES


1. Trinka E, Cock H, Hesdorffer D, et al. A definition and classification of status epilepticus—Report of the ILAE Task Force on Classification of Status Epilepticus. *Epilepsia*. 2015;56(10):1515–1523.
2. Synowiec AS, Singh DS, Yenugadhati V, et al. Ketamine use in the treatment of refractory status epilepticus. *Epilepsy Res*. 2013;105(1–2):183–188.
3. Gaspard N, Foreman B, Judd LM, et al. Intravenous ketamine for the treatment of refractory status epilepticus: a retrospective multicenter study. *Epilepsia*. 2013;54(8):1498–1503.
4. Ilvento L, Rosati A, Marini C, et al. Ketamine in refractory convulsive status epilepticus in children avoids endotracheal intubation. *Epilepsy Behav*. 2015;49:343–346.
5. Shearer P, Riviello J. Generalized convulsive status epilepticus in adults and children: treatment guidelines and protocols. *Emerg Med Clin North Am*. 2011;29:51–64.
6. Rossetti AO, Reichhart MD, Schaller MD, et al. Propofol treatment of refractory status epilepticus: a study of 31 episodes. *Epilepsia*. 2004;45:757–763.

Chapter 39

# The Geriatric Patient

Katren R. Tyler and Stephen Bush

## THE CLINICAL CHALLENGE

Comorbid illnesses are common in the older population, and for any given illness or injury, older adults have a worse outcome than younger adults. Aging causes progressive deterioration in physiologic reserve often exacerbated by preexisting chronic conditions, so the elderly are at increased risk of peri-intubation adverse events.

Advanced age affects airway management decision making in four principal areas. Cardiovascular morbidity, pulmonary pathology, frailty syndromes, and chronic underlying conditions are particularly relevant in avoiding the pitfalls of airway management in geriatric patients.

Older patients requiring emergency airway management are likely to have significant comorbidities. Older adults are also increasingly obese and paradoxically most likely to be malnourished. Older adults may require airway management for multiple reasons; however, their expected clinical course is often the most important factor in deciding to intubate in the emergency department (ED). Even without an immediate threat to oxygenation, ventilation, or airway protection, the geriatric patient often has a more prolonged and complex clinical course requiring airway support as part of their therapy. Conversely, the use of noninvasive ventilation techniques may provide an important ventilator bridge during information gathering, medical decision making and family discussions.

### Decreased Cardiorespiratory Reserve

Age-related changes in the lungs impair gas exchange, reducing oxygen tension at baseline. The normal $Pa_{O_2}$ falls by 4 mm Hg per decade after the age of 20. Total lung capacity does not change significantly, but functional residual capacity (FRC) and closing volume (CV) increase with age. CV increases more than FRC, leading to atelectasis, especially in the supine position. Reduced sensitivity of central respiratory drive, weakened respiratory muscles, and altered chest wall mechanics impair the ability of the older adult to respond to hypoxia and hypercarbia. Consequently, oxygen saturation may fall rapidly in the face of a respiratory threat. Older patients are also at risk of pulmonary aspiration because of blunted airway reflexes, swallowing disorders, drug effects, and delayed gastric emptying. Older patients with chronic obstructive pulmonary disease (COPD) or obstructive sleep apnea may live with partially compensated respiratory insufficiency, be on home oxygen, or require respiratory support at baseline through nasal continuous positive airway pressure (CPAP) machines.

The aging heart has reduced contractility and limited coronary blood flow, and dysrhythmias, such as atrial fibrillation, further impair the ability to increase cardiac output. $\beta$-blockers and calcium channel blockers may limit responses to physiologic stresses by preventing compensatory elevations in heart rate. A relatively fixed cardiac output impairs the physiologic response to the hypotensive effects of intubation drugs. Finally, the presence of cardiovascular or cerebrovascular disease reduces the patient's tolerance of hypoxemia or hypotension.

The elderly are more prone to postintubation hypotension, which may be persistent and severe. In addition to age, patients presenting with an elevated shock index (heart rate divided by systolic blood pressure), respiratory failure, or history of end-stage renal failure and chronic renal insufficiency are at increased risk. Circulatory collapse would be expectedly more common in elderly patients. Postintubation cardiac arrest occurs in about 4% of patients immediately following rapid sequence intubation (RSI), with pulseless electrical activity (PEA) being the most common rhythm. Patients with postintubation hypotension are at highest risk of progressing to cardiac arrest. In hemodynamically vulnerable patients, aggressive volume resuscitation and blood pressure support in advance of intubation, if time allows, is advisable.

Older patients are more likely to present to the ED in cardiac arrest. The optimal airway management strategy in primary cardiac arrest has come under scrutiny recently. Definitive airway placement is not required in the immediate arrest period. Providers should focus on quality chest compressions and limiting overventilation, which can impede venous return. This is discussed in more detail in the Evidence section. Nonetheless, if intubation is performed, a patient in cardiac arrest is generally a technically straightforward intubation as they are flaccid and without protective reflexes. Management should follow the crash airway algorithm as discussed in Chapter 3.

### Increased Incidence of Difficult Airway

Advanced age is a marker for difficult bag-mask ventilation (BMV) (see Chapter 2). Older patients also have an increased incidence of difficult direct laryngoscopy, although this is not a factor of age itself, but rather a result of impairment of neck mobility and mouth opening. A fixed flexion deformity of the neck may be unrecognized until the pillow is removed prior to intubation; intubation with conventional laryngoscopy is challenging under these conditions and patients with rheumatoid arthritis may have unstable upper cervical spines. The mucosa of older adults is more friable, often desiccated, and less elastic, making them more vulnerable to damage. Similarly, changes associated with aging and the cumulative effects of disease cause difficulty with the insertion of extraglottic devices (EGDs) and provision of a surgical airway. For all of these reasons, maximizing the opportunity for first-attempt success through proper positioning, robust preoxygenation, and the liberal use of intubating introducers and videolaryngoscopy is recommended.

### Ethical Considerations

In airway management, as in all other aspects of resuscitation, the patient's preferences regarding therapeutic interventions must be respected. Advanced age in and of itself is not a contraindication to advanced airway intervention. Poor outcomes relate more to functional limitation and comorbidities rather than to chronologic age. In cases where life-sustaining interventions are either inappropriate or not desired, noninvasive positive pressure ventilation can provide respiratory assistance and comfort. CPAP or bilevel positive airway pressure can also act as a temporizing measure when data are lacking and information about advanced directives is gathered prior to intubation.

## APPROACH TO THE AIRWAY

As the elderly tolerate hypoxia poorly, intubation should be considered early in their management. A careful preintubation assessment will identify difficult airway predictors, such as poor mouth opening, absent teeth, stiff lungs, and reduced cervical spine range of motion. Most often, the operator will be confident with respect to laryngoscopy, particularly if a videolaryngoscope is used, and with respect to oxygenation using a bag and mask or EGD, so RSI is usually the technique of choice. Regardless of the results of a bedside assessment for difficulty, in older patients, one should be prepared for an unexpected difficult airway. This requires planning, communication, and preparation of rescue airway devices.

Preoxygenation is particularly important as older patients may desaturate quickly because of age-associated changes in the heart and lungs and preexisting disease. For the same reasons, preoxygenation may not be as effective as in a younger, healthier patient. Passive breathing through a bag and mask apparatus, use of facemask oxygen at a flush flow rate of at least 40 L per minute, and apneic oxygenation should be considered early if preoxygenation through more traditional means is not adequate (see Chapter 5). BMV may be required to maintain oxygen saturation >90% after the induction agent and neuromuscular blocking agent (NMBA) are given, particularly if more than one laryngoscopic attempt is required.

During BMV, the mask seal may be problematic because of facial wasting and edentulousness, and a two-handed two-person technique, with a nasal or oral airway, is advisable. Well-fitting dentures should be left in place during BMV and removed for intubation. If the dentures are displaced, poorly fitting, or already acting as a foreign body, they should be removed. Loss of elastic tissues promotes collapse and partial obstruction of the upper airway. Obesity adds to the redundant tissue in the upper airway, which may precipitate a functional obstruction with loss of tone. Older patients may have oropharyngeal obstruction because of hematoma or cancer of the head and neck. Reduced lung compliance and chest wall stiffness may make oxygenation using a bag and mask or EGD difficult, and this may be worsened by coexisting COPD or heart failure.

When preintubation assessment identifies a difficult airway, the operator should choose the best possible device (usually a videolaryngoscope) and ensure optimal patient positioning to create the greatest likelihood of success. Alternative airway approaches, including awake flexible endoscopy, may be chosen over RSI, as guided by the difficult airway algorithm (Chapter 3).

Surgical cricothyrotomy is the appropriate choice in a "can't intubate, can't oxygenate" situation, but this procedure may be difficult in the elderly as they are more likely to have distortion of the tissues as a result of cancer or radiotherapy or limited access as in the case of a fixed flexion deformity involving the cervical spine.

## Drug Dosage and Administration

### *Preintubation Optimization*

In general, geriatric patients have less physiologic reserve than younger adults and are more susceptible to the hypotensive effects of sedative agents. With this in mind, preintubation optimization endeavors to maximize the patient's cardiovascular physiology and abort profound hypotension or circulatory collapse that can happen even with modest doses of induction drugs.

Delayed sequence intubation, discussed in Chapter 20, may be particularly well suited to the geriatric population who are more likely to be acutely confused and agitated prior to intubation and are at greater risk of hypoxemia than younger adults. The use of a dissociative dose of ketamine (1 mg per kg IV) to reduce agitation and oxygen consumption and increase compliance with oxygen delivery results in less frequent and severe hypoxemic events. Although initial experiences have been positive, robust evidence to support this has yet to be published, and it may not be appropriate in all practice settings. Similarly, there is little evidence regarding the use of vasoconstrictors or inotropes prior to administration of induction agents to prevent hypotension and consequent cerebral and coronary hypoperfusion. However, it is reasonable in high-risk patients to administer a pressor agent in an attempt to mitigate peri-intubation hemodynamic adverse events.

### *Paralysis with Induction*

Etomidate is the preferred agent in older patients because of its superior hemodynamic stability, although in profoundly compromised patients a full induction load may still precipitate hypotension. The standard induction dose should be reduced by half in geriatric patients and a two thirds reduction is advisable if significant hemodynamic compromise exists. Propofol may cause significant hypotension in critically ill patients and is not recommended as the primary induction agent for older patients requiring RSI.

Ketamine causes less cardiovascular instability and is useful in reactive airways disease; however, its sympathomimetic properties may be problematic in patients with ischemic heart disease, cerebrovascular disease, elevated intracranial pressure, or Parkinson's disease.

Older adults are more likely to have an acquired contraindication to succinylcholine, predominantly a neurologic injury (typically recent stroke), or a degenerative neuromuscular disorder (multiple sclerosis). If the decision is made to use succinylcholine in geriatric patients, contraindications should be sought by history from the patient, prehospital providers or family members, physical examination (especially for neurologic disability), and review of clinical records, if possible. For example, a recent denervating stroke (3 days to 6 months) is associated with a risk of receptor-mediated hyperkalemia. Chronic renal disease, including renal failure, is not a contraindication to succinylcholine use. Many providers now use rocuronium as their primary NMBA, especially in elderly patients. The dose is the same as in younger adults.

## POSTINTUBATION MANAGEMENT

The principles of postintubation management, set out in Chapters 7 and 20, are appropriate to the aging adult. Anticipate greater sensitivity to both the sedative and hemodynamic effects of sedatives (e.g., midazolam and propofol) and analgesics (e.g., morphine, fentanyl, and alfentanil) and titrate accordingly. Neuromuscular blockade is rarely required. If used, the NMBA should also be given in reduced doses and with increased intervals between doses. Ventilator settings are not usually affected by age, but reduced compliance may increase ventilation pressures. In COPD, it is advisable to limit peak pressure and allow a prolonged expiratory phase, although severe respiratory acidosis should be avoided in ischemic heart disease. Positive pressure ventilation, particularly with high levels of positive end-expiratory pressure, can cause hypotension, particularly if hypovolemia is present, and may exacerbate the hypotensive effects of sedative drugs. Pressure-controlled ventilation is the preferred mode.

## TIPS AND PEARLS

- Older patients have an increased incidence of both anatomic and physiologic difficulties. These challenges are identified and managed in generally the same fashion as for the younger patient. RSI is usually the procedure of choice.
- Elderly patients desaturate quickly, placing a premium on preoxygenation. Passive oxygenation during apnea (oxygen at 15 L per minute by nasal cannula) may delay desaturation, and BMV may be required after induction or between intubation attempts. Delayed sequence intubation may be useful in older adults because of agitation and delirium.
- Age-related cardiovascular changes, preexisting disease, and drug interactions enhance the hypotensive response to induction, and reduced doses of sedatives and hypnotics should be used. Reduced cardiac output prolongs the arm–brain circulation time, and a delayed onset of action should be anticipated for all intravenous drugs.

## EVIDENCE

- **What is the cardiovascular risk of intubation in elderly patients?** Geriatric patients are at risk for adverse hemodynamic consequences following intubation, both from the cardiovascular effects of induction drugs and also from the decreased venous return that accompanies positive pressure ventilation. Elderly patients are more likely to be malnourished and dehydrated, resulting in lower intravascular volumes.[1] Peri-intubation hypotension is common, occurring in as many as 25% of all patients.[2,3] ED-based intubation registries have shown an association between age and postintubation hypotension, with age > 70 years being an independent predictor.[3] Patients experiencing peri-intubation hypotension were nearly 15 times more likely to die during their hospitalization.[4] From that same registry, it was found that hypotension progressed to postintubation cardiac arrest in approximately 4% of encounters, with PEA being the most common rhythm.[4] In another large observational study, preintubation hypotension (SBP < 90 mm Hg) was the strongest predictor of postintubation cardiac arrest.[5] Initiation of a shock-sensitive intubation protocol that focuses on appropriate fluid loading, early use of vasopressors, and cardiostable drug selection can lower rates of refractory shock and cardiac arrest.[6] When time allows, vulnerable patients requiring intubation should have aggressive volume resuscitation, reduced dose induction agent use, and support with vasopressors to mitigate hemodynamic compromise.

- **Is older age a predictor of difficult intubation or complications of intubation?** Older age is an independent predictor of difficult intubations and adverse peri-intubation events.[7] Patients older than 80 years and those with predicted difficult airways such as Mallampati class III and IV are more likely to sustain an airway injury during anesthesia.[8] However, the decision to proceed with intubation is more appropriately based on the original indications for intubation (failure to ventilate, failure to protect airway, and the anticipated clinical course) rather than on age. Survival following emergency airway management is more likely to be a product of the acute illness and background comorbidities rather than the act of intubation.[9]
- **Which muscle relaxant should be used for RSI in the elderly?** Older patients are more likely to have an acquired contraindication to succinylcholine, most commonly a recent stroke; however, any upper or lower motor neuron defect at least 72 hours old puts the patient at risk for postsynaptic receptor upregulation and hyperkalemia.[10] Disuse atrophy is also a risk factor in the older age group. Theoretically, the risk of massive release of intracellular potassium is only present between 3 days and about 6 months after an acute stroke, when acetylcholine receptors proliferate at the neuromuscular end plate. However, given that many ED patients requiring emergent intubation are unable to provide a full and complete history, many emergency physicians will opt to use rocuronium instead of succinylcholine for RSI in older patients.[11]

## REFERENCES


1. Pereira GF, Bulik CM, Weaver MA, et al. Malnutrition among cognitively intact, noncritically ill older adults in the emergency department. *Ann Emerg Med*. 2015;65(1):85–91.
2. Hasegawa K, Hagiwara Y, Imamura T, et al. Increased incidence of hypotension in elderly patients who underwent emergency airway management: an analysis of a multi-centre prospective observational study. *Int J Emerg Med*. 2013;6(1):12.
3. Heffner AC, Swords D, Kline JA, et al. The frequency and significance of postintubation hypotension during emergency airway management. *J Crit Care*. 2012;27(4):417.e9–417.e13.
4. Heffner AC, Swords DS, Nussbaum ML, et al. Predictors of the complication of postintubation hypotension during emergency airway management. *J Crit Care*. 2012;27(6):587–593.
5. Kim WY, Kwak MK, Ko BS, et al. Factors associated with the occurrence of cardiac arrest after emergency tracheal intubation in the emergency department. *PLoS One*. 2014;9(11):e112779.
6. Jabre S, Jung B, Corne P, et al. An intervention to decrease complications related to endotracheal intubation in the intensive care unit: a prospective, multiple-center study. *Intensive Care Med*. 2010;36(2):248–255.
7. Johnson KN, Botros DB, Groban L, et al. Anatomic and physiopathologic changes affecting the airway of the elderly patient: implications for geriatric-focused airway management. *Clin Interv Aging*. 2015;10:1925–1934.

8. Hua M, Brady J, Li G. The epidemiology of upper airway injury in patients undergoing major surgical procedures. *Anesth Analg*. 2012;114(1):148–151.
9. Theodosiou CA, Loeffler RE, Oglesby AJ, et al. Rapid sequence induction of anaesthesia in elderly patients in the emergency department. *Resuscitation*. 2011;82(7):881–885.
10. Martyn JA, Richtsfeld M. Succinylcholine-induced hyperkalemia in acquired pathologic states: etiologic factors and molecular mechanisms. *Anesthesiology*. 2006;104(1):158–169.
11. Brown CA 3rd, Bair AE, Pallin DJ, et al. Techniques, success, and adverse events of emergency department adult intubations. *Ann Emerg Med*. 2015;65(4):363–370.

# Chapter 40

# The Morbidly Obese Patient

Megan L. Fix and Richard D. Zane

## THE CLINICAL CHALLENGE

The World Health Organization and the National Institutes of Health define a person to be overweight when he or she has a body mass index (BMI) between 25 and 29.9 kg per $m^2$, and a person to be obese when BMI is >30 kg per $m^2$. Morbid obesity is variably defined as a BMI > 35 or 40 kg per $m^2$. The National Health and Nutrition Examination Survey for 2011 to 2012 estimates that 69.0% of the adults in the United States over the age of 20 are either overweight or obese (33.9% overweight, 35.1% obese). After a long period of rise, the prevalence of obesity has leveled somewhat in the last 5 years. The 2014 Behavioral Risk Factor Surveillance System, a state-based cross-sectional random survey of the adult population of the United States, showed considerable differences in the prevalence of obesity across states. The United Kingdom's fourth National Audit Project (NAP4) reported that morbidly obese patients are at a fourfold higher risk of major complications (death, brain damage, emergency surgical airway, unanticipated or prolonged ICU admission) when compared to nonobese patients.

## APPROACH TO THE AIRWAY

As for all patients, managing the airway of obese patients requires a structured, methodical assessment to identify the specific predictors of difficult bag-mask ventilation (BMV), cricothyrotomy, extraglottic device (EGD) placement, and tracheal intubation. It is controversial whether obesity alone is a predictor of difficult laryngoscopy, or whether obese patients tend to have a higher incidence of other markers of difficult intubation. Patient attributes differ, and some obese patients may have multiple anatomical risk factors for airway difficulty in addition to obesity, whereas others may not. Nevertheless, morbidly obese patients develop both physiologic and anatomic changes that can make airway management particularly challenging because morbidly obese patients have excess adipose tissue not only on the breast, neck, thoracic wall, and abdomen but also internally in the mouth and pharynx. When compared with lean patients, this excess tissue makes accessing the airway (intubation and tracheostomy) and maintaining patency (during sedation or mask ventilation) of the upper airway more difficult.

The degree of pathologic, physiologic, and anatomical changes correlates with the degree and extent of obesity and comorbidities common with obese patients. The physiologic and anatomical changes associated with morbid obesity are listed in **Box 40-1**. The main effects of obesity on airway management are (1) rapid arterial desaturation, secondary to a decreased functional residual capacity (FRC) and increased oxygen consumption; (2) difficult airway management, specifically difficult BMV, resulting from increased risk of obstruction from excess pharyngeal adipose tissue and increased resistance resulting from the weight of the chest wall and the mass of abdominal contents limiting diaphragmatic excursion; and (3) difficult laryngoscopy, intubation, and cricothyrotomy.

Obesity affects almost every aspect of normal physiology, most notably the respiratory and cardiovascular systems. Obese patients often have baseline hypoxemia with a widened alveolar–arterial oxygen gradient primarily because of ventilation–perfusion (V/Q) mismatching. Lung volumes develop a restrictive pattern with multiple disturbances, the most important of which is decreased FRC. Notably, these indices change exponentially with the degree of obesity. The decline in FRC has been ascribed to "mass loading" of the abdomen and splinting of the diaphragm. FRC may be reduced to the extent that it falls within the range of closing capacity, thus leading to small airway closure and V/Q mismatch. The FRC declines further when the individual assumes the supine position, resulting in worsening of the V/Q mismatch, right-to-left shunt, and arterial hypoxemia. Although the vital capacity, total lung capacity (TLC), and FRC may be maintained in mild obesity, they can be reduced by up to 50% in severely obese patients. The decreased FRC causes rapid oxyhemoglobin desaturation during the apneic phase of rapid sequence intubation (RSI), even in the setting of adequate preoxygenation (see Chapter 5).

The work of breathing (WOB) is increased 30% to 400% in morbidly obese patients because of decreased chest wall compliance, increased airway resistance, and an abnormal diaphragmatic position. These changes limit the maximum ventilatory capacity (MVC). The obese patient has elevated oxygen consumption and carbon dioxide ($CO_2$) production because of the metabolic activity of the excess body mass.

Cardiovascular changes in obesity include increased extracellular volume, cardiac output, left ventricular end diastolic pressure, and left ventricular hypertrophy (LVH). The absolute total blood volume (BV) is increased, but it is relatively less on a volume/weight basis when compared with lean patients (50 vs. 75 mL per kg). Cardiac morbidity, including hypertension (HTN), ischemic heart disease, and cardiomyopathy, correlates with progressive obesity.

Other changes include an increase in renal blood flow (RBF) and glomerular filtration rate (GFR), fatty infiltration of the liver, and a propensity for diabetes mellitus and obstructive sleep apnea (**Box 40-1**).

Increased chest wall weight, increased facial girth, and redundant pharyngeal tissue all contribute to defining obesity as an independent risk factor for difficult BMV (see Chapter 2). Obese patients tend to have a smaller pharyngeal space because of deposition of adipose tissue in the tongue, tonsillar pillars, and aryepiglottic folds. Patients with obesity have an increased risk of obstructive sleep apnea, another independent risk factor for difficult BMV. Difficult BMV should be anticipated in the obese patient, often requiring a two-person technique with both oral and nasopharyngeal airways in place. In severe or superobese patients, BMV may simply be impossible as the mask seal pressure required to overcome the increased weight and resistance may be far in excess of that possible with a bag and mask. In addition, challenging BMV is associated with difficult intubation in 30% of the cases. Intubation difficulty is also associated with increased neck circumference and high Mallampati scores. Cricothyrotomy is more difficult because of the increase in neck circumference, the thickness of the subcutaneous tissues, anatomical distortions, and adipose tissue obscuring landmarks, often requiring deeper and longer incisions. EGDs may not be able to overcome the high resistance of the weighted chest wall and restricted diaphragms. Second-generation EGDs, such as the LMA supreme, can provide higher leak pressures (25 to 30 cm $H_2O$) and may be more successful in obese patients.

BOX 40-1

**Physiologic and anatomical changes associated with obesity.**

| Physiologic Changes Associated with Obesity According to System | Anatomical Changes Associated with Obesity |
|---|---|
| **Pulmonary** | |
| ▪ Increased intrathoracic pressure with a restrictive respiratory pattern: ↓FRC, ↓ERV, ↓TLC | ▪ Increased facial girth<br>▪ Increased tongue size<br>▪ Smaller pharyngeal area |
| ▪ Increased WOB, decreased MVC | ▪ Redundant pharyngeal tissue (risk of obstructive sleep apnea) |
| ▪ V/Q mismatch (predisposes to hypoxemia) | ▪ Increased neck circumference |
| ▪ Risk of pulmonary HTN | ▪ Increased chest girth |
| ▪ Obesity hypoventilation syndrome | ▪ Increased breast size<br>▪ Increased abdominal girth |
| **Cardiac**<br>▪ Increased cardiac output<br>▪ Increased BV, SV<br>▪ HTN, LVH<br>▪ Increased metabolic rate: ↑$Vo_2$, ↑$CO_2$ production | |
| **Renal**<br>▪ Increased RBF and GFR | |
| **Hepatic/gastrointestinal**<br>▪ Fatty infiltration of the liver<br>▪ Increased intra-abdominal pressure<br>▪ Risk for hiatal hernia, GERD | |
| **Endocrine**<br>▪ Increased risk of diabetes<br>▪ Hyperlipidemia | |
| **Hematologic**<br>▪ Increased risk of DVT<br>▪ Polycythemia (with chronic hypoxemia) | |
| **Musculoskeletal**<br>▪ Degenerative joint disease<br>▪ Decubital changes | |

ERV, expiratory reserve volume; SV, stroke volume; $Vo_2$, oxygen consumption; GERD, gastroesophageal reflux; DVT, deep venous thrombosis; BV, blood volume; LVH, left ventricular hypertrophy.

## TECHNIQUE

Morbidly obese patients vary with respect to airway difficulty, and a methodical LEMON assessment is essential to anticipate and plan appropriately for intubation (see Chapter 2). When the airway appears particularly difficult, the difficult airway algorithm advocates for careful preparation and an awake approach with topical anesthesia and, if necessary, light sedation.

Proper positioning is essential in obese patients in order to ensure adequate preoxygenation as well as the best attempt at direct laryngoscopy and tracheal intubation. Ideally, the patient should be placed in a "ramped" position—propped up on linens or on a commercially available pillow, from the midpoint of the back to the shoulders and head for proper positioning, as shown in **Figure 40-1**. To confirm proper positioning, the patient should be viewed from the side, and an imaginary horizontal line should be able to be drawn from the external auditory meatus to the sternal notch. This position facilitates more effective preoxygenation and prolongs the duration of time before arterial desaturation with apnea.

The importance of effective preoxygenation is paramount in obese patients as they desaturate at a much faster rate than other patients. Although 3 minutes of tidal volume breathing or eight vital capacity breaths with 100% $FIO_2$ (best achieved using flush rate oxygen) are recommended in the general population, in the obese population, further efforts may be required. Noninvasive positive pressure ventilation (NIV) and positive end-expiratory pressure (PEEP) can be used if ambient pressure oxygenation is suboptimal. Preoxygenation is challenging in the supine position and, unless contraindicated, obese patients should be upright or in the reverse Trendelenberg position. Similarly, apneic oxygenation, provided by nasal cannula at 15 L per minute flow, should be used routinely to hopefully extend the period of safe apnea.

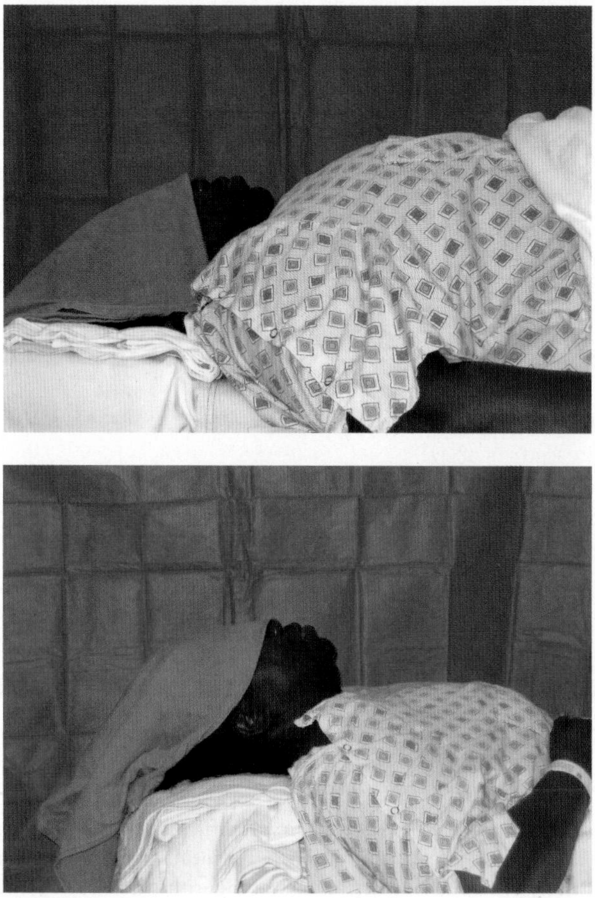

A

B

● **FIGURE 40-1. A:** Patient is supine with the weight of the breast/chest obstructing access to the airway. **B:** Patient is propped on linens to establish better anatomical landmarks and remove the weight of the breasts/chest off the airway. Here, it is possible to draw an imaginary horizontal line from the external auditory meatus to the angle of Louis.

To determine the best technique, the risks and benefits of managing the airway with the patient awake versus unconscious are weighed. When time and conditions permit, particularly in the morbidly obese patient, or the obese patient with additional markers of difficult laryngoscopy, an awake technique with either flexible endoscopy or video laryngoscopy is the preferred method. No matter which route is chosen, proper airway equipment must be available and checked for proper functioning and, ideally, help is readily available in the event intubation proves to be exceedingly difficult. Video laryngoscopy is preferred because it has a greater likelihood of providing an excellent view of the glottis. When performing direct laryngoscopy, a short-handled laryngoscope will be easier to insert because the chest prevents the longer handle from gaining blade access to the mouth. During ventilation by BMV or using an EGD, placing the patient in reverse Trendelenberg or a semi-upright position reduces upward pressure against the diaphragm by the abdominal contents and may also mitigate some of the "weight effect" of chest wall tissues, such as the breasts. Both the standard and the intubating laryngeal mask airway have been shown to be effective in providing ventilation, with the latter also serving as a conduit for tracheal intubation. Rigid fiber-optic intubating devices and video laryngoscopy have been shown to be successful in managing the airway of the obese patient as well. During direct laryngoscopy, the bougie may be helpful when only the arytenoids or the tip of the epiglottis is visible.

BMV often requires two providers using two-handed bilateral jaw thrust and mask seal, with oropharyngeal and nasopharyngeal airways in place and the airway pressure relief valve and mask seal set so that continuous positive airway pressure (5 to 15 cm $H_2O$) is delivered to the pharynx. Relaxation of the upper airway muscles during RSI will often cause collapse of the adipose-laden, soft-walled pharynx between the uvula and epiglottis, making BMV and tracheal intubation more difficult. This greatly reinforces the need to use oral and nasal airways, augmented by positioning the patient semi-upright, as described earlier.

Cricothyrotomy may be extremely challenging in the severely obese patient because the chin may be directly contiguous with the chest wall, making identification of and access to anatomical landmarks difficult. Care must be taken to ensure that landmarks are found. Bedside ultrasound can be used to identify the cricothyroid membrane, and if time permits, the skin can be "dotted" or "marked" with a pen prior to starting the intubation attempt. During the procedure, one or two assistants whose sole role is to hold or retract neck, facial, and chest fat folds may also be required. As in all patients, cricothyrotomy is a tactile procedure. Finally, due to increased neck diameter, many tracheostomy tubes will not be long enough for the morbidly obese patient and an endotracheal tube (ETT) can be advanced through the cricothyrotomy incision for definitive airway placement.

## Drug Dosage and Administration

Obesity, along with any associated comorbidities, affects all aspects of the pharmacodynamic and pharmacokinetic properties of medications, including absorption, onset, volume of distribution ($V_d$), protein binding, metabolism, and clearance. In the obese patient, there is not only an increase in adipose tissue, but also an increase in lean body mass of approximately 30% of the total excess weight. The ratio of fat to lean mass increases, however, causing a relative decrease in the percentage of lean mass and water in obese patients when compared with lean patients. In addition, there is an increase in BV and cardiac output. The $V_d$ for a particular agent is affected by the combination of these obesity-associated factors, along with the specific lipophilicity of the drug. Protein binding is affected by an increased concentration of lipids, which limit the binding of some drugs, thus increasing the free plasma concentration. In contrast, increased $\alpha_1$-glycoprotein may increase protein binding of other drugs, thus decreasing the free plasma concentration. For most agents that undergo hepatic metabolism, there is minimal change in effective half-life despite the high incidence of fatty infiltration of the liver. Agents handled by the kidney, however, have accelerated clearance because of increased GFR. These pharmacokinetic and pharmacodynamic changes can make the net effect of these agents somewhat unpredictable and dosage adjustment may be required.

In general, the lipophilicity of the agent can indicate the dosage requirement. Most anesthetic agents are lipophilic, thus an increase in $V_d$ and dose of the drug is expected, but this is not consistently demonstrated in pharmacologic studies because of factors such as end-organ clearance or protein binding. Less lipophilic agents such as neuromuscular blockers stay in the water compartment and have little or no change in $V_d$. This argues, in general, for ideal body weight (IBW) dosing. However, in the context of emergency RSI, optimal intubating conditions created by appropriate sedation and neuromuscular blockade are paramount. Succinylcholine is a total body weight (TBW) drug, despite it's hydrophilic nature. This has been very well studied (see Chapter 22) and is related to enhanced pseudocholinesterase activity in morbidly obese patients. The same is true for rocuronium. IBW dosing has been shown to be *adequate* to manage obese patients in the controlled environment of the OR; however, in the ED, it could create a worst case scenario of an incompletely paralyzed difficult emergency intubation. In this scenario, a low dose of rocuronium could result in ineffective or absent intrinsic ventilatory drive, yet inadequate mouth opening to permit laryngoscopy. TBW dosing will prolong rocuronium's activity, but with a baseline duration of action of 45 minutes, there is little downside to this approach. In addition, the manufacturer's recommendation is TBW dosing. Therefore, for emergency RSI, we advocate for TBW dosing for all neuromuscular blockers in an effort to *avoid underdosing* and the resultant suboptimal intubating conditions. For induction agents (when given in overdose can produce cardiovascular depression), dosing should aim to *avoid overdose* and be based on lean body weight (LBW) or IBW in the morbidly obese patient (see later). Table 40-1 summarizes dosing adjustment recommendations for common RSI medications.

Drug dosing for obese patients can be difficult to remember, given that some drugs are dosed using IBW, some using LBW, and some using TBW. IBW must be estimated or looked up in a table or nomogram, based on the patient's height and sex. TBW may be reported by the patient, or obtained using a bed scale. LBW can be thought of as IBW plus 30% of the difference between TBW and IBW. In other words, for every pound or kilogram the patient is overweight, about one-third of this contributes to lean body mass.

**TABLE 40-1 Dosing Recommendations for Drugs Commonly Used in Airway Management**

| Drug | Dosing | Comments |
|---|---|---|
| Propofol | IBW | Lipophilic, systemic clearance and $V_d$ at steady state correlate well with TBW. High affinity for excess fat and other well-perfused organs. High hepatic extraction and conjugation relates to TBW. Cardiovascular depression limits dosage to IBW for use in induction. Maintenance dosing may be initiated at TBW but titrated to effect using sedation scales |
| Midazolam | IBW | Lipophilic, increased $V_d$, prolonged sedative effect due to accumulation in adipose tissue and inhibition of cytochrome P450 3A4 by other drugs or obesity itself |
| Succinylcholine | TBW | Hydrophilic, increased plasma cholinesterase activity increases in proportion to body weight |
| Vecuronium | TBW | Hydrophilic, $V_d$ increased and clearance decreased; however, optimal intubating conditions argue for TBW dosing |
| Rocuronium | TBW | Hydrophilic, $V_d$ increased and clearance decreased; however, optimal intubating conditions argue for TBW dosing |
| Fentanyl | LBW | Lipophilic, increased $V_d$ and elimination half-life, distributes extensively in excess body mass. Respiratory depression limits dosing to LBW. Maintenance dosing is initiated at LBW but should be titrated using a sedation scale |
| Etomidate | LBW | Increased $V_d$, dose may need to be decreased with liver disease |

## POSTINTUBATION MANAGEMENT

The changes in the anatomy and physiology of obese patients have important implications for ventilator management. The initial tidal volume should be calculated based on IBW and then adjusted according to airway pressures, with the success of oxygenation and ventilation indicated by pulse oximetry and capnography, or arterial blood gas monitoring. Generally, the use of at least 5 to 10 cm $H_2O$ of PEEP is recommended to prevent end-expiratory airway closure and atelectasis. In severe obesity, it may be necessary to ventilate the patient in the semierect position to move the weight of the breasts, abdominal fat, or pannus off the chest wall.

Portable bedside radiographs are usually of poor quality in the obese patient, limiting their clinical value, although one can usually determine if the ETT is in a mainstem bronchus.

When considering extubation of the obese patient, a conservative approach should be taken. Review documentation regarding the difficulty of BMV and tracheal intubation, and consider the possibility of the patient requiring emergent reintubation.

## TIPS AND PEARLS

- The predicted difficulty in intubation combined with the decreased physiologic reserve in obese patients makes timely airway management important, and the decision to intubate cannot be delayed.
- For many obese patients, an awake technique, usually awake flexible endoscopy or video laryngoscopy, is the preferred method of intubation. If RSI is performed, rescue strategy should be well laid out, and the necessary equipment immediately available.
- Decreased FRC predisposes obese patients to rapid desaturation and hypoxemia. This may be mitigated with careful planning utilizing techniques such as head up or "ramped" positioning, NIV and PEEP for preoxygenation, good two-person BVM technique, and application of PEEP postintubation.

## EVIDENCE

- **Is obesity an independent risk factor for difficult intubation?** Classically, morbid obesity has been described as an independent predictor of difficult intubation, but it is not clear if it is obesity itself or more commonly described predictors of difficult intubation that contribute. Both neck circumference and increased BMI have been found to be independent predictors of difficult intubation. Obesity also proves to be a risk factor for difficult intubation in the prehospital environment. In 2011, Holmberg et al.[1] found obesity to be an independent risk factor for difficult intubation after reviewing >800 prehospital intubations.
- **Is video laryngoscopy superior to direct laryngoscopy in obese patients?** Optimal positioning as described earlier will augment intubation attempts using any technique or device. A few studies have looked at video versus direct laryngoscopy in obese patients and found that video-assisted techniques result in significantly better glottic visualization. In morbidly obese patients, GlideScope laryngoscopy provided better glottic views and lower intubation difficulty scores compared to the Macintosh laryngoscope, with only slightly longer time to intubation.[2]
- **What is the role of position for preoxygenation and apneic oxygenation in the intubation of the obese patient?** Not only is intubation more difficult in obese patients but so is bag mask ventilation. In addition, obese patients desaturate more rapidly than nonobese patients, making preoxygenation challenging as well. Positioning with the head elevated anterior to the shoulders aligning the external auditory meatus with the sternal notch or angle (**Fig. 40-1**) has been shown to make both oxygenation and intubation easier. Oxyhemoglobin desaturation was

significantly delayed and fewer patients desaturated <90% when oxygen was continuously administered at 5 L per minute by nasal cannulae during the apneic phase of intubation.[3]

- **What is the role of NIV and recruitment maneuvers (RMs) in the obese patient?** Obese patients have greater risk for hypoxemia and atelectasis during induction and intubation, and some have advocated for further techniques to improve oxygenation such as NIV and a RM. NIV aims to increase the recruitment of collapsed alveoli and RM, which consists of a transient increase in inspiratory pressure after intubation (40 cm $H_2O$ for 40 seconds), with a goal of decreasing atelectasis. This was evaluated in 66 morbidly obese patients randomized to three groups: conventional preoxygenation, preoxygenation with NIV, and preoxygenation with NIV + postintubation RM. This study found that the combination of preoxygenation with NIV and RM improved $Pao_2$ and end expiratory lung volume compared to conventional preoxygenation.[4]
- **Can ultrasound accurately identify the cricothyroid membrane in obese patients?** As described earlier, the increased neck circumference and impalpable landmarks can make an emergency cricothyroidotomy challenging in the obese patient. A few studies have looked at the use of ultrasound to identify the cricothyroid membrane with promising results.[5,6] One randomized trial found that the use of ultrasound in human cadavers with poorly defined landmarks significantly reduced the complications (e.g., laryngeal trauma) from 74% to 25% and increased the risk of a correct insertion by a factor of 5.[6]

## REFERENCES


1. Holmberg TJ, Bowman SM, Warner KJ, et al. The association between obesity and difficult prehospital tracheal intubation. *Anesth Analg*. 2011;112:1132–1138.
2. Andersen LH, Rovsing L, Olsen KS. GlideScope videolaryngoscope vs. Macintosh direct laryngoscope for intubation of morbidly obese patients: a randomized trial. *Acta Anaesthesiol Scand*. 2011;55:1090–1097.
3. Ramachandran SK, Cosnowski A, Shanks A, et al. Apneic oxygenation during prolonged laryngoscopy in obese patients: a randomized, controlled trial of nasal oxygen administration. *J Clin Anesth*. 2010;22:164–168.
4. Futier E, Constantin JM, Pelosi P, et al. Noninvasive ventilation and alveolar recruitment maneuver improve respiratory function during and after intubation of morbidly obese patients. *Anesthesiology*. 2011;114:1354–1363.
5. Dinsmore J, Heard AM, Green RJ. The use of ultrasound to guide time-critical cannula tracheotomy when anterior neck airway anatomy is unidentifiable. *Eur J Anaesthesiol*. 2011;28:506–510.
6. Siddiqui N, Arzola C, Friedman Z, et al. Ultrasound improves cricothyrotomy success in cadavers with poorly defined neck anatomy: a randomized control trial. *Anesthesiology*. 2015;123:1033–1041.

Chapter 41

# Foreign Body in the Adult Airway

Ron M. Walls and Erik G. Laurin

## THE CLINICAL CHALLENGE

Airway obstruction caused by a foreign body presents a unique series of challenges to the practitioner. First, when incomplete obstruction is present, there exists the possibility that a particular action, or the failure to take specific action, could aggravate the situation by converting a partial obstruction to a complete obstruction. Second, when complete obstruction is present, instinctive interventions, such as bag-mask ventilation, have the potential to make the situation worse, for example, by causing a supraglottic obstruction to move below the cords making retrieval more difficult or impossible. Third, a common maneuver, such as the endotracheal intubation with bag ventilation, may meet with an unexpected result, such as the complete inability to move any air, defying the provider's attempts to find a solution to a problem perhaps never before encountered. Finally, the completely or partially obstructed airway is a unique clinical situation, unlike other airway threats, and requires a specific set of evaluations and interventions, often in a very compressed period of time.

The patient with a foreign body in the airway may present with signs of upper airway obstruction or may present comatose and apneic, with only the history of onset to provide clues as to the cause of the crisis. The obstruction may be complete, as in the patient who aspirates a food bolus, and is unable to move sufficient air to phonate. Although these situations usually arise in the out-of-hospital setting, they may occasionally present to the emergency department (ED), usually when an incomplete obstruction converts to a complete obstruction. A partially obstructing foreign body will cause symptoms and signs of incomplete upper airway obstruction, specifically stridor, altered phonation, subjective difficulty breathing, and often a sense of fear or panic on the part of the patient. In many cases, there will be a preceding condition that has increased the risk of aspiration. Many patients who aspirate food are physically or mentally impaired, elderly, or intoxicated with drugs or alcohol.

## APPROACH TO THE AIRWAY

Management of the suspected or known foreign body in the adult airway follows similar rationale to that used in the pediatric patient (see Chapter 27) and depends on the location of the foreign body and whether the obstruction is incomplete or complete. Location may be supraglottic, infraglottic, or distal to the carina. Because the precise location of the foreign body is usually not known, the following discussion focuses on the approach to the foreign body whose location is uncertain.

## Incomplete Obstruction by a Foreign Body

When the patient presents with an incompletely obstructing foreign body, the objective is to reestablish a fully patent airway and prevent the conversion of a partial obstruction to a complete obstruction. If the patient is cooperative, breathing spontaneously and oxygen saturation adequate (possibly with supplemental oxygen), then the best approach often is to have emergency airway equipment immediately accessible in case the patient deteriorates while efforts are made to rapidly mobilize the necessary providers for prompt removal in the operating room (OR). Some foreign bodies are obviously accessible and can be removed in the ED. There is risk, however, with an incompletely obstructing supraglottic foreign body, that attempts at removal in the ED might result in displacement of the foreign body into the trachea, where it is no longer amenable to removal with common ED instruments. If transfer to the OR is not an option (e.g., because it would require transfer to another hospital), then a decision must be made as to whether the foreign body should be removed in the ED. If so, the best approach is to handle the airway much as one would handle awake laryngoscopy for a difficult intubation (see Chapter 23). The operator assembles the appropriate equipment, preoxygenates the patient, explains the procedure to the patient, and administers titrated sedation and topical anesthesia recognizing that either may trigger total obstruction. With the patient sedated, the operator carefully inserts the laryngoscope with the left hand, inspecting at each level of insertion before advancing to ensure that the foreign body is not pushed farther down by the tip of the laryngoscope. Either a conventional or a video laryngoscope may be used. The technique is one of "lift and look" followed by a small advance (perhaps 1 cm), and then another lift and look, and so on. It may be necessary to take a break to allow the patient to reoxygenate or to administer more sedation or anesthesia. When the foreign body is identified, the best instrument for removal (Magill forceps, tenaculum, or towel clip) is selected. Some foreign bodies, such as smooth-surfaced objects, cannot be grasped well with the Magill forceps. After the object is grasped and successfully removed, laryngoscopy is again performed to ensure that no additional foreign body remains in the airway. The patient should then be observed until fully recovered from the sedation and topical anesthesia to ensure that symptoms have resolved and there are no other issues. Some patients may require a longer period of observation or admission to hospital if the provider suspects additional small foreign bodies below the vocal cords, significant aspiration, symptoms of upper airway edema after removal of the foreign body, or if there is concern about the patient's comorbidities (e.g., chronic health issues and intoxication).

Upper airway foreign body causing incomplete obstruction should be considered a true emergency, and an early decision is required regarding the appropriateness of removal in the ED versus expedited transfer to the OR. If, at any point, the airway becomes completely obstructed, then the patient is managed as described in the following section.

## Complete Obstruction of the Airway

When airway obstruction is complete, the patient is unable to breathe or phonate and may hold his or her neck with one or both hands, the so-called universal choking sign. The patient may appear terrified and will be making attempts at inspiration. In general, after complete obstruction of the airway with ensuing apnea, oxygen saturation will rapidly fall to levels incompatible with consciousness.

Initial management is dictated by whether the patient is conscious or unconscious. If the patient is conscious, the abdominal thrust maneuver should immediately and repeatedly be applied until either the foreign body is expelled or the patient loses consciousness (see algorithm, **Fig. 41-1**). Whether the maneuver is called the abdominal thrust maneuver or the Heimlich maneuver is of no importance; they are one and the same. There is no point in attempting instrumented removal of an upper airway foreign body while the patient is still conscious, as a struggling and uncooperative patient in extremis will likely result in inability to grasp the foreign body, or even worse, displacement of the foreign body further down the airway. If the abdominal thrust maneuver is successful in expelling

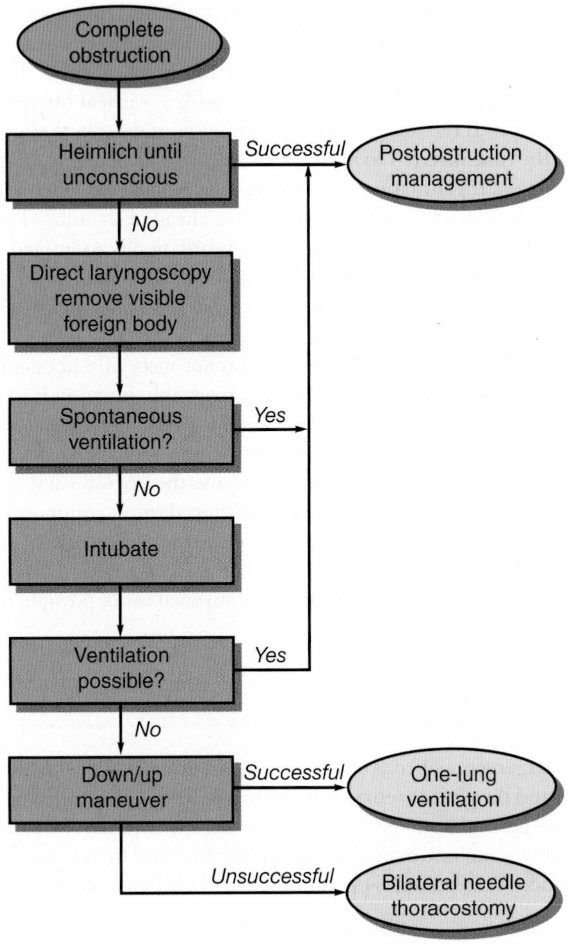


● **FIGURE 41-1.** Management of Complete Obstruction by a Foreign Body. See text for explanation.

the foreign body, and the patient can phonate and breathe normally, then observation for a few hours is sufficient, and it is not mandatory to visualize the airway if the patient remains asymptomatic. If the abdominal thrust maneuver is unsuccessful in removing the foreign body and the patient loses consciousness, a rapid series of chest thrusts (equivalent to those used during CPR) may be tried.

Thereafter, the first step is immediate direct or video laryngoscopy *before any attempts at bag-mask ventilation, which may cause the foreign body to move from a supraglottic to an infraglottic position.* Generally, the patient will be flaccid, and it will not be necessary to administer a neuromuscular blocking agent. Time should not be lost waiting for an intravenous line to be established. Under direct or video laryngoscopy, a foreign body above the glottis is easily identifiable. Again, Magill forceps, a tenaculum, a towel clip, or any other suitable device can be used to remove the foreign body. After removal of the foreign body, the larynx is inspected through direct or video laryngoscopy to ensure that there is no residual foreign material. When the foreign body is removed, the patient may begin spontaneous ventilation immediately. If the patient does not begin to breathe spontaneously, immediate intubation and initiation of positive-pressure ventilation is indicated and can be performed during the same laryngoscopy (**Fig. 41-1**).

If laryngoscopy does not identify a foreign body, and the glottis is clearly visualized, then either there is no foreign body or the foreign body is below the vocal cords. In this case, the patient should immediately be intubated and ventilated. If ventilation is successful, then resuscitation proceeds as for any other patient. If bag ventilation through the endotracheal tube meets with total resistance (no air movement and no end-tidal carbon dioxide detection), then the trachea is completely obstructed. The stylet should immediately be replaced into the endotracheal tube, the cuff deflated, and the tube advanced all the way to its hilt in an attempt to push a tracheal foreign body into the right (or left) mainstem bronchus. If the foreign material is thought to be soft, then an attempt at ventilation can be made with the tube inserted to its deepest extent, on the basis that the tube may have passed through the obstruction. If ventilation is not successful, then the foreign body is assumed to be solid and to have been pushed into the mainstem bronchus ahead of the tube. The tube is withdrawn to its normal level, and the cuff is reinflated, and then ventilation is attempted. The strategy here is to try to convert an obstructing tracheal foreign body (which will be lethal) to an obstructing mainstem bronchus foreign body (which can be removed in the OR). Thus, the patient can be kept alive by ventilating one lung while the other lung is obstructed.

If the down-then-up maneuver just described is not successful in establishing one-lung ventilation, there are two clinical possibilities. The only reversible situation is when the patient has one obstructed mainstem bronchus and a tension pneumothorax on the other side. Pneumothorax can occur in foreign body cases because of the abnormally high pressures generated both by the patient, while conscious, and by the rescue maneuvers. Because the operator has no way of knowing into which mainstem bronchus the foreign body was advanced (most commonly the right, but possibly the left), bilateral needle thoracostomy should be performed, in the hope of identifying a tension pneumothorax. If a pneumothorax is not identified, the second clinical possibility is complete bilateral mainstem obstruction, a condition from which survival is not possible regardless of treatment.

## POSTINTUBATION MANAGEMENT

Postintubation management depends on the clinical circumstances. If the foreign body has been successfully removed and the patient remains obtunded, perhaps from posthypoxemic encephalopathy, then ventilation and general management are as for any other postarrest patient. If the foreign body has been pushed down into one mainstem bronchus, the other lung must be ventilated carefully at low rates with reduced tidal volumes to minimize the risk of barotrauma while waiting for the OR.

## TIPS AND PEARLS

1. If the obstruction is incomplete and the patient is stable, usually the best approach is to wait for definitive removal in the OR under a double setup. If you are forced to act, move cautiously and deliberately to ensure that you do not convert a supraglottic obstruction into an infraglottic obstruction.
2. If the obstructing foreign body is above the vocal cords and cannot be removed, cricothyrotomy is indicated.
3. If the obstructed foreign body is distal to the vocal cords and cannot be seen from above by direct laryngoscopy, it is extremely unlikely that cricothyrotomy will place an airway below the level of the obstruction, and therefore cricothyrotomy is not indicated.
4. A rapid series of abdominal thrust maneuvers is a reasonable first step in any case of complete obstruction and is the only maneuver that can be performed on a patient with a complete obstruction who is awake and responsive. In the unconscious patient, chest thrusts may help, but plan to proceed quickly to direct laryngoscopy.
5. If the patient is unconscious and does not regain spontaneous ventilations when supraglottic foreign bodies are cleared, then tracheal intubation should be performed and ventilations established.
6. If ventilations are impossible through the endotracheal tube, then the "down-then-up" maneuver should be performed with the endotracheal tube with hopes of advancement of an obstructing tracheal foreign body into a mainstem bronchus, withdrawal of the endotracheal tube into its usual mid-tracheal position, and oxygenation and ventilation of the other lung.

## EVIDENCE

- **When should I use abdominal thrust maneuvers versus back blows?** There are no completely sound studies comparing the effectiveness of various methods for expelling an obstructing foreign body. There is no clear evidence to establish the superiority of chest compressions over abdominal thrusts or vice versa. The American Heart Association (AHA), in its 2010 guidelines for emergency cardiac care, recommends a progression of airway clearing maneuvers in the conscious patient, beginning with back blows and progressing to abdominal thrusts.[1] There was no significant change to this approach in the 2015 AHA guideline update. If the abdominal thrust maneuver is not successful despite repeated attempts, and the patient is unconscious, then chest thrusts can be tried, but there is no evidence that they will be more successful than abdominal thrusts. For obese patients or women late in pregnancy, chest thrusts are preferred. A cadaver study indicates that greater airway pressures can be developed using chest thrusts than with abdominal thrusts when the patient is unconscious, and this evidence is reflected in the AHA recommendations.[2]

## REFERENCES

1. Berg RA, Hemphill R, Abella BS, et al. 2010 American Heart Association guidelines for cardiopulmonary resuscitation and emergency cardiovascular care. *Circulation*. 2010;122:S685–S705.
2. Langhelle A, Sunde K, Wik L, et al. Airway pressure with chest compressions versus Heimlich manoeuvre in recently dead adults with complete airway obstruction. *Resuscitation*. 2000;44:105–108.

# Chapter 42

# Safe Extubation of the Emergency Patient

Justen Naidu and Laura V. Duggan

## THE CLINICAL CHALLENGE

Extubation is an uncommon procedure in emergency medicine. However, certain scenarios, such as a rapidly recovering polysubstance overdose patient may make extubation desirable. The fourth National Audit Project found that nearly one-third of reported major airway complications occurred at extubation, which has led the Difficult Airway Society guidelines (see Evidence section). Although these guidelines focus on perioperative medicine, many of the principles of a comprehensive planned approach to extubation apply.

With the changing scope of practice, emergency medicine physicians may be involved increasingly in the process of extubating patients. The recognition of the potentially difficult extubation, creation of an extubation strategy, and execution of a safe extubation procedure are all important elements that emergency physicians should be familiar with.

Although extubation is a vital component in airway management, it receives significantly less attention than endotracheal intubation. A recent Medline search comparing the ratio of intubation to extubation articles found the ratio to be 57:1. The same meticulous planning and communication involved with endotracheal intubation should also be practiced with removal of the endotracheal tube (ETT). Similar to intubation, recognition of the potentially difficult extubation is instrumental in the planning process. Despite these important factors, the body of literature on extubation is significantly less comprehensive than intubation. On a positive note, this deficit in the literature is an opportunity for extubation research and publication, especially in emergency medicine.

## PLANNING FOR EXTUBATION

A morbidly obese 55-year-old restrained driver is brought into the ED from a single-passenger, single-vehicle incident 30 minutes prior during severe winter weather. He was intubated in the field because of decreased level of consciousness. Four attempts using both direct and video-based laryngoscopy were required prior to intubation success secondary to a cervical collar, short neck, and redundant soft tissue.

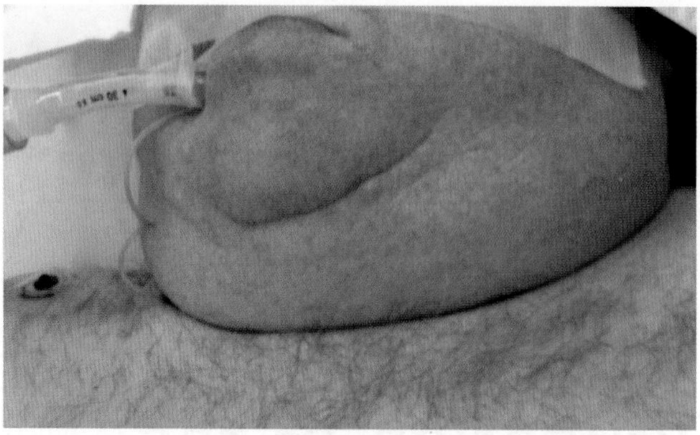

● **FIGURE 42-1.** Intubated morbidly obese 55-year-old restrained driver brought into emergency department.

CT scan reveals a single lung contusion but no flail segment or other significant injuries. The patient's hemodynamics are within normal limits and aside from a high blood alcohol level, initial and repeated blood work results are stable. It is now 8 hours after the incident and the patient remains in the ED. He is responsive to command, moving all extremities, and is becoming more agitated. He now requires 4-point restraints in addition to escalating doses of sedation. His tongue is large and bruised. Some bruising was noted over the anterior chest on secondary survey. A total of 2 L of crystalloid has been infused, but no blood products. An arterial blood gas on minimal vent settings (pressure support with an $F_{IO_2}$ of 30%) shows a $P_{O_2}$ of 100 mm Hg, $O_2$ saturation of 98%, $P_{CO_2}$ of 43 mm Hg.

The nurses would like to know if you would like to extubate him, or continue to escalate his sedation (**Fig. 42-1**). How should you proceed?

## EXTUBATION CRITERIA

Fortunately, there are defined general principles to follow when considering a patient for extubation. Unlike intubation, extubation is *always* an elective procedure. In a busy ED environment, there are always the pressures of time and bed-space. It is helpful to have a written "checklist approach" to allow bedside nurses and other health care workers to assess a patient's readiness for extubation prior to physician attendance for the final decision making. **Table 42-1** highlights minimal recommendations to consider when evaluating a patient for extubation. Some institutions have implemented evidence-based checklists and have reduced the incidence of extubation failure. Having a consistent, predictable approach should be the overall goal of the airway provider and emergency system.

## RISK STRATIFICATION

Once the decision to extubate has been made, focus shifts to the identification of which airways may be at increased risk. The Difficult Airway Society recommends risk-stratifying of patients into *low risk* vs. *high risk* of extubation failure (see **Tables 42-2** and **42-3**). This helps to narrow the focus to the *at-risk* group in order to identify those patients who require additional planning. Some of the general risk factors that are highlighted in the at-risk group for extubation are listed in.

Special attention should be placed on the airway risk factors section because this can be difficult to identify prior to extubation. Interventions since intubation, such as extensive fluid resuscitation,

**TABLE 42-1 Extubation Criteria**

| | |
|---|---|
| Reversal of underlying process | ▪ No further need for mechanical ventilation identified<br>▪ No expected need in immediate hospital course |
| Level of consciousness | ▪ Alert patient<br>▪ Sedation medications discontinued |
| Ability to oxygenate | ▪ Spontaneous breathing<br>▪ Tidal volume > 5–7 mL/kg<br>▪ $Spo_2$ > 92 with $Fio_2$ 30 |
| Ability to ventilate | ▪ PEEP < 8 mm Hg<br>▪ Peak voluntary negative pressure >20 cm $H_2O$ |
| Predictors of impending airway loss | ▪ Protecting own airway<br>▪ Reversal of neuromuscular blockade (TOF > 90)<br>▪ PEF > 60 L/min (cough assessment)<br>▪ Difficult intubation?<br>▪ Difficult bag-mask ventilation? |
| Pulmonary secretions | ▪ Oropharyngeal secretions minimal<br>▪ Risk of aspiration minimal |

**TABLE 42-2 DAS Risk Stratification**

| | |
|---|---|
| Low risk | ▪ Fasted?<br>▪ Uncomplicated airway<br>▪ No general risk factors |
| At risk | ▪ Ability to oxygenate uncertain<br>▪ Reintubation potentially difficult<br>▪ General risk factors (Table 42-3) |

From Mitchell V, Dravid R, Patel A, et al. Difficult Airway Society Guidelines for the management of tracheal extubation. *Anaesthesia*. 2012;67(3):318–340.

**TABLE 42-3 General Risk Factors**

| | |
|---|---|
| Airway risk factors | ▪ Known difficult airway<br>▪ Airway deterioration (trauma, edema, bleeding)<br>▪ Restricted airway access<br>▪ Obesity/OSA<br>▪ Aspiration risk |
| General risk factors | ▪ Cardiovascular<br>▪ Respiratory<br>▪ Neurologic<br>▪ Metabolic<br>▪ Special surgical requirements<br>▪ Special medical requirements |

may have resulted in airway edema and could predispose the airway to extubation failure because of obstruction. Anticipated course of disease also plays a role; burns or infection to the face or neck may be more difficult to reintubate than initially recorded.

Failure of extubation is usually due to one of two issues, or both: upper airway obstruction or respiratory failure. Upper airway obstruction, including laryngospasm, is associated with immediate respiratory distress and hypoxia. On the other hand, respiratory failure, or a gradual decline in the ability of the patient to breathe on his/her own without support, is a much more common issue in the ICU. Immediate upper airway collapse and obstruction is more common in the postoperative setting than in the ICU, but gradual respiratory failure remains the most common cause of the need to reintubate the patient. In emergency medicine, the characteristics of patients failing extubation are unknown.

## ADDITIONAL TESTING

If a patient is identified as having an *at-risk* airway, the emergency physician must first decide whether extubation should even be attempted in the ED. If extubation remains part of the plan after taking into consideration the patient's high-risk features, intubation history, and availability of difficult airway tools and specialty support, then additional testing may be needed in order to determine whether conditions are safe enough to extubate. If suspicious for the possibility of upper airway obstruction, a cuff leak test may be performed (see **Box 42-1**). What does a cuff leak, or lack thereof, really predict? A cuff leak test predicts postextubation stridor in children intubated for croup. Cuff leak does *not* necessarily predict success of extubation, but can be used with a number of other criteria to judge

BOX
**42-1**

### Cuff leak test.

*What is the Cuff Leak Test*? The cuff leak test is used to predict the population that may be at increased risk of postoperative stridor. It is a measurement of the cuff leak volume, which is equal to the difference between the inspiratory tidal volume and the average expiratory tidal volume while the cuff around the endotracheal tube is deflated.

*How is it performed*? There are variable methodologies described in the literature. The most common is to set the assist control mode with the fixed tidal volumes of 10 to 12 mL per kg. The inspiratory tidal volume with the cuff inflated is then measured. The cuff is then deflated and a brief period of coughing usually proceeds. Following the resolution of coughing, four to six breaths are given, and the average value of the three lowest expiratory tidal volumes is computed. The difference between the inspiratory tidal volume with the cuff inflated and the averaged expiratory tidal volume with the cuff deflated is used to calculate the cuff leak volume.

*Application to practice*: The cuff leak volume of $<$130 mL is generally accepted as indicating a cuff leak is absent (positive test) and places the patient at risk for postextubation stridor and extubation failure. The absence of a cuff leak should therefore alert the airway manager to the potential for a postextubation complication and a plan should be devised accordingly.

the likelihood of success (see Evidence section). Adding to this is the use of the terms "negative" and "positive" cuff leak test. Both terms have been used when there is a cuff leak present, and when there isn't, creating confusion. The authors believe the terms positive and negative should be abandoned. Communicating that a cuff leak is present or absent is much clearer.

An absent cuff leak should alert the airway manager to the potential for postextubation stridor and, therefore, the potential for airway obstruction. The airway can be evaluated by direct laryngoscopy, videolaryngoscopy, or nasopharyngoscopy. Nasopharyngoscopy can be achieved with pediatric bronchoscope or nasopharyngoscope and 3 to 4 sprays of 4% lidocaine nasally. If nasopharyngoscopy is chosen, the patient should be sitting up and asked to flex his or her neck forward ("like a chicken") to maximally open the hypopharyngeal space and allow for best visualization. The ETT cuff can be deflated, and breathing around the ETT can be assessed by direct inspection. Videolaryngoscopy has the advantage of creating a "shared mental model," with health care professionals taking care of the patient being able to also visualize the airway. Topicalization of the posterior pharynx including the vallecula is usually required for either video or direct laryngoscopy. Sedation may also be required. Assessment of cough can also be completed by performing a peak expiratory flow. Values of less than 60 L per minute have been associated with an increased incidence of extubation failure.

## PROCESS OF EXTUBATION

### General Extubation

Extubation is an elective procedure that should be planned and prepared well. Overall, the goal should be maintenance of oxygenation, maintenance of ventilation, and a well-laid-out plan in the event extubation failure occurs. An awake, spontaneously breathing patient can accomplish several of the overall goals during extubation independently. They are able to protect their airway, maintain patency with muscular tone, and facilitate gas exchange with spontaneous breathing. This is significantly different to the heavily sedated patient. For this reason, extubation is generally recommended in an awake state. This corresponds well with the extubation criteria highlighted in Table 42-1. The general process of extubation in a *low-risk* situation follows the stepwise process described in Table 42-4.

### Complications

The majority of low-risk extubation procedures are completed without significant complications. However, vigilance during this period of transition from a controlled situation is imperative as

TABLE 42-4 General Steps

| General Steps |
|---|
| 1. Extubation criteria met (Table 42-1) |
| 2. Deliver 100% oxygen |
| 3. Suction of airway |
| 4. Insert soft bite block |
| 5. Position patient with head up |
| 6. Untie/tape tube |
| 7. Deflate cuff |
| 8. Apply positive pressure while removing ETT |
| 9. Transfer to facemask |
| 10. Confirm continued ventilation/oxygenation |

TABLE 42-5 Extubation Complications

| |
|---|
| Hypoventilation |
| Upper airway obstruction |
| Laryngospasm (**Box 42-2**) |
| Bronchospasm |
| Vocal cord damage |
| Negative pressure pulmonary edema |
| Pulmonary aspiration |
| Coughing |
| Hemodynamic alterations (tachycardia, hypertension, dysrhythmias, ACS) |

hypoxic insults are not uncommon during this time. This was further highlighted by the fourth National Audit Project from the United Kingdom where approximately one-third of the major airway incidences occurred at extubation (Evidence section). Complications that can occur during extubation are listed in Table 42-5. A component in the planning process for extubation is to mitigate the risk factors that lead to complications. Even with the low risk, one should still be able to handle the complications of extubation should they occur (**Box 42-2** and Table 42-6).

## ADJUNCTS TO EXTUBATION

### *Airway Exchange Catheter*

Patients deemed at *high risk* of extubation failure may require adjuncts added to the airway plan. A common technique is the use of an airway exchange catheter (AEC) for maintenance of continuous

BOX 42-2

**Laryngospasm.**

*What is laryngospam?* Laryngospasm is an exaggerated prolongation of the normal glottis closure reflex triggered by mechanical or chemical (aspiration, secretions) stimulus.

*What are the risk factors?* The risk factors for laryngospasm can be broken into patient or procedure factors. Patient factors that increase the risk of laryngospasm include young age (children), smokers, and recent respiratory infection. Procedural factors include airway manipulation (intubation/extubation), stimulation during the transition period between deep anesthetic/awake state and the presence of debris in the airway (blood, secretions).

*Management*: The first step in management is reduction of the risk factors associated with laryngospasm. This includes suctioning of the airway prior to extubation and avoiding extubation when transitioning from the plane of deep anesthetic to awake state. If laryngospasm does occur, prompt recognition followed by treatment is imperative (Table 42-6).

TABLE 42-6 Treatment of Laryngospasm

| | |
|---|---|
| 1. | Call for help |
| 2. | Apply continuous positive pressure and administer 100% $F_{IO_2}$ in an attempt to "break" spasm |
| 3. | Larson's maneuver: place middle fingers posterior to mandible and anterior to mastoid process. Combine with jaw thrust forward |
| 4. | Low-dose propofol 0.25 mg/kg, if persists high-dose propofol 1–2 mg/kg |
| 5. | Succinylcholine 1 mg/kg IV if severe hypoxia, with persistent cord closure if propofol ineffective. Consider atropine 1 mg should bradycardia occur |
| 6. | No resolution? "cannot intubate, cannot ventilate" algorithm |

access to the airway. AECs are thin, hollow tubes with a blunt end located distally. They are supplied with a 15 mm connector compatible with a breathing circuit as well as a luer lock connectors for high-pressure (jet) ventilation (**Fig. 42-2**). The most commonly available AECs are made by Cook Medical (Bloomington, Indiana, www.cookmedical.com). The Cook 11F and 14F AECs are commonly used in adults, are tolerated well in the awake patient, and are compatible with ETTs with internal diameters greater than 4 mm and 5 mm, respectively; 19F AECs are also available, but are only tolerated in awake patients 50% of the time and depends on keeping the tip of the AEC above the very sensitive carina. Therefore, the numbers on the AEC should be aligned with the ETT numbers accordingly. No lidocaine is required through or around the AEC as this has not been shown to increase tolerance of the device. Patients can phonate with an 11F or 14F AEC in place. The method for using an AEC is highlighted in **Table 42-7** and **Figure 42-3**.

Complications associated with AECs include pneumothorax, pneumoperitoneum, hypoxia during airway management, perforation of the lower airways, and unintended esophageal misplacement potentially also leading to perforation. Supplemental oxygen postextubation should be maintained with a facemask, nasal prongs, or continuous positive airway pressure (CPAP), although oxygen insufflation and jet ventilation through an AEC is possible. The use of oxygen insufflation and jet ventilation through AEC can be complicated by life-threatening barotrauma and should be avoided except in a can't intubate can't oxygenate (CICO) situation. If this occurs, low flow rates (1 to 2 L per minute) while prepping the neck for surgical airway access are preferred.

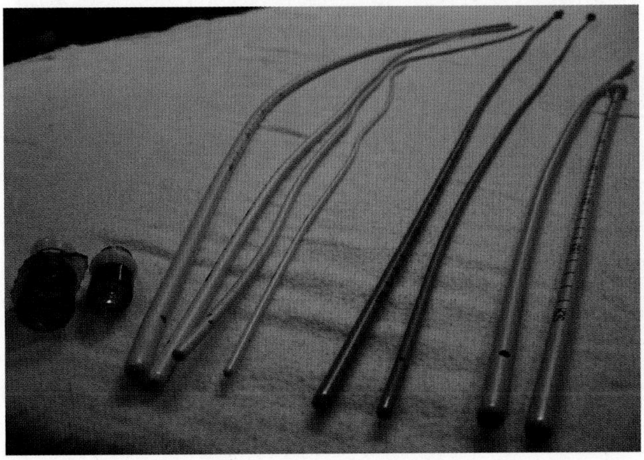

● **FIGURE 42-2.** Examples of airway exchange catheters, Aintree catheters, and Rapid Fit connectors.

**TABLE 42-7 Airway Exchange Catheter**

| | |
|---|---|
| 1. | Selection of AEC 11F or 14F |
| 2. | Decide how far to insert AEC. If any doubt that tip will lay above carina, examination of endotracheal tube depth should be completed with a fiber-optic scope prior to insertion |
| 3. | Oxygen insufflation through the catheter should NOT be used except in life-threatening situations by an expert trained in the technique. Use alternative methods for oxygenation |
| 4. | Insert lubricated catheter through endotracheal tube to predetermined depth (usually 20–22 cm). Never advance against resistance |
| 5. | Oropharyngeal suctioning prior to removal. |
| 6. | Proceed with extubation over AEC while maintaining in fixed position. |
| 7. | Secure AEC in place with tape on side of mouth/forehead (**Fig. 42-3**) |
| 8. | Transfer to facemask with capnography for detection of possible obstruction |
| 9. | Clearly label AEC so as not to be confused with nasogastric tube |
| 10. | If extubation fails, reintubate over catheter with either direct or video-assisted laryngoscopy (**Table 42-8**) |

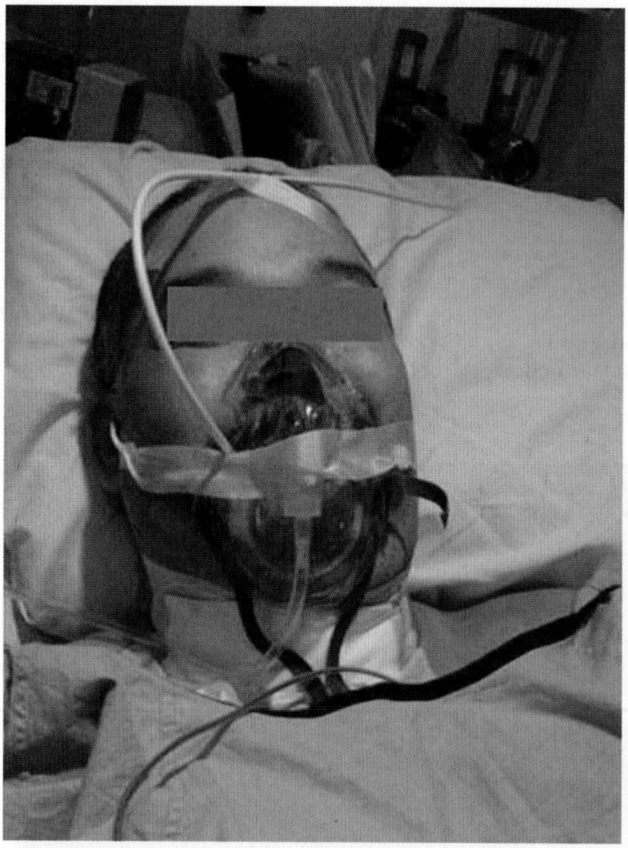

● **FIGURE 42-3.** Patient with AEC taped to forehead. Note the use of facemask for supplemental oxygen. (From Duggan LV, Law JA, Murphy MF. Brief review: supplementing oxygen through an airway exchange catheter: efficacy, complications, and recommendations. *Can J Anesth*. 2011;58(6):560–568.)

TABLE **42-8** **AEC for Reintubation (DAS Algorithm)**

| | |
|---|---|
| 1. | Position of patient: Sitting up as much as possible. Oro- and hypopharynx suctioned |
| 2. | Apply 100% oxygen with CPAP via facemask, or apply high-flow nasal prongs |
| 3. | Select small endotracheal tube with soft tip blunt tip |
| 4. | Administer anesthetic or topicalization as indicated |
| 5. | Use direct or indirect laryngoscopy to retract the tongue and railroad the endotracheal tube (with bevel facing anteriorly) over the AEC |
| 6. | Confirm position of the tube with capnography if time allows |

The timing to remove an AEC postextubation is the subject of much debate and should be individualized to the patient's respiratory reserve, potential for difficult reintubation, and clinical course. They can be left in the airway for 24 hours and longer.

Reintubation over an AEC should be performed using a videolaryngoscope as it has a higher first-pass success rate when compared to direct laryngoscopy. Railroading an ETT over an AEC *without* a laryngoscope, either video or direct laryngoscopy, is associated with a high failure rate including dislodgment of the AEC.

The patient should be in the semi-sitting position to allow for soft tissues to fall away from the glottis. Suction is very useful prior and during reintubation and should be under the pillow of the patient. The patient's head, if possible, should be extended. The operator should be high above the head of the bed, either on step stools or the bedframe (this also gets the attention of everyone in the room!). Reintubation can be performed with topicalization only, sedation, or complete induction. Dexmedetomidine (Precedex) can be a useful adjunct, especially in the agitated patient. Table 42-8 highlights a sequence for the use of AEC for resecuring the airway. Similar to the approach to intubation, a well-laid-out plan in the event of failure is crucial.

ETT that "hugs" the sides of the AEC should be chosen. In other words, this is a time for oxygenation, not ICU preferences for a larger ETT.

The proximity between the sidewalls of the AEC and the inner wall of the ETT will make the difference between success and failure of this technique. If there is a significant space between them, the glottic structures can become "hung up" in this space, preventing passage of the ETT and potentially dislodging the AEC. Solutions to this issue include choosing a smaller ETT size or "increasing" the size of the AEC with an Aintree© catheter (**Fig. 42-4**).

As the glottis is reached with the ETT, a counterclockwise twist of the ETT will aid in its passage. The leading edge of the ETT is on the right side of the ETT, and this will move it away from the right-sided glottic structures. Small maneuvers such as the ones described above will increase the success rate of reintubation over an AEC.

Finally, like any other procedure, the use of an AEC as part of a staged extubation plan requires some experience and practice. The authors recommend inviting anesthesia or ICU colleagues with experience using these devices for consultation until the practitioner is comfortable.

## NONINVASIVE VENTILATION

Extubation to noninvasive ventilation (NIV) has been evaluated in the adult ICU population as a useful adjunct in individuals at increased risk of failure, especially in patients with chronic obstructive pulmonary disease (COPD), obesity, and high-risk features for extubation failure (see Evidence section). Immediate application of bilevel positive airway pressure (BiPAP) following extubation with initial inspiratory positive airway pressure ranging from 8 to 16 cm $H_2O$ and expiratory positive airway pressure ranging from 4 to 6 cm $H_2O$ is recommended. The settings are then adjusted according to $Pao_2$ and $Paco_2$. If used, a minimum of 24 hours is required to confer benefit. At the current time, it is unknown whether the short-term application of nasal intermittent positive

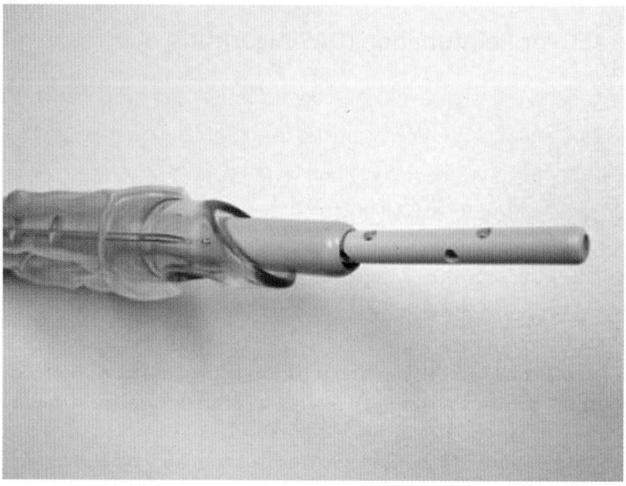

● **FIGURE 42-4.** 11F Airway exchange catheter (AEC) sheathed in Aintree© 19F catheter to assist in preventing soft tissues from catching between the AEC and endotracheal tube. (From Law JA, Duggan LV. Extubation guidelines: anaesthetists' use of airway exchange catheters. *Anaesthesia*. 2012;67(8):918–919.)

pressure ventilation as an adjunct to ED extubation results in decreased failure rates. However, due to the overall benefits demonstrated in the ICU population, and the postoperative benefits for obstructive sleep apnea and obese patients, consideration for extubation to BiPAP should be included as part of the airway plan when clinically indicated.

## SEDATION DURING EXTUBATION

Intubation and positive pressure ventilation can be uncomfortable for patients leading to ventilator dyssynchrony, potential patient and health care worker safety issues (and the need for physical or chemical restraints). The goal during extubation is a calm cooperative patient who can follow commands and is capable of meeting their own respiratory requirements. Postextubation sedation should be considered carefully weighing multiple factors such as the patient's agitation and delirium, high-risk features, and access to appropriate medication. If sedation is required, agents that both facilitate patient compliance, yet have minimal affect on ventilatory drive and protective airway reflexes should be used. Dexmedetomidine has been found to be helpful in the management of postextubation agitation and delirium. Dexmedetomidine does not negatively influence respiratory drive, unlike many other sedative agents.

## CASE SUMMARY

This patient was able to follow commands, but was intermittently agitated. Dexmedetomidine infusion was begun with 1 mcg/kg/hour for the first hour then decreased to 0.5 mcg/kg/hour thereafter in order to facilitate cooperation. The patient was sitting up and the oropharynx and ETT was suctioned. There was a cuff leak on quantitative assessment of >130 mL. With topicalization of atomized 4% lidocaine, gentle videolaryngoscopy was performed to assess the extent of upper airway soft tissue swelling. The patient was asked to take several breaths to assess movement of the upper airway soft tissues.

A 14F AEC was placed through the ETT, aligning it to the ETT markings. Care was taken not to advance it too far into the airway and potentially impinge on the carina. The AEC was taped to the oxygen facemask. The patient was able to speak with the AEC in place.

The patient was observed for 4 hours with the AEC in place, such as can be seen in the photo of a separate patient in **Figure 42-3**. No signs of upper airway collapse occurred, and the patient showed no signs of respiratory failure. The AEC was removed uneventfully.

Developing an approach to extubating patients in the ED will become an increasingly important part of practice. The ability to identify the *at-risk* airway and plan accordingly is imperative. Written criteria for safe extubation is helpful in assisting all health care workers use a common language in extubation planning and assessment. Being comfortable with the adjuncts to extubation including AECs and transition from extubation to immediate NIV are a worthwhile skill to have in one's repertoire.

## EVIDENCE

- **What makes a patient high risk to extubate and is there evidence to guide safe extubation in emergency patients?** There are no quality ED studies on this topic. Much of our recommendations are extrapolated from the perioperative literature.[1] The fourth National Audit Project found that nearly one-third of reported major airway complications occurred at extubation.[2] Analysis of the American Society of Anesthesiology Closed Claims Project database showed that 17% (26/156) of the cases resulting in death or brain death occurred at the time of extubation.[3,4] Accepted criteria for extubation from the anesthesia literature include: resolution of the underlying disease process, appropriate levels of alertness, adequate intrinsic ventilator drive, minimal secretions, and an oxygen saturation >92% with spontaneous breathing.[5] One pilot study in trauma patients showed that institution of an extubation checklist decreased the rate of extubation failure.[6] High-risk patients include those with a known difficult airway, obesity, compromised oxygenation, and poor physiology and cardiovascular reserve.[7] Extubation failure is typically the result of either periextubation obstruction and laryngospasm or progressive hypoxic respiratory failure; the latter is most commonly seen in ICU patients.[8] Patients who exhibit high-risk features should either remain intubated or undergo extubation with specialty support from anesthesia or otolaryngology.
- **If a cuff leak is present, what does that mean?** A cuff leak is the difference between the inspiratory tidal volume and the average expiratory tidal volume while the cuff around the ETT is deflated. Lack of an adequate cuff leak (positive test) is variably defined in the literature, but a volume difference <110 to 130 mL is considered a positive result. In a recent meta-analysis of nine studies evaluating the cuff leak test (lack of adequate leak) as a predictor of postextubation airway obstruction, patients with a positive test were four times more likely to have airway obstruction. The pooled sensitivity was 63%, with a specificity of 86%.[9] Additionally, peak inspiratory flows <60 L per minute have been associated with an increased incidence of extubation failure.[10]
- **What is the role of AECs during extubation?** AECs have been shown to increase the first-pass success rate in patients with known or suspected difficult airways requiring reintubation. Mort et al.[11] found an overall success rate of reintubation over an AEC of 92%, with 87% occurring on the first pass. The use of AECs has been shown to be well tolerated by awake patients, as long as they do not touch the sensitive carina.[11] Oxygen insufflation and jet ventilation through AECs can be complicated by barotrauma and should be avoided except in CICO situations. Low oxygen flow rates of 1 to 2 L per minute are recommended.[12] Intubation over an AEC should be performed using a videolaryngoscope as it results in the highest chance of first-pass success.[11]
- **Should noninvasive positive pressure ventilation be used after extubation?** There is evidence that extubation to NIV helps reduce the rate of reintubation, ICU mortality, and ICU length of stay.[13] This is most beneficial in patients with COPD, chronic respiratory disorders, and those identified at high risk of extubation failure.[13–15] The length of BiPAP application that has shown to be beneficial at reducing the rate of reintubation has ranged from 24 to 48 hours. One study evaluated extubation to BiPAP for a duration of 12 hours and did not show a significant difference in the rate of reintubation. In obese patients, extubation to CPAP

following general anesthetic or in the recovery room has been shown to decrease the incidence of postoperative respiratory complications.[16] For patients with obstructive sleep apnea, the American Society of Anesthesiology has recommended the continuous use of CPAP or BiPAP in the postoperative period.[17]

## REFERENCES


1. Mitchell V, Dravid R, Patel A, et al. Difficult Airway Society Guidelines for the management of tracheal extubation. *Anaesthesia*. 2012;67(3):318–340.
2. Difficult T, Society A. *Major Complications of Airway Management in the United Kingdom*; 2011.
3. Murphy C, Wong DT. Airway management and oxygenation in obese patients. *Can J Anesth*. 2013;60(9):929–945.
4. Strauss RA. Management of the difficult airway. *Atlas Oral Maxillofac Surg Clin NA*. 2010;18(1):11–28.
5. Gray SH, Ross JA, Green RS. How to safely extubate a patient in the emergency department: a user's guide to critical care. *Can J Emerg Med*. 2013;15(5):303–306.
6. Howie WO, Dutton RP. Implementation of an evidence-based extubation checklist to reduce extubation failure in patients with trauma: a pilot study. *AANA J*. 2012;80(3):179–184.
7. Thille AW, Boissier F, Ben Ghezala H, et al. Risk factors for and prediction by caregivers of extubation failure in ICU patients. *Crit Care Med*. 2014;(8):1.
8. Cavallone LF, Vannucci A. Extubation of the difficult airway and extubation failure. *Anesth Analg*. 2013;116(2):368–383.
9. Ochoa ME, Marin Mdel C, Frutos-Vivar F, et al. Cuff-leak test for the diagnosis of upper airway obstruction in adults: a systematic review and meta-analysis. *Intensive Care Med*. 2009;35(7):1171–1179. doi:10.1007/s00134-009-1501-9.
10. Su WL, Chen YH, Chen CW, et al. Involuntary cough strength and extubation outcomes for patients in an ICU. *Chest*. 2010;137(4):777–782. doi:10.1378/chest.07-2808.
11. Mort TC. Continuous airway access for the difficult extubation: the efficacy of the airway exchange catheter. *Anesth Analg*. 2007;105(5):1357–1362.
12. Duggan LV, Law JA, Murphy MF. Brief review: supplementing oxygen through an airway exchange catheter: efficacy, complications, and recommendations. *Can J Anesth*. 2011;58(6):560–568. doi:10.1007/s12630-011-9488-4.
13. Bajaj A, Rathor P, Sehgal V, et al. Efficacy of noninvasive ventilation after planned extubation: a systematic review and meta-analysis of randomized controlled trials. *Hear Lung J Acute Crit Care*. 2015;44(2):1–8. doi:10.1016/j.hrtlng.2014.12.002.
14. Ferrer M, Valencia M, Nicolas JM, et al. Early noninvasive ventilation averts extubation failure in patients at risk: a randomized trial. *Am J Respir Crit Care Med*. 2006;173(2):164–170. doi:10.1164/rccm.200505-718OC.
15. Ferrer M, Sellarés J, Valencia M, et al. Non-invasive ventilation after extubation in hypercapnic patients with chronic respiratory disorders: randomised controlled trial. *Lancet*. 2009;374(9695):1082–1088. doi:10.1016/S0140-6736(09)61038-2.
16. Neligan PJ, Malhotra G, Fraser M, et al. Continuous positive airway pressure via the Boussignac system immediately after extubation improves lung function in morbidly obese patients with obstructive sleep apnea undergoing laparoscopic bariatric surgery. *Anesthesiology*. 2009;110(4):878–884. doi:10.1097/ALN.0b013e31819b5d8c.
17. American Society of Anesthesiologists Task Force on Perioperative Management of patients with obstructive sleep apnea. Practice guidelines for the perioperative management of patients with obstructive sleep apnea. *Anesthesiology*. 2014;120(2):268–286.

# Index

**Note**: Pages followed by *f* indicate figures; pages followed by *t* indicate tables; pages followed by *b* indicate boxes

## B

## D

## E

## N



## O

## P

## Q



## R

## S

## T

# onal Airway Management Resources

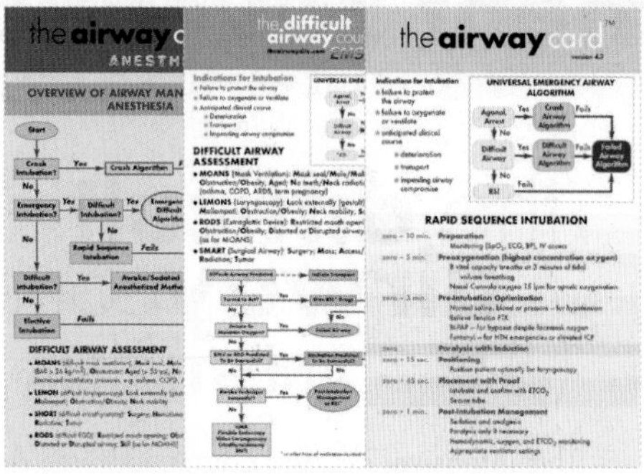


**The Airway Cards** are the definitive pocket reference guides containing essential information including airway algorithms, mnemonics and drug dosing. These include: The Airway Card™, The Airway Card Anesthesia™, and The Airway Card EMS™.

Available for purchase at *www.theairwaysite.com.*

**The Difficult Airway App™** is an essential tool for clinicians who manage emergency airways. The app features easy, yet sophisticated adult and pediatric drug dosing, decision-making support, rapid sequence intubation guidelines and educational resources including illustrations and videos.

For more information, visit *www.theairwaysite.com.*

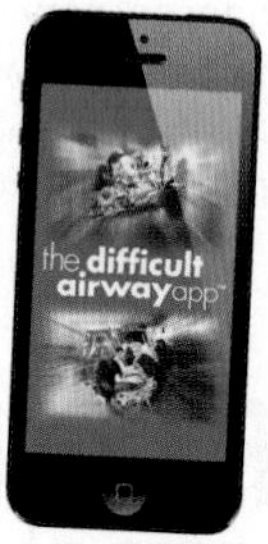


SimStore™
Making Simulation Easier
OFFICIAL DEVELOPER

**Airway Management Simulations:** Airway Management Education Center is an official simulation developer for the Laerdal/HealthStream SimStore. To find our simulation sets and supporting curricular materials, search "Airway Management Education Center" at *mysimcenter.com.*

**The Airway Site** (*www.theairwaysite.com*) is the on-line home for The Difficult Airway Course™ family of courses. Visit to learn more about each of the courses, to register for a course, and for links to other valuable airway resources.

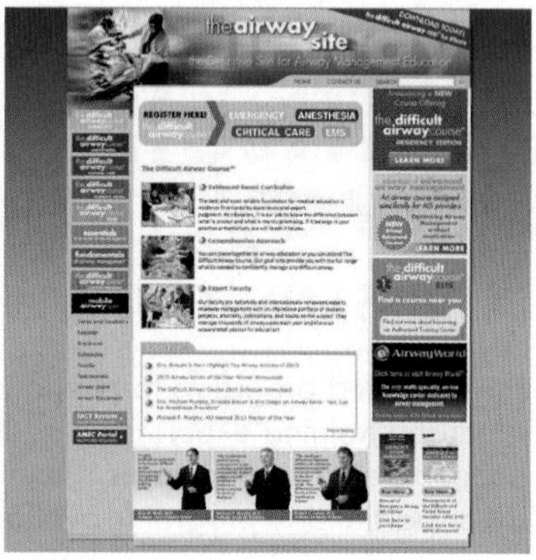


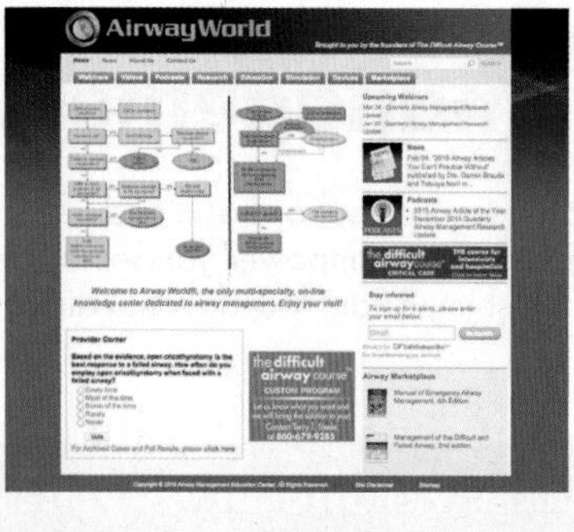


**Airway World** is an online multi-specialty website dedicated to airway management. In Airway World you will find free webinars, instructional videos, podcasts, research summaries, sentinel articles and much more! Visit *www.airwayworld.com* to get started.

RBS1704